# The Philadelphia Guide: Inpatient Pediatrics

### Second Edition

# The Philadelphia Guide: Inpatient Pediatrics

## Second Edition

**Edited by**

**Samir S. Shah, MD, MSCE**
Director, Division of Hospital Medicine
James M. Ewell Endowed Chair
Attending Physician in Hospital Medicine & Infectious Diseases
Cincinnati Children's Hospital Medical Center
Professor, Department of Pediatrics
University of Cincinnati College of Medicine
Cincinnati, Ohio

**Lisa B. Zaoutis, MD**
Associate Professor of Clinical Pediatrics
Department of Pediatrics
Perelman School of Medicine of the University of Pennsylvania
Director, Pediatrics Residency Program
The Children's Hospital of Philadelphia
Philadelphia, Pennsylvania

**Marina Catallozzi, MD, MSCE**
Assistant Professor of Pediatrics and Population and Family Health
at Columbia University Medical Center
New York, New York

**Gary Frank, MD**
Chief Quality and Patient Safety Officer
Children's Healthcare of Atlanta
Adjunct Associate Professor of Pediatrics
Department of Pediatrics
Emory University School of Medicine
Atlanta, Georgia

McGraw Hill Education

New York   Chicago   San Francisco   Athens   London   Madrid   Mexico City
Milan   New Delhi   Singapore   Sydney   Toronto

This book is printed on acid-free paper.

McGraw-Hill Education books are available at special quantity discounts to use as premiums and sales promotions or for use in corporate training programs. To contact a representative, please visit the Contact Us pages at www.mhprofessional.com

The Philadelphia Guide: Inpatient Pediatrics, 2ed.

1 2 3 4 5 6 7 8 9 0   DOC/DOC   20 19 18 17 16 15

ISBN 978-0-07-182921-2
MHID 0-07-182921-0

This book was set in Minion Pro.

The editors were Alyssa Fried and Christie Naglieri.
The production supervisor was Richard Ruzycka.
Project Management was provided by Asheesh Ratra, MPS Ltd.
The index was prepared by Julie Grady.
RR Donnelley was printer and binder.

This book is printed on acid-free paper.

**Library of Congress Cataloging-in-Publication Data**

The Philadelphia guide
   Inpatient pediatrics / edited by Samir S. Shah, Lisa B. Zaoutis, Gary
Frank, Marina Catallozzi. — Second edition.
       p. ; cm.
   Includes bibliographical references and index.
     ISBN 978-0-07-182921-2 (pbk. : alk. paper) — ISBN 0-07-182921-0 (pbk. : alk. paper)
   I. Shah, Samir S., editor.   II. Zaoutis, Lisa B., editor.   III. Frank, Gary, 1971- , editor.
IV. Catallozzi, Marina, editor.   V. Title.
     [DNLM: 1. Pediatrics—Handbooks. WS 39]
   RJ61
   618.92—dc23

                                                                            2015011413

*To our mentors for sharing their wisdom and knowledge*
*To our families for providing love and support for all of our endeavors*
*To our patients for teaching us and to their families for trusting us*

# Contents

Contributors . . . . . . . . . . . . . . . . . . . . . . . . . . . . . . . . . . . . . . . . . . . . . . . . . . . . . . ix
Foreword . . . . . . . . . . . . . . . . . . . . . . . . . . . . . . . . . . . . . . . . . . . . . . . . . . . . . . . . . . xv
Preface—*Inpatient Pediatrics*, 2nd Edition . . . . . . . . . . . . . . . . . . . . . . . . . . . . . . . xvii
List of Abbreviations . . . . . . . . . . . . . . . . . . . . . . . . . . . . . . . . . . . . . . . . . . . . . . . . . xix

1 Adolescent Medicine . . . . . . . . . . . . . . . . . . . . . . . . . . . . . . . . . . . . . . . . . . . . . . .1
   *Christopher B. Renjilian, MD, MBE, Krishna Wood White, MD, MPH, and
   Leonard J. Levine, MD*

2 Allergy and Asthma . . . . . . . . . . . . . . . . . . . . . . . . . . . . . . . . . . . . . . . . . . . . . . .11
   *Irene Fung, MD, Solrun Melkorka Maggadottir, MD, and
   Terri Brown-Whitehorn, MD*

3 Analgesia and Sedation . . . . . . . . . . . . . . . . . . . . . . . . . . . . . . . . . . . . . . . . . . . .25
   *Arul M. Lingappan, MD, F. Wickham Kraemer III, MD, and
   Melissa Desai Patel, MD, MPH*

4 Calculations . . . . . . . . . . . . . . . . . . . . . . . . . . . . . . . . . . . . . . . . . . . . . . . . . . . . 34
   *Barbara-Jo Achuff, MD, FAAP, Vanessa N. Madrigal, MD, and
   Donald L. Boyer, MD, MSEd, FAAP*

5 Cardiology . . . . . . . . . . . . . . . . . . . . . . . . . . . . . . . . . . . . . . . . . . . . . . . . . . . . . .41
   *Javier J. Lasa, MD, Chitra Ravishankar, MD, and
   Joseph Rossano, MD, MS, FAAP, FAAC*

6 Dermatology . . . . . . . . . . . . . . . . . . . . . . . . . . . . . . . . . . . . . . . . . . . . . . . . . . . .73
   *Leslie Castelo-Soccio, MD, PhD, and Kara N. Shah, MD, PhD*

7 Emergency Medicine . . . . . . . . . . . . . . . . . . . . . . . . . . . . . . . . . . . . . . . . . . . . . .90
   *Margaret Samuels-Kalow, MD, MPhil, and Angela Ellison, MD, MSc*

8 Endocrinology . . . . . . . . . . . . . . . . . . . . . . . . . . . . . . . . . . . . . . . . . . . . . . . . . . 100
   *Christine T. Ferrara, MD, PhD, Amanda M. Ackermann, MD, PhD, and
   Andrew A. Palladino, MD*

9 Fluids and Electrolytes . . . . . . . . . . . . . . . . . . . . . . . . . . . . . . . . . . . . . . . . . . . . 121
   *Sonal Bhatnagar, MD, and Lawrence Copelovitch, MD*

10 Gastroenterology . . . . . . . . . . . . . . . . . . . . . . . . . . . . . . . . . . . . . . . . . . . . . . . . 132
   *Benjamin Sahn, MD, MS, and Petar Mamula, MD*

11 Genetics . . . . . . . . . . . . . . . . . . . . . . . . . . . . . . . . . . . . . . . . . . . . . . . . . . . . . . . 155
   *Elizabeth Bhoj, MD, PhD, Rebecca Ahrens-Nicklas, MD, PhD, and
   Tara L. Wenger, MD, PhD*

12 Hematology . . . . . . . . . . . . . . . . . . . . . . . . . . . . . . . . . . . . . . . . . . . . . . . . . . . . 169
   *Erin Blevins, MD, MSCE, and Char Witmer, MD, MSCE*

13 Human Immunodeficiency Virus Infection . . . . . . . . . . . . . . . . . . . . . . . . . . . . . 189
   *Daniel H. Reirden, MD, AAHIVMS*

# Contents

**14** Immunology .............................................. 219
Gita Ram, MD, and Soma Jyonouchi, MD

**15** Infectious Diseases ....................................... 237
Katie Chiotos, MD, Lori Handy, MD, MSCE, Salwa Sulieman, DO, and
Jeffrey S. Gerber, MD, PhD

**16** Metabolism .............................................. 303
Rebecca Ganetzky, MD, and Can Ficicioglu, MD, PhD

**17** Neonatology.............................................. 327
Elisabeth Raab, MD, MPH, Tawia A. Apenteng, MD,
Jennifer M. Brady, MD, and Mary Catherine Harris, MD

**18** Nephrology .............................................. 344
Joann Spinale Carlson, MD, and Rebecca L. Ruebner, MD, MSCE

**19** Neurology................................................ 359
Annapurna Poduri, MD, MPH, Renée A. Shellhaas, MD, Dennis J. Dlugos, MD,
Peter H. Berman, MD, and Gihan I. Tennekoon, MD

**20** Nutrition................................................. 389
Jamie Merves, MD, Diane Barsky, MD, and Maria R. Mascarenhas, MBBS

**21** Oncology ................................................ 401
Jason L. Freedman, MD, Benjamin R. Oshrine, MD, and Naomi Balamuth, MD

**22** Ophthalmology........................................... 434
Gil Binenbaum, MD, MSCE, and Stefanie L. Davidson, MD

**23** Orthopedics.............................................. 444
Christian Turner, MD, Matthew Grady, MD, and Theodore Ganley, MD

**24** Otolaryngology........................................... 454
Pamela Mudd, MD, and John Germiller, MD, PhD

**25** Procedures .............................................. 468
Mercedes M. Blackstone, MD, Jeannine Del Pizzo, MD, and Sarah Fesnak, MD

**26** Psychiatry................................................ 484
Rahim Rahemtulla, MD, and Amy Kim, MD

**27** Pulmonology............................................. 490
Kelly Adams, DO, Stamatia Alexiou, MD, and Howard B. Panitch, MD

**28** Rheumatology............................................ 508
Elaine Ramsay, MD, Alysha Taxter, MD, and Jon Burnham, MD, MSCE

**29** Surgery ................................................. 526
Jesse D. Vrecenak, MD, and Michael L. Nance, MD

**30** Toxicology ............................................... 548
Ruth Abaya, MD, MPH, and Diane Calello, MD

**Appendix A** ................................................. 577
**Appendix B** ................................................. 579
**Index** ...................................................... 585

# Contributors

**Ruth Abaya, MD, MPH,** Attending Physician, Division of Emergency Medicine, The Children's Hospital of Philadelphia; and Assistant Professor of Pediatrics, Perelman School of Medicine at the University of Pennsylvania, Philadelphia, Pennsylvania

**Barbara-Jo Achuff, MD, FAAP,** Assistant Professor, Department of Pediatrics, Cardiac Critical Care Baylor College of Medicine, Texas Children's Hospital, Houston, Texas

**Amanda M. Ackermann, MD, PhD,** Clinical Fellow in Pediatric Endocrinology and Diabetes, Division of Endocrinology and Diabetes, The Children's Hospital of Philadelphia, Philadelphia, Pennsylvania

**Kelly Adams, DO,** Fellow, Pediatric Pulmonology, The Children's Hospital of Philadelphia, Philadelphia, Pennsylvania

**Rebecca Ahrens-Nicklas, MD, PhD,** Resident, The Children's Hospital of Philadelphia, Philadelphia, Pennsylvania

**Stamatia Alexiou, MD,** Fellow, Pediatric Pulmonology, The Children's Hospital of Philadelphia, Philadelphia, Pennsylvania

**Tawia A. Apenteng, MD,** Attending Neonatologist, The Children's Hospital of Philadelphia Newborn Care at Pennsylvania Hospital, Philadelphia, Pennsylvania

**Naomi Balamuth, MD,** Attending Physician, Division of Oncology, Children's Hospital of Philadelphia; and Assistant Professor of Pediatrics, Perelman School of Medicine at the University of Pennsylvania, Philadelphia, Pennsylvania

**Diane Barsky, MD,** Attending Physician, Medical Director, Home Parenteral Nutrition Service, Division of Gastroenterology, Hepatology and Nutrition, The Children's Hospital of Philadelphia, Instructor of Pediatrics, Clinical Assistant Professor of Pediatrics, Perelman School of Medicine at the University of Pennsylvania, Philadelphia, Pennsylvania

**Peter H. Berman, MD,** Senior neurologist, The Children's Hospital of Philadelphia; and Professor Emeritus, Perelman School of Medicine at the University of Pennsylvania, Philadelphia, Pennsylvania

**Sonal Bhatnagar, MD,** Assistant Professor of Pediatrics, Division of Pediatric Nephrology and Hypertension, The University of Texas Health Science Center at Houston, Houston, Texas

**Elizabeth Bhoj, MD, PhD,** Fellow, Division of Human Genetics and Molecular Biology, The Children's Hospital of Philadelphia, Philadelphia, Pennsylvania

**Gil Binenbaum, MD, MSCE,** Attending Surgeon, Division of Pediatric Ophthalmology, The Children's Hospital of Philadelphia, Philadelphia, Pennsylvania

**Mercedes M. Blackstone, MD,** Attending Physician, Pediatric Emergency Medicine, The Children's Hospital of Philadelphia, Associate Professor of Clinical Pediatrics, Perelman School of Medicine at the University of Pennsylvania, Philadelphia, Pennsylvania

**Erin Blevins, MD,** Attending Physician, Department of Pediatrics, Hematology and Oncology, Naval Medical Center San Diego, San Diego, California

**Donald L. Boyer, MD, MSEd, FAAP,** Attending Physician, Pediatric Critical Care Medicine, The Children's Hospital of Philadelphia, Assistant Professor, Department of Anesthesiology & Critical Care Medicine, Perelman School of Medicine at the University of Pennsylvania, Philadelphia, Pennsylvania

**Jennifer M. Brady, MD,** Assistant Professor of Pediatrics, Division of Neonatology, Cincinnati Children's Hospital Medical Center, Cincinnati, Ohio

**Terri Brown-Whitehorn, MD,** Associate Professor of Clinical Pediatrics, Perelman School of Medicine at the University of Pennsylvania, The Children's Hospital of Philadelphia, Philadelphia, Pennsylvania

**Jon Burnham, MD, MSCE,** Attending Physician, Division of Rheumatology, The Children's Hospital of Philadelphia; Associate Professor of Pediatrics, Perelman School of Medicine at the University of Pennsylvania, Philadelphia, Pennsylvania

**Diane Calello, MD,** Robert Wood Johnson University Hospital, New Brunswick, New Jersey

**Leslie Castelo-Soccio, MD, PhD,** Section of Dermatology, The Children's Hospital of Philadelphia, Assistant Professor of Pediatrics and Dermatology, Perelman School of Medicine at the University of Pennsylvania, Philadelphia, Pennsylvania

**Marina Catallozzi, MD, MSCE,** Assistant Professor of Pediatrics and Population and Family Health at Columbia University Medical Center, New York, New York

**Katie Chiotos, MD,** Fellow, Divisions of Infectious Diseases and Critical Care Medicine, The Children's Hospital of Philadelphia, Philadelphia, Pennsylvania

**Lawrence Copelovitch, MD,** Assistant Professor of Pediatrics, Division of Nephrology, The Children's Hospital of Philadelphia, Perelman School of Medicine at the University of Pennsylvania, Philadelphia, Pennsylvania

**Stefanie L. Davidson, MD,** Attending Surgeon, Division of Pediatric Ophthalmology, The Children's Hospital of Philadelphia, Philadelphia, Pennsylvania

**Jeannine Del Pizzo, MD,** Attending Physician, Division of Emergency Medicine, The Children's Hospital of Philadelphia; and Assistant Professor of Clinical Pediatrics, Perelman School of Medicine at the University of Pennsylvania, Philadelphia, Pennsylvania

**Dennis J. Dlugos, MD,** Professor of Neurology, Perelman School of Medicine at the University of Pennsylvania, and Attending Physician, Division of Neurology, The Children's Hospital of Philadelphia, Philadelphia, Pennsylvania

**Angela Ellison, MD, MSc,** Assistant Professor of Pediatrics, Division of Emergency Medicine, The Children's Hospital of Philadelphia, Perelman School of Medicine, University of Pennsylvania, Philadelphia, Pennsylvania

**Christine T. Ferrara, MD, PhD,** Clinical Fellow in Pediatric Endocrinology and Diabetes, Division of Endocrinology and Diabetes, The Children's Hospital of Philadelphia, Philadelphia, Pennsylvania

**Sarah Fesnak, MD,** Fellow, Division of Emergency Medicine, The Children's Hospital of Philadelphia, Philadelphia, Pennsylvania

**Can Ficicioglu, MD, PhD,** Associate Professor of Pediatrics, Perelman School of Medicine at the University of Pennsylvania; Attending Physician, Division of Metabolism, Director of the Newborn Metabolic Screening Program, The Children's Hospital of Philadelphia, Philadelphia, Pennsylvania

**Jason L. Freedman, MD,** Clinical Instructor, Division of Oncology, The Children's Hospital of Philadelphia, Philadelphia, Pennsylvania

**Irene Fung, MD,** Fellow, Division of Allergy and Immunology, The Children's Hospital of Philadelphia, Philadelphia, Pennsylvania

**Rebecca Ganetzky, MD,** Fellow, Division of Metabolism, The Children's Hospital of Philadelphia, Philadelphia, Pennsylvania

**Theodore Ganley, MD,** Director of Sports Medicine, The Children's Hospital of Philadelphia, Associate Professor of Orthopaedic Surgery, Perelman School of Medicine at the University of Pennsylvania, Philadelphia, Pennsylvania

**Jeffrey S. Gerber, MD, PhD,** Assistant Professor of Pediatrics, Perelman School of Medicine at the University of Pennsylvania, Division of Infectious Diseases, The Children's Hospital of Philadelphia, Philadelphia, Pennsylvania

**John Germiller, MD, PhD,** Attending Surgeon, Division of Pediatric Otolaryngology, The Children's Hospital of Philadelphia; and Associate Professor of Clinical Otorhinolaryngology/Head and Neck Surgery, Perelman School of Medicine at the University of Pennsylvania, Philadelphia, Pennsylvania

**Matthew Grady, MD,** Fellowship Director, Primary Care Sports Medicine, The Children's Hospital of Philadelphia, Assistant Professor of Clinical Pediatrics, Perelman School of Medicine at the University of Pennsylvania, Philadelphia, Pennsylvania

**Lori Handy, MD, MSCE,** Attending Physician, Division of Pediatric Infectious Diseases, Nemours/Alfred I. duPont Hospital for Children, Wilmington, Delaware

**Mary Catherine Harris, MD,** Professor of Pediatrics, Division of Neonatology, The Children's Hospital of Philadelphia, Perelman School of Medicine at the University of Pennsylvania, Philadelphia, Pennsylvania

**Soma Jyonouchi, MD,** The Children's Hospital of Philadelphia, Assistant Professor, Division of Allergy and Immunology, Philadelphia, Pennsylvania

**Amy Kim, MD,** Assistant Professor of Clinical Psychiatry, Perelman School of Medicine at the University of Pennsylvania; Attending Physician, Department of Child and Adolescent Psychiatry and Behavioral Sciences, The Children's Hospital of Philadelphia, Philadelphia, Pennsylvania

**F. Wickham Kraemer III, MD,** Assistant Professor of Anesthesiology and Critical Care, Section Chief, Acute and Chronic Pain Management, The Children's Hospital of Philadelphia, Perelman School of Medicine at the University of Pennsylvania, Department of Anesthesiology and Critical Care, Philadelphia, Pennsylvania

**Javier J. Lasa, MD,** Attending Physician, Divisions of Critical Care and Cardiology, Texas Children's Hospital, Assistant Professor of Pediatrics, Baylor College of Medicine, Houston, Texas

**Leonard J. Levine, MD,** Associate Professor of Pediatrics, Drexel University College of Medicine, Attending Physician, Division of Adolescent Medicine, St. Christopher's Hospital for Children, Philadelphia, Pennsylvania

**Arul M. Lingappan, MD,** Pediatric Anesthesiology Attending, The Children's Hospital of Philadelphia, Perelman School of Medicine at the University of Pennsylvania, Department of Anesthesiology and Critical Care, Philadelphia, Pennsylvania

**Vanessa N. Madrigal, MD,** Attending Physician, Pediatric Critical Care Medicine, Children's National Medical Center, Assistant Professor, Department of Pediatrics, George Washington University, Washington, Washington DC

**Solrun Melkorka Maggadottir, MD,** Allergy/Immunology Fellow, The Children's Hospital of Philadelphia, Philadelphia, Pennsylvania

**Petar Mamula, MD,** Division of GI, Hepatology & Nutrition, The Children's Hospital of Philadelphia, Professor of Pediatrics, Perelman School of Medicine at the University of Pennsylvania, Philadelphia, Pennsylvania

**Maria R. Mascarenhas, MBBS,** Section Chief, Nutrition, Division of Gastroenterology, Hepatology and Nutrition, The Children's Hospital of Philadelphia, Associate Professor of Pediatrics, Perelman School of Medicine at the University of Pennsylvania, Philadelphia, Pennsylvania

**Jamie Merves, MD,** Attending Physician, Division of Gastroenterology, Hepatology and Nutrition, The Children's Hospital of Philadelphia, Assistant Professor of Clinical Pediatrics, Perelman School of Medicine at the University of Pennsylvania, Philadelphia, Pennsylvania

**Pamela Mudd, MD,** Division of Pediatric Otolaryngology, The Children's Hospital of Philadelphia, Department of Otorhinolaryngology, Perelman School of Medicine at the University of Pennsylvania, Philadelphia, Pennsylvania

**Michael L. Nance, MD,** Professor of Surgery, Perelman School of Medicine at the University of Pennsylvania, Josephine J. and John M. Templeton, Jr. Chair in Pediatric Trauma, Director of the Pediatric Trauma Program, The Children's Hospital of Philadelphia, Philadelphia, Pennsylvania

**Benjamin R. Oshrine, MD,** Division of GI, Hepatology & Nutrition, The Children's Hospital of Philadelphia, Philadelphia, Pennsylvania

**Andrew A. Palladino, MD,** Division of Endocrinology and Diabetes, The Children's Hospital of Philadelphia, Philadelphia, Pennsylvania

**Howard B. Panitch, MD,** Professor of Pediatrics, Perelman School of Medicine at the University of Pennsylvania, Director of Clinical Programs, Division of Pulmonary Medicine, The Children's Hospital of Philadelphia, Philadelphia, Pennsylvania

**Melissa Desai Patel, MD, MPH,** Assistant Professor of Pediatrics, Perelman School of Medicine at the University of Pennsylvania, Medical Director of  Sedation Services, Attending Physician, Division of General Pediatrics, The Children's Hospital of Philadelphia, Philadelphia, Pennsylvania

**Annapurna Poduri, MD, MPH,** Director, Epilepsy Genetics Program, and Associate in Neurology, Boston Children's Hospital; and Associate Professor of Neurology, Harvard Medical School, Cambridge, Massachusetts

**Elisabeth Raab, MD, MPH,** Attending Neonatologist, Pediatrix Medical Group, Huntington Memorial Hospital, Pasadena, California

**Rahim Rahemtulla, MD,** Clinical Assistant Professor, Department of Child and Adolescent Psychiatry, New York University School of Medicine; Attending Physician, Lincoln Hospital and Mental Health Center, Department of Psychiatry, New York, New York

**Gita Ram, MD,** Assistant Physician, Division of Allergy and Immunology, The Children's Hospital of Philadelphia, Philadelphia, Pennsylvania

**Elaine Ramsay, MD,** Rheumatology Fellow, Division of Rheumatology, The Children's Hospital of Philadelphia, Philadelphia, Pennsylvania

**Chitra Ravishankar, MD,** Associate Professor of Pediatrics, Division of Cardiology, The Children's Hospital of Philadelphia, Perelman School of Medicine at the University of Pennsylvania, Philadelphia, Pennsylvania

**Daniel H. Reirden, MD, AAHIVMS,** Associate Professor of Pediatrics and Internal Medicine, Adolescent Medicine and Infectious Disease; Director of Internal Medicine-Pediatric Residency; and Medical Director, CHIP Youth Clinic, University of Colorado School of Medicine and Children's Hospital Colorado, Denver, Colorado

**Christopher B. Renjilian, MD, MBE,** Fellow, The Craig-Dalsimer Division of Adolescent Medicine, The Children's Hospital of Philadelphia, Philadelphia, Pennsylvania Resident, Pediatrics, The Children's Hospital of Philadelphia, Philadelphia, Pennsylvania

**Joseph Rossano, MD, MS, FAAP, FAAC,** Attending Cardiologist, Cardiac Center and the Cardiac Intensive Care Unit (CICU), Medical Director, Pediatric Heart Transplant and Heart Failure, Assistant Professor of Pediatrics, Perelman School of Medicine at the University of Pennsylvania, The Children's Hospital of Philadelphia, Division of Cardiology, Philadelphia, Pennsylvania

**Rebecca L. Ruebner, MD, MSCE,** Attending Physician, Division of Nephrology, The Children's Hospital of Philadelphia; Assistant Professor of Pediatrics, Perelman School of Medicine at the University of Pennsylvania, Philadelphia, Pennsylvania

**Benjamin Sahn, MD, MS,** Assistant Professor of Pediatrics, Hofstra North Shore-LIJ School of Medicine Division of Pediatric Gastroenterology & Nutrition Steven & Alexandra Cohen Children's Medical Center of New York North Shore - Long Island Jewish Health System New Hyde Park, New York, New York

**Margaret Samuels-Kalow, MD, MPhil,** Instructor, Division of Emergency, Medicine, Department of Pediatrics, The Children's Hospital of Philadelphia, Perelman School of Medicine at the University of Pennsylvania, Philadelphia, Pennsylvania

**Kara N. Shah, MD, PhD,** Director, Division of Dermatology, Cincinnati Children's Hospital, Associate Professor of Pediatrics and Dermatology, University of Cincinnati College of Medicine, Cincinnati, Ohio

**Renée A. Shellhaas, MD,** Assistant Professor, Pediatrics, C.S. Mott Children's Hospital, University of Michigan Health System, Ann Arbor, Michigan

**Joann Spinale Carlson, MD,** Division of Pediatric Nephrology and Hypertension, Rutgers/ Robert Wood Johnson Medical School, New Brunswick, New Jersey

**Salwa Sulieman, DO,** Assistant Professor of Pediatrics, University of Missouri-Kansas City, Division of Infectious Diseases, Children's Mercy Hospital, Kansas City, Missouri

**Alysha Taxter, MD,** Rheumatology Fellow, Division of Rheumatology, The Children's Hospital of Philadelphia, Philadelphia, Pennsylvania

**Gihan I. Tennekoon, MD,** Attending Physician, Division of Neurology, The Children's Hospital of Philadelphia; and Professor of Neurology, Perelman School of Medicine at the University of Pennsylvania, Philadelphia, Pennsylvania

**Christian Turner, MD,** Primary Care Sports Medicine Fellow, The Children's Hospital of Philadelphia, Philadelphia, Pennsylvania

**Jesse D. Vrecenak, MD,** Fellow, Division of General and Thoracic Surgery, Department of Surgery, The Children's Hospital of Philadelphia, Perelman School of Medicine at the University of Pennsylvania, Philadelphia, Pennsylvania

**Nicole Washington, MD,** Pediatric Chief Resident, 2014–2015, The Children's Hospital of Philadelphia, Philadelphia, Pennsylvania

**Tara L. Wenger, MD, PhD,** Assistant Professor, Division of Craniofacial Medicine, Department of Pediatrics, Seattle Children's Hospital, Seattle, Washington

**Krishna Wood White, MD, MPH,** Director, Adolescent Medicine Program, Clinical Assistant Professor of Pediatrics, Thomas Jefferson University, Nemours/A.I. DuPont Hospital for Children, Wilmington, Delaware

**Char Witmer, MD, MSCE,** Attending Physician, Division of Hematology, The Children's Hospital of Philadelphia; and Assistant Professor of Pediatrics, Perelman School of Medicine at the University of Pennsylvania, Philadelphia, Pennsylvania

# Foreword

Having started my training in pediatrics at The Children's Hospital of Philadelphia, and then continuing my training and practice at other major academic medical centers, I came to appreciate the premier care that patients receive when knowledge and dedication come together. When I was a young trainee at CHOP, a welcomed resource to inpatient care was a series of resident handouts. These were prepared by senior residents and passed along from one year to the next, each senior class updating and improving on the work of their predecessors. Twenty-five years after leaving CHOP, I had the privilege to return in a leadership role for the Department of Pediatrics. Among the many welcomed surprises since my return, I was delighted to see the valued handouts that had served me so well as a trainee have been developed into *The Philadelphia Guide: Inpatient Pediatrics*. The practical information that guided me back then is now available in this concise and well-organized book. It provides effective management of the lion's share of patients admitted to the hospital and is a reliable source for efficient and fact-filled teaching on rounds.

Increasingly, patient care is evidence-based, often operationalized through clinical pathways. These pathways may be informed by national committees with broad representation and multidisciplinary input, or from similar local efforts, institutional experience, and application of the literature. It is in this spirit that this book was created. The authors and editors have assembled the second edition of *The Philadelphia Guide: Inpatient Pediatrics* to carry on the tradition of learning, improving, and then sharing knowledge that I first encountered as a resident at CHOP. I am especially proud that the authors, from all across the country, all share a connection to CHOP. They are trainees, young faculty, and more senior leaders in their fields who enjoy carrying on the practice of life-long learning and advancement of knowledge. I am confident that this book will serve as an important guide to diagnostic and therapeutic decisions in the pediatric inpatient setting and a valuable tool for all of us involved in delivering care to children and adolescents.

Joseph W. St. Geme, III, MD
Physician-In-Chief
The Children's Hospital of Philadelphia
Chairman, Department of Pediatrics
Perelman School of Medicine, University of Pennsylvania

# Preface—*Inpatient Pediatrics,* 2nd Edition

Care of the hospitalized child has evolved dramatically since publication of the first edition of *The Philadelphia Guide: Inpatient Pediatrics.* Conditions that previously required prolonged hospitalization are now often treated exclusively in the outpatient setting or with only a brief hospitalization. Advances in medical technology have improved the survival rate of premature infants and those with chronic medical conditions. Further, changes in healthcare delivery have placed renewed emphasis on value, with an expectation of better outcomes at lower cost. As a result, the type of physician caring for these patients has also changed. At many institutions, hospital-based specialists, or "hospitalists," now provide care for the majority of patients admitted to general pediatric wards, leading to the evolution of pediatric hospital medicine as a new specialty.

As we prepared the second edition, Hospital Medicine remained our core focus. We believe that *Inpatient Pediatrics* should provide clinicians with the vital information necessary to make management decisions in the care of hospitalized children. Once again, we were fortunate that over 75 leading experts in pediatric hospital medicine and pediatric subspecialty care, many with roots at The Children's Hospital of Philadelphia, share their collective wisdom by contributing to this book.

Designed to be an invaluable resource on the hospital wards, *Inpatient Pediatrics* features:

• Practical diagnostic strategies
• Extensive differential diagnosis suggestions
• Up-to-date treatment and management guidelines
• Alphabetical organization within chapters for rapid access
• Structured format with consistent headings throughout
• Bulleted format for efficient and effective presentation of relevant information
• Print and electronic versions to maximize portability and ensure access to information whenever and wherever necessary

Appendices cover normal vital signs, neonatal codes, and PALS algorithms as well as rapid access to pediatric dosages for emergency, airway, and rapid sequence intubation medications, and cardioversion.

A formulary was omitted with the understanding that pediatric dosing information is now accessible through most institutional formularies and widely available mobile apps.

As many clinicians are involved in the care of children, this book is ideal for practitioners of all levels, from students to attending physicians, physician assistants, advanced practice nurses, pediatric nurses, and health practitioners from all disciplines involved in the care of the hospitalized child.

The goal of this book is to provide a single reference with sufficient detail to guide diagnostic and therapeutic decisions for a wide range of conditions. We believe that the consistent format, detailed focus on diagnosis and management, and comprehensive coverage of topics have accomplished that goal, enabling you to give the best possible care to your patients. We hope you think so, too.

Samir S. Shah
Lisa B. Zaoutis
Marina Catallozzi
Gary Frank
November 2015

# List of Abbreviations

| | |
|---|---|
| AIN: | acute interstitial nephritis |
| AKI: | acute kidney injury |
| ALCL: | anaplastic large cell lymphoma |
| ALK: | anaplastic lymphoma kinase |
| ALL: | acute lymphoblastic leukemia |
| Alph1-AT: | alpha-1 antitrypsin |
| AMKL: | acute megakaryocytic leukemia |
| AML: | acute myeloid leukemia |
| ANA: | antinuclear antibody |
| ANC: | absolute neutrophil count |
| ANCA: | anti-neutrophil cytoplasmic antibody |
| Anti-SMA: | anti-smooth muscle antibody |
| APGAR: | appearance, pulse, grimace, activity, respiration |
| APML: | acute promyelocytic leukemia |
| ASCA: | anti-*Saccharomyces cerevisiae* antibody |
| ASD: | atrial septal defect |
| ATN: | acute tubular necrosis |
| ATRA: | all-trans retinoic acid |
| BP: | blood pressure |
| BWS: | Beckwith–Wiedemann syndrome |
| CBD: | common bile duct |
| CCK: | cholecystokinin |
| CD: | Crohn's disease |
| CGD: | chronic granulomatous disease |
| CHD: | congenital heart disease |
| CHF: | congestive heart failure |
| CINV: | chemotherapy-induced nausea vomiting |
| CML: | chronic myelogenous leukemia |
| CMV: | cytomegalovirus |
| CNS: | central nervous system |
| CRT: | cardiac resynchronization therapy |
| CXR: | chest x-ray |
| DBP: | diastolic blood pressure |
| DISIDA scan: | diisopropyl iminodiacetic acid labeled with 99m-technetium |
| DVT: | deep venous thrombosis |
| EBV: | Epstein–Barr virus |

| | |
|---|---|
| ECG: | electrocardiogram |
| ECMO: | extracorporeal membrane oxygenation |
| EPS: | extrapyramidal symptoms |
| ETT: | via endotracheal tube |
| FENa: | fractional excretion of sodium |
| FISH: | fluorescence in situ hybridization |
| GAS: | group A streptococcus |
| GER: | gastroesophageal reflux |
| GERD: | gastroesophageal reflux disease |
| GFR: | glomerular filtration rate |
| GI: | gastrointestinal |
| GN: | glomerulonephritis |
| GNR: | gram negative rods |
| GVHD: | graft-versus-host disease |
| HELLP: | hemolysis, elevated liver enzymes, low platelets |
| HHV6: | human herpesvirus 6 |
| HLA: | human leukocyte antigen |
| HLH: | hemophagocytic lymphohistiocytosis |
| HLHS: | hypoplastic left heart syndrome |
| HOCM: | hypertrophic obstructive cardiomyopathy |
| HSCT: | hematopoietic stem cell transplantation |
| HSP: | Henoch–Schönlein purpura |
| HSV: | herpes simplex virus |
| HUS: | hemolytic uremic syndrome |
| IBD: | inflammatory bowel disease |
| IBS: | irritable bowel syndrome |
| IC: | indeterminate colitis |
| ICU: | intensive care unit |
| IM: | intramuscular |
| IN: | intranasal |
| IV: | intravenous |
| JDM: | juvenile dermatomyositis |
| JIA: | juvenile idiopathic arthritis |
| JMML: | juvenile myelomonocytic leukemia |
| LA: | left atrium |
| LDH: | lactate dehydrogenase |
| LES: | lower esophageal sphincter |
| LGBTQ: | lesbian, gay, bisexual, transgender, and questioning |
| LKM: | liver-kidney-microsomal |

| | |
|---|---|
| LLSB: | left lower sternal border |
| LSD: | D-lysergic acid diethylamide |
| LV: | left ventricle |
| LVAD: | left ventricular assist device |
| LVNC: | left ventricular noncompaction |
| MAS: | Macrophage activation syndrome |
| MDS: | myelodysplastic syndrome |
| MLL: | mixed lineage leukemia |
| MPGN: | membranoproliferative glomerulonephritis |
| MRS: | magnetic resonance spectroscopy |
| NEMO: | a primary immunodeficiency syndrome caused by genetic mutations in the X-linked NEMO gene |
| NHL: | non-Hodgkin Lymphoma |
| NMDA: | N-methyl-D-aspartate |
| NPO: | nothing by mouth |
| NS: | nephrotic syndrome |
| NSAIDs: | nonsteroidal anti-inflammatory drugs |
| PAC: | premature atrial contraction |
| PCA: | patient controlled analgesia |
| PCP: | phencyclidine |
| PDA: | patent ductus arteriosus |
| PDD: | pervasive developmental delay |
| PG: | prostaglandin |
| Pi: | protease inhibitor |
| PICC: | peripherally inserted central catheters |
| PMBCL: | primary mediastinal B-cell lymphoma |
| PNET: | peripheral neuroectodermal issue |
| PO: | by mouth |
| PPI: | proton pump inhibitor |
| PR: | per rectum |
| PRSA: | post-streptococcal reactive arthritis |
| PTLD: | post-transplant lymphoproliferative disease |
| PUCAI: | pediatric ulcerative colitis activity index |
| PUD: | peptic ulcer disease |
| PVC: | premature ventricular contraction |
| PVR: | pulmonary vascular resistance |
| RA: | right atrium |
| RCM: | restrictive cardiomyopathy |
| RTA: | renal tubular acidosis |

## List of Abbreviations

| | |
|---|---|
| RUQ: | right upper quadrant |
| RV: | right ventricle |
| SaO$_2$: | oxygen saturation |
| SBP: | systolic blood pressure |
| SC: | subcutaneous |
| SCID: | severe combined immunodeficiency |
| SCT: | stem cell transplantation |
| SI: | suicidal ideation |
| SIRS: | systemic inflammatory response syndrome |
| SLA: | soluble liver antigen |
| SLE: | systemic lupus erythematosus |
| SMS: | superior mediastinal syndrome |
| STEC: | Shiga toxin-producing *Escherichia coli* |
| SVCS: | superior vena cava syndrome |
| SVR: | systemic vascular resistance |
| SVT: | supraventricular tachycardia |
| TAPVR: | total anomalous pulmonary venous return |
| TD: | tardive dyskinesia |
| TGA: | transposition of the great arteries |
| TMD: | transient myeloproliferative disorder |
| TPN: | total parenteral nutrition |
| TTP: | thrombotic thrombocytopenic purpura |
| UAG: | urine anion gap |
| UC: | ulcerative colitis |
| URI: | upper respiratory infection |
| UTI: | urinary tract infection |
| VADs: | ventricular assist devices |
| VIP: | vasoactive intestinal peptide |
| VOD: | veno-occlusive disease |
| VSD: | ventricular septal defect |
| VT: | ventricular tachycardia |
| VZV: | varicella zoster virus |
| WAS: | Wiskott–Aldrich syndrome |
| WBC: | white blood cell |
| WPW: | Wolff–Parkinson–White syndrome |
| XRT: | radiotherapy |

# The Philadelphia Guide: Inpatient Pediatrics

Second Edition

# 1

# Adolescent Medicine

*Christopher B. Renjilian, MD, MBE*
*Krishna Wood White, MD, MPH*
*Leonard J. Levine, MD*

## ANOREXIA NERVOSA

### DSM-V CRITERIA* FOR ANOREXIA NERVOSA ARE SUMMARIZED BELOW

- Restriction of calories compared to requirements which leads to significantly low weight
- Intense fear of gaining weight
- Disturbance in the way in which one's body weight or shape is experienced
- *Restricting type:* During the prior 3 months with anorexia nervosa, the person has not achieved weight loss through being regularly engaged in binge eating or purging behavior (self-induced vomiting, use of laxatives/diuretics/enemas) but through dieting and excessive exercise
- *Binge eating/Purging type:* During the prior 3 months with anorexia nervosa, the person has regularly engaged in binge eating or purging behavior (self-induced vomiting, use of laxatives/diuretics/enemas)

*\*Note:* DSM-V no longer sets a specific percent of ideal body weight but states that "significantly low weight" is less than is minimally normal or normally expected (for children and adolescents). DSM-V removes amenorrhea as a criterion for anorexia as it did not apply to males, females on contraceptives, or pre-menarchal females. Also, patients that meet all of the criteria except amenorrhea have the same clinical course as those who meet all four criteria.

### EPIDEMIOLOGY

- 1% of adolescent females; female:male = 20:1
- Age at presentation ranges from 10 to 25 years
- Increasing incidence in adolescent males, nonwhite populations, and lower socioeconomic groups; more common among individuals involved in sports or activities where size and body shape impact their success
- Bimodal age of onset at 14 and 18 years corresponding with life transitions (i.e., puberty, moving from high school to college or work)
- Mortality rates range from 1.8% to 5.9% (usually because of cardiac complications or suicide)

### ETIOLOGY

- *Genetic:* Increased risk in first-degree relatives with an eating disorder
- *Neurotransmitters:* Serotonin and its relationship to hunger and satiety
- *Psychologic:* Theories range from perfectionism, identity conflicts, history of abuse, negative comments from others about weight or appearance, enmeshed families, and sociocultural influences

### CLINICAL MANIFESTATIONS

- Menstrual disorders are the most common presentation
- Frequently, patients do not have complaints, but family members are concerned about significant weight loss, secondary amenorrhea, dizziness, lack of energy, gastrointestinal complaints (e.g., constipation), and/or pale skin

- Depending on amount of weight loss, clinical findings can range from normal to findings of orthostasis, bradycardia, hypothermia, hypotension, dry skin, lanugo hair, thinning hair, brittle nails, peripheral edema, acrocyanosis, and findings suggestive of purging such as eroded tooth enamel, scars on knuckles, or parotid enlargement
- External evidence of self-harm, such as scars from cutting on the extremities

## DIAGNOSTICS

- Must consider the differential diagnosis for weight loss and exclude malabsorption and catabolic states
- Clinical information is vital. Questions should focus on disordered thinking and behavior. Screening questions (e.g., SCOFF questionnaire) can be helpful:
  ✓ Do you make yourself *sick* because you feel uncomfortably full?
  ✓ Do you worry you have lost *control* over how much you eat?
  ✓ Have you recently lost more than *one* stone (6.3 kg [14 lb]) in a 3-month period?
  ✓ Do you believe yourself to be *fat* when others say you are too thin?
  ✓ Would you say that *food* dominates your life?

*Give one point for every yes; scores of 2 or more indicate anorexia nervosa or bulimia*

- Laboratory studies are not diagnostic of anorexia nervosa. Table 1-1 suggests tests to obtain in the initial assessment of a patient suspected of having anorexia nervosa. Further tests should be ordered based on clinical suspicion for other diseases
- *ECG:* Indicated for bradycardia less than 50 bpm to rule out prolonged QTc or dysrhythmias. Low voltage, ST segment depression, or conduction abnormalities may also be seen
- *DEXA:* Evaluate bone density in patients who are amenorrheic greater than 6 months
- *Imaging:* Chest x-ray, brain magnetic resonance imaging, barium enema, and upper gastrointestinal series with small bowel follow-through should be considered based on clinical concern for other conditions as an explanation for symptoms

## MANAGEMENT

- *Indications for inpatient treatment are listed in* Table 1-2
- *Interdisciplinary team:* Comprised of a physician, dietician, and mental health professional should generate a coordinated consistent plan of care and be available for team meetings with patient and family; recent studies highlight importance of family-based therapy
- *Fluids/Electrolytes/Nutrition:*
  ✓ Correction of dehydration
  ✓ Blind weights with the patient wearing only a gown at same time and on the same scale each day are best. Expected rate of weight gain is 0.9–1.4 kg (2–3 lb) per week
- *Refeeding syndrome:* Constellation of cardiac, neurologic, and hematologic complications as phosphate shifts from extracellular to intracellular compartments in patients with total body phosphate depletion secondary to malnutrition
  ✓ *Pathophysiology:* Catabolic→anabolic state→energy used as adenosine triphosphate (ATP)→phosphorus→erythrocyte 2,3 diphosphoglycerate (2,3 DPG)→tissue hypoxia
  ✓ *Risk factors:* Moderate to severe anorexia (less than 10% below ideal body weight)
  ✓ *Prevention:* Slow refeeding with or without phosphorous supplementation (in patients with normal renal function)
  ✓ *Monitoring:* Telemetry, frequent vital signs, and electrolytes especially phosphorus, potassium, and magnesium
  ✓ *Clinical manifestations:* Cardiac arrest, delirium, congestive heart failure
- *Cardiovascular:* Telemetry for patients with significant bradycardia, dysrhythmias, and electrolyte abnormalities until resolution of conditions

| TABLE 1-1 | Laboratory Studies in Anorexia Nervosa |
|---|---|
| **Study** | **Rationale/Interpretation** |
| Serum chemistries | Hyponatremia—water loading or inappropriate regulation of ADH |
| | Hypophosphatemia—severe malnutrition |
| | Hypokalemic, hypochloremic metabolic alkalosis—vomiting |
| | Acidosis—laxative abuse |
| | Hypoglycemia |
| | High blood urea nitrogen and creatinine—dehydration +/− purging |
| Complete blood cell count | High hemoglobin—dehydration |
| | Anemia—chronic disease and/or iron deficiency |
| | Leukopenia and thrombocytopenia |
| Liver function tests (including prealbumin) | Prealbumin and albumin—evaluate nutritional status |
| | Abnormal liver enzymes—fatty liver infiltration |
| Cholesterol, triglycerides | Elevated due to abnormal lipoprotein metabolism |
| ESR | Normal to low in anorexia |
| Urinalysis | Low specific gravity—water loading |
| Morning cortisol level | Rule out adrenal insufficiency |
| Thyroid function tests | Euthyroid sick sinus syndrome—normal or low thyroid-stimulating hormone and normal thyroxine |
| | Rule out hyper- or hypothyroidism |
| β-HCG | Rule out pregnancy |
| Prolactin | Rule out prolactinoma |
| LH and FSH | Rule out ovarian failure |

ADH, antidiuretic hormone; ESR, erythrocyte sedimentation rate; FSH, follicle-stimulating hormone; HCG, human chorionic gonadotropin; LH, luteinizing hormone.

| TABLE 1-2 | Criteria for Hospital Admission for Children, Adolescents, and Young Adults with Anorexia Nervosa |
|---|---|

**Criteria for Hospital Admission**

<75% of ideal body weight or ongoing weight loss despite intensive management

Refusal to eat

Body fat <10%

Heart rate <50 beats per minute daytime; <45 beats per minute nighttime

Systolic pressure >90 mm Hg

Orthostatic changes in pulse (20 beats per minute or blood pressure <10 mm Hg)

Temperature <96°F

Arrhythmia

Adapted with permission from Rosen DS; American Academy of Pediatrics Committee on Adolescence: Identification and management of eating disorders in children and adolescents, *Pediatrics* 2010 Dec;126(6): 1240–1253.

- *Gastrointestinal:* Control of constipation with stool softeners (avoid laxatives). Metoclopramide may be helpful with bloating and constipation secondary to delayed gastric emptying
- *Endocrinology:*
  - ✓ *Osteopenia:* Weight gain is best therapy; a multivitamin with 400 IU of vitamin D and 1200–1500 mg/day of elemental calcium is recommended. Estrogen or estrogen/progestin replacement therapy should be considered
  - ✓ *Amenorrhea:* Menses will resume with adequate weight gain and improved nutritional status; no hormonal therapy required
- *Psychiatry:*
  - ✓ *Safety and compliance:* 1:1 observation by qualified staff with experience with eating disorders is required, especially in the beginning of treatment
  - ✓ Mental status abnormalities improve with correction of malnourished state. Most interventions should begin after patient is medically stable
  - ✓ *Psychotherapy:* Cognitive behavioral therapy is the most effective form of therapy
  - ✓ *Pharmacotherapy:* Indicated only for treatment of comorbid disorders (i.e., depression, obsessive compulsive disorder). There is no FDA-approved drug for treatment of anorexia nervosa

## ABNORMAL UTERINE BLEEDING

**Bleeding from the uterine endometrium unrelated to an anatomic lesion. Abnormal bleeding can be identified as menstrual cycles that occur less than 21 or more than 45 days apart, bleeding lasting more than 8 days, or blood loss greater than 80 mL/cycle.**

### ETIOLOGY

- Anovulatory cycles (over 75% of cases)
  - ✓ Commonly occurs in first few years after menarche
  - ✓ Hypothalamic-pituitary-ovarian axis not fully mature→ovarian estrogen production doesn't consistently reach level needed to trigger luteinizing hormone (LH) surge→failure to ovulate each month
  - ✓ No ovulation→estrogen unopposed because no corpus luteum or progesterone secretion→continuously stimulated endometrium without stromal support→lining outgrows blood supply→endometrium breaks down with variable shedding, necrosis, and irregular bleeding

### DIFFERENTIAL DIAGNOSIS

- *Anovulatory cycles:* Immaturity of hypothalamic-pituitary-ovarian (HPO) axis
- *Pregnancy:* Ectopic, threatened or incomplete abortion, placenta previa, hydatidiform mole
- *Sexually transmitted infection (STI):* vaginitis (e.g., *Trichomonas*), cervicitis (e.g., gonorrhea, *Chlamydia*), pelvic inflammatory disease (i.e., endometritis)
- *Endocrinopathy causing anovulation:* Thyroid disease (hypothyroidism, hyperthyroidism), hyperprolactinemia (e.g., prolactinoma, dopamine antagonists), adrenal disorders (e.g., Addison disease, Cushing disease), polycystic ovary syndrome (PCOS), or other disorder of androgen excess
- *Systemic disease causing anovulation:* Chronic renal failure, systemic lupus erythematosus
- *Hematologic disorder:* Thrombocytopenia (e.g., idiopathic thrombocytopenic purpura, leukemia), defects in platelet function (e.g., von Willebrand disease), coagulation disorders
- *Medications:* Direct effect on hemostasis (e.g., warfarin, chemotherapeutic agents), indirect effect by altering hormone levels (e.g., breakthrough bleeding with hormonal contraception)

- *Trauma:* Laceration to vaginal mucosa or cervix
- *Foreign body:* Retained tampon or condom
- Endometriosis
- *Structural abnormalities (rare):* Uterine polyps, myoma, cervical hemangioma, arteriovenous malformation, neoplasm

## CLINICAL MANIFESTATIONS

- Bleeding pattern can help guide evaluation
  - ✓ Consider hematologic disorder if normal cyclic intervals with increased bleeding during each cycle, especially if occurs since menarche
  - ✓ Normal intervals with bleeding between cycles may suggest infection pregnancy, or foreign body
  - ✓ Endocrinopathy, anovulatory cycles, and medication effects are suggested by lack of any cycle regularity
- Physical exam may be unremarkable, especially if due to anovulatory cycles
- May have evidence of anemia (e.g., pallor, lethargy) or hypovolemia, depending on amount of blood loss
- Signs and symptoms will reflect underlying etiology. For example:
  - ✓ *Prolactinoma:* Headaches, visual changes, nipple discharge
  - ✓ *Thyroid disease:* Diarrhea or constipation, palpitations, skin changes, heat or cold intolerance
  - ✓ *Bleeding disorder:* Epistaxis and gingival bleeding, easy bruising
  - ✓ *Sexually transmitted infection:* Fever, abdominal pain, vaginal discharge, dysuria
  - ✓ *Retained foreign body:* Foul smelling odor and discharge
  - ✓ *PCOS:* Acne, hirsutism, acanthosis nigricans

## DIAGNOSTICS

### Clinical Assessment

- *Obtain menstrual history:* Age of menarche, interval between menses, duration of flow, frequency of tampon/pad changes, with or without cramping (cramping often is a marker for ovulatory cycles due to progesterone secretion), last menstrual period
- Obtain sexual history in confidential manner
- Ask about symptoms of anemia (e.g., dizziness or lightheadedness)
- Assess hemodynamic stability
- *Special attention to:* nutritional status, visual fields (i.e., pituitary lesions), thyroid size, breast exam (for galactorrhea), evidence of androgen excess (hirsutism, acne), ecchymoses or petechiae, Sexual Maturity Rating
- Pelvic exam if ever been sexually active (including bimanual exam) or to visualize source of bleeding

### Studies

- *Pregnancy test:* On every adolescent female presenting with vaginal bleeding
- Complete blood count with differential
- *STI testing:* Wet prep for white blood cells or *Trichomonas*, nucleic acid amplification testing for *N. gonorrhea* and *C. trachomatis* (urine or cervical swabs)
- PT/PTT
- Depending on history, may also consider von Willebrand studies, thyroid-stimulating hormone, prolactin level, LH, follicle-stimulating hormone, serum androgens (e.g., free testosterone, dehydroepiandrosterone-S, androstenedione)

- Pelvic ultrasound (if mass palpated on bimanual exam or if concerned for structural abnormalities)

## MANAGEMENT

- Depends on severity of bleeding and degree of anemia
- *Hormonal therapy is the mainstay of treatment:* Usually oral contraceptive pill (OCP) used to provide hemostasis (estrogen) and to stabilize the endometrium (progesterone). *Note:* Must ask about contraindications to estrogen use specified in the Center for Disease Control's Medical Eligibility Criteria for Contraceptive Use (2012) and if category 3 or 4 use progesterone only (http://www.cdc.gov/reproductivehealth/UnintendedPregnancy/USMEC.htm)
- Address underlying pathology (e.g., infection, endocrinopathy)
- *Adjunct management:* Menstrual diaries, iron supplementation, NSAIDs
- Mild dysfunctional uterine bleeding (DUB) (hemoglobin greater than 12 g/dL, no active bleeding)
  ✓ Prolonged menses or shortened cycles
  ✓ Reassurance and observation
- *Moderate DUB (hemoglobin 10-12 WITHOUT active bleeding):* Combined OCP with 30–35 μg ethinyl estradiol (EE) plus progestin
  ✓ One pill daily for 6 months, then reevaluate
  ✓ If estrogen contraindicated, use oral progesterone only: Medroxyprogesterone acetate 10 mg orally for 10 days, repeat monthly
- Moderate DUB (hemoglobin 10-12 WITH active bleeding)
  ✓ Combined OCP with 30–35 μg EE plus progestin
  ✓ One pill twice a day until bleeding stops, then once daily
- Severe DUB (hemoglobin less than 10 WITH active bleeding)
  ✓ Combined OCP with higher dose of estrogen (50 μg EE (preferred) or 35 μg EE if not available)
  ✓ One pill four times daily for 4 days, then three times daily for 3 days, then twice daily for 2 days, then once daily
  ✓ If not tolerating oral medications or if hemodynamically unstable, can use high-dose conjugated estrogen (Premarin) given intravenously every 4 hours up to 24 hours to control bleeding, then add oral progesterone or switch to OCP as soon as possible to avoid heavy estrogen withdrawal bleed
  ✓ Give antiemetics when estrogen given in multiple doses per day. Table 1-2 lists antiemetics
  ✓ Blood transfusions are rarely necessary in the management of AUB
  ✓ May require hospitalization if actively bleeding; requires close outpatient follow-up once stabilized

## EMERGENCY CONTRACEPTION

**Emergency contraception is a method of contraception where a drug or intrauterine device is used after unprotected intercourse.**

## INDICATIONS

- Pregnancy prevention following unprotected vaginal intercourse, contraceptive failure (e.g., broken condom, missed or late doses of hormonal contraceptives), sexual assault
- Most effective within 72 hours or less since aforementioned event; additional data supports effectiveness within 120 hours

## OPTIONS

- Three general classes of hormonal emergency contraception (EC) are currently approved for use in the United States (see Table 1-3):
  - ✓ Progestin-only oral regimens including levonorgestrel (e.g., *Plan B, Next Choice*)
  - ✓ Novel progestin receptor agonist/antagonist oral regimens including ulipristal (*Ella*)
  - ✓ Combination estrogen and progestin oral regimens using alternative dosing of combination OCPs, also known as the Yuzpe method
- Nonhormonal methods of EC are currently limited to insertion of the copper intrauterine device (IUD). Copper IUD is currently the most effective method of EC

| TABLE 1-3 | Emergency Contraception Regimens[*] | | |
|---|---|---|---|
| **Regimen Name** | **Pills per Dose/Color (Repeat Once in 12 Hours)** | **Advantages of Regimen[†]** | **Disadvantages of Regimen** |
| **Yuzpe Regimen (Combined Estrogen/Progestin)** | | | |
| *Preven* | 2 blue | • 75% efficacy | • 72-hour window |
| *Ovral, Ogestrel* | 2 white | | |
| *Alesse, Levlite* | 5 pink | • *Preven* comes with patient info book and urine pregnancy test | • Side effects including nausea/vomiting common |
| *Aviane* | 5 orange | | |
| *Nordette, Levlen* | 4 light-orange | • Patient may already have OCPs | • Cannot be used in individuals in which estrogen is contraindicated (refer to Center for Disease Control's Medical Eligibility Criteria for Contraceptive Use [2012])[**] |
| *Levora, Lo/Ovral* | 4 white | | |
| *Low-Ogestrel* | 4 yellow | • Established safety/efficacy | |
| *Triphasil, Tri-Levlen, Trivora* | 4 pink | • Can continue as contraception | |
| **Progestin Only** | | | |
| *Plan B* | 1 white | • 89% efficacy | • 72-hour window |
| *Ovrette* | 20 yellow | • *Plan B* comes with patient info kit | |
| | | • More effective than combined | |
| | | • Less side effects | |
| **IUD** | NA | • 99% efficacy | • Contraindicated for those with or at risk of STDs, other pelvic infections, anatomic anomalies, and in immunocompromised patients |
| | | • Can be inserted up to 5 days after unprotected sex | |
| | | • Can continue as contraception | |

[*]Most effective when given in first 12 hours of unprotected sex.
[†]Applies to medications with a particular regimen unless specifically noted.
[**]http://www.cdc.gov/reproductivehealth/UnintendedPregnancy/USMEC.htm
IUD, intrauterine device; NA, not applicable; OCPs, oral contraceptive pills; STDs, sexually transmitted diseases.

## CONTRAINDICATIONS

- *All regimens*: Pregnancy; hypersensitivity to drug components; undiagnosed vaginal bleeding
- *Method-specific contraindications*
  - ✓ *Progestin-only oral regimens:* No contraindications
  - ✓ *Progestin receptor agonist/antagonist:* Unclear if can be used safely in pregnancy
  - ✓ *Combination OCPs:* Same as above, but also include contraindications to estrogen exposure (e.g., history of thrombophilia, thromboembolic disease, migraine with aura or neurologic changes; refer to Center for Disease Control's Medical Eligibility Criteria for Contraceptive Use [2012])
  - ✓ *Copper IUD*: Abnormal genital tract anatomy, infection at the time of insertion

## MECHANISM OF ACTION

- Inhibit or delay ovulation
- Disrupt follicular development
- Impairment of corpus luteum
- Create unfavorable environment for sperm function
- Copper IUD also alters endometrium, likely interfering with implantation; unclear if such alteration also occurs with hormonal emergency contraception

## ADVERSE EFFECTS

- *Occur mostly with combined EC (containing estrogen):* Nausea/vomiting; dizziness; fatigue; breast tenderness, altered menstrual cycle
- Copper IUD may cause cramping or increased menstrual flow; also low risk of uterine perforation upon insertion

## SAFETY

- Short course of therapy leads to few complications

## ANTICIPATORY GUIDANCE

- *Nausea/vomiting:* Common in combined regimen; can be reduced by pretreatment with oral anti-emetic (e.g., metoclopramide 10 mg or meclizine 25–50 mg) given 1 hour before EC
- *Effect on menstrual cycle:* Next menses may be early or late but should come within 21 days
- *Effect on pregnancy:* Levonorgestrel and combined OCP regimens do not affect established pregnancy or lead to birth anomalies; data on progestin receptor agonist/antagonist and pregnancy still unclear
- *Follow-up:* Not required but recommended for contraceptive counseling and/or pregnancy testing if no menses in 21 days

## PELVIC INFLAMMATORY DISEASE

Clinical condition referring to infection and inflammation involving the female upper genital tract including endometritis, salpingitis, tubo-ovarian abscess, and pelvic peritonitis. Pelvic inflammatory disease (PID) is a common and morbid complication of some sexually transmitted infections (STIs), in particular *Chlamydia trachomatis* (most commonly) and *Neisseria gonorrhoeae*.

## EPIDEMIOLOGY

- Affects 8% of US women during reproductive years
- Approximately 1 million US women are diagnosed with PID each year. The true incidence of PID and its complications have been difficult to ascertain because no national surveillance or reporting requirements exist, national estimates are limited by insensitive clinical diagnosis criteria, and definitive diagnosis can be challenging
- Major cause of other reproductive health problems including infertility, ectopic pregnancy, abscess formation, and chronic pelvic pain
- Risk factors for PID include adolescence, history of PID, current or past infection with gonorrhea or chlamydia, male partner with gonorrhea or chlamydia, multiple partners or partner with multiple partners, douching, IUD insertion with previous 3 weeks, bacterial vaginosis, low socioeconomic status (may be surrogate marker for decreased access to care)
- Sexually active women younger than 25 years old are most at risk because the immature cervix (i.e., cervical ectopy) is more likely to be infected with an STI

## ETIOLOGY

- Microorganisms ascend from the lower genital tract (cervix) to infect the upper genital tract (uterus, fallopian tubes, etc.)
- Most cases of PID are considered to be polymicrobial
- *C. trachomatis* and *N. gonorrhoeae* are the most commonly implicated organisms
- Several microorganisms that comprise the vaginal flora (anaerobes, *Gardnerella vaginalis, Haemophilus influenzae, Streptococcus agalactiae,* enteric gram-negative organisms) and other pathogens (genital mycoplasmas, cytomegalovirus, and *Ureaplasma urealyticum*) have also been associated with PID
- Pathogenesis is a complicated and poorly understood process involving interactions between genetics, immunology, and bacterial virulence factors

## CLINICAL MANIFESTATIONS

- Symptoms can range from none to severe
- Lower abdominal pain is the most common presentation
- Other symptoms may include fever, abnormal vaginal discharge, dyspareunia, dysuria, DUB, right upper quadrant pain (consistent with perihepatitis or Fitz–Hugh–Curtis syndrome secondary to capsular inflammation)

## DIAGNOSTICS

- The clinical diagnosis of acute PID is imprecise. The most common clinical presentations (e.g., lower abdominal pain) are nonspecific, but the use of diagnostic criteria to increase specificity has a significant impact on sensitivity. Because of the high risk of adverse outcomes with untreated PID, it is recommended that health care providers maintain a low threshold for the diagnosis of PID and err on the side of overtreatment
- *Minimum criteria in women with lower abdominal pain:* Uterine tenderness, adnexal tenderness, or cervical motion tenderness on bimanual examination
- *Additional criteria to increase specificity:* WBCs on vaginal wet preparation, abnormal cervical or vaginal mucopurulent discharge, temperature (oral) greater than 38.3°C, elevated erythrocyte sedimentation rate or C-reactive protein, laboratory documentation of infection with *C. trachomatis* or *N. gonorrhoeae*
- PID is less likely if no WBCs are found on the wet preparation of the vaginal secretions

- *Most specific criteria for the diagnosis of PID include:* Endometrial biopsy with evidence of endometritis, transvaginal ultrasound or MRI demonstrating thickened fallopian tubes or tubo-ovarian complex/abscess, and laparoscopic abnormalities consistent with PID
- Laparoscopy is the gold standard, but is not frequently warranted

## MANAGEMENT

- Regardless of laboratory results, treatment for PID must include coverage of *C. trachomatis*, *N. gonorrhoeae*, anaerobes, gram-negative organisms, and streptococci
- Because early treatment is an important part of the strategy to prevent adverse outcomes from PID, many clinical situations may warrant empiric therapy even while an evaluation for other causes of the presenting illness is still underway
- *Criteria for hospitalization:* Pregnancy; poor clinical response to oral therapy; failure to follow or tolerate outpatient oral therapy; severe illness evidenced by nausea, vomiting, or high fever; tubo-ovarian abscess (TOA); inability to rule out a surgical abdomen (e.g., appendicitis). Note that adolescence is no longer a criterion for hospitalization
- *Parenteral regimens (adapted from the CDC STD treatment guidelines):*
  ✓ *Regimen A:* Cefotetan 2 g IV every 12 hours OR cefoxitin 2 g IV every 6 hours PLUS doxycycline 100 mg orally (preferable because of pain with infusion and same bioavailability) or IV every 12 hours; discontinue IV therapy 24 hours after clinical improvement and complete total of 14 days of doxycycline; for TOA, can add clindamycin or metronidazole for increased anaerobic coverage
  ✓ *Regimen B:* Clindamycin 900 mg IV every 8 hours PLUS gentamycin loading dose IV or IM (2 mg/kg of body weight) followed by a maintenance dose (1.5 mg/kg) every 8 hours; discontinue IV therapy 24 hours after clinical improvement and complete total of 14 days of doxycycline 100 mg orally twice a day or clindamycin 450 mg orally four times a day (clindamycin has better anaerobic coverage for a TOA)
  ✓ Alternative parenteral regimens exist but have not been as well studied
- *Outpatient regimens (adapted from the CDC STD treatment guidelines):*
  ✓ Ceftriaxone 250 mg IM in a single dose OR cefoxitin 2 g IM in a single dose (given with probenecid 1 g orally) OR other parenteral third-generation cephalosporin (ceftizoxime or cefotaxime) PLUS doxycycline 100 mg orally twice a day for 14 days
  ✓ Additional anaerobic coverage may be provided by adding metronidazole 500 mg orally twice a day for 14 days to the above regimen
  ✓ Alternative oral regimens using fluoroquinolones are no longer recommended due to changing resistance patterns for *N. gonorrhoeae*. However, if parenteral cephalosporin therapy is not feasible, use of fluoroquinolones (levofloxacin 500 mg orally once daily or ofloxacin 400 mg twice daily for 14 days) can be considered low community prevalence and individual risk for gonorrhea
  ✓ Expect clinical improvement within 3 days of initiating outpatient treatment; if no improvement, patient may require hospitalization, additional testing, or surgical intervention
- Partners who have had sexual contact with the patient during the 60 days before symptoms occurred should be treated empirically for *C. trachomatis* and *N. gonorrhoeae*
- Instruct patients to abstain from sexual intercourse until patient and current partner have both completed treatment regimen and are free from symptoms
- All women diagnosed with PID should be offered HIV testing at the time of diagnosis
- Repeat screening of all women who have been diagnosed with chlamydia or gonorrhea is recommended 3–6 months after treatment
- Prevent PID by screening high-risk women, treating any suspected PID, avoiding douching, treating bacterial vaginosis (because of the association with PID), and promoting condom use

# 2 | Allergy and Asthma

*Irene Fung, MD*
*Solrun Melkorka Maggadottir, MD*
*Terri Brown-Whitehorn, MD*

## ANAPHYLAXIS

Anaphylaxis is an acute, potentially life-threatening systemic allergic reaction. It is most commonly triggered by interaction of an allergen with specific IgE antibody bound to mast cells and basophils leading to cell activation and mediator release. Non-IgE-mediated direct mast cell degranulation results in mediator release.

### EPIDEMIOLOGY

- Lifetime prevalence for all triggers is 0.05–2%
- Food is the most common cause of anaphylaxis, affecting up to 8% of young children and 3–4% of adults
- Drugs are the second most common cause of anaphylaxis
- Anaphylaxis leads to 500–1000 deaths per year in the United States

### ETIOLOGY

- Major causes are *food* (milk, egg, soy, wheat, peanut, tree nut, fish, and shellfish); *medications* (antibiotics, aspirin, nonsteroidal anti-inflammatory drugs (NSAIDs), biologics, chemotherapeutics, muscle relaxants, blood products, radiocontrast media); *latex; insect stings* (especially bees and wasps); and *allergy immunotherapy*
- Rare causes include exercise-induced and idiopathic forms

### DIFFERENTIAL DIAGNOSIS

- Other causes of shock (hypovolemic, cardiogenic, and septic), myocardial infarction, pulmonary embolism, status asthmaticus, pneumothorax, vasovagal reaction, serum sickness, hereditary angioedema, scombroid poisoning, carcinoid syndrome, pheochromocytoma, and underlying systemic mastocytosis (which increases risk of anaphylaxis)

### PATHOPHYSIOLOGY

- Previous exposure to an allergen (antigen) leads to allergen-specific IgE antibody production. IgE binds to the surface of mast cells and basophils. Upon subsequent exposure, the antigen binds cell-bound IgE, triggering cell activation and degranulation. At times, there is no known prior allergen exposure and reaction occurs on first known exposure
- Mediators involved include histamine, arachidonic acid derivatives (prostaglandins and leukotrienes), tryptase, bradykinin, and platelet-activating factor. These mediators cause smooth muscle spasm (bronchi, coronary arteries, and GI tract), increased vascular permeability, vasodilation, and complement activation. Patients therefore develop urticaria, angioedema, wheezing, emesis, diarrhea, and hypotension
- Nonimmunologic (previously known as anaphylactoid) reactions result from non-IgE-mediated degranulation of mast cells and basophils. This can occur with radiocontrast media, NSAIDs, opiates, and other agents

## HISTORY

- Exposure to a known allergen and/or prior history of anaphylaxis is helpful but not always present
- Onset is typically within 30 minutes from exposure to allergens. Symptoms typically progress very rapidly. At times, reactions may occur up to 2 hours post exposure
- When treated, symptoms usually resolve within a few hours. However, biphasic responses can occur in up to 20% of cases with recurrence of symptoms 8–10 hours later

## CLINICAL MANIFESTATIONS

- *Cutaneous (80–90% of patients):* Urticaria, pruritus, flushing, and angioedema. Patients with severe manifestation of anaphylaxis do not always present with skin findings
- *Respiratory (60% of patients):* Lower airway symptoms include wheezing, cough, stridor, chest tightness, and dyspnea. Upper airway symptoms include: sneezing, congestion/rhinorrhea, dysphonia, laryngeal edema (drooling), and hoarseness
- *Gastrointestinal (45% of patients):* Nausea, vomiting, abdominal pain, diarrhea
- *Cardiovascular (45% of patients):* Chest pain, palpitations, tachycardia or bradycardia, dysrhythmia, hypotension, shock, cardiac arrest
- *CNS (15% of patients):* Feeling of "impending doom," anxiety, headache, confusion, and/or behavior changes. In younger children, this may manifest as irritability, fatigue, or cessation of play
- Anaphylaxis can progress within minutes to shock, arrhythmia, and cardiac arrest. Death is most often from upper and/or lower airway obstruction or cardiovascular collapse

## DIAGNOSTIC TESTING

- Diagnosis is clinical and early intervention is life-saving. Treatment should never be withheld while awaiting laboratory/imaging results
- Plasma tryptase level is elevated if obtained <4 hours of start of symptoms. Tryptase is often normal in food-induced anaphylaxis
- ECG may show dysrhythmia, ischemic changes, or signs of myocardial infarction and cardiac enzymes can be elevated

## MANAGEMENT

### First Line

- ABCs, airway management as needed, supplemental oxygen
- Epinephrine 1:1000, 0.01 mL/kg IM per dose (maximum 0.5 mL per dose) or epinephrine auto-injector; repeat in 5–15 minutes as needed. Auto-injectors are recommended to decrease risk of error. Administer epinephrine IM as soon as anaphylaxis is recognized
- Isotonic intravenous fluid resuscitation for hypotension, progressing to volume expanders and/or vasoactive infusions if inadequate response to epinephrine IM
- Trendelenburg position

### Second Line

- Diphenhydramine liquid (H1-antihistamine) 1 mg/kg IV/PO (maximum 50 mg per dose); every 6 hours (maximum 300 mg/day) OR Cetirizine liquid (H2-antihistamine) daily
- Nebulized albuterol (β-adrenergic agonist) 2.5–5 mg/3 mL for wheezing/chest tightness if not resolved after epinephrine administration
- Ranitidine ($H_2$-antihistamine) 1 mg/kg IV/PO (maximum 50 mg per dose); every 6 hours (maximum 300 mg/day)

- Hydrocortisone 2 mg/kg IV (maximum 60 mg) once, then 1 mg/kg IV every 6 hours. Alternatives: methylprednisolone 1–2 mg/kg IV, then 1 mg/kg/dose every 6 hours; or oral prednisone 2 mg/kg once then 1 mg/kg/dose (maximum 60 mg). There is no evidence to support glucocorticoid treatment beyond the acute setting
- If patient is taking a β-agonist medication and symptoms not responsive to epinephrine IM consider giving glucagon
- There is no definitive length of time for therapy. If a patient is being discharged from the hospital, 24 hours of antihistamines and oral steroids should be sufficient. However, if a patient is admitted to the hospital to manage a severe reaction, it is reasonable to continue therapy at least until symptoms have completely resolved

## HOSPITAL ADMISSIONS

- Admissions to the hospital for observation should include patients with one or more of the following:
  - ✓ Current severe reaction with hypotension or need for >1 dose of epinephrine
  - ✓ History of severe reaction or biphasic reaction
  - ✓ History of severe asthma or in a current asthma exacerbation

## FOLLOW UP

- Patients that do not require hospitalization should be observed at least 8 hours
- Upon discharge
  - ✓ Prescribe an epinephrine auto-injector and train patient/caregivers in its proper use
  - ✓ Develop an anaphylaxis action plan and review with patient/caregivers
  - ✓ Educate patient/family around allergen avoidance if an allergen has been identified
  - ✓ List identified allergen in the medical record
  - ✓ Recommend a medical alert bracelet/necklace
  - ✓ Make a referral for an allergy follow-up appointment

## ANGIOEDEMA AND URTICARIA

**Urticaria refers to transient, raised, pruritic, erythematous, blanching skin lesions. Angioedema is a transient, often asymmetric swelling in the deep dermis and subcutaneous or submucosal tissues with little or no pruritus. Angioedema and urticaria often occur together. A hereditary form of isolated angioedema also exists.**

## EPIDEMIOLOGY

- Acute urticaria/angioedema, lasting <6 weeks, is seen in up to 20% of the population
- Chronic urticaria/angioedema, lasting >6 weeks, is seen in 0.5% of the population

## ETIOLOGY

### Acute Urticaria/Angioedema

- Causes of acute urticaria/angioedema include infections (most often viral, but has been associated with parasites and certain bacteria), foods, contact reaction, environmental allergen exposure (dog, rolling in grass), medications (NSAID, aspirin, angiotensin converting enzyme [ACE] inhibitors), insect stings, activities which increase body temperature (cholinergic), and physical triggers (cold, heat, water, vibration, and sunlight)

### Chronic Urticaria and Angioedema

- A specific cause of chronic urticaria and angioedema is rarely found, especially in pediatrics. Rare causes include underlying autoimmune urticaria, malignancy, or mast cell disease, such as urticaria pigmentosa or systemic mastocytosis

## PATHOPHYSIOLOGY

- *IgE-mediated:* Previous allergen (antigen) exposure leads to production of allergen-specific IgE antibody. IgE binds to surface of mast cells and basophils. Upon subsequent exposure, the antigen binds cell-bound IgE, leading to cell activation and degranulation, resulting in urticaria and/or angioedema
- *Non-IgE-mediated:* Nonspecific activation and degranulation of mast cells and/or basophils. Triggers are physical stimuli (e.g., cold, heat, pressure, vibration, water, sunlight), complement factors (e.g., C3a, C4a, and C5a), and some medications (e.g., NSAIDs, opiates)
- *Autoimmune urticaria:* Chronic idiopathic urticaria is a diagnosis of exclusion. In 30–40% of cases an auto-antibody against the IgE receptor on mast cells and basophils is identified. Rarely, anti-IgE antibodies are demonstrated. Thyroid auto-antibodies can be seen but only have value in the context of abnormal thyroid hormone levels

## DIFFERENTIAL DIAGNOSIS

- Viral exanthem, contact dermatitis, papule urticaria, erythema multiforme, urticarial vasculitis, and systemic lupus erythematosus (SLE)

## CLINICAL MANIFESTATION

- Individual urticarial lesions are transient lasting <2–3 hours, resolve, and reappear in another area. Each individual lesion does not last >24 hours. Dermatographism may be seen when stroking of skin leads to linear wheals (occurs in 2–5% of population)

## DIAGNOSTICS

- Diagnosis is clinical
- Allergy testing for acute urticaria is useful if a specific food or environmental trigger is suspected based on history. If hives last longer than 24 hours, a "hidden" food allergy is unlikely
- Extensive studies to determine infectious etiology are not often recommended as they do not typically change management
- Consider a skin biopsy and dermatology referral when individual urticarial lesions persist >24 hours or are atypical in appearance
- Laboratory workup should be considered for chronic urticaria if there are additional concerning symptoms (e.g., joint pain/swelling, fatigue, fever, weight loss) that may be suggestive of autoimmune, myeloproliferative, oncologic, endocrine or vasculitis disorder or a family history of angioedema

## MANAGEMENT

- If a trigger is identified, avoidance is advised
- Acute cases usually self-resolve. Treatment is aimed at decreasing pruritus and providing comfort. First- or second-generation (non-sedating) antihistamines (e.g., cetirizine, fexofenadine) are used for primary management. First-generation antihistamines may cause sedation and do not last as long. If symptoms are not well controlled, high-dose non-sedating antihistamines are used in combination with $H_2$ antihistamines (e.g., ranitidine). If symptoms recur after antihistamine administration, scheduled dosing of antihistamines for 2-5 days may be considered
- In chronic urticaria additional medications may be considered, including leukotriene-receptor antagonists (e.g., montelukast), biologics (e.g., omalizumab), alternative anti-inflammatory medications (e.g., sulfasalazine, dapsone), or immunosuppressive medications (e.g., cyclosporine, tacrolimus)
- Glucocorticoids can reduce symptoms; however, they are not recommended long term as acute worsening of symptoms may occur when stopped

- Cyproheptadine is useful in cold-induced urticaria
- Initial acute urticaria may progress to anaphylaxis and epinephrine would be warranted. Observation for a few hours may be indicated in select cases

## ANGIOEDEMA—HEREDITARY FORMS

### EPIDEMIOLOGY

- Hereditary angioedema (HAE) is a rare disease, accounting for about 2% of angioedema cases. Its prevalence is about 1/10,000–1/50,000
- Autosomal dominant inheritance. However, family history can be negative

### ETIOLOGY

- *Type I (85%):* Low or absent the protein C1-inhibitor (INH)
- *Type II (15%):* Normal/high levels of C1-INH but the protein is nonfunctioning
- *Type III:* Rare, more severe, and more common in women. Underlying mediator remains unidentified, but has been associated with estrogen and coagulation factor XII mutations. Level and function of C1-INH may be normal

### PATHOPHYSIOLOGY

- Without proper levels or function of C1-INH, there is unopposed activation of the first component of the classical complement pathway. Angioedema occurs due to formation of bradykinin and complement factors
- Acquired forms exist where a lymphoproliferative disorder leads to production of a monoclonal antibody that neutralizes existing C1-INH

### DIFFERENTIAL DIAGNOSIS

- Allergic reactions, malignancy, allergic urticaria/angioedema, rheumatologic disease, ACE-inhibitor-induced angioedema

### CLINICAL MANIFESTATIONS

- Angioedema, without urticaria, lasting 1–4 days
- A prodromal reticular rash may present prior to onset
- Affected areas include the skin and mucous membranes, larynx, and bowel wall
- Episodes are often spontaneous but known triggers include trauma, surgery (including dental work), emotional stress, infection, exogenous estrogen, and menstruation

### DIAGNOSTICS

- Serum C4 level is the best screening test and is low due to consumption. The sample should be placed on ice, otherwise complement levels can be falsely low
- C1-INH level and function can also be measured and can differentiate among the forms of HAE

### MANAGEMENT

#### Acute Treatment

- Plasma-derived C1-INH (Berinert®)
- Recombinant kallikrein inhibitor (Ecallintide®), for patients >16 years of age
- Recombinant bradykinin-2 receptor inhibitor (Icatibant®), for patients >18 years of age
- If the above are not available, consider fresh frozen plasma (FFP) as it contains C1-INH

- Aminocaproic acid and tranexamic acid can be useful but take hours to exert an effect
- Intravenous fluids and pain medications (perhaps avoid opiates, which can cause nonimmune-mediated mast cell degranulation)

### Chronic/Prophylactic Treatment

- Androgens (danazol or stanozolol); increase hepatic C1-INH synthesis
- Plasma-derived C1-INH (Cinryze®) infusions every 3–4 days

### Short-Term Prophylaxis Prior to Surgery/Trauma

- Fresh frozen plasma (FFP) the night prior to or on the day of surgery
- Plasma-derived C1-INH on the day of surgery
- Androgen medication started 3–4 days prior to surgery

## DRUG ALLERGY

### CLASSIFICATION

- Modified Gel-Coombs Classification of Hypersensitivity reactions (Table 2-1)
- *Nonimmunologic-mediated (pseudoallergic) reactions:* Due to nonimmune degranulation of mast cells and basophils (e.g., vancomycin, radiocontrast dye, opiates, NSAID-induced urticaria)

### HISTORY

- Hives, angioedema, and anaphylaxis-type symptoms occurring within minutes to hours suggest Type I hypersensitivity
- Cough within 10 days of drug administration (e.g., nitrofurantoin) with peripheral eosinophilia and migratory infiltrates suggests pulmonary drug hypersensitivity

| TABLE 2-1 | Classification of Hypersensitivity Reactions | |
| --- | --- | --- |
| **Classification Type** | **Immunoreactants** | **Clinical Presentation** |
| I | Mast cell-mediated, IgE dependent | Anaphylaxis, urticaria, angioedema, asthma, allergic rhinitis |
| IIa | Antibody-mediated cytotoxic reaction) | Immune cytopenias |
| IIb | Antibody-mediated cell-stimulating reactions | Graves disease, chronic idiopathic urticaria |
| III | Immune complex-mediated | Serums sickness, vasculitis |
| IVa | Th1 cell-mediated, macrophage activation | Type 1 diabetes Contact dermatitis (also IVc) |
| IVb | Th2 cell-mediated, eosinophilic inflammation | Persistent asthma and allergic rhinitis |
| IVc | Cytotoxic T cell-mediated (perforin, granzyme B) | Stevens–Johnson syndrome, toxic epidermal necrolysis syndrome(TENS) |
| IVd | T-cell-mediated, neutrophilic inflammation | Acute generalized exanthematous pustulosis (AGEP), Behçet disease |

Data from Uzzaman A and Cho SH. *Allergy Asthma Proceedings* 2012 33:S96–S99; and Ditto AM. Drug allergy. In: Grammer LC and Greenberger PA, eds. *Patterson's Allergic Diseases* 7th ed. Philadelphia, PA: Wolters Kluwer, Lippincott, Williams & Wilkins; 2009.

- Maculopapular exanthem days after drug administration (e.g., amoxicillin) suggests a T-cell-mediated reaction
- Skin reaction always occurring in the same area suggests a fixed drug eruption
- Lichenification/eczema occurring 1–3 days after drug administration (e.g., hydrochloro-thiazide) suggests photo-allergic reaction
- Fine pustules, fever, and neutrophilia occurring after days of drug administration suggest acute generalized exanthematous pustulosis (AGEP)
- Rash and fever with lymphadenopathy, arthralgia, gastrointestinal symptoms, and protein-uria occurring after 1–3 weeks after drug administration suggest serum sickness or serum sickness-like reaction
- Rash and fever with eosinophilia, facial edema, and organ involvement (e.g., liver, kidney, lymph nodes) 2–8 weeks after drug administration suggest drug reaction with eosinophilia and systemic symptoms (DRESS)
- Mucosal erosion, target lesions, epidermal necrosis, and multi-organ involvement occur-ring days to weeks after drug administration suggest Stevens–Johnson Syndrome/Toxic Epidermal Necrolysis (SJS/TEN)

## RISK FACTORS FOR DRUG ALLERGY

- Host factors include patient's genetics, history of prior allergic reaction, underlying con-comitant diseases (e.g., HIV, cystic fibrosis), and female sex
- Drug factors include high dose, repetitive courses, large molecular weight of drug, and intravenous administration

## DIAGNOSTICS

- Serum tryptase
  ✓ High positive predictive value (PPV) but low negative predictive value (NPV) in peri-operative anaphylaxis
- *Skin-prick testing and specific IgE testing:*
  ✓ For patients who have reaction to penicillin, skin testing is available
  ✓ Skin testing to other drugs is not validated but may be helpful
  ✓ Neither skin nor specific IgE tests are diagnostic for cytotoxic, immune-complex, or cell-mediated drug-induced allergic reactions

## MANAGEMENT

- Stop the medication. If anaphylaxis occurs, follow treatment as outlined in Anaphylaxis section
- Drug avoidance
- Drug desensitization is used when there is history of immediate reaction, there are no alter-native drugs, and the drug is medically necessary. This is best performed by an allergist in a critical care setting as the patient may develop anaphylaxis

## COMMONLY IMPLICATED DRUGS

- Antibiotics
  ✓ Penicillin can cause all types of reactions, from Type I to Type IV
  ✓ Sulfa antibiotics
    ▪ The majority of reactions are cytotoxic, although 30% of reactions are Type I
    ▪ Patients with HIV have a higher risk of reacting to sulfonamides
- Chemotherapeutics
  ✓ Type I reactions are reported for almost all commonly used agents, and range from mild skin reactions to severe anaphylaxis

✓ Paclitaxel and docetaxel produce non-IgE-mediated (anaphylactoid) reactions in up to 42% of patients on first administration, but rarely with subsequent cycles

✓ Platinum compounds (cisplatin, carboplatin) can produce Type I reactions

- Asparaginase can produce Type I and pseudo-allergic reactions
- Local anesthetics
  ✓ Allergy testing is available
- Muscle relaxants
  ✓ Can cause an IgE or pseudo-allergic reaction
- Natural Rubber Latex (NRL)
  ✓ High-risk groups include those with history of multiple surgeries (especially genitourinary and abdominal surgery), and those with occupations where latex gloves are frequently used
  ✓ Positive skin-prick test to a reliable crude NRL extract is more sensitive than specific IgE to latex to confirm diagnosis
- Nonsteroidal anti-inflammatory drugs (NSAIDs) and aspirin
  ✓ For patients with history of urticaria or angioedema to NSAIDs, avoidance is recommended. If required, graded challenge protocol may be used
  ✓ Aspirin exacerbated respiratory disease (AERD) is characterized by aspirin- or NSAID-induced respiratory reaction in patients with underlying asthma
- Radiocontrast media
  ✓ Can cause a non-IgE-mediated reaction that is unpredictable. If there is a history of prior reaction, pretreatment protocols may prevent reaction: a corticosteroid (e.g., prednisone) given at 13, 7, and 1 hour prior to procedure and an antihistamine (e.g., diphenhydramine) given 1 hour prior. Reaction is not related to underlying shellfish allergy

## NON-IgE-MEDIATED FOOD ALLERGY

**A food allergy is an abnormal reaction to a food or food additive. Reactions can be divided into IgE- and non-IgE-mediated. IgE-mediated reactions have been described earlier in this chapter. This section focuses on non-IgE-mediated reactions seen in the inpatient setting including food protein-induced colitis, food protein-induced enterocolitis (or food protein-induced enterocolitis syndrome [FPIES]), and eosinophilic esophagitis.**

### FOOD PROTEIN-INDUCED COLITIS

#### Clinical Manifestations

- Healthy appearing infants who present with streaks of blood or mucous in stools without fissure or identifiable cause. Unlike those with food protein-induced enterocolitis, these babies are well and are often managed as outpatients

#### Epidemiology

- Food protein-induced colitis is thought to occur in 2–6% of infants in developed countries. Approximately 60% are breast fed. The most common foods triggers are milk and soy

#### Diagnostics

- Diagnosis of food protein-induced colitis is made by history
- Elimination of food from diet (maternal and/or infant) resolves symptoms

#### Treatment/Prognosis

- Stop offending food(s)—most often milk and/or soy
- Consider reintroduction of food around 12 months of age, as typical natural history is resolution by this time

## FOOD PROTEIN-INDUCED ENTEROCOLITIS (FPIES)

### Clinical Manifestations

- *Acute:* Ill appearing infant who presents 2 hours after ingestion of a food with severe vomiting and lethargy, often followed by diarrhea; may also have hypotension (15–20% may present with hypovolemic shock) and hypothermia
- *Chronic:* Ill appearing infant who presents with more chronic symptoms of abdominal pain, vomiting, failure to thrive, and abnormal stools (chronic diarrhea that may contain mucous or blood)

### Differential Diagnosis

- *Acute FPIES:* Sepsis, surgical abdomen, malrotation, other causes of shock
- *Chronic FPIES:* Structural abnormalities, gastroesophageal reflux disease, infection, cyclic vomiting, metabolic disorder, inflammatory bowel disease, behavioral issues

### Epidemiology

- FPIES is thought to occur in 0.16% of infants. The majority have symptoms when ingesting food directly rather than through breast milk after the mother's ingestion. Most common triggers are milk, soy, rice, and oats in the United States. Other sources include chicken, fish, and sweet potatoes

### Diagnosis

- Made by history. There is no confirmatory test. At times, an elevated white blood cell count with neutrophilia is observed
- If the diagnosis is unclear, special food challenge is recommended

### Treatment/Prognosis

- *Acute management:*
  - ✓ *Rehydration:* Normal saline fluid boluses intravenously or orally
  - ✓ Supportive care
  - ✓ Epinephrine traditionally does NOT help
  - ✓ Ondansetron has been used with success in some patients
  - ✓ Avoidance
  - ✓ Slow introduction of new foods
- *Chronic management:*
  - ✓ Avoidance of known triggers
  - ✓ Elemental formula may be necessary
  - ✓ Slow introduction of foods
- Most children will outgrow these issues by school age (sometimes by 3 years of age)
- Food challenge in a hospital setting may be appropriate

## EOSINOPHILIC ESOPHAGITIS

### Clinical Manifestations

- *Infants:* Gastroesophageal reflux disease (GERD), at times failure to thrive (FTT)
- *Children:* Abdominal pain, GERD, FTT
- *Adolescent/adults:* Difficulty swallowing, food or pill impaction

### Epidemiology

- 1 in 2000 patients in developed countries
- 5–10% of pediatric patients with poorly controlled gastroesophageal reflux

## Differential Diagnosis

- Proton pump inhibitor (PPI)-responsive esophageal eosinophilia, eosinophilic gastroenteritis, Crohn disease, inflammatory bowel disease, celiac disease, medication, infection, hypereosinophilic syndrome, graft-versus-host disease

## Diagnosis

- Diagnosis is made when patient has persistent esophageal eosinophilia (minimum of 15 eosinophils per high powered field) despite use of high-dose PPI (1–2 mg/kg/day for 8 weeks prior to endoscopy) with good compliance

## Treatment/Prognosis

- If food or medication impaction is present, removal is top priority
- This disorder is often co-managed by gastroenterology, allergy, and nutrition
- *Dietary therapy:* Food elimination based on most common causes of eosinophilic esophagitis (milk, soy, egg, and/or wheat) or allergy testing, or switch to elemental formula
- *Medical management:* Systemic steroids for severe symptoms for short-term therapy. Alternative option for management includes swallowed steroids (viscous budesonide or inhaled steroids). When used, patients should not eat or drink for 30 minutes after dosing
- May require esophageal dilatation if severe narrowing (confirmed by barium swallow)
- Repeat endoscopy following either dietary or medical management to assess progress

## ASTHMA

**Asthma is diffuse, chronic inflammatory disease of large and small airways punctuated by acute exacerbations of airflow obstruction which are at least partially reversible.**

### EPIDEMIOLOGY

- Affects approximately 1 in 11 children in the United States
- Nearly 1 in 5 children with asthma will present to the ER for asthma-related care
- Prevalence higher in African Americans, Hispanics, and inner-city youth

### PATHOPHYSIOLOGY

- *Triggers:* Allergic (e.g., pet dander, dust mites, pollen), nonspecific stimuli (e.g., smoke, exercise, chemical spray), and infections (e.g., viral, bacterial, fungal)
- *Mast cells in airway mucosa release mediators (e.g., histamine, leukotrienes, platelet-activating factor) that cause biphasic immune response:*
  ✓ *Early (begins within minutes):* Bronchoconstriction
  ✓ *Late (begins 6–8 hours later):* Hypersecretion of mucus, airway edema, epithelial desquamation, and infiltration of inflammatory cells
- Airway obstruction with nonuniform ventilation and atelectasis leads to ventilation/perfusion (V/Q) mismatch. Hyperinflation leads to decreased compliance and increased work of breathing. Increased intra-thoracic pressure impairs venous return and reduces cardiac output

### HISTORY

- Acute episodes of cough, wheeze, shortness of breath, increased work of breathing
- Symptoms can occur outside of viral illness (triggers: exercise, emotional upset, weather change, allergen)
- Family history of asthma and/or atopy is common

- Relief from asthma medications in the past may be helpful
- *Comorbid conditions can aggravate flares:* Sinusitis, rhinitis, gastroesophageal reflux disease (GERD), obstructive sleep apnea (OSA), allergic bronchopulmonary aspergillosis (ABPA)

## DIFFERENTIAL DIAGNOSIS OF WHEEZING

- *Anatomic:* Extrinsic (e.g., bronchial or tracheal stenosis, tracheomalacia, vascular ring, lymphadenopathy, tumor); intrinsic to airway (e.g., foreign body, laryngeal web, pulmonary sequestration, bronchial adenoma)
- *Inflammatory/infectious:* Allergic rhinitis and sinusitis, viral or obliterative bronchiolitis, atypical pneumonia, hypersensitivity pneumonitis, pulmonary hemosiderosis
- *Genetic/metabolic:* Cystic fibrosis, primary immune deficiency, ciliary dysfunction, alpha 1-antitrypsin deficiency
- *Other:* Vocal cord dysfunction, aspiration from swallowing dysfunction or gastroesophageal reflux, habit cough, heart disease

## PHYSICAL EXAM

- *General:* Well appearing versus ill or toxic-looking, cough, audible wheeze
- *Vital signs:* Tachycardia, tachypnea, pulsus paradoxus (systolic BP drop >10 mm Hg with inspiration); decreased pulse oximetry level
- *Respiratory:* Nasal flaring, accessory muscle use, prominence of ribs or clavicles with inspiration, increase in chest wall diameter, wheezing, decreased breath sounds, prolonged expiratory phase

## DIAGNOSTICS

### Acute Exacerbation

- *ABG* (consider obtaining if there is concern for respiratory insufficiency/failure)
  - ✓ *Early or mild/moderate exacerbation:* Elevated pH, low $pCO_2$, normal or low $pO_2$ (respiratory alkalosis)
  - ✓ Respiratory insufficiency is suggested by normal pH and $pCO_2$ with low $pO_2$
  - ✓ Respiratory failure is suggested by low pH with elevated $pCO_2$ (respiratory acidosis) and low $pO_2$
- *Chest x-ray (obtain only if there is concern for another diagnosis or complication)*
  - ✓ Typical findings include hyperinflation, peribronchial thickening, atelectasis
  - ✓ *Other diagnoses or complications may be identified:* For example, pneumonia, aspirated foreign body, or pneumothorax

### Outpatient Setting

- *Spirometry (in children ≥5 years)*
  - ✓ Values are compared to age, height, sex, and race-matched references
  - ✓ *Obstruction:* Decreased $FEV_1$ and $FEV_1/FVC$ (whereas normal or increased $FEV_1/FVC$ with reduced FVC suggests restriction)
  - ✓ In severe cases, FVC can also be reduced due to air trapping
  - ✓ *Reversibility:* Increase in $FEV_1$ ≥12% and ≥10% of predicted after short-acting bronchodilator
  - ✓ Like $FEV_1/FVC$, decreased $FEF_{25-75\%}$ correlates with poorer $PC_{20}$, PEF variability, and bronchodilator response, but has more variability
- *Peak expiratory flow (PEF):* Spirometry is recommended over PEF for diagnosis as there is wide variability in published PEF values. It may be useful in the acute setting to compare to patient's personal best value

- *Bronchoprovocation (methacholine, histamine, cold air, exercise):* Useful if asthma suspected and spirometry is equivocal
- *Methacholine challenge:* Helpful to rule out asthma if negative
  - ✓ $PC_{20}$ is the methacholine concentration causing a 20% fall in FEV1. A cut-off of 8–16 mg/mL is used as an optimal cutoff point to identify asthmatics
  - ✓ A positive test is seen in asthma, but also in allergic rhinitis, cystic fibrosis, and COPD
- *Skin testing or immunoCAP® testing:* To identify potential triggers
- *Management of Acute Exacerbation:* Close monitoring of symptoms is needed as they can change over time (Table 2-2 and Figure 2-1)

## Medications

- *Albuterol:* Metered-dose inhaler (MDI) 4–8 puffs or nebulized 2.5 mg/dose (<20 kg) or 5 mg/dose (>20 kg) every 20 minutes × 3 doses
- *Ipratropium bromide:* 0.25–0.5 mg nebulized, every 20 minutes × 3 doses with initial albuterol treatments. Has additive effect with beta-agonists, and reduces likelihood of admission from emergency department (ED). Once hospitalized, no reduction in length of hospital stay has been demonstrated with ongoing therapy with this medication

| TABLE 2-2 | Classifying Asthma Severity in the Urgent Care Setting | | |
|---|---|---|---|
| | **Symptoms and Signs** | **Initial PEF or FEV$_1$ (% Predicted or Personal Best)** | **Clinical Course** |
| **Mild** | Dyspnea only with activity (assess tachypnea in young children) | ≥70% | • Usually care at home<br>• Prompt relief with inhaled SABA<br>• Possible short course OCS |
| **Moderate** | Dyspnea interferes or limits usual activity | 40–69% | • Usually needs office or ED visit<br>• Relief from frequent SABA<br>• OCS; some symptoms last for 1–2 days after treatment is begun |
| **Severe** | Dyspnea at rest; interferes with conversation | <40% | • Usually requires ED visit; likely admission<br>• OCS; some symptoms last for >3 days after treatment begun<br>• Adjunctive therapies helpful |
| **Subset: Life-threatening** | Too dyspneic to speak; perspiring | <25% | • ED/admission; possibly ICU<br>• Minimal or no relief from frequent SABA<br>• IV corticosteroids<br>• Adjunctive therapies helpful |

Adapted with permission from NAEPP Expert Panel Report: Guidelines for the Diagnosis and Management of Asthma—Update on Selected Topics 2007 NIH publication no. 08-5846; originally printed October, 2002.
ED, emergency department; FEV1, forced expiratory volume in 1 second; ICU, intensive care unit; OCS, oral corticosteroids; PEF, peak expiratory flow; SABA, short-acting beta2-agonist.

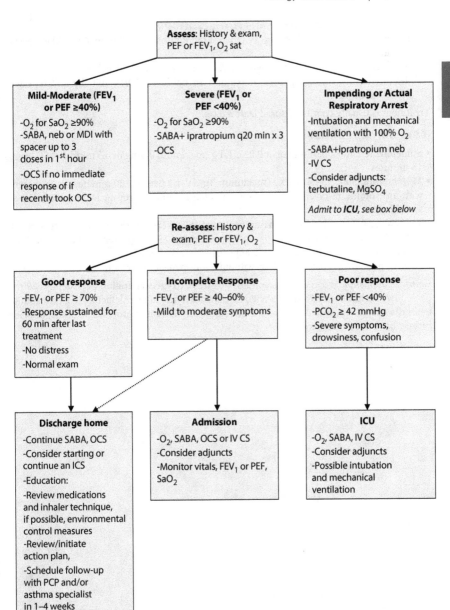

FIGURE 2-1 **Management of asthma exacerbation in the ER and Hospital.** (Adapted with permission from NAEPP Expert Panel Report 3: Guidelines for the Diagnosis and Management of Asthma—Update on Selected Topics 2007 NIH publication no. 08-5846; originally printed October, 2007.)

- *Systemic corticosteroids (for moderate to severe exacerbations):*
  - ✓ methylprednisolone 1–2 mg/kg IV, then 1 mg/kg/dose (maximum 60 mg/day) every 6 hours; or
  - ✓ oral prednisone 2 mg/kg once then 1 mg/kg/dose (maximum 60 mg); or
  - ✓ dexamethasone 0.6 mg/kg/dose (maximum 16 mg/dose) PO/IV initially and repeated 12–18 hours later)

Treatment is usually continued for at least 5 days.

## If Severely Ill, Consider

- Epinephrine 1:1000, 0.01 mg/kg or 0.01 mL/kg (maximum 0.3 mg or 0.3 mL/dose) SC every 15 minutes
- *Magnesium sulfate:* 25–50 mg/kg (maximum 2 g) IV/IO over 15–30 minutes. Pretreatment with an isotonic intravenous fluid bolus is often helpful to prevent hypotension due to vasodilation
- Terbutaline 0.01 mg/kg/dose (maximum 0.4 mg) SC every 10–15 minutes for two doses. For an IV infusion, bolus with 10 mcg/kg (maximum 750 mcg) over 5 minutes and then start an infusion at 0.4 mcg/kg/min (range 0.4–3 mcg/kg/min)
- Positive pressure ventilation with or without endotracheal intubation

*Consider admission if:* Persistent respiratory distress, oxygen saturation persistently <90%, peak flow rate less than 50% of predicted levels, underlying high-risk factors (e.g., congenital heart disease, neuromuscular disease, cystic fibrosis), ED visit in previous 24 hours, or prior history of severe exacerbation.

# 3 Analgesia and Sedation

*Arul M. Lingappan, MD*
*F. Wickham Kraemer III, MD*
*Melissa Desai Patel, MD, MPH*

## ANALGESIA

### ANALGESIA IS THE DIMINUTION OR ELIMINATION OF PAIN IN THE CONSCIOUS PATIENT.

- Even neonates demonstrate behavioral and hormonal changes in response to painful procedures
- Children do not have to understand the meaning of pain nor do they have to communicate pain to experience pain
- Preemptive analgesia may decrease post-injury opioid requirements

## ASSESSMENT OF PAIN

- *Observational-behavioral measures*
  - ✓ Useful in infants and toddlers (who do have physiologic and behavioral responses to pain, such as increased heart rate, blood pressure, respiratory rate, crying, flushing, facial expressions, and body movements)
  - ✓ Example: FLACC (Face, Leg, Activity, Cry, Consolability) Behavioral Pain Scale (Merkel SI, et al. The FLACC: A behavioral scale for scoring postoperative pain in young children. *Pediatr Nurs.* 1997;23(3):293–297)
- *Self-report*
  - ✓ OUCHER scale combines numeric and faces scales, making it appropriate for young children (available at http://www.oucher.org)
  - ✓ *Faces scale:* The child is asked to point to the face that best describes his/her own pain (available at http://www.wongbakerfaces.org)
  - ✓ *Verbal numeric pain rating:* Useful in developmentally normal children 6–7 years of age (or older). Pain is rated from 0 to 10 (0 is no pain and 10 is the worst pain imaginable)

## LOCAL ANESTHESIA

### EUTECTIC MIXTURE OF LOCAL ANESTHETICS (EMLA)

- 2.5% Lidocaine/2.5% Prilocaine
- Apply to intact skin; complete anesthesia in 60–90 minutes
- Use for blood drawing/IV placement, bone marrow aspiration, lumbar puncture in non-emergent settings
- May use liposomal lidocaine (LMX) for faster onset; topical lidocaine only; anesthesia in 30 minutes
- *Contraindications:* Methemoglobinemia, age less than 1 month

### LIDOCAINE, EPINEPHRINE, TETRACAINE (LET)

- Used for dermal lacerations; apply to open wound
- Contraindicated in areas supplied by end-arteries (digits, pinna, nose, penis)

## VISCOUS LIDOCAINE

- For older children who can expectorate
- Combine with diphenhydramine and Maalox in equal parts (1:1:1) to create "magic mouthwash" (can also exclude lidocaine if mouth sores create a concern for systemic absorption)
- *Usual dose:* 15 mL of undiluted mixture to "swish and spit" (not swallow); maximum dose is 4.5 mg/kg or 300 mg of lidocaine component (up to every 3 hours). Smaller amounts work well

## LIDOCAINE JELLY

- Used for nasogastric tube placement and urethral catheterizations

## INJECTABLE LOCAL ANESTHETIC

- Buffer with 1 mL (1 meq/mL) sodium bicarbonate ($NaHCO_3$) per 9 mL lidocaine or 0.1 mL $NaHCO_3$ per 10 mL bupivacaine to reduce pain associated with injection
- Enhance efficacy and duration by using in combination with epinephrine
- Contraindicated in areas supplied by end arteries (digits, pinna, nose, penis)

## NARCOTIC ANALGESICS

- All doses referred to here are equianalgesic doses
- All opioids can be reversed with naloxone hydrochloride (Narcan) 0.01 mg/kg IV/IM/SC/ETT; naloxone can be repeated every 2 minutes as needed to maximum of 10 mg
- All narcotics may have side effects of sedation, nausea, vomiting, pruritus, and constipation

## CODEINE

- Codeine is metabolized into morphine by cytochrome P450 2D6, but this enzyme is absent in up to 10% of the population
- No longer recommended for use in children due to variable metabolism where non-metabolizers will have minimal to no analgesia, and ultra-rapid metabolizers will be at risk for excessive sedation, respiratory depression, and death

## FENTANYL

- 0.001 mg/kg/dose IV with onset in 1–2 minutes; duration: 0.5–1 hour (repeat or higher dosing may result in increased context-sensitive half-life)
- 0.01 mg/kg/dose transmucosal with onset in 15 minutes (FDA approved for cancer pain only)
- The transdermal patch is used in chronic pain management for opioid tolerant patients with expected pain management needs of several weeks
- *Caution:* Chest wall rigidity may occur with high doses and rapid IV push; reversible with naloxone or neuromuscular paralysis/endotracheal intubation

## HYDROMORPHONE

- 0.015 mg/kg/dose IV/SC (usual adult dose 0.4–0.8 mg) with onset in 5–10 minutes; duration: 3–4 hours
- 0.02–0.08 mg/kg/dose PO with onset in 30–60 minutes (usual adult dose 2–4 mg); duration: 3–4 hours
- Has no active metabolites

## MEPERIDINE

- Rarely used for analgesic purposes due to severe drug interactions (MAO inhibitors)
- Occasionally used to treat postoperative shivering or medication-induced shaking (e.g., amphotericin-related rigors)
- *Side effects:* Tachycardia, seizures, worsens bronchospasm, serotonin syndrome
- Active metabolite, normeperidine, may accumulate and induce seizures

## METHADONE

- 0.1 mg/kg/dose IV with onset in 15–30 minutes; duration: 12–24 hours
- 0.1 mg/kg/dose PO with onset in 30–60 minutes; duration: 12–24 hours
- Commonly used as an opioid taper
- Due to drug accumulation with long half-life, respiratory side effects may not appear until days after drug initiation
- Baseline ECG is necessary as methadone may prolong QT interval

## MORPHINE

- 0.1 mg/kg/dose IV (usual adult dose 2–4 mg) with onset in 5–10 minutes; duration: 3–4 hours
- 0.1–0.2 mg/kg/dose SC with onset in 10–30 minutes; duration: 4–5 hours
- 0.3–0.5 mg/kg/dose PO with onset in 30–60 minutes; duration: 4–5 hours
- *Side effects:* Nausea, sedation, pruritus, constipation, seizures (in neonates—due to decreased elimination of active metabolite morphine-3-glucuronide)
- *Contraindications:* Renal failure (active metabolites may accumulate to cause profound sedation and/or respiratory depression)

## NALBUPHINE

- 0.1 mg/kg/dose (usual adult dose 5 mg) with onset in 5–10 minutes; duration: 6 hours
- Partial opioid agonist, resulting in plateau of analgesic effects but also minimizing risk of respiratory depression
- May be used to treat opioid-related side effects (e.g., pruritus, nausea/vomiting) by the partial opioid antagonism at the mu receptor
- Relatively contraindicated in patients on chronic opioids as nalbuphine may precipitate acute opioid withdrawal

## OXYCODONE

- 0.1 mg/kg/dose PO with onset in 30–60 minutes; duration: 4–6 hours
- Active metabolite, oxymorphone, can accumulate in renal failure
- When oxycodone is made with acetaminophen, this limits its utility in young children due to the toxicity of acetaminophen

## NON-NARCOTIC ANALGESICS

### ACETAMINOPHEN

- Antipyretic; weak analgesic
- *Side effects:* Hepatic necrosis (overdosage)
- *Usual dose:* 10–15 mg/kg PO or rectally every 4–6 hours; adult dose: 325 mg$^{-1}$ g/dose
- *Maximum dose:* 4 g/day (adults); 90 mg/kg/day (children)
- Acetaminophen should be administered in a separate formulation from an opioid to reduce the toxic potential of an acetaminophen overdose

## NONSTEROIDAL ANTI-INFLAMMATORY DRUGS

- Useful for inflammatory pain
- *Side effects:* Platelet inhibition, gastrointestinal irritation, nephrotoxicity
- *Ibuprofen:* 5–10 mg/kg PO every 6–8 hours with a maximum of 40 mg/kg/day; adult dose 200–400 mg/dose, maximum 1.2 g/day
- *Ketorolac:* 0.5 mg/kg/dose IV/IM every 6 hours with maximum 30 mg every 6 hours which is usual adult dose (avoid if post conceptual age <44 weeks versus <6 months depending on institutional protocol)
- *Naproxen:* 5–10 mg/kg/dose PO every 8–12 hours with maximum 1000 mg/day; adult dose 250–500 mg/dose; maximum 1000 mg/day

## ASPIRIN

- No longer routinely used for analgesia due to side effects, but continues to be utilized for anti-platelet effects in specific situations (e.g., Kawasaki disease, vascular shunts, etc.)
- *Side effects:* Reye's syndrome (avoid in children with varicella or influenza)

## KETAMINE

- Low dose infusions of 0.1–0.2 mg/kg/h may utilized for analgesia (especially in patients on chronic opioids as part of a weaning regimen) and higher dose infusions (e.g., 0.5–2 mg/kg/h) or boluses (2 mg/kg IV or 4 mg/kg IM) may be used for sedation
- *Side effects:* Excess salivary secretions (prevent with glycopyrrolate pretreatment), nystagmus, increased ICP (though cerebral perfusion pressure maintained given increased mean arterial pressure), emergence delirium

## DIAZEPAM

- 0.05–0.1 mg/kg/dose IV every 6–8 hours for muscle spasms and anxiolysis
- 0.1–0.2 mg/kg/dose PO every 6–8 hours (usual adult dosing 2–10 mg)
- Prolonged half-life can lead to late onset of side effects which are sedation, respiratory depression, and hypotension and can be worsened by coadministration of opioids

## NON-PHARMACOLOGIC METHODS OF ANALGESIA

- Distraction, music, play
- Acupuncture, massage, and hypnosis are other methods of analgesia usually requiring trained practitioners

## PATIENT-CONTROLLED ANALGESIA

- Indicated for acute/chronic pain of known etiology as well as preemptive pain management. Cardiorespiratory monitoring is required. Six or 7 years is minimum age to control a Patient-Controlled Analgesia (PCA). Parents and nurses can also be trained to administer a PCA for younger patients or those with developmental delay
- Minimum developmental age of about 7 years to self-administer PCA
  - ✓ Parents and nurses can also be trained to administer PCA to younger patients and those with developmental delay
- *Route:* IV or rarely SC
- Dosing for PCA:
  - ✓ *Morphine:* Basal dose 10–20 µg/kg/h; bolus dose 10–20 µg/kg; lockout 8–10 minutes, four to six boluses per hour; maximum dose per hour: 100–150 µg/kg

✓ *Hydromorphone:* Basal dose 3–4 µg/kg/h; bolus dose 3–4 µg/kg/h; lockout 8–10 minutes, four to six boluses per hour; maximum dose per hour: 15–20 µg/kg
✓ *Fentanyl:* Basal dose 0.25–1 µg/kg/h; bolus dose 0.25–1 µg/kg; lockout 8–10 minutes, two to three boluses per hour; maximum dose per hour: 2 µg/kg

## SEDATION

### SEDATION IS A CONTINUUM

- *Minimal Sedation (anxiolysis):* A drug-induced state in which cognitive function and coordination may be impaired. Patients respond normally to verbal commands. Protective airway reflexes are maintained. Ventilatory and cardiovascular functions are unaffected
- *Moderate Sedation:* A drug-induced state of depressed consciousness. Patients respond purposefully to verbal commands, either alone or accompanied by light tactile stimulation. There is significant loss of orientation to environment, with moderate impairment of gross motor function. Protective airway reflexes are maintained. Ability to maintain patient airway and cardiovascular function are usually maintained. There may be mild alterations in ventilatory responsiveness
- *Deep Sedation:* A drug-induced state of depressed consciousness or unconsciousness from which a patient is not easily aroused. Patients may respond purposefully to painful stimulation. May be accompanied by a partial or complete loss of protective reflexes, which may include the inability to maintain a patent airway independently and respond purposefully to physical stimulation or verbal command. Spontaneous ventilation may be inadequate. Cardiovascular function is usually maintained
- *General Anesthesia:* Drug-induced loss of consciousness with loss of protective reflexes, inability to maintain patent airway, and loss of purposeful response. Cardiovascular function may be impaired

## PREPARATION FOR SEDATION

### PATIENT-RELATED FACTORS

- *Pre-sedation Assessment* (Table 3-1 and Figure 3-1): Essential to identify high-risk patient populations to both anticipate and reduce adverse sedation events
- *NPO Guidelines (American Society of Anesthesiology [ASA]):*
  ✓ No clear liquids for 2 hours before sedation
  ✓ No breast milk for 4 hours prior to sedation
  ✓ No formula for 6 hours prior to sedation
  ✓ No solids/milk for 8 hours prior to sedation
  ✓ In an emergency situation: Delay sedation if possible or use lightest possible level of sedation. Consider elective intubation for airway protection
- *ASA Classification:*
  - I: Normal healthy patient
  - II: Mild systemic disease
  - III: Severe systemic disease
  - IV: Severe systemic disease associated with significant dysfunction and potential threat to life
  - V: Critical medical condition where operative intervention is critical to survival

### PROCEDURAL CONSIDERATIONS

- Duration of procedure
- Painful versus nonpainful

| TABLE 3-1 | Pre-Sedation Assessment |
|---|---|

- History
  - ✓ Allergies and adverse reactions
  - ✓ Current medications
  - ✓ Indication for procedure
  - ✓ Previous sedation/anesthesia history
  - ✓ History of upper airway problems, OSA, snoring
  - ✓ Prematurity and corrected gestational age (if applicable)
  - ✓ Major medical illnesses, physical abnormalities (e.g., facial dysmorphisms, scoliosis, syndromes, etc.), neurologic problems, developmental delays
  - ✓ Review of systems addressing active pulmonary, cardiac, renal, hepatic, and metabolic concerns
  - ✓ Current or recent illnesses (e.g., upper respiratory infection, fever, anemia, etc.)
  - ✓ Relevant family hx (e.g., anesthesia-related complications)
- Examination
  - ✓ Age
  - ✓ Weight
  - ✓ Vital signs (including blood pressure, heart rate, respiratory rate, oxygen saturation)
  - ✓ Cardiovascular exam
  - ✓ Lung exam
  - ✓ Neurologic exam
  - ✓ Mental status
  - ✓ Airway status (see Figure 3-1 for Mallampati Classification)

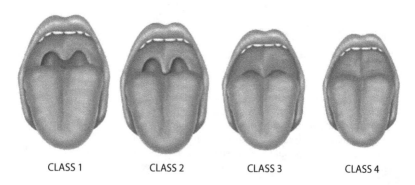

| CLASS 1 | CLASS 2 | CLASS 3 | CLASS 4 |

MALLAMPATI CLASSIFICATION

CLASS 1 : Soft palate, fauces, uvula, pillars
CLASS 2 : Soft palate, fauces, portion of uvula
CLASS 3 : Soft palate, base of uvula
CLASS 4 : Hard palate only

FIGURE 3-1 **Mallampati Classification of pharyngeal structures.** (Reproduced with permission from Bruncardi FC, Anderson DK, Billar TR, et.al. *Schwartz's Principles of Surgery*, 10th ed. New York, NY: McGraw Hill; 2014.)

- Position for procedure
- Need for immobility
- Age and ability to cooperate with instructions

## PROVIDER-RELATED FACTORS

- Dedicated sedation providers. Require at least two providers—one to administer sedation and one to monitor the sedation
  - ✓ Providers require airway skills, advanced life support skills, experience managing complications, and ability to rescue patient from a level of sedation which is deeper than anticipated
  - ✓ Traditionally administered by anesthesiologists, intensivists, and emergency medicine physicians with RN, CRNA, NP, or PA support
  - ✓ Increasing number of pediatric hospitalists performing sedation within a dedicated sedation program and with similar outcomes and complication rates
- Equipment (can use SOAPME acronym)
  - ✓ **S**uction—Apparatus including catheters (Tonsil, Yankauer)
  - ✓ **O**xygen—Supply and age-appropriately sized positive pressure oxygen delivery system
  - ✓ **A**irway—Size-appropriate equipment (nasopharyngeal and oropharyngeal airways, facemask, bag-valve-mask, etc.)
  - ✓ **P**harmacy—Medications for sedation, sedative antagonists and resuscitation, intravenous fluids
  - ✓ **M**onitors—Pulse oximeter, blood pressure, end-tidal $CO_2$ detector, stethoscope
  - ✓ **E**xtra equipment—Special equipment or drugs for the given case
- *Monitoring:*
  - ✓ Continuous pulse oximetry, heart rate, and end-tidal monitoring
  - ✓ Vital signs with blood pressure monitored every 15 minutes for minimal sedation and every 5 minutes for moderate or deep sedation
  - ✓ Consider full cardiorespiratory monitoring for specific cases (e.g., ketamine)
  - ✓ *Backup system for emergencies:* Highly trained and reliable (e.g., code team, 911)

## OVERVIEW OF SEDATIVE DRUGS

- Anxiolytics—Make patients more comfortable
  - ✓ *Benzodiazepines (e.g., diazepam, midazolam, lorazepam):* Provide anxiolysis and amnesia. Often used as premedication or as adjunct with analgesics. Administered PO, IV, IN, IM, or PR
  - ✓ *Nitrous oxide:* Anxiolytic with some analgesia effect. Administered via inhaled delivery system
- Analgesics—Achieve pain control
  - ✓ *Lidocaine (e.g., LMX):* Local analgesia at the procedure site. Administered topically or SQ
  - ✓ *Opioid agonists (e.g., fentanyl, morphine):* Dose-dependent analgesia and sedation. Often used in conjunction with anxiolytics or hypnotics. Administered PO, IV, or IN
  - ✓ *Ketamine:* Dissociative sedative with analgesic and amnestic properties. Administered PO, IV, or IM
- Hypnotics—Achieve sleep/immobility, especially useful for noninvasive procedures
  - ✓ *Chloral hydrate:* Produces sleep with mild to moderate respiratory depression. Currently with limited manufacturing resources. Administered PO or PR
  - ✓ *Barbiturates (e.g., pentobarbital):* Potent sedative, hypnotic and anesthetic properties. Administered PO, IV, or PR

✓ *Central α2 adrenergic agonists (e.g., clonidine, dexmedetomidine):* Sedative, anxiolytic, and sometimes analgesic properties. Administered PO, IN, or IV
✓ *Etomidate:* Short-acting anesthetic and amnestic. Especially useful in settings of hemodynamic instability. Administered IV
✓ *Propofol:* Sedative, hypnotic, and anesthetic properties. Administered IV
• Sedative antagonists
✓ *Flumazenil:* Short-acting agent that reverses benzodiazepine-induced sedation (use cautiously in patients with seizure disorders, as benzodiazepine reversal can induce seizures)
✓ *Naloxone:* Short-active agent that reverses opiate-induced sedation

## SEDATION-RELATED COMPLICATIONS

• Airway obstruction
• Laryngospasm
• Hypoventilation and apnea
• Vomiting/Aspiration
• Cardiovascular instability

## POST-SEDATION RECOVERY AND DISCHARGE

• Patient recovery should be monitored with vital signs at regular intervals until patient is awake and interactive
• Patients should only be discharged once specific criteria have been met: Stable vital signs, adequate pain control, return to level of consciousness that is similar to baseline for that patient, adequate head control and muscle strength to maintain patent airway, adequate hydration (tolerates oral challenge), and nausea/vomiting should be controlled

## PROCEDURE-SPECIFIC SEDATION

### COMPUTED TOMOGRAPHY (CT) SCAN

• Need for relative immobility but not analgesia
• Young infants often can be swaddled and may not require sedation. Patients 6 weeks–3 years old are the most likely age group to require sedation
• *Option 1:* PO Pentobarbital 2–4 mg/kg PO 30 minutes before procedure; repeat ½ dose 20–30 minutes after initial dose if patient still moving. Maximum dose: 100 mg or 8 mg/kg. Works well in infants <10 kg who do not require an IV for the procedure. Can use in conjunction with IN versed or fentanyl if need additional sedation
• *Option 2:* IV Pentobarbital 2–3 mg/kg slow IV push with titration to response. Give in increments of 1–3 mg/kg IV. Time to sedation is 2–5 minutes and time to recovery is 1–2 hours. Maximum 100 mg/dose or about 10 mg/kg
• Midazolam and fentanyl are unreliable in producing sedation with immobility but can be used as an adjunct to hypnotics to decrease total dose of longer acting medications

### MAGNETIC RESONANCE IMAGING (MRI)

• Need for relative immobility but not analgesia. Study typically lasts >45 minutes
• Young infants can often be swaddled or placed in an immobilizer device and may not require sedation. Children often require sedation until 6–8 years of age but older children, especially those with developmental delays, claustrophobia, ADHD, and/or anxiety, may require sedation as teenagers

• IV Pentobarbital 2–3 mg/kg; maximum dose 100 mg/dose with titration to response. Give in increments of 1–3 mg/kg. Can use in conjunction with IV midazolam (0.05–0.1 mg/kg with maximum of 2.5 mg max/dose) and fentanyl (1 µg/kg with maximum of 100 µg/dose) to reduce total pentobarbital dose required

## LUMBAR PUNCTURE

• Infants younger than 2 months are not routinely sedated for this procedure
• Midazolam 0.05–0.1 mg/kg IV given 3–5 minutes before lumbar puncture significantly decreases anxiety in older children. Repeat 0.1 mg/kg IV doses as needed to achieve adequate sedation. Maximum 2.5 mg/dose
• Fentanyl 1–2 µg/kg IV given via slow push over 3–5 minutes can provide analgesia. Repeat 1 µg/kg IV doses as needed to achieve adequate sedation. Maximum dose 100 µg/dose
• Can use midazolam and fentanyl together to achieve moderate to deep sedation as indicated. Can consider adding ketamine or pentobarbital as needed, depending on patient-specific characteristics (see options below)

## PAINFUL PROCEDURES SUCH AS FRACTURE REDUCTION/INCISION AND DRAINAGE/BURN DEBRIDEMENT/CENTRAL VENOUS LINE

• *Option 1:* Midazolam IV (0.05–0.1 mg/kg with maximum of 2.5 mg/dose) plus fentanyl (1–2 µg/kg with maximum dose of 100 µg/dose). Titrate additional doses as needed to achieve adequate sedation
• *Option 2:* Ketamine (0.5–2 mg/kg with maximum of 100 mg/dose) slow IV push. Titrate additional doses as needed to achieve adequate sedation. Consider atropine or glycopyrrolate premedication to decrease secretions. Can use midazolam and fentanyl adjuncts if needed to reduce total ketamine dose
• *Option 3 (for longer procedures, ≥30 minutes):* Midazolam IV (0.05–0.1 mg/kg with maximum of 2.5 mg/dose) plus fentanyl (1 µg/kg with maximum dose of 100 µg/dose) plus pentobarbital IV (2–3 mg/kg with maximum dose of 100 mg/dose)
• When using combination of sedatives/analgesics, start with lowest dose possible and give additional doses as needed to achieve desired depth of sedation. The rate of complications increases with polypharmacy

# Calculations*

4

CHAPTER

Barbara-Jo Achuff, MD, FAAP
Vanessa N. Madrigal, MD
Donald L. Boyer, MD, MSEd, FAAP

## ALVEOLAR-ARTERIAL OXYGEN GRADIENT (A-a GRADIENT)

$$A\text{-}a \text{ gradient} = PAO_2 - PaO_2$$
$$PAO_2 = F_iO_2(P_{atm} - P_{H_2O}) - (PaCO_2/R)$$

$PAO_2$ = Alveolar partial pressure of $O_2$ [mm Hg]
$PaO_2$ = Arterial partial pressure of $O_2$ [mm Hg]
$FiO_2$ = Fraction of inspired $O_2$ (0.21 in room air)
$P_{atm}$ = Atmospheric pressure (about 760 mm Hg at sea level)
$P_{H_2O}$ = Partial pressure of water vapor (about 47 mm Hg at 37°C)
$PaCO_2$ = Arterial partial pressure of $CO_2$ [mm Hg]
$R$ = Respiratory quotient, reflecting basal metabolic rate describing amount of $CO_2$ production for a given $O_2$ consumption (ranges from 0.7 to 1; usually 0.8 is used)

- Measure of the efficiency of the oxygenation of blood
- The normal A-a gradient varies with age. A helpful calculation is [age(years)+10]/4
- Normal A-a gradient ranges from 7 to 14 mm Hg when breathing room air; 20–65 mm Hg when on 100% $O_2$. As the gradient value increases, it is reflective of a worsening condition
- Gradient is affected by ventilation/perfusion (V/Q) or diffusion abnormalities but unaffected by hyper- or hypoventilation
- If $PaO_2$ corrects with supplemental $O_2$, consider asthma or other conditions associated with V/Q mismatch
- If $PaO_2$ does not correct with supplemental $O_2$, consider shunt

## ABSOLUTE NEUTROPHIL COUNT (ANC)

$$ANC = WBC \times (Polys/100 + Bands/100)$$

$WBC$ = White blood cell count [cells/mm³]
$Polys$ = Percentage of polymorphonuclear neutrophils
$Bands$ = Percentage of band forms

- Neutropenia generally defined as an ANC less than 1500 cells/mm³
- Severe neutropenia (ANC <500 cells/mm³) is associated with a high risk of infection

---

*Note: Commonly used conversions are listed separately and may be referred to as needed in the "Conversions of Units" section of this chapter.

## ANION GAP (SERUM)

$$\text{Serum AG} = [Na^+] - ([Cl^-] + [HCO_3^-])$$

$AG$ = Anion Gap
$[Na^+]$ = Serum concentration of sodium ions [mEq/L]
$[Cl^-]$ = Serum concentration of chloride ions [mEq/L]
$[HCO_3^-]$ = Serum concentration of bicarbonate ions [mEq/L]
- Aids in classifying metabolic acidosis
- Normal anion gap is 8–12 mEq/L
- Elevated anion gap is caused by an increase in unmeasured anions which may be any of the following:

"MUD PILES": Methanol; Uremia; Diabetic ketoacidosis; Paraldehyde or Phenformin; Iron, Infection, or INH; Lactic acidosis; Ethanol or Ethylene glycol; and Salicylates
- Acidosis with a normal anion gap ("non-anion gap acidosis") is generally caused by a loss of $HCO_3^-$ which can be associated with multiple causes, including the following:

"HARD-UP": Hyperalimentation; Acetazolamide; Renal tubular acidosis; Diarrhea; Ureteroenteric fistula; Pancreaticoduodenal fistula

Note: Hypoalbuminemia leads to underestimation of the AG and requires the following correction: Corrected AG=AG+0.25(40−Alb)

## ARTERIAL OXYGEN CONTENT (CaO₂)

$$CaO_2 = (Hb \times 1.36 \times SaO_2) + (0.0031 \times PaO_2)$$

Hb: Hemoglobin concentration [g/dL]
$SaO_2$: Saturation of hemoglobin with oxygen [0.99%]
$PaO_2$: Arterial partial pressure of $O_2$ [mm Hg]
(1 g Hb can carry 1.36 mL of oxygen [mL/g])
0.0031: Oxygen solubility coefficient [$O_2$/dL/mm Hg]
- Directly reflects the total number of oxygen molecules in the arterial blood, both bound and unbound to hemoglobin
- The $SaO_2$, or Pulse oximetry, is reflective of the oxygen bound by hemoglobin
- Note that the contribution of dissolved oxygen (as reflected in the latter portion of the equation [$0.0031 \times PaO_2$]) is very small
- Normal $CaO_2$ range: 17–24 mL/dL

## BIOSTATISTICS

|        | +Disease | −Disease |
|--------|----------|----------|
| +Test  | TP       | FP       |
| −Test  | FN       | TN       |

TP, True positive; FP, false positive; FN, false negative; TN, true negative.

- Prevalence: Proportion of people with disease in an entire population
  {(TP + FN)/(TP + FP + FN + TN)}
  Remember that "incidence" is the number of new cases in a time frame (often a year) and prevalence is the number of people with disease in the total population at any one time

- *Sensitivity*: Proportion of people with disease who will have a positive result
  ✓ Sens = {TP/(TP+FN)}
- *Specificity*: Proportion of people without the disease who will have a negative result
  ✓ Spec = {TN/(FP+TN)}
- *Positive predictive value (PPV)*: Proportion of people with a positive test result who actually have the disease
  ✓ PPV = {TP/(TP+FP)}
- *Negative predictive value (NPV)*: Proportion of people with a negative test result who do not have disease
  ✓ NPV = {TN/(FN+TN)}
- *Odds ratio (OR)*: Evaluates whether the odds of a certain event or outcome is the same for two groups
  ✓ OR= (TP×TN)/(FN×FP)
- *Relative risk reduction (RRR)*: Measures how much the risk (rate of some outcome) is reduced in the experimental group compared to the control group
  ✓ RRR=CER−EER/CER where CER is the control group event rate and EER is the experimental event rate
- *Absolute risk reduction (ARR)*: The difference on outcome rates between the control and the treatment groups
  ✓ ARR=CER−EER
- *Number needed to treat (NNT)*: The number of patients that would need to be treated to prevent one bad outcome
  ✓ NNT = 1/ARR or 1/(CER−EER)
- *Likelihood ratio* for a test result is defined as the ratio between the probability of observing that result in patients with the disease in question, and the probability of that result in patients without the disease

$$\text{Likelihood Ratio, positive} = \text{Sens}/(1 - \text{Spec})$$

$$\text{Likelihood Ratio, negative} = (1 - \text{Sens})/\text{Spec}$$

## BODY MASS INDEX (BMI)

$$\text{Body Mass Index} = \text{Weight}/\text{Height}^2$$

*Weight [kg]*
*Height [m]*
- *Adult values*: Normal is 18–25; overweight is 25–30; obese is greater than 30
- Pediatric norms vary by age and according to growth charts

## BODY SURFACE AREA (BSA [MOSTELLER METHOD])

$$\text{Body Surface Area} = \sqrt{\text{Weight} \times \text{Height}/3600}$$

*Body Surface Area [m²]*
*Weight [kg]*
*Height [cm] (notice difference from BMI calculation which is in meters)*
- Used to calculate dosages for certain medications (e.g., steroids, chemotherapeutic agents)
- Other formulas for BSA have been derived (Boyd, Dubois, and Haycock)

## CEREBRAL PERFUSION PRESSURE

$$CPP = MAP - CVP$$

or

$$CPP = MAP - ICP$$

*(use whichever equation refers to a higher "downstream" pressure [CVP or ICP] for the given patient, reflecting the pressure driving gradient)*
*CPP: Cerebral perfusion pressure [mm Hg]*
*CVP: Central venous pressure (direct measure) [mm Hg]*
*MAP: Mean arterial pressure (calculated or direct measure) [mm Hg]*
*ICP: Intracranial pressure (direct measure) [mm Hg]*
- Maintenance of CPP reduces mortality after severe brain injury
- ICP monitoring is recommended in most comatose patients with severe head injury and is considered a central part of critical care management
- A CPP>60 mm Hg and ICP<20 are desired for patients recovering from a brain injury. Note that in a hypotensive patient even small increases in ICP can be detrimental
- MAP can be calculated by doubling the diastolic blood pressure and then adding it to the systolic blood pressure and dividing that sum by 3 (see MAP calculation)
- If the CPP gets too low, then the brain may not get enough oxygen and the patient can suffer hypoxic brain injury

## CHANGE IN SERUM SODIUM (ΔSODIUM)

$$\Delta Sodium = Infusate\ Na^+ + Infusate\ K^+ - (Serum\ Na^+/(TBW + 1))$$

*Infusate $Na^+$: Amount of sodium in infusion [mmol/L]*
*Infusate $K^+$: Amount of potassium in infusion [mmol/L]*
*Serum $Na^+$: Serum sodium [mmol]*
*TBW: Total body water (Liters)*

| TBW Watson Formula*: | Male TBW | $2.447 - (0.09 \times age) + (0.11 \times height) + (0.34 \times weight)$ |
|---|---|---|
| | Female TBW | $-2.1 + (0.11 \times height) + (0.25 \times weight)$ |

*Generally estimated at 60% of total body weight (kg); age measured in years; height measured in centimeters; weight measured in kilograms higher (about 70%) in neonates and infants.

- Calculation of change in serum sodium helps predict sodium changes associated with a given infusion. May be used to limit the risk of demyelinating encephalopathy due to rapid correction of hypo- or hypernatremia

## CONVERSIONS OF UNITS

Degrees Fahrenheit = 1.8 × degrees Celsius + 32
1 inch = 2.54 centimeters (cm)
1 teaspoon = 5 milliliters (mL)
1 tablespoon = 15 milliliters (mL)
1 fluid ounce = 30 milliliters (mL)

1 deciliter (dL) = 0.1 liter (L)
1 dry ounce = 30 grams (g)
1 atmosphere = 760 mm Hg = 760 torr (1 torr = 1 mm Hg)
2.2 pounds = 1 kilogram (kg)
1 milligram (mg) = 0.001 gram (g)
1 microgram (mcg or μg) = 0.001 milligrams (mg)

## CORRECTED QT INTERVAL (QT$_c$ [BAZETT])

$$QT_c = QT/\sqrt{RR}$$

*QT = Measured QT interval [seconds]*
*RR = Preceding RR interval [seconds]*
*1 box width = 0.04 seconds (when paper runs at 25 mm/sec)*
- QT$_c$ > 0.44 seconds is concerning for long QT syndrome
- Certain electrolyte abnormalities and medications may increase the QT$_c$

## CORRECTED SERUM CALCIUM (FOR HYPOALBUMINEMIA)

$$\text{Corrected Calcium} = (ALB_n - ALB_p) \times 0.8 + Ca_p$$

*$ALB_n$ = Normal plasma alb = 4.0 g/dL*
*$ALB_p$ = Measured plasma alb [g/dL]*
*$Ca_p$ = Measured plasma calcium concentration [mg/dL]*
- Corrects the measured plasma calcium concentration for hypoalbuminemia
- Measuring an ionized calcium level may be more accurate

## CORRECTED SERUM SODIUM (FOR HYPERGLYCEMIA)

$$\text{Corrected Sodium} = Na_p^+ + (Gluc_p - 100) \times 1.6/100$$

*$Na_p^+$ = Plasma sodium concentration [mmol/L]*
*$GL_p$ = Measured plasma glucose concentration [mmol/L]*

## CREATININE CLEARANCE (FROM TIMED URINE SPECIMEN)

$$CrCl = (U_{Cr} \times U_{vol})/(P_{Cr} \times T_{min})$$
$$\text{Corrected CrCl} = CrCl \times 1.73/BSA$$

*CrCl = Creatinine clearance [mL/min]*
*Corrected CrCl = Corrected to a body surface area of 1.73 m² [mL/min/1.73 m²]*
*$U_{Cr}$ = Urine creatinine [mg/dL]*
*$U_{vol}$ = Urine volume [mL]*
*$P_{Cr}$ = Plasma creatinine concentration [mg/dL]*
*$T_{min}$ = Time of urine collection [minutes]*
- Represents the volume of plasma cleared of creatinine per unit time
- Creatinine is freely filtered, not reabsorbed, and minimally secreted by the kidneys. Thus, creatinine clearance is an estimate of glomerular filtration
- Clearance can be normalized to 1.73 m² in order to compare it to reference values

## CREATININE CLEARANCE (SCHWARTZ METHOD)

$$CrCl = K \times Height/P_{Cr}$$

*CrCl = Creatinine clearance [mL/min]*
*K (age-dependent constant) = 0.33 for low birth weight infants; 0.45 for term infants; 0.55 for children; 0.55 for adolescent girls; 0.7 for adolescent boys*
*Height [cm]*
$P_{Cr}$ *= Plasma creatinine concentration [mg/dL]*
- A simple estimate of GFR in children derived from body length and serum creatinine
- GFR can be used to screen for kidney disease, follow disease progression, confirm need for definitive treatment (e.g., dialysis, transplantation), and help determine appropriate medication doses for patients with kidney injury or disease

## FRACTIONAL EXCRETION OF SODIUM (FE$_{Na}$)

$$FE_{Na} = 100 \times (U_{Na} \times P_{Cr})/(U_{Cr} \times P_{Na})$$

$U_{Na}$ *= Urine sodium concentration [mEq/L]*
$P_{Cr}$ *= Plasma creatinine concentration [mg/dL]*
$U_{Cr}$ *= Urine creatinine concentration [mg/dL]*
$P_{Na}$ *= Plasma sodium concentration [mEq/L]*
- $FE_{Na} < 1.0\%$ concerning for prerenal azotemia
- $FE_{Na} > 2.0\%$ concerning for acute tubular necrosis

## FREE WATER DEFICIT

$$FWD = Coeff \times Weight \times (Na_{p}/140 - 1)$$

*FWD [L]*
*Weight [kg]*
$Na_{p}$ *= Measured plasma sodium concentration [mEq/L]*
*Coeff: 0.6 for children and nonelderly men; 0.5 for nonelderly women and elderly men; 0.45 for elderly women.*
- Provides an adequate estimate of the water deficit in patients with hypernatremia caused by pure water loss. (See Change in Serum Na$^+$ formula)
- Used to determine the amount of free water needed to treat hypernatremia (usually corrected over a period of hours to days dependent on the acuity of onset)

## GLUCOSE INFUSION RATE (GIR)

$$GIR = \%Glucose \times Daily\ Rate/144 = (\%Glucose \times Hourly\ Rate)/(6 \times Weight)$$

*Glucose infusion rate (GIR) [mg/kg/min]*
*%Glucose = Percent glucose in intravenous fluid (e.g., D10W contains 10% glucose)*
*Daily Rate = Fluid administration rate [mL/kg/day]*
*Hourly Rate = Fluid administration rate [mL/h]*
*Weight [kg]*
- Used in the management of hypoglycemia, especially in neonates
- Glucose utilization of healthy neonates is approximately 5–8 mg/kg/min

## MEAN ARTERIAL PRESSURE (MAP)

$$MAP = \frac{Systolic\,Pressure + (2 \times Diastolic\,Pressure)}{3}$$

- Based on assumption that diastole lasts approximately twice as long as systole

## OSMOLALITY (SERUM)

$$Calc\,Serum\,Osm = (2 \times Na^+) + \frac{GLC}{18} + \frac{BUN}{2.8}$$

$Na^+$ = Serum sodium concentration [mEq/L]
GLC = Serum glucose concentration [mg/dL]
BUN = Serum urea nitrogen concentration [mg/dL]
- Normal serum osmolality is approximately 285–295 mOsm/L
- Osmolal gap = Measured Osm−Calculated Osm (normal $\leq$10)
- If the measured serum osmolality is more than 10 mOsm/L above the calculated serum osmolality, consider causes for an osmolal gap due to unmeasured osmotically active substances such as mannitol, ethanol, methanol, and ethylene glycol

## P/F RATIO

$$P/F = PaO_2/FiO_2$$

$PaO_2$= Arterial partial pressure of $O_2$ [mm Hg]
$FiO_2$= Fraction of inspired oxygen
- Index of severity of hypoxemia; lower number indicates shunt
- Used as part of the definition of Acute Lung Injury (ALI) and Acute Respiratory Distress Syndrome (ARDS)
- For ALI, P/F = 200–300 mm Hg
- For ARDS, P/F <200 mm Hg

## WINTER'S FORMULA

$$PaCO_2 = 1.5(HCO_3^-) + 8 \pm 2$$

$PaCO_2$ = Arterial partial pressure of $CO_2$ [mm Hg]
$[HCO_3^-]$ = Serum concentration of bicarbonate ions [mEq/L]
- Calculates the expected $PaCO_2$ in pure metabolic acidosis (respiratory compensation)
- The patient's actual (measured) $PaCO_2$ is then compared to this
  - ✓ If the two values correspond, respiratory compensation can be considered to be adequate
  - ✓ If the measured $PaCO_2$ is higher than the calculated value, there is also a primary respiratory acidosis
  - ✓ If the measured $PaCO_2$ is lower than the calculated value, there is also a primary respiratory alkalosis

# Cardiology

*Javier J. Lasa, MD*
*Chitra Ravishankar, MD*
*Joseph Rossano, MD, MS, FAAP, FAAC*

## CONGENITAL HEART DISEASE

### AORTIC STENOSIS

**A form of acyanotic congenital heart disease (CHD) in which obstruction of the left ventricular outflow tract leads to a systolic pressure gradient between the left ventricle (LV) and the aorta.**

- *Aortic valve stenosis:* Most common form of aortic stenosis; frequently due to bicuspid aortic valve; identified in up to 2% of adults
- *Subvalvular stenosis:* Due to fibromuscular ring or shelf below the aortic valve; may be associated with malalignment ventricular septal defect (VSD) or aortic coarctation
- *Supravalvular stenosis:* Least common form of aortic stenosis; may be localized or diffuse; may be associated with Williams syndrome

### EPIDEMIOLOGY

- 3–6% of congenital heart defects; male:female = 4:1

### PATHOPHYSIOLOGY

- *Critical aortic stenosis:* High pressure gradients across the aortic valve may result in LV failure, low cardiac output, and pulmonary edema
- Pressure gradient may increase as cardiac output increases with growth during childhood
- Abnormal diastolic filling is due to LV hypertrophy

### CLINICAL MANIFESTATIONS

- Often asymptomatic in infancy, but can present with irritability, paleness, tachycardia, tachypnea, retractions, and rales; symptoms depend on severity and location of obstruction
- Heart failure is most common in neonates with critical disease or in adults with untreated disease
- Ventricular arrhythmias and sudden death may occur
- *Physical examination:* Early systolic ejection click at the apex; harsh ejection systolic murmur at the base radiates to the neck; palpable left ventricular lift; precordial systolic thrill at base

### DIAGNOSTICS

- *Chest x-ray (CXR):* May show cardiomegaly (evidence of LV hypertrophy) and pulmonary edema with critical obstruction
- *ECG:* LV hypertrophy or LV strain in severe disease
- *Echocardiography:* Defines anatomy and hemodynamic severity of the lesion
- *Cardiac catheterization:* Required to establish severity and measure pressure gradient across aortic valve, and for treatment of aortic stenosis

## MANAGEMENT

### Medical

- Prostaglandin $E_1$ (PGE$_1$) dilates the ductus arteriosus to augment systemic output in severely ill neonates with critical obstruction
- Inotropic support with dopamine or epinephrine may also be required to maintain adequate cardiac output both before and after the intervention

### Surgical or Catheter-based Interventions

- *Aortic valve stenosis:* Percutaneous balloon aortic valvuloplasty is the preferred approach for aortic stenosis; surgical valvotomy; aortic valve replacement with pulmonary autograft or Ross procedure (preferred in infants and young children) prosthetic valve or aortic homograft
- *Subaortic stenosis:* Surgical removal of fibromuscular shelf or membrane, myomectomy may be required for muscular tunnel-like obstruction (Konno procedure)
- *Supravalvular stenosis:* Surgery to widen or repair stenotic segment

## ATRIAL SEPTAL DEFECT

A form of acyanotic CHD characterized by openings in the atrial septum at one of the following four locations:

- *Ostium secundum:* Located at site of foramen ovale; accounts for 50–70% of all atrial septal defects (ASDs)
- *Ostium primum:* Located low in the septum; also called incomplete atrioventricular canal defect or endocardial cushion defect, and always associated with cleft in mitral valve
- *Sinus venosus:* Located high in the septum near the superior vena cava or located low in the septum near the inferior vena cava (least common); associated with anomalous pulmonary venous return
- *Coronary sinus septal defect:* A portion of the coronary sinus roof is missing, causing blood to shunt from the left atrium into the coronary sinus and then into the right atrium; least common type of ASD

### EPIDEMIOLOGY

- 5–10% of CHD; male:female = 1:2; 1 in 1500 live births

### PATHOPHYSIOLOGY

- Small defects may close spontaneously
- Magnitude of left-to-right shunt depends on size of the defect and pulmonary and systemic vascular resistance, and relative compliance of the ventricles
- Results in right atrial and right ventricular volume overload; if unrepaired pulmonary vascular disease can develop in adulthood

### CLINICAL MANIFESTATIONS

- Often asymptomatic in childhood and cardiac evaluation is prompted by murmur; may not present until adulthood
- Occasionally presents in childhood with fatigue, dyspnea, respiratory infections, and congestive heart failure (CHF)
- CHF is more common if the ASD is associated with borderline left sided structures such as mitral valve abnormalities or mild coarctation

- Atrial dysrhythmias including fibrillation and supraventricular tachycardia are more common in adults
- Pulmonary hypertension is more common in adults
- Paradoxical emboli may occur
- *Physical exam:* $S_1$ is loud or normal; $S_2$ is widely split and fixed; prominent right ventricular cardiac impulse; midsystolic pulmonary ejection murmur; diastolic murmur at left lower sternal border (LLSB) may represent flow across the tricuspid valve if pulmonary to systemic flow ratio (Qp:Qs) is greater than 2:1

## DIAGNOSTICS

- *CXR:* Right atrial enlargement, right ventricular hypertrophy (RVH), dilated pulmonary artery, and increased pulmonary vasculature
- *ECG:* Right axis deviation and RVH
- *Echocardiography:* Reveals location, size, and associated anomalies
- *Cardiac catheterization:* May be used to confirm presence of the defect and determine pulmonary to systemic flow ratio (Qp:Qs)

## MANAGEMENT

### Medical

- Heart failure symptoms may be managed with digoxin and diuretics (e.g., furosemide)
- Occasional arrhythmias may require medical management
- Secundum ASDs close spontaneously in about 40–50% of patients

### Surgical or Catheter-based Interventions

- Usually recommended if pulmonary:systemic flow ratio (Qp:Qs) is greater than 2:1, patient is symptomatic, or ASD is moderate or large in size
- Uncomplicated ASDs are often closed between 2 and 4 years of age
- Defect is sutured or a patch is applied, often under cardiopulmonary bypass, though closure devices deployed by transvenous catheterization are increasingly used

## COARCTATION OF THE AORTA

**A form of acyanotic CHD in which there is narrowing of the aorta, most commonly just beyond the origin of the left subclavian artery.**

- May occur in isolation or in association with other cardiac defects

## EPIDEMIOLOGY

- 5–8% of congenital heart defects; male:female = 2:1
- Often associated with Turner syndrome

## PATHOPHYSIOLOGY

- Degree of symptoms and timing of presentation depends on severity of coarctation
- Decreased blood flow to lower extremities and lower half of the body may occur, especially after closure of the ductus arteriosus
- LV outflow tract obstruction leads to LV hypertrophy and increased systolic pressures; eventually LV dysfunction may develop, causing low output cardiac failure and pulmonary edema
- Extensive collateral circulation may develop in older children and young adults who are not diagnosed early in life

## CLINICAL MANIFESTATIONS

- *Neonates:* May present in the first 3 weeks of life (especially after closure of the ductus arteriosus) with tachypnea, poor feeding, diaphoresis, CHF, cardiogenic shock, and/or decreased femoral pulses
- *Older children:* Upper extremity hypertension and claudication
- *On exam:* Decreased or absent femoral pulses; systolic murmur at left sternal border between third and fourth intercostal space radiating to left infrascapular area; ejection click if bicuspid aortic valve is present

## DIAGNOSTICS

- *Four-extremity blood pressures (BPs):* Differential in BP (>10 mm Hg) between right upper extremity and lower extremities
- *CXR:* Cardiomegaly and pulmonary edema is usually seen in neonates and infants, rib notching noted in children over 6 years of age
- *ECG:* LV hypertrophy and possible left atrial (LA) enlargement in older children; RV hypertrophy in neonates
- *Echocardiography:* Reveals segment of coarctation and associated anomalies
- *Cardiac catheterization:* May be performed to delineate affected segment and potentially for treatment in older children, adolescents, and adults
- *MRI:* May help define lesion and identify collateral vessels; used for serial follow-up

## MANAGEMENT

### Medical

- $PGE_1$ maintains patency of ductus to help provide distal perfusion in severely affected neonates. Inotropic support may be required for those presenting in extremis
- Rebound hypertension is common in the immediate postoperative period and may require antihypertensive medication, especially in older children

### Surgical

- Timing depends on age of diagnosis, severity of disease, and related defects
- Surgery is usually preferred for neonates and infants. Techniques include end-to-end anastomosis, patch augmentation, and subclavian flap repair. Percutaneous balloon angioplasty or stent angioplasty for native coarctation is usually reserved for recurrent coarctation or primary therapy in older children, adolescents, or adults

## ENDOCARDIAL CUSHION DEFECT

**A form of acyanotic CHD in which there is malformation of the endocardial cushion resulting in defects in the interatrial and/or interventricular septum. Defects may be partial or incomplete (e.g., ostium primum atrial septal defect, common atrium, posterior ventricular septal defect) or complete (e.g., complete atrioventricular canal).**

- *Complete atrioventricular canal:* One large atrioventricular valve, and both ASD and VSD

## EPIDEMIOLOGY

- 4–5% of CHD; 0.19 in 1000 live births
- 30% of children with complete endocardial cushion defects have Down syndrome; 20–25% of children with Down syndrome have endocardial cushion defects

## PATHOPHYSIOLOGY

- Varying degrees of left-to-right shunt result in CHF and recurrent pneumonia. The hemodynamic effect of the lesion depends on the specific location of the defect, the degree of shunting, and valvular incompetence

## CLINICAL MANIFESTATIONS

- Usually present within the first few weeks of life with failure to thrive, tachypnea, tachycardia, respiratory infections, and/or heart failure
- Untreated defects may lead to Eisenmenger syndrome (irreversible pulmonary arterial hypertension resulting from long-standing excessive pulmonary blood flow)
- Physical exam findings depend on the extent of the lesion and may include hyperdynamic precordium with palpable thrill at LLSB; accentuated pulmonic component of $S_2$; variable systolic murmur may be inaudible or grade 3–4/6 and holosystolic; signs of heart failure

## DIAGNOSTICS

Findings depend on the extent of the lesion and may include:

- *CXR:* Cardiomegaly, pulmonary vascular congestion, prominent main pulmonary artery
- *ECG:* Left or superior deviation of QRS axis (−40 to −150 degrees), ventricular hypertrophy (right and/or left)
- *Echocardiography:* Helps define size of the defects, size of the ventricles, and anatomy of the valve
- *Cardiac catheterization:* May be used to evaluate pulmonary hypertension and to look for additional VSDs

## MANAGEMENT

### Medical

- *Anti-congestive medications:* Digoxin, diuretics, ACE inhibitors

### Surgical

- Definitive surgical treatment is usually recommended before 6 months of age, particularly in infants with Down syndrome
- Palliative pulmonary artery banding is usually reserved for cases in which more definitive surgical options are challenging (e.g., prematurity)

## HYPOPLASTIC LEFT HEART SYNDROME

**A form of cyanotic CHD characterized by underdevelopment of the LV and ascending aorta. The mitral and aortic valves are atretic or critically stenosed. Systemic circulation is dependent on a patent ductus arteriosus (PDA).**

## EPIDEMIOLOGY

- 1% of CHD, more common in males
- Most common cause of cardiac death in the first month of life
- Chromosomal abnormalities in up to 25% of patients

## PATHOPHYSIOLOGY

- Blood returning from the lungs passes through a patent foramen ovale or an ASD into the right atrium (RA) and RV

- If a VSD is present and the aortic valve is not completely stenotic, a small amount of blood may enter the aorta directly. Otherwise, there is complete mixing of systemic and pulmonary blood, which enters the pulmonary artery and passes through a PDA into the systemic circulation, including retrograde flow in the ascending aorta
- As the PDA closes, systemic output decreases and metabolic acidosis ensues

## CLINICAL MANIFESTATIONS

- Most present within 48–72 hours of life as the ductus arteriosus closes
- Cyanosis, dyspnea, poor feeding, heart failure, hepatomegaly, poor perfusion, decreased peripheral pulses, shock
- A minority with a restrictive ASD or intact atrial septum present immediately after birth with profound cyanosis, respiratory failure, and circulatory collapse
- *On exam:* Right parasternal lift; single, loud $S_2$; soft, nonspecific systolic ejection murmur

## DIAGNOSTICS

- *Prenatal ultrasound:* Allows for antenatal diagnosis, counseling, and time to consider treatment options; increasingly predominant method for diagnosis in current era
- *CXR:* Cardiomegaly, pulmonary venous congestion, pulmonary edema
- *ECG:* RV hypertrophy
- *Echocardiography:* Defines anatomy
- *Cardiac catheterization:* Rarely needed in the current era except for diagnosis and treatment of restrictive ASD

## MANAGEMENT

### Medical

- Without intervention, hypoplastic left heart syndrome (HLHS) is fatal within the first month of life
- $PGE_1$ maintains ductal patency and systemic perfusion
- Ratio of pulmonary vascular resistance (PVR) to systemic vascular resistance (SVR) is actively managed to assure adequate oxygenation and systemic output. Generally, oxygen saturation ($SaO_2$) greater than 70% is adequate and $SaO_2$ greater than 90% is undesirable because it indicates pulmonary overcirculation. *Supplemental oxygen is usually NOT required*

### Surgical

- *Norwood Procedure:* First stage in a three-staged surgical palliation of HLHS. While survival has improved, there is still a substantial risk of death during childhood
- *Hybrid:* Consisting of bilateral pulmonary artery bands and stenting of the PDA is the preferred neonatal palliation in some centers
- *Orthotopic Heart Transplantation:* Will be needed in many HLHS patients, though rare as a primary therapy; requires lifelong immunomodulatory therapy; shortage of available donors

## TETRALOGY OF FALLOT

A form of cyanotic CHD resulting from a malaligned infundibular/subpulmonary septum and characterized by (1) overriding aorta; (2) right ventricular outflow tract obstruction; (3) malalignment VSD; and (4) RV hypertrophy.

## EPIDEMIOLOGY

- 5–7% of CHD; incidence: 1 in 2700
- 15% of patients with TOF have DiGeorge syndrome; 50% of patients with DiGeorge syndrome have TOF

## PATHOPHYSIOLOGY

- Pulmonary valve annulus has variable size and helps determine degree of RV outflow tract obstruction
- Severity of symptoms determined by degree of RV outflow tract obstruction (related to subvalvular pulmonary stenosis) and right-to-left shunt; degree of shunt depends on PVR, SVR, and presence or absence of a PDA
- VSD is usually large and unrestrictive
- Mild cases may have imperceptible cyanosis ("pink tet")

## CLINICAL MANIFESTATIONS

- *Paroxysmal Hypercyanotic Attacks ("Tet spells")*
  - ✓ Characterized by the sudden onset of increased cyanosis, dyspnea, and change in mental status (often with irritability)
  - ✓ Due to sudden increased ratio of pulmonary to SVR resulting in increased right-to-left shunting across the VSD and reduction in pulmonary blood flow
  - ✓ May lead to severe hypoxemia, metabolic acidosis, and death
  - ✓ Onset generally between 2 and 9 months of age
- If untreated, cyanosis is observed in most patients by 1 year of age; dyspnea with exertion; clubbing and tendency to assume a "knee-to-chest" or squatting position are seen in older children
- *On exam:* RV impulse harsh systolic ejection murmur at left sternal border; single second heart sound

## DIAGNOSTICS

- *CXR:* "Boot-shaped" heart, clear lung fields, possible right aortic arch
- *ECG:* Right axis deviation, RV hypertrophy, dominant R-wave or RSR' pattern in precordial leads
- *Echocardiography:* Defines anatomy
- *Cardiac catheterization:* May rarely be required to delineate coronary artery anatomy

## MANAGEMENT

### "Tet" Spells

- Remove restrictive clothing, calm patient, and place the baby in parent's lap in knee-to-chest position
- Oxygen
- Morphine
- Phenylephrine or IV beta-blocker rarely required

### Medical

- In neonates, avoid stressors such as cold, and monitor blood glucose levels
- If RV outflow tract obstruction is severe, infants may be dependent on a PDA and require $PGE_1$
- Oral propranolol may decrease frequency and severity of "Tet" spells

## Surgical

- *Palliative surgery:* Systemic-to-pulmonary artery shunt (e.g., modified Blalock–Taussig shunt) can augment pulmonary blood flow in severely affected infants
- *Total surgical correction:* Often done during infancy

## TOTAL ANOMALOUS PULMONARY VENOUS RETURN

**A form of cyanotic CHD in which the pulmonary veins drain anomalously into systemic veins. There are four types of total anomalous pulmonary venous return (TAPVR):**

1. *Supracardiac:* Pulmonary veins course superiorly to a "vertical vein," which drains into the innominate vein. Blood then flows to the superior vena cava and the RA

2. *Infracardiac:* Pulmonary veins course inferiorly through a descending vein, which drains into the portal system. Blood then flows to the hepatic veins, inferior vena cava, and RA. Pulmonary venous obstruction may occur at multiple levels in the descending vein

3. *Cardiac:* Pulmonary veins insert directly into the coronary sinus and RA

4. *Mixed:* Combination of other types

### EPIDEMIOLOGY

- 1–2% of congenital heart defects; male > female
- Most common supracardiac > infracardiac > cardiac > mixed

### PATHOPHYSIOLOGY

- Because pulmonary venous return enters systemic venous circulation, mixing through an ASD or a patent foramen ovale must occur for survival
- Right atrial, ventricular, and pulmonary artery dilation are common due to volume overload
- If pulmonary venous obstruction exists (common with infracardiac TAPVR), pulmonary congestion and pulmonary hypertension develop. In this case, neonates will be profoundly cyanotic and show signs of respiratory distress immediately after birth
- If there is no pulmonary venous obstruction and the ASD is not restrictive, then oxygen saturations above 90% are common. These patients are still at risk for right heart failure

### CLINICAL MANIFESTATIONS

- If pulmonary venous obstruction exists, patients present at 24–48 hours of life with cyanosis, tachypnea, and tachycardia
- If pulmonary venous obstruction does not exist, patients present with mild cyanosis, failure to thrive, dyspnea, and/or CHF
- *With pulmonary venous obstruction:* Single, loud $S_2$; gallop; faint or no murmur
- *Without pulmonary venous obstruction:* Increased right ventricular impulse; $S_2$ widely split and fixed; 2/6–3/6 systolic ejection murmur at left upper sternal border; middiastolic rumble at LLSB

### DIAGNOSTICS

- *CXR:* If pulmonary venous obstruction exists, pulmonary edema is seen. If pulmonary venous obstruction does not exist, cardiomegaly is seen
- *ECG:* RV hypertrophy
- *Echocardiography:* Large RV, compressed LV, ASD, or patent foramen ovale

- *MRI:* May be used to confirm diagnosis and help define anatomy
- *Cardiac catheterization and angiography:* Helps define anatomy, ratio of pulmonary to systemic flow, and degree of pulmonary hypertension

## MANAGEMENT

- Supplemental oxygen
- $PGE_1$ may decrease venous obstruction in infracardiac TAPVR by maintaining patency of the ductus venosus. However, $PGE_1$ carries a risk of worsening pulmonary congestion by increasing left to right shunt through a PDA
- In obstructive type of TAPVR, emergent surgery will relieve pulmonary venous obstruction. In the absence of obstruction, surgery is generally recommended in infancy
- Goal of surgery is to redirect/connect pulmonary venous return to the LA

## TRANSPOSITION OF THE GREAT ARTERIES

**A form of cyanotic CHD whereby the aorta arises from the morphological RV and the pulmonary artery arises from the morphological LV.**

- The most common form is dextra-transposition of the great arteries (d-TGA) in which the aorta is anterior and to the right of the pulmonary artery
- Associated abnormalities include VSD, pulmonary stenosis, and coarctation of the aorta

### EPIDEMIOLOGY

- 5% of CHD; male:female = 3:1

### PATHOPHYSIOLOGY

- TGA results in two parallel circuits such that deoxygenated blood is carried by the aorta to the body, while oxygenated blood is carried by the pulmonary artery to the lungs
- To sustain life, mixing must occur through an associated PDA, VSD, or ASD, with the best mixing occurring at the level of the ASD
- If untreated, TGA is usually fatal in the neonatal period

### CLINICAL MANIFESTATIONS

- Cyanosis immediately after birth is typical in TGA with intact ventricular septum
- *On exam:* Often, no murmur is appreciated; murmur of VSD may be noted; single, loud $S_2$

### DIAGNOSTICS

- *Hyperoxia Test:* 100% oxygen is administered via oxyhood for 10 minutes. If $PaO_2$ increases above 100 mm Hg, parenchymal lung disease is suspected, whereas a $PaO_2$ less than 50 indicates cyanotic heart disease
- *CXR:* Mild cardiomegaly, "egg-on-a-string" appearance of cardiac silhouette, pulmonary vascular congestion
- *ECG:* Right axis deviation, RV hypertrophy
- *Echocardiography:* Confirms anatomy and associated defects; helps estimate degree of mixing
- *Cardiac catheterization:* Angiogram may be used to define coronary anatomy; may be accompanied by balloon atrial septostomy as initial palliative procedure for adequate mixing

### MANAGEMENT

#### Medical

- *$PGE_1$:* Maintains patency of the ductus arteriosus in order to augment mixing
- Oxygen

**Surgical**

- *Balloon Atrial Septostomy (Rashkind Procedure):* Increases interatrial mixing and indicated in the presence of cyanosis and a restrictive ASD
- *Arterial Switch Operation (ASO):* Restores LV as the systemic pump
- *Atrial Switch Operation (Mustard or Senning technique):* Risk of late RV failure and arrhythmias and rarely used in the current era

## TRICUSPID ATRESIA

**A form of cyanotic CHD in which there is no outlet from the RA to the RV and the RV is hypoplastic. The entire systemic blood flow enters the LA via a patent foramen ovale or an ASD.**

### EPIDEMIOLOGY

- 1% of congenital heart defects

### PATHOPHYSIOLOGY

**A VSD is usually present. The pathophysiology in tricuspid atresia depends on whether the great arteries are normally related or transposed, and whether there is any obstruction to pulmonary or systemic blood flow.**

### CLINICAL MANIFESTATIONS

- In the presence of pulmonary atresia or severe pulmonary stenosis, presentation is within 24–48 hours
- Most patients present by 2 months of age with cyanosis and tachypnea
- Occasionally, patients with TGA develop pulmonary overcirculation and present with CHF
- Rarely, older patients present with cyanosis, dyspnea on exertion, polycythemia, and easy fatigability
- *On exam:* May have holosystolic murmur at left sternal border or ejection systolic murmur at left upper sternal border; single $S_2$; increased LV impulse

### DIAGNOSTICS

- *CXR:* May see pulmonary undercirculation or overcirculation
- *ECG:* Left axis deviation, RA enlargement, LV hypertrophy
- *Echocardiography:* Usually sufficient to delineate anatomic features

### MANAGEMENT

**Medical**

- $PGE_1$ in severely cyanotic infants (e.g., pulmonary atresia or severe pulmonic stenosis and subpulmonic stenosis) maintains patency of ductus arteriosus and promotes pulmonary blood flow
- Treatment of CHF may be necessary in patients with high pulmonary flow

**Surgical**

- If pulmonary blood flow is diminished, initial palliative procedures may include balloon atrial septostomy, Blalock–Taussig shunt, or surgical septectomy
- If pulmonary blood flow is increased, pulmonary arterial banding may be beneficial
- Ultimate goal is staged palliation to Fontan completion

## TRUNCUS ARTERIOSUS

**A form of cyanotic CHD in which a single arterial trunk arising from the heart supplies the coronary, pulmonary, and systemic, circulations.**

- One semilunar valve with two to seven septal leaflets, which may be stenotic or regurgitant
- Large VSD

### EPIDEMIOLOGY

- 1–3% of congenital heart defects
- May be associated with 22q11 microdeletion/DiGeorge syndrome

### PATHOPHYSIOLOGY

- Because blood leaves the heart through a single trunk, complete mixing occurs and cyanosis may be minimal
- Degree of arterial $SaO_2$ depends on the ratio of SVR to PVR
- As PVR decreases postnatally, pulmonary blood flow increases and heart failure often develops
- Associated anomalies may include truncal stenosis, truncal insufficiency, and interrupted aortic arch

### CLINICAL MANIFESTATIONS

- Usually present with mild cyanosis, and tachypnea in the first month of life
- Neonates with truncus and interrupted aortic arch present within the first 24–48 hours when the ductus arteriosus constricts
- Features of 22q11 microdeletion/DiGeorge syndrome
- *On physical exam:* Bounding pulses; systolic ejection click; single $S_2$; harsh systolic murmur; diastolic decrescendo murmur if truncal insufficiency

### DIAGNOSTICS

- *CXR:* Cardiomegaly, boot-shaped heart, pulmonary congestion, possible right aortic arch
- *ECG:* LV hypertrophy, RV hypertrophy
- *Echocardiography:* Usually sufficient to delineate anatomy

### MANAGEMENT

- Prostaglandin for truncus with interrupted aortic arch
- Surgery is recommended in the neonatal period

#### Surgical

- Patch closure of the VSD, placement of a conduit from the RV to the pulmonary arteries after separating them from the truncus
- In the past, surgical banding of pulmonary arteries was used to limit pulmonary overcirculation; this strategy is no longer used due to the high incidence of pulmonary hypertension

## VENTRICULAR SEPTAL DEFECT

**A form of acyanotic CHD characterized by an opening in the ventricular septum in one of four locations:**

1. *Perimembranous or conoventricular:* Defect involving the membranous septum beneath the aortic valve; 70% of VSDs

2. *Muscular (trabecular):* Defect within the muscular septum between the LV and RV; often involves multiple, small defects which may be difficult to repair surgically; 5–20% of VSDs
3. *Outlet (supracristal, subpulmonary, malalignment, conoseptal hypoplasia, subarterial):* Defect beneath the pulmonic valve which communicates with the RV outflow tract; 5–7% of VSDs
4. *Inlet or canal type:* Located posteriorly and inferiorly to perimembranous VSDs; 5–8% of VSDs; often associated with endocardial cushion defects

## EPIDEMIOLOGY

• Two to six per 1000 live births; 25% of CHD
• Most common form of CHD

## PATHOPHYSIOLOGY

• Small defects (restrictive) are not usually hemodynamically significant
• Large defects (unrestrictive) allow significant left-to-right shunting as the PVR declines, causing pulmonary overcirculation, and heart failure
• Large, unrepaired defects can lead to pulmonary vascular obstructive disease and Eisenmenger's syndrome
• Complications include pulmonary vascular obstructive disease, RV outflow tract obstruction, aortic regurgitation, and endocarditis

## CLINICAL MANIFESTATIONS

• May be asymptomatic and present with a murmur
• Symptomatic VSDs often present at 4–6 weeks of age as PVR decreases and may present with dyspnea, poor growth, feeding difficulties, sweating, fatigue
• VSDs are often silent in the newborn period while PVR is similar to SVR
• Physical exam findings vary depending on size and location of the VSD as well as the degree of PVR and may include loud, harsh, blowing holosystolic murmur at LLSB; palpable thrill at LLSB with parasternal lift and apical thrust; $S_3$ and a middiastolic rumble may be present. Small defects may be associated with loud murmurs

## DIAGNOSTICS

• *CXR:* May be normal or may reveal cardiomegaly and increased pulmonary vasculature
• *ECG:* May be normal or may reveal evidence of LV hypertrophy, LA hypertrophy, and biventricular hypertrophy
• *Echocardiography:* Reveals the size and location of the VSD
• *Cardiac catheterization:* Rarely indicated in the current era

## MANAGEMENT

### Medical

• Small VSDs are often well tolerated
• Approximately 70% of VSDs close spontaneously. Small, muscular defects are most likely to close spontaneously
• If signs of heart failure, consider diuretics, ACE inhibitors, or digoxin

### Surgical

• Indications for surgery include uncontrolled heart failure, development of aortic regurgitation, RV outflow tract obstruction
• Surgical closure with a Dacron or Gortex patch
• Pulmonary arterial palliative banding is usually reserved for complicated cases and premature infants

## SURGERIES FOR CONGENITAL HEART DISEASE

### ARTERIAL SWITCH OPERATION (OF JATENE)

- *Indication:* Transposition of the great arteries (TGA)
- *Definition:* The coronary arteries are reimplanted into the pulmonary artery (neoaorta). The pulmonary artery and aorta are transected above the sinus of Valsalva, the pulmonary artery is usually brought in front of the neo-aorta (Lecompte maneuver), and reattached

### BLALOCK–TAUSSIG SHUNT

- *Indication:* Tetralogy of Fallot, tricuspid atresia, pulmonary atresia
- *Definition:* Direct anastomosis of the subclavian artery to the ipsilateral pulmonary artery, thereby creating a systemic to pulmonary shunt

### BLALOCK–TAUSSIG SHUNT, MODIFIED

- *Indication:* Tetralogy of Fallot, tricuspid atresia, pulmonary atresia
- *Definition:* A Gortex graft connects the subclavian artery to the ipsilateral pulmonary artery, thereby creating a systemic to pulmonary shunt

### NORWOOD PROCEDURE OR STAGE I

- *Indication:* Usually first stage for single ventricle heart disease (e.g., HLHS and variants)
- Reconstruction of the hypoplastic ascending aorta and the aortic arch using the main pulmonary artery and homograft patch, placement of a Blalock–Taussig shunt or shunt from RV to the pulmonary artery (Sano modification), and removal of the atrial septum

### BIDIRECTIONAL GLENN SHUNT OR HEMI-FONTAN (4–6 MONTHS)

- *Indication:* Usually second stage for single ventricle heart disease (e.g., tricuspid atresia, HLHS)
- *Definition:* Direct connection of the superior vena cava to undivided right pulmonary artery, allowing blood flow to both lungs

### FONTAN PROCEDURE (2–4 YEARS)

- *Indication:* Usually third stage for single ventricle heart disease
- *Definition:* Connection of the inferior vena cava to the right pulmonary artery. Modifications include lateral tunnel and extracardiac conduit with or without fenestration

### MUSTARD AND SENNING PROCEDURE

- *Indication:* Transposition of the great arteries (TGA)
- *Definition:* Use of native atrial or prosthetic baffles to divert pulmonary venous blood to the RV and systemic venous blood to the LV

### PULMONARY ARTERY BANDING

- *Indication:* Single ventricle heart disease with increased pulmonary blood flow, complicated VSD
- *Definition:* Constriction of the pulmonary artery to reduce pulmonary blood flow

### ROSS PROCEDURE

- *Indication:* Aortic stenosis, aortic regurgitation, or mixed aortic valve disease
- *Definition:* Replacement of diseased aortic valve and root with patient's own pulmonary valve and root (autograft). A homograft is placed into the position of the pulmonary valve, and the coronary arteries are reimplanted into the autograft

## ACQUIRED HEART DISEASE

## HEART FAILURE

**Heart failure occurs when oxygen delivery by the heart is impaired secondary to an inability of the heart to fill or eject blood.**

### ETIOLOGY

- *Congenital cardiac causes of heart failure (symptoms generally arise from excessive blood flow to the lungs in left to right shunting lesions):* Atrioventricular septal defect, coarctation of the aorta, critical aortic or pulmonary stenosis, PDA, TGA, tricuspid atresia, HLHS, truncus arteriosus, VSD, and TAPVR
- *Acquired cardiac causes of heart failure:* Arrhythmias, Kawasaki disease, viral myocarditis, rheumatic heart disease, metabolic disorder, muscular dystrophy, chemotherapy (e.g., doxorubicin), idiopathic dilated cardiomyopathy, hypertrophic cardiomyopathy, restrictive cardiomyopathy (RCM)
- *Noncardiac causes of heart failure:* Acute hypertension, anemia, hyper- and hypothyroidism, obstructive sleep apnea

### CLINICAL MANIFESTATIONS

- *Infants:* Failure to thrive, increased work of breathing, feeding difficulties, excessive perspiration
- *Children and adolescents:* Shortness of breath, reduced exercise tolerance, peripheral edema, cough, orthopnea
- *On exam:* Hepatomegaly, rales, tachypnea, tachycardia, gallop rhythm

### DIAGNOSTICS

- *CXR:* Helps assess degree of cardiomegaly and pulmonary edema
- *ECG:* May demonstrate increased voltages, abnormal ST segments, T-wave inversions, Q-waves, and/or rhythm disturbances. The ECG is rarely normal in advanced cardiomyopathy or heart failure
- *Echocardiography:* Helps define congenital heart defects, ventricular size, ventricular function, shortening fraction, ejection fraction, and evidence of diastolic dysfunction

### MANAGEMENT

- *General measures:* Treatment of precipitating factors such as fluid overload, fever, anemia, infection, hypertension, and arrhythmias
- *Diuretics:*
  - ✓ *Loop diuretics* (e.g., furosemide) are considered first-line therapy for heart failure. Electrolyte abnormalities (e.g., hypokalemia, hypochloremia) are common
  - ✓ *Thiazide diuretics* (e.g., chlorothiazide, hydrochlorothiazide) work at the distal tubule and are often used to complement loop diuretics
  - ✓ *Spironolactone* is potassium sparing and is often used in combination with loop or thiazide diuretics
- *Digoxin* increases cardiac contractility; toxicities include bradycardia, heart block, and ventricular arrhythmias
- *Afterload Reducing Agents:*
  - ✓ Reduction in afterload results in increased stroke volume and improved cardiac output
  - ✓ *ACE Inhibitors (e.g., captopril, enalapril):* Reduce PVR by blocking the conversion of angiotensin I to angiotensin II. ACE inhibitors are also thought to have a positive effect on myocardial remodeling

✓ *Intravenous afterload reducing agents* such as milrinone, nitroprusside, and hydralazine are usually reserved for intensive care unit (ICU) patients with decompensated heart failure and low cardiac output
- *Intravenous Inotropic Agents:* Dopamine, dobutamine, and milrinone are generally reserved for ICU patients with decompensated HF and evidence of life-threatening low cardiac output

## CARDIOMYOPATHIES

**Cardiomyopathies are broadly defined as diseases of the heart muscle.**

The common cardiomyopathies encountered in childhood are dilated cardiomyopathy, hypertrophic cardiomyopathy, left ventricular noncompaction (LVNC), and RCM.

### DILATED CARDIOMYOPATHY

#### EPIDEMIOLOGY
- The most common cardiomyopathy of childhood, characterized by an enlarged (dilated) ventricle with depressed ventricular function. The incidence is 0.6–0.7 per 100,000 children

#### ETIOLOGY
- Multiple etiologies including cytoskeletal protein abnormalities, metabolic diseases, myocarditis, endocrinopathies, though most cases are idiopathic

#### CLINICAL MANIFESTATIONS
- Often leads to heart failure and need for heart transplantation. Transplant-free survival only about 50% at 5 years in pediatric dilated cardiomyopathy patients

#### MANAGEMENT
- Medical treatment often includes inhibition of the renin-angiotensin-aldosterone system (e.g., ACE-inhibitors, angiotensin receptor blockers, and aldosterone antagonists), beta-adrenergic receptor blockade, diuretics, and digoxin
- Device therapy may include implantable cardioverter-defibrillators with or without the ability to perform cardiac resynchronization therapy (CRT), and ventricular assist devices (VADs)

### HYPERTROPHIC CARDIOMYOPATHY

#### EPIDEMIOLOGY
- The second most common cardiomyopathy diagnosed in childhood, characterized by a thickened (hypertrophied) non-dilated LV, with the observed hypertrophy not occurring secondary to another disease (e.g., aortic valve stenosis)

#### ETIOLOGY
- Most cases caused by a mutation of genes encoding for sarcomeric proteins. However, other etiologies including glycogen storage diseases, Noonan's syndrome, and mitochondrial diseases can also lead to the hypertrophic cardiomyopathy phenotype

#### CLINICAL MANIFESTATIONS
- LV outflow tract obstruction can occur from subaortic hypertrophy and systolic anterior motion of the mitral valve
- The most common disease leading to sudden death with athletics in the United States
- Symptoms can include chest pain, palpitations, arrhythmias, and heart failure. However, many patients are asymptomatic

## OTHER CARDIOMYOPATHIES

### EPIDEMIOLOGY

- Left ventricular noncompaction
  - ✓ Increasingly recognized cardiomyopathy characterized by prominent trabeculations in the LV giving a characteristic "spongy" appearance to the myocardium
  - ✓ True incidence and prevalence of LV noncompaction is unknown and may be associated with other disorders such as Barth's syndrome, chromosomal abnormalities, and mitochondrial disorders
- Restrictive cardiomyopathy
  - ✓ Least common cardiomyopathy encountered in childhood with an estimated incidence of 0.03–0.04 per 100,000 children

### CLINICAL MANIFESTATIONS

- Left ventricular noncompaction
  - ✓ Wide variability in disease ranging from coexisting with complex CHD, associated with a dilated or hypertrophied ventricle, to normal LV size and function
  - ✓ Prognosis is variable but arrhythmias, dilation, hypertrophy, and dysfunction portend a worse prognosis
- Restrictive cardiomyopathy
  - ✓ Characterized by a severe abnormality in the diastolic functioning of the myocardium. The systolic function is usually preserved
  - ✓ Poor prognosis with most children not surviving 2–3 years after the diagnosis. There is a high risk of sudden death, pulmonary hypertension, and thromboembolism

### MANAGEMENT

- Restrictive cardiomyopathy
  - ✓ No known effective medical therapies; heart transplantation is often recommended in newly diagnosed patients

## MYOCARDITIS

**Myocarditis is inflammation of the myocardium with myocellular necrosis.**

### EPIDEMIOLOGY

- Typically sporadic, but occasionally epidemic
- Infants usually have more acute and fulminant course
- Has been implicated in sudden infant death syndrome

### ETIOLOGY

- Viral is most common (e.g., parvovirus, coxsackievirus, adenovirus)
- *Other infectious agents:* Bacterial, fungal, parasitic, *Borrelia burgdorferi*
- *Trypanosoma cruzi* (Chagas disease) and *Clostridium diphtheriae* are common outside the United States
- Collagen vascular disease
- *Immune mediated:* Kawasaki disease, rheumatic fever
- Toxin induced (e.g., cocaine)
- *Giant cell myocarditis:* Rare, but often severe and fatal

## PATHOPHYSIOLOGY

- Involves damage to the myocardium from the initial infection, as well as the subsequent immune response
- May result in dilated cardiomyopathy

## CLINICAL MANIFESTATIONS

- Often preceded by a flu-like illness
- May present with new onset CHF or arrhythmias
- Dyspnea, exercise intolerance, fevers
- May be acute and fulminant or chronic
- *On exam:* Fever, tachycardia, tachypnea, gallop, signs of CHF, murmur of mitral insufficiency

## DIAGNOSTICS

- *CXR:* Cardiomegaly +/− pulmonary edema
- *ECG:* Tachycardia, low QRS voltages, ST/T-wave changes, arrhythmias
- *Echocardiography:* Enlarged chambers, impaired LV function, mitral regurgitation
- *Laboratory studies:* ESR, CRP, cardiac enzymes, serum viral titers
- *Endomyocardial biopsy:* Gold standard for diagnosis. Viral polymerase chain reaction (PCR) on biopsy sample is more sensitive than serum PCR
- *MRI:* Increasingly utilized for the diagnosis. Can demonstrate myocardial inflammation and quantitative function

## MANAGEMENT

### Medical

- *Heart Failure:* Afterload reduction and diuretics. Inotropic agents should be used with caution as the damaged myocardium is more sensitive to arrhythmias and reserved for patients with poor perfusion
- *Immunosuppression may be appropriate depending on etiology:* IVIG (2 g/kg) and occasionally corticosteroids
- *Outcome:* Approximately one-third of patients recover, one-third have residual dysfunction, and one-third develop chronic heart failure requiring transplant

### Surgical

- Transplant may be necessary
- LVAD (left ventricular assist device) and ECMO (extracorporeal membrane oxygenation) may be used as a bridge to recovery or transplant

## PERICARDITIS

**Pericarditis is defined as inflammation of the pericardium.**

## EPIDEMIOLOGY

- Infectious type is more common in younger children
- Incidence slightly higher in males

## ETIOLOGY

- *Viral:* Echovirus and coxsackie B most common
- Bacterial, including *Mycoplasma tuberculosis*

- *Collagen vascular:* Rheumatoid arthritis, systemic lupus erythematosus
- Uremia
- Neoplastic or radiation induced
- Drug induced (e.g., procainamide, hydralazine)
- *Post-pericardiotomy syndrome:* Seen in about 10% of children 1–4 weeks after cardiac surgery

## PATHOPHYSIOLOGY

- Deposits of infectious material or an inflammatory infiltrate results in an immune response and leads to changes in pericardial membrane function
- A pericardial effusion may result if altered hydrostatic and/or oncotic pressure leads to fluid accumulation
- *Tamponade:* An increase in intrapericardial pressure results in restriction of ventricular filling and a decrease in cardiac output
- *Constrictive pericarditis* is the late result of earlier pericarditis and is characterized by a thick, fibrotic, calcified pericardium
- *Post-pericardiotomy syndrome:* A nonspecific hypersensitivity reaction after manipulation of the pericardial space

## CLINICAL MANIFESTATIONS

- Fever, dyspnea
- Chest pain often radiates to the back or left shoulder, is worse with lying down, and is alleviated by leaning forward
- *On exam:* Fever, tachypnea, tachycardia, friction rub, muffled heart sounds (if an effusion is present)
- With tamponade, may have signs of CHF, *pulsus paradoxus* (exaggerated decrease in systolic BP by greater than 10 mm Hg with inspiration), or *Kussmaul's sign* (paradoxical rise in jugular venous pressure during inspiration)

## DIAGNOSTICS

- *CXR:* Cardiomegaly with "water bottle" appearance if effusion present
- *ECG:* Tachycardia, diffuse ST elevation, T-wave inversion; may see *electrical alternans* if effusion present (variation of QRS axis with each beat due to movement of the heart within the pericardial fluid)
- *Echocardiogram:* With effusion, will see fluid in the pericardial space. In tamponade: RV collapse in early diastole, atrial collapse in end-diastole and early systole

## MANAGEMENT

- *Viral:* Usually self-limited. Treatment includes rest, analgesia, anti-inflammatory medications
- *Bacterial:* Open drainage and aggressive antibiotic therapy
- *Collagen vascular:* Steroids and salicylates often used
- *Post-pericardiotomy:* Rest, nonsteroidal anti-inflammatory agents
- *Constrictive pericarditis:* Pericardial stripping
- *Pericardiocentesis:* Indications include hemodynamic compromise, bacterial pericarditis, and as a diagnostic aid; send pericardial fluid for cell count, culture, and cytology; complications can include arrhythmias and hemopericardium

## ENDOCARDITIS

**Infection/inflammation of the cardiac endothelium with associated immunologic response.**

### EPIDEMIOLOGY

- Incidence is increasing due to IV drug use, survivors of cardiac surgery, patients taking immunosuppressants, and chronic IV catheters
- More common with CHD associated with a steep pressure gradient: PDA, restrictive VSD, left-sided valvular disease, systemic-pulmonary communications

### ETIOLOGY

- *Common organisms: Streptococcus viridans* group (about 50%); *Staphylococcus aureus* (about 30%)
- *Other organisms:* For example, fungal, HACEK group (*Haemophilus* spp., *Actinobacillus actino-mycetemcomitans, Cardiobacterium hominis, Eikenella corrodens, Kingella* spp.)
- *Common associations:* CHD: *S. aureus*; dental procedures: *S. viridans* group; bowel/GU surgery: *group D Strep*; IV drug use: *Pseudomonas* spp., *Serratia* spp.; cardiac surgery: *Candida* spp.

### PATHOPHYSIOLOGY

- Turbulent blood flow damages the endothelium
- Damaged site serves as nidus for adherence of bacteria
- Platelets and fibrin form a vegetation that may embolize
- Immune response produces systemic symptoms

### CLINICAL MANIFESTATIONS

- Fevers, chills, night sweats, dyspnea, arthralgias, central nervous system manifestations, chest/abdominal pain
- *On exam:* Tachycardia; new or changing murmur; splenomegaly; manifestations of heart failure; Roth spots (pale retinal lesions surrounded by hemorrhage); Janeway lesions (flat, painless, on palms and soles); Osler nodes (painful nodes on pads of fingers and toes)

### DIAGNOSTICS

- Blood cultures drawn from two separate sites
- Elevated erythrocyte sedimentation rate and C-reactive protein
- Leukocytosis, anemia, hypogammaglobulinemia
- Hematuria may result from immune complex glomerulonephritis with hypocomplementemia and positive rheumatoid factor (10–70%)
- *Echocardiography:* Can detect vegetations greater than 2–3 mm; may detect valvular dysfunction; transesophageal echocardiography is more sensitive

#### Modified Duke Criteria

- *Major criteria:* Positive blood culture (typical microorganism from two different blood cultures; enterococcus without primary focus; positive serology for Q fever) or echocardiographic evidence
- *Minor criteria:* Predisposing condition, temperature greater than 38.0°C, vascular or immunologic phenomena on physical exam, laboratory studies suggestive of infection
- *Definite endocarditis:* Pathologic diagnosis, 2 major, 1 major and 3 minor, or 5 minor
- *Possible endocarditis:* 1 major and 1 minor or 3 minor
- *Rejected:* Alternate diagnosis accounts for symptoms, resolution of manifestations with ≤4 days of antibiotic therapy, or no pathologic evidence at surgery

## MANAGEMENT

*Empiric therapies based on American Heart Association guidelines (therapy may be tailored based on susceptibilities):*

- *S. viridans group:* Penicillin G for 4–6 weeks
- *S. aureus:* Nafcillin for 6–8 weeks
- *HACEK group:* Third generation cephalosporin for 4 weeks
- Culture-negative: Ceftriaxone and gentamycin (add nafcillin or vancomycin if high level of suspicion for staphylococcal endocarditis) for 4–6 weeks
- *Fungal:* Amphotericin B; surgery often indicated
- *Indications for surgery:* Intracardiac abscess, severe valvular regurgitation, recurrent embolic disease, heart failure, infected prosthetic material
- *Outcome:* Most relapses occur in 1–8 weeks after therapy; mortality is 20–25% with antibiotics; serious morbidity (e.g., heart failure, systemic, or pulmonary emboli) in 50–60% of patients

## ENDOCARDITIS PROPHYLAXIS

Adapted from *Prevention of Infective Endocarditis : Guidelines from the American Heart Association: A Guideline from the American Heart Association Rheumatic Fever, Endocarditis, and Kawasaki Disease Committee, Council on Cardiovascular Disease in the Young, and the Council on Clinical Cardiology, Council on Cardiovascular Surgery and Anesthesia, and the Quality of Care and Outcomes Research Interdisciplinary Working Group. Circulation.* 2007;116(15):1736–1754.

Infective endocarditis prophylaxis for dental procedures is reasonable only for patients with underlying cardiac conditions associated with the highest risk of adverse outcome from infective endocarditis from dental procedures. The administration of prophylactic antibiotics solely to prevent endocarditis is no longer recommended for patients who undergo GU or GI tract procedures, including diagnostic esophagogastroduodenoscopy or colonoscopy.

### High-Risk Patients

- Prosthetic cardiac valve or prosthetic material used for cardiac valve repair
- Previous infectious endocarditis
- Cardiac transplantation recipients with cardiac valvular disease
- Congenital heart disease only in the following categories:
  - ✓ Unrepaired cyanotic CHD, including palliative shunts and conduits
  - ✓ Completely repaired congenital heart defect with prosthetic material or device, whether placed by surgery or by catheter intervention, during the first 6 months after the procedure
  - ✓ Repaired CHD with residual defects at the site or adjacent to the site of a prosthetic patch or prosthetic device (which inhibit endothelialization)

## PROPHYLAXIS RECOMMENDATIONS
### Dental and Oral Procedures

- *Regimen:* Single dose 30–60 minutes before procedure
- *Oral:* Amoxicillin 50 mg/kg (children) or 2 g (adult)
- Cephalexin, clindamycin, or azithromycin are acceptable alternatives for penicillin allergic patients

## ELECTROCARDIOGRAPHY

### PRECORDIAL LEAD PLACEMENT

V1: 4th intercostal space (ICS) ICS, right sternal border (RSB)
V2: 4th ICS, LSB
V3: Equidistant between V2 and V4
V4: 5th ICS, left MCL
V5: Horizontal to V4, left AAL
V6: Horizontal to V4, left MAL
V3R, V4R, V5R, V6R: Mirror image to V3, V4, V5, and V6 on the right side of the chest.

*Note*: ICS, intercostal space; RSB, right sternal border; LSB, left sternal border; MCL, midclavicular line; AAL, anterior axillary line; MAL, midaxillary line; MCL, midclavicular line

### RATE

- On a standard ECG, paper moves at 25 mm/sec
- Each small square is 1 mm (0.04 seconds) and each large square is 5 mm (0.2 seconds) (Figure 5-1)
- Heart rate can be estimated by counting the number of large boxes between QRS intervals where 1 box = 300 bpm, 2 boxes = 150 bpm, 3 boxes = 100 bpm, 4 boxes = 75 bpm, 5 boxes = 60 bpm, and 6 boxes = 50 bpm

### RHYTHM

- The cardiac rhythm may be determined by examining the rhythm strip that appears at the bottom of a standard 12-lead ECG

### AXIS

- The QRS axis represents the net direction of electrical activity during ventricular systole (Figure 5-2 and Table 5-1)

### P-WAVE

- Represents sinus node depolarization (Figure 5-1)
- Best seen in leads II and $V_1$
- In children, P-wave is normally less than 2.5 mm tall and 0.10 seconds in duration
- Tall P-waves may represent right atrial enlargement whereas wide P-waves may represent LA enlargement

### PR INTERVAL

- From beginning of P-wave to beginning of QRS complex
- Refer to Table 5-2 for PR Interval Norms

### QRS COMPLEX

- Represents ventricular depolarization (see Table 5-2)

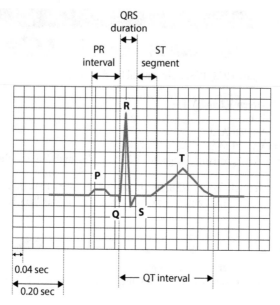

FIGURE 5-1 **Segments and Intervals.** (Reproduced with permission from Ewtry EH, Jeon C, Ware MG: *Blueprints Cardiology*, 2nd edition. Philadelphia, PA: Lippincott Williams & Wilkins; 2006.)

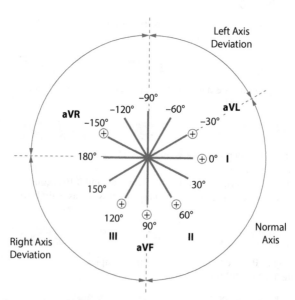

FIGURE 5-2 **Axis.** (Modified with permission from Ewtry EH, Jeon C, Ware MG: *Blueprints Cardiology*, 2nd edition. Philadelphia, PA: Lippincott Williams & Wilkins; 2006.)

| TABLE 5-1 | Normal QRS Axis by Age | |
|---|---|---|
| Age | Mean (Degrees) | Range (Degrees) |
| 1 week–1 month | +110 | +30 to +180 |
| 1–3 months | +70 | +10 to +125 |
| 3 months–3 years | +60 | +10 to +110 |
| >3 years | +60 | +20 to +120 |
| Adult | +50 | −30 to +105 |

Reproduced with permission from Park MK: *Pediatric Cardiology for Practitioners*. 4th ed. St. Louis, MO: Mosby; 2002.

| TABLE 5-2 | QRS Duration Norms and PR Interval Norms in Seconds | | | |
|---|---|---|---|---|
| | QRS Duration Norms | | PR Interval Norms | |
| Age | Mean | Upper Limit | Mean | Upper Limit |
| 0–1 month | 0.05 | 0.065 | 0.09–0.10 | 0.11–0.12 |
| 1–6 months | 0.05 | 0.07 | 0.09–0.11 | 0.11–0.14 |
| 6 months–1 year | 0.05 | 0.07 | 0.10–0.11 | 0.11–0.14 |
| 1–3 years | 0.06 | 0.07 | 0.10–0.12 | 0.12–0.15 |
| 3–8 years | 0.07 | 0.08 | 0.12–0.15 | 0.14–0.17 |
| 8–12 years | 0.07 | 0.09 | 0.14–0.16 | 0.15–0.18 |
| 12–16 years | 0.07 | 0.10 | 0.15–0.16 | 0.16–0.19 |
| Adult | 0.08 | 0.10 | 0.15–0.17 | 0.17–0.21 |

Modified with permission from Park M, Guntheroth WG: *How to Read Pediatric ECGs*. 3rd ed. St Louis, MO: Mosby; 1992.

## QT INTERVAL

- Measured from beginning of QRS complex to end of T-wave
- QT interval varies with heart rate and is corrected by Bazett's formula as follows:

$$QT_c = \frac{QT}{\sqrt{RR \text{ preceding}}}$$

- $QT_c$ greater than 0.44 seconds may be abnormal (see "Long QT syndrome")

## ST SEGMENT

- Segment between the end of the QRS complex and beginning of the T-wave
- Displacement by more than 1–2 mm from the isoelectric line may represent myocardial injury, pericarditis, or a repolarization abnormality

| TABLE 5-3 | R and S Voltage Norms in $V_1$ and $V_6$: Mean (Upper Limit) in Millimeters | | | |
|---|---|---|---|---|
| Age | R in $V_1$ | R in $V_6$ | S in $V_1$ | S in $V_6$ |
| 0–1 month | 15 (25) | 6 (21) | 10 (20) | 4 (12) |
| 1–6 months | 11 (20) | 10 (20) | 7 (18) | 2 (7) |
| 6 months–1 year | 10 (20) | 13 (20) | 8 (16) | 2 (6) |
| 1–3 years | 9 (18) | 12 (24) | 13 (27) | 2 (6) |
| 3–8 years | 7 (18) | 14 (24) | 14 (30) | 1 (5) |
| 8–12 years | 6 (16) | 14 (24) | 16 (26) | 1 (4) |
| 12–16 years | 5 (16) | 14 (22) | 15 (24) | 1 (5) |
| Young adult | 3 (14) | 10 (21) | 10 (23) | 1 (13) |

Modified with permission from Park M, Guntheroth WG: *How to Read Pediatric ECGs*. 3rd ed. St Louis, MO: Mosby; 1992.

## T-WAVE

- Represents ventricular repolarization
- Normally upright in leads I and II and inverted in aVR
- Abnormalities may represent ischemia or electrolyte abnormalities

## LEFT VENTRICULAR HYPERTROPHY, ECG SIGNS

- Left axis deviation (Table 5-3)
- R-wave in I, II, III, aVL, V5, or V6 greater than upper limit of normal
- S-wave in V1 or V2 greater than upper limit of normal
- *Signs of volume overload*: Q-wave in V5 and V6 5 mm or greater and tall, symmetric T-waves
- *Signs of strain*: Inverted T-waves in leads I or aVF, V5–V6

## RIGHT VENTRICULAR HYPERTROPHY, ECG SIGNS

- Right axis deviation
- R-wave in V1, V2, or aVR greater than upper limit of normal
- S-wave in I or V6 greater than upper limit of normal
- Q-wave in V1
- *Signs of strain*: T axis outside normal range (0 to −90 degrees), inverted in V1

## ARRHYTHMIAS

### ATRIAL FIBRILLATION

An ectopic atrial foci leads to an extremely fast atrial rate (350–600 bpm). The ventricular response is usually fast (greater than 100 bpm) and "irregularly irregular." The fast, disorganized ventricular response may lead to decreased cardiac output. Atrial fibrillation is much more common in adults than in children.

### ETIOLOGY

- Structural heart disease, dilated atria, myocarditis, digitalis toxicity, cardiac surgery

## MANAGEMENT

- For sustained atrial fibrillation (>48 hours), consider anticoagulation with warfarin or heparin and echocardiogram to look for thrombus
- Digoxin with or without beta-blockers may control the ventricular rate
- Termination of atrial fibrillation may be achieved through direct current cardioversion (especially in unstable patients) or with antiarrhythmic medications (e.g., amiodarone)

## ATRIAL FLUTTER

**An intra-atrial reentrant circuit leads to a rapid atrial rate around 300 bpm with a characteristic sawtooth pattern on ECG. Because the ventricles cannot respond at 300 bpm, there is often 2:1, 3:1, or 4:1 block.**

### ETIOLOGY

- Structural heart disease, myocarditis, digitalis toxicity, cardiac surgery, dilated atria with mitral insufficiency

### MANAGEMENT

- To prevent thromboembolism, consider anticoagulation with warfarin or heparin before cardioversion
- Vagal maneuvers or adenosine may produce a temporary slowing of the heart rate, but do not terminate the rhythm
- Procainamide or amiodarone may terminate the rhythm
- Digoxin slows the ventricular rate by increasing the AV block
- Direct current cardioversion often restores normal sinus rhythm

## ATRIOVENTRICULAR BLOCK

**AV block ("heart block") occurs when conduction through the atrioventricular node is impaired.**

### FIRST-DEGREE AV BLOCK

- *Definition:* Indicates that the PR interval is above the upper limit of normal for age
- *Etiology:* Rheumatic fever, cardiomyopathy, ASD, Ebstein's anomaly, infectious diseases, ischemic heart disease, hyperkalemia, digitalis toxicity, other medications
- *Management:* Generally asymptomatic and does not require treatment

### SECOND-DEGREE AV BLOCK, MOBITZ TYPE I (WENCKEBACH)

- *Definition:* Progressive lengthening of PR interval with eventual dropped beat
- *Etiology:* Myocarditis, cardiomyopathy, myocardial infarction, congenital heart defect, cardiac surgery, digitalis toxicity, other medications
- *Management:* Usually does not progress and does not require treatment

### SECOND-DEGREE AV BLOCK, MOBITZ TYPE II

- *Definition:* Normal PR intervals are followed by episodes of heart block (i.e., P-wave is not conducted to the ventricles)
- *Etiology:* Myocarditis, cardiomyopathy, myocardial infarction, congenital heart defect, cardiac surgery, digitalis toxicity, other medications
- *Management:* May progress to complete heart block; may require pacemaker

## THIRD-DEGREE AV BLOCK

- *Definition:* Complete dissociation of atrial and ventricular activity (i.e., no relationship between P-wave and QRS complex)
- *Etiology:* Isolated anomaly, maternal SLE, Sjögren syndrome, congenital heart defect, cardiac surgery, myocarditis, endocarditis, Lyme carditis, acute rheumatic fever, cardiomyopathy, myocardial infarction, certain drug overdoses
- *Management:* Patients are often unstable and may require transcutaneous pacing, atropine, or isoproterenol. A transvenous or permanent pacemaker is often required

## LONG QT SYNDROME

**A cardiac repolarization abnormality characterized by prolongation of the QT interval, which can result in torsades de pointes and sudden cardiac death.**

- Corrected QT interval is calculated by Bazett's formula (see above)

### ETIOLOGY

#### Hereditary Causes of Long QT Syndrome

- *Jervell–Lange-Nielsen Syndrome:* Autosomal recessive, congenital deafness
- *Romano–Ward Syndrome:* Autosomal dominant transmission, normal hearing
- Sporadic mutations in potassium and sodium channels

#### Acquired Causes of a Prolonged QT Interval

- *Electrolyte Abnormalities:* Hypokalemia, hypomagnesemia, hypocalcemia
- *Drugs:* Antiarrhythmics, tricyclic antidepressants, erythromycin, antihistamines, phenothiazine, cocaine, organophosphates
- *Other:* Stroke, subarachnoid hemorrhage, myocardial ischemia, liquid protein diets

### PATHOPHYSIOLOGY

- Lengthening of ventricular repolarization leads to R on T phenomena and precipitation of torsades de pointes
- Congenital long QT syndrome may result from a variety of mutations that affect transmembrane ion channels responsible for cardiac repolarization

### CLINICAL MANIFESTATIONS

- Often presents with unexplained syncope or sudden cardiac death brought on by exercise or fright
- May present with presyncope, seizures, dizziness, and palpitations

### DIAGNOSTICS

- *Family History:* Long QT syndrome or unexplained sudden cardiac death
- *ECG:* Increased $QT_c$, torsades de pointes, T-wave alternans, notched T-waves, low resting heart rate
- *Corrected QT interval:* $QT_c$ greater than 440 msec is suspicious and $QT_c$ greater than 460 msec is concerning
- *Exercise Stress Test:* Prolongation of $QT_c$ seen with exercise
- *24 Holter Monitor:* May demonstrate arrhythmia

## MANAGEMENT

### Short Term

- Immediate cardioversion of torsades de pointes
- Magnesium bolus and infusion
- Maintain high normal level of potassium
- Temporary cardiac pacing
- Withdrawal of offending drugs
- Correction of electrolyte abnormalities
- Isoproterenol in cases of acquired long QT

### Long Term

- Beta-blockers
- Left thoracic sympathectomy
- Permanent pacemaker and cardioverter-defibrillator
- May have to avoid sports and stressful activities

## PREMATURE ATRIAL CONTRACTION (PAC)

**An atrial beat arising from an ectopic stimulus in the left or right atrium, which occurs before the next normal sinus beat is due.**

- The P-wave has a different shape than the normal sinus P-wave
- If the PAC is conducted, the QRS complex is generally the same as the QRS complex of preceding beats
- Occasionally, the PAC is conducted aberrantly through the ventricles causing a wide QRS complex
- If the PAC reaches the AV node while it is still refractory, the PAC may not be conducted to the ventricles

### ETIOLOGY

- PACs are very common in normal people and do not necessarily indicate the presence of disease
- *Other causes:* Emotional stress, hyperthyroidism, caffeine, structural heart disease, medications (epinephrine, theophylline)

### MANAGEMENT

- Medical management generally not required if PACs are an isolated finding

## PREMATURE VENTRICULAR CONTRACTION

**A premature ventricular contraction (PVC) is a ventricular beat arising from an ectopic ventricular stimulus, which occurs before the next normal sinus beat is due.**

- Wide QRS complex (greater than 0.08 seconds in infants, greater than 0.12 seconds in children)
- Two PVCs in a row are called a "couplet" or a "pair"
- Three PVCs in a row define ventricular tachycardia
- PVCs may be uniform indicating they arise from a single focus

- Multiform PVCs may arise from different foci or from the same focus and often signify underlying heart disease
- *R on T Phenomenon:* When PVCs occur during the T-wave of the preceding beat, they may precipitate ventricular tachycardia or ventricular fibrillation

## ETIOLOGY

- PVCs often occur in normal hearts
- *Other causes:* Anxiety, caffeine, hypoxemia, sympathomimetics, myocardial infarction, electrolyte abnormalities, and structural heart disease

## MANAGEMENT

- PVCs are often benign and usually do not require treatment
- Correction of underlying abnormalities (e.g., electrolyte abnormalities) may reduce the frequency of PVCs
- Medications such as beta-blockers or antiarrhythmics are occasionally considered

## SUPRAVENTRICULAR TACHYCARDIA (SVT)

**A reentrant supraventricular rhythm may occur when there are two conducting pathways, unidirectional block in one pathway, and slow conduction in the other pathway. SVT may also be due to an automatic atrial rhythm. The two most common forms of reentrant SVT are:**

- *Atrioventricular nodal reentry tachycardia:* The AV node consists of a slow, posterior pathway and a fast, anterior pathway. Onset may be triggered by a premature atrial impulse, which reaches the AV node when the fast pathway is still refractory. The premature impulse conducts anterogradely through the slow pathway and then retrogradely through the fast pathway. Atrioventricular nodal reentry tachycardia is more common in teens and young adults
- *Atrioventricular reentry tachycardia:* An accessory pathway exists outside of the AV node. Anterograde conduction typically occurs via the AV node and retrograde conduction via the accessory pathway (orthodromic). This results in a normal QRS complex. Anterograde conduction occasionally occurs via the accessory pathway and retrograde conduction via the AV node (antidromic). This results in a wide QRS complex, which may be difficult to differentiate from ventricular tachycardia. Atrioventricular reentry tachycardia is common in Wolff–Parkinson–White (WPW) syndrome and is more common in infants and toddlers

## CLINICAL MANIFESTATIONS

- Rapid, regular heart rate, usually 150–250 bpm
- Palpitations, syncope, near-syncope, lightheadedness, shortness of breath

## DIAGNOSTICS

- *Laboratory studies:* Consider electrolytes
- *CXR:* May show infection, cardiomyopathy, pulmonary edema
- *Echocardiogram:* If structural heart defect suspected
- *ECG during SVT:* Heart rate 150–250 bpm, P-wave may be within or after QRS, typically narrow QRS, occasionally wide QRS
- *ECG after termination of the SVT:* May show a delta wave (upsloping QRS complex) in WPW syndrome
- *Adenosine:* May terminate the arrhythmia

## MANAGEMENT

### Short Term

- *If unstable, direct current cardioversion:* (0.5 J/kg increased in steps to 2 J/kg)
- *Vagal maneuvers:* Ice to face, Valsalva, carotid sinus massage
- Adenosine by rapid IV push (initial dose 0.1 mg/kg [max 6 mg], increase by 0.05 mg/kg if unsuccessful to maximum of 0.35 mg/kg or 12 mg)
- Calcium channel blockers (avoid in infants less than 1 year old), class IC agents, digoxin (controversial), and amiodarone may also be effective

### Long Term

- *Antiarrhythmic drug therapy:* Propranolol, verapamil, amiodarone, procainamide, quinidine, flecainide, digoxin
- Radiofrequency catheter ablation is often successful in ablating the accessory pathway
- No treatment is sometimes an acceptable alternative
- Digoxin and calcium channel blockers are contraindicated in WPW syndrome

## SYNCOPE

**Syncope is transient loss of consciousness and postural tone due to inadequate cerebral perfusion.**

### EPIDEMIOLOGY

- 15% of children and adolescents between ages 8 and 18 experience syncope
- Unusual under age 6 except in the setting of seizure disorders, breath-holding, and cardiac abnormalities

### ETIOLOGY

- *Neurocardiogenic syncope (vasodepressor, vasovagal):*
  - ✓ Most common type of syncope; may be provoked by increased vagal tone during micturition, defecation, cough, or hair brushing; may be provoked by peripheral vasodilation during "fight or flight" response, warm temperature, anxiety, or blood drawing
  - ✓ Decreased cardiac filling leads to increased cardiac contractility and activation of stretch receptors. A reflex increase in vagal tone further compromises cardiac output, resulting in syncope
- *Cardiac syncope:*
  - ✓ Dysrhythmias may include SVT, ventricular tachycardia (VT), heart block, WPW, long QT syndrome
  - ✓ *Outflow tract obstruction:* Hypertrophic obstructive cardiomyopathy (HOCM), pulmonary hypertension
  - ✓ *Inflow obstruction:* Restrictive cardiomyopathy, effusion
  - ✓ May be accompanied by brief seizure (*Stokes–Adams syndrome*)
- *Neuropsychiatric syncope:* Seizures, migraines, hypoglycemia, "hysterical" syncope, hyperventilation (e.g., panic attack)

### CLINICAL MANIFESTATIONS

- Symptoms of "presyncope" may include diaphoresis, lightheadedness, palpitations, and tunnel vision
- Cardiac symptoms may include palpitations, shortness of breath, chest pain, and color changes

- Family history may be notable for sudden death, arrhythmias, CHD, seizures, metabolic disorders, and psychiatric history
- Significant physical exam findings are uncommon in children
- Vital signs may demonstrate orthostasis
- Systolic ejection murmur that increases with Valsalva or standing is concerning for HOCM
- Loud second heart sound may indicate pulmonary hypertension

## DIAGNOSTICS

- ECG recommended regardless of cardiac symptoms
- *If concern for seizure activity or trauma:* Neurology referral, EEG, head CT
- *If concern for cardiac disease:* ECG, CXR, echocardiogram, exercise stress test, Holter monitor
- Tilt table testing may help diagnose neurocardiogenic syncope

## MANAGEMENT

### Acute Management

- Keep patient supine until fully recovered
- For an arrhythmia, consider pharmacologic treatment, defibrillation, or cardioversion as per Pediatric Advanced Life Support protocols

### Cardiac Syncope

- *Congenital heart disease present:* Treat underlying cause
- *Arrhythmia present:* May need internal defibrillator, medication, radiofrequency ablation in catheterization laboratory (e.g., WPW syndrome)
- Exercise stress test and electrophysiologic testing in catheterization laboratory may aid in diagnosis

### Neurocardiogenic Syncope

- *Volume expansion:* Encourage fluid and salt intake
- Mineralocorticoids (e.g., Florinef) increase circulating volume and help maintain cerebral perfusion pressure. Efficacy is approximately 60–80%
- Beta-blockers modify the abnormal feedback loop and prevent increased vagal output

## VENTRICULAR FIBRILLATION

**An uncoordinated, chaotic ventricular rhythm with QRS complexes of varying size and shape. Ventricular fibrillation is a pulseless rhythm without effective cardiac output and is terminal unless an effective ventricular beat is restored.**

## ETIOLOGY

- Hyperkalemia, severe hypoxia, surgery, myocarditis, myocardial infarction
- *Drugs and toxins:* Digitalis, quinidine, catecholamines, anesthetics

## MANAGEMENT

- CPR, airway, oxygen, IV or IO access
- Defibrillate up to three times (2 J/kg, 4 J/kg, 4 J/kg) and then with 4 J/kg 30–60 seconds after each medication
- Epinephrine (first dose: 0.1 mL/kg of 1:10,000 IV/IO or 0.1 mL/kg of 1:1000 via ETT; subsequent doses 0.1 mL/kg of 1:1000 IV/IO/ETT)
- Amiodarone (5 mg/kg IV/IO)
- Lidocaine (1 mg/kg IV/IO)

## VENTRICULAR TACHYCARDIA

**Ventricular tachycardia (VT) is defined as at least three premature ventricular beats in a row at a rate above 120 bpm (varies by age) characterized by wide QRS complexes.**

- Sustained VT lasts longer than 30 seconds

### ETIOLOGY

- Cardiomyopathy, myocarditis, cardiac surgery, electrolyte abnormalities, drugs and toxins, long QT syndrome, anomalous left coronary artery

### MANAGEMENT

#### Ventricular Tachycardia with Pulses

- Early cardiology consultation is recommended
- The following medications may be considered: amiodarone (5 mg/kg IV over 20–60 minutes), procainamide (15 mg/kg over 30–60 minutes), or lidocaine (1 mg/kg over 2–4 minutes)
- If signs of shock are present, immediate synchronized cardioversion is indicated (0.5–1 J/kg initially, up to 2 J/kg)
- Magnesium (25 mg/kg over 10–20 minutes) is indicated if torsades de pointes is suspected

#### Pulseless Ventricular Tachycardia

- CPR, airway, oxygen, IV or IO access
- Defibrillate up to three times (2 J/kg, 4 J/kg, 4 J/kg) and then with 4 J/kg 30–60 seconds after each medication
- Epinephrine (first dose: 0.1 mL/kg of 1:10,000 IV/IO or 0.1 mL/kg of 1:1000 via ETT; subsequent doses 0.1 mL/kg of 1:1000 IV/IO/ETT)
- Amiodarone (5 mg/kg IV/IO)
- Lidocaine (1 mg/kg IV/IO)
- Magnesium (25 mg/kg over 10–20 minutes) is indicated if torsades de pointes is suspected

## WOLFF–PARKINSON–WHITE SYNDROME (WPW)

**A form of ventricular pre-excitation in which an accessory pathway bypasses the AV node leading to a variety of supraventricular tachyarrhythmias.**

### EPIDEMIOLOGY

- Affects 0.1–3% of general population
- Occasionally inherited in an autosomal dominant pattern
- May be associated with Ebstein anomaly or corrected transposition

### PATHOPHYSIOLOGY

- Atrial impulses bypass the AV node through the accessory pathway causing pre-excitation
- Paroxysmal SVT in WPW usually results from antegrade conduction through the AV node and retrograde conduction through the accessory pathway (orthodromic)
- Paroxysmal SVT may result from antegrade conduction through the accessory pathway and retrograde conduction through the AV node (antidromic). In this case, the QRS complex is wide and the rhythm may be difficult to distinguish from VT
- Patients are also at risk for atrial fibrillation, atrial flutter, and ventricular fibrillation (rare)

## CLINICAL MANIFESTATIONS

• Palpitations, dizziness, syncope, chest discomfort, shortness of breath

## DIAGNOSIS

• *Family History:* WPW, SVT, sudden cardiac death, unexplained early death (e.g., car accidents, drownings)
• *ECG:* Shortening of the PR interval, widening of the QRS complex, slurred upstroke of the QRS complex (delta wave)

## MANAGEMENT

• Vagal maneuvers such as ice to face, Valsalva, carotid sinus massage (hemodynamically stable patients)
• *Adenosine:* Initial drug of choice (initial dose: 0.1 mg/kg IV; maximum 6 mg)
• *Other potential agents:* Calcium channel antagonists, beta-blockers, digoxin, procainamide; however, caution should be used with digoxin and calcium channel blockers, which may increase the ventricular rate during atrial fibrillation and can lead to ventricular fibrillation
• Radiofrequency catheter ablation is the treatment of choice in symptomatic and high-risk patients

# 6 Dermatology

*Leslie Castelo-Soccio, MD, PhD*
*Kara N. Shah, MD, PhD*

## BLISTERING DISORDERS

### NECROTIZING FASCIITIS

**An acute, rapidly progressive, necrotizing, life-threatening infection of the subcutaneous tissues, often associated with septic shock or Streptococcal toxic shock syndrome.**

• Can be rapidly fatal if not recognized and treated promptly and appropriately

#### EPIDEMIOLOGY

• Rare in children; estimated 500–1500 cases per year in the United States
• Can be seen at any age, including neonates
• Most children with invasive Group A β-hemolytic Streptococcus (GABHS) infection are otherwise healthy; more than 50% of children with non-GABHS necrotizing fasciitis have at least one risk factor
• *Risk factors:* Antecedent varicella infection (with GABHS-related cases); recent surgery or trauma; intramuscular injection; chronic medical conditions (diabetes mellitus, malnutrition, obesity, immunosuppression). In neonates, circumcision, omphalitis, history of scalp electrode placement, necrotizing enterocolitis

#### ETIOLOGY

• Inoculation of bacteria into the subcutaneous tissues with resultant proliferation and release of destructive enzymes and exotoxins results in extensive tissue necrosis, thrombosis of blood vessels, and rapid progression along fascial planes
• *Common:* GABHS. Typically involves the groin or lower extremities
• *Less common:* Aerobic and non-aerobic organisms, including *Staphylococcus aureus*, anaerobic streptococci, group B *Streptococcus*, *Proteus vulgaris*, *Escherichia coli*, *Pseudomonas aeruginosa*, and *Bacteroides fragilis*. May be polymicrobial. Usually involves the abdominal wall, perianal or genital area, or a postoperative wound

#### DIFFERENTIAL DIAGNOSIS

• Cellulitis, erysipelas, pyoderma, staphylococcal scalded skin syndrome, toxic shock syndrome, burns

#### CLINICAL MANIFESTATIONS

• Initial symptoms may be nonspecific and include localized pain, fever, chills, vomiting, pharyngitis, malaise, altered mental status, and myalgias
• Skin manifestations are toxin-mediated, typically seen with GABHS-related necrotizing fasciitis, and present with erythematous ill-defined patch(es) or plaque(s)
• Associated signs and symptoms include severe pain out of proportion to clinical findings, extreme tenderness involving both affected and clinically unaffected areas, numbness, edema, and murky dishwater-like discharge

- Rapid progression to purpuric patch(es) or plaque(s) with or without blistering, followed by the development of ulceration and gangrene. Crepitus may be appreciated in non-GABHS-related necrotizing fasciitis
- Systemic toxicity that may include features of septic shock or, in the case of invasive GABHS, toxic shock syndrome with hypotension and multisystem organ failure
- *Fournier's gangrene:* Involvement of the genital and perianal area; typically polymicrobial

## DIAGNOSTICS

- Clinical diagnosis requires high level of suspicion
- Cultures of blood, wound, and deep tissue (incisional biopsy)
- Histology of incisional biopsy reveals tissue necrosis
- *CBC:* Leukocytosis
- *CRP, ESR:* Elevated
- *Metabolic panel:* Hyponatremia, elevated blood urea nitrogen, metabolic acidosis, hypocalcemia, elevated serum creatine phosphokinase
- Ultrasound may demonstrate fascial thickening and fluid collections
- MRI is more sensitive than CT but may overestimate involvement; a negative MRI can exclude necrotizing fasciitis

## MANAGEMENT

- Prompt surgical consultation and surgical exploration with wide excision of necrotic tissue; delay results in higher mortality. Surgical reexploration and repeat debridement may be required 24–48 hours later
- *Wound care:* Vacuum-assisted wound closure, flap reconstruction, and split-thickness skin grafting may be required
- Pain management
- Broad spectrum antibiotics should be started empirically and adjusted based on culture results. For GABHS-related cases: penicillin plus clindamycin. For non-GABHS-related cases: clindamycin plus a third generation cephalosporin or ampicillin, gentamycin, and metronidazole are recommended
- Intravenous immunoglobulin (IVIG) may benefit patients with GABHS-related necrotizing fasciitis and toxic shock syndrome.
- Hyperbaric oxygen therapy may be helpful where available
- In children, mortality is about 5% and highest in those with comorbid medical conditions, non-GABHS-related disease, septic shock, multisystem organ failure, and young age
- The risk of secondary invasive GABHS infection is significantly elevated in household contacts and approaches 200 times that of the general population; therefore, chemoprevention should be considered for close contacts

## STAPHYLOCOCCAL SCALDED SKIN SYNDROME

**Staphylococcal scalded skin syndrome (SSSS) is a bacterial toxin-mediated exfoliative rash characterized by areas of erythema and superficial desquamation, resembling a superficial burn.**

## EPIDEMIOLOGY

- Generally occurs in children who lack neutralizing antibodies to staphylococcal toxins, including neonates and children younger than 5 years of age or older children and adults with renal impairment or immunosuppression

- Outbreaks of SSSS may occur in nurseries and neonatal units as a result of asymptomatic carriage by staff
- Occult or apparent infection or colonization with *Staphylococcus aureus* strains harboring exfoliative exotoxin, typically belonging to phage group II

## ETIOLOGY

- Exfoliative toxins ETA and ETB are produced by certain strains of *Staphylococcus aureus* and act as serine proteases that degrade a specific keratinocyte cell adhesion molecule, desmoglein-1, resulting in the formation of a superficial, substratum corneum blister at the stratum granulosum
- Nidus of infection typically involves head or neck or circumcision site (neonates) but may not be clinically apparent
- Exotoxin dissemination via the bloodstream results in generalized blistering and may result in part from delayed renal clearance of exotoxin and/or lack of anti-exotoxin antibodies

## DIFFERENTIAL DIAGNOSIS

- Thermal burn, toxic epidermal necrolysis, Kawasaki disease, toxic shock syndrome, toxin-mediated perineal erythema, erythema multiforme, Stevens–Johnson syndrome, epidermolysis bullosa

## CLINICAL MANIFESTATIONS

- Prodrome of fever (low-grade), malaise, irritability, rhinorrhea, pharyngitis and/or conjunctivitis
- Tender, erythematous patches develop initially in intertriginous zones and on face, may become more generalized
- Superficial, flaccid bullae develop in involved areas and often rupture spontaneously, revealing moist, denuded areas resembling burns
- *Nikolsky sign:* Extension of blister with applied lateral pressure along edge of blister
- Perioral, periocular, and perinasal erythema and crusting are characteristic
- Involved areas eventually desquamate and heal without scarring within 2–3 weeks

## DIAGNOSTICS

- *Bacterial Gram stain and culture:* Nares/nasopharynx, perianal/perineum, conjunctivae, umbilicus (neonates), blood (rarely positive); rarely, source may be osteomyelitis, septic arthritis, pyomyositis, pneumonia, or other non-cutaneous infection. Toxin-induced blisters or areas of exfoliation are generally culture-negative
- *Skin biopsy:* Rarely necessary but can differentiate SSSS from toxic epidermal necrolysis (TEN), skin biopsy for frozen section can be performed rapidly to differentiate superficial split within granular layer of epidermis (SSSS) from deeper, full-thickness epidermal involvement (TEN)

## MANAGEMENT

- Most patients have an excellent prognosis if identified and treated promptly
- Parenteral antibiotics are recommended. Use oxacillin, nafcillin, or cefazolin for empiric therapy. Methicillin resistance is rare in exotoxin-producing strains of *Staphylococcus aureus*. Clindamycin may be added to decrease exotoxin production
- *Localized or limited involvement may respond to oral antibiotics:* Clindamycin, penicillinase-resistant penicillin, first- or second-generation cephalosporin
- Topical and/or systemic corticosteroids are contraindicated
- Therapy should be continued for a minimum of 7–10 days

- *Wound care:* Leave bullae intact. Denuded areas may be covered with petrolatum gauze or other non-adherent contact layer dressing. Minimize friction. Monitor for secondary infection
- Cool compresses applied to areas of facial crusting and application of ophthalmic antibiotic ointment may be helpful
- Patients require supportive therapy with pain management, nutrition, temperature control, and hydration

## STEVENS–JOHNSON SYNDROME AND TOXIC EPIDERMAL NECROLYSIS

**Stevens–Johnson syndrome (SJS) and toxic epidermal necrolysis (TEN) are rare hypersensitivity reactions within the spectrum of severe cutaneous adverse reactions (SCAR). Predominantly drug-related, they share a common pathophysiology. They are dermatologic emergencies with significant morbidity and mortality.**

- SJS manifests as atypical targetoid lesions associated with erosions involving two or more mucous membranes. Bullous lesions may be present. Skin involvement is limited to 10% or less of body surface area (BSA)
- SJS/TEN overlap shares features of SJS and TEN with involvement of 10–30% BSA in association with mucous membrane involvement
- TEN manifests as extensive skin erythema, pain, and sloughing involving >30% BSA, usually in association with mucous membrane erosions

### EPIDEMIOLOGY

- Estimated incidence of 2 per 1 million in the general population

### ETIOLOGY

- Proposed pathogenesis involves activation of cytotoxic T-cells by drug antigens and elaboration of inflammatory cytokines and circulating pro-apoptotic factors, including Fas ligand and granulysin, which leads to keratinocyte apoptosis, skin necrosis, and skin detachment
- Genetic susceptibility has been demonstrated in some populations in association with specific HLA alleles, including HLA-B*1502 and carbamazepine-induced SJS in Han Chinese
- *Most common drugs implicated:* Antibiotics (aminopenicillins, sulfonamides), allopurinol, NSAIDS of the oxicam type, and aromatic anticonvulsants (phenobarbital, phenytoin, carbamazepine). Other drugs: antibiotics (cephalosporins, tetracyclines, macrolides, quinolones), NSAIDS of the acetic acid type
- SJS may also occur with *Mycoplasma pneumoniae* infection; the clinical presentation often manifests as mucositis without significant cutaneous manifestations (*M. pneumoniae*-associated mucositis)
- In some cases, no clear etiology can be identified

### DIFFERENTIAL DIAGNOSIS

- *Exanthematous erythematous macules and papules:* Viral exanthems, morbilliform/exanthematous drug eruption, urticarial hypersensitivity, urticarial vasculitis, drug reaction with eosinophilia and systemic symptoms (DRESS)/drug-induced hypersensitivity syndrome (DIHS)
- *Targetoid lesions:* Annular urticaria, erythema multiforme
- *Bullous lesions:* Bullous impetigo, linear IgA disease (chronic bullous dermatosis of childhood), childhood bullous pemphigoid, childhood pemphigus vulgaris, generalized bullous fixed drug eruption

- *Skin peeling and sloughing:* SSSS, toxic shock syndrome, Kawasaki disease, paraneoplastic pemphigus, acute generalized exanthematous pustulosis acute cutaneous graft versus host disease
- *Mucositis:* Herpetic gingivostomatitis, aphthous stomatitis, pemphigus vulgaris, acute genital ulceration/idiopathic vulvar aphthosis

## CLINICAL MANIFESTATIONS

- Generally develops within 2 months of drug initiation, and often within first 1–4 weeks
- Prodrome of fever, malaise, pharyngitis, and eye pain may be noted
- Cutaneous manifestations typically begin on the torso and face and may rapidly generalize
- *SJS:* Primary lesions are discrete, atypical targetoid lesions, often violaceous and/or blistered. Lesions may coalesce, in particular on face and torso
- *TEN:* Primary lesions are tender, erythematous patches and plaques that develop large bullae that coalesce and rapidly slough, leaving large denuded areas of skin. Positive Nikolsky sign: extension of blister with applied lateral pressure along edge of blister
- Mucositis (oropharyngeal, conjunctivae, urethral, genital, perirectal) often results in pain, poor oral intake, and dehydration
- Ocular manifestations include conjunctivitis, eyelid edema, blepharitis, corneal erosions, symblepharon, and corneal scarring, which is a major cause of long-term morbidity and may result in blindness
- Rarely, gastrointestinal and respiratory epithelia may become involved
- Severe cutaneous involvement may result in cutaneous dyschromia and scarring. Nail dystrophy and alopecia may occur. Areas of mucous membrane involvement, including the oropharynx, vagina, urethra, and esophagus, are at risk for scarring, adhesions, and strictures. Long-term sequelae are reported in approximately 50% of children

## DIAGNOSTICS

- Usually a clinical diagnosis but skin biopsy can be helpful if the diagnosis is uncertain. *SJS:* intense interface reaction along the dermal–epidermal junction with central necrosis or blister formation. *TEN:* can be performed as a frozen section and reveals full-thickness epidermal necrosis and a subepidermal split

## MANAGEMENT

- Dermatology consultation recommended
- Prompt discontinuation of all possible inciting medications or treatment of etiologic underlying infection (e.g., *Mycoplasma*)
- *Supportive care:* Pain management, nutritional support, maintain isothermia, maintain hydration and electrolyte balance (hyponatremia, hypokalemia, and hypophosphatemia are common)
- Close surveillance for infection/sepsis and impending respiratory failure, which increase the risk of death. Hypovolemia and septicemia may result in shock and multisystem organ failure
- *Wound care:* Bullae should be left intact but may be drained via sterile technique. Application of petrolatum gauze or other non-adherent contact layer. Judicious use of topical antibiotics. Use of specialized mattress to minimize pressure can be helpful. Frequent application of bland emollients/lubricating ointments to involved mucosa. Oral hygiene may be assisted by use of an oral disinfectant rinse such as chlorhexidine
- *Appropriate consultation for mucous membrane involvement:* Eyes (Ophthalmology); urethral (Urology); gastroesophageal, intestinal, rectal (Gastroenterology); tracheobronchial tree (Pulmonology)

- Systemic corticosteroids are of uncertain benefit. Short-term early use may moderate disease progression, but prolonged use is contraindicated
- Use of IVIG appears to be effective at arresting progression of the disease for both SJS and TEN. For progressive disease, especially if recognized early within first 2–3 days of presentation, IVIG 1 mg/kg/day for 3–4 days may be beneficial. Other therapeutic agents that have been used include cyclosporine and infliximab

## EXANTHEMS

## DRUG REACTION WITH EOSINOPHILIA AND SYSTEMIC SYMPTOMS (DRESS)/DRUG-INDUCED HYPERSENSITIVITY SYNDROME (DIHS)

**A distinct and potentially life-threatening severe adverse drug reaction characterized by a morbilliform cutaneous eruption with fever, lymphadenopathy, hematologic abnormalities, and multiorgan manifestations.**

### EPIDEMIOLOGY

- Incidence is unknown but some report overall population risk ranging from 1 in 1000 to 1 in 10,000 drug exposures
- Incidence may be as high as 10–50 per 100,000 individuals on anticonvulsants such as phenytoin and carbamazepine and 1 per 100 children on lamotrigine
- Individuals with specific human leukocyte antigen haplotypes (HLA types) are predisposed; HLA alleles are necessary but not sufficient to elicit a drug response

### ETIOLOGY

- Considered a severe systemic hypersensitivity reaction to a medication and its reactive drug metabolites; although specific pathophysiology is not known, appears to be mediated by activation of CD4-positive and CD8-positive T-lymphocytes
- Eosinophilia may play a role in visceral complications
- Aromatic anticonvulsants (phenobarbital, carbamazepine, phenytoin, and lamotrigine), minocycline, and sulfonamide antibiotics are most common causes but antibiotics including ampicillin, cefotaxime, streptomycin, and vancomycin have also been implicated
- Antivirals including abacavir and nevirapine, antidepressants including bupropion and fluoxetine, antihypertensives including amlodipine and captopril, nonsteroidal anti-inflammatory drugs (NSAIDs) including celecoxib and ibuprofen, as well as miscellaneous medications including allopurinol, ranitidine, epoetin alfa, and mexiletine have also been implicated
- Most often occurs between 2 and 6 weeks after initiation of a medication but reaction can occur more quickly upon reexposure to a medication
- Individuals with specific human leukocyte antigen haplotypes (HLA types) are predisposed; HLA alleles are necessary but not sufficient to elicit a drug response
- HLA-B*5701 allele has been associated with abacavir-induced DRESS
- HLA-A*3101 is associated with carbamazepine drug reactions including DRESS and SJS/TEN syndrome in Japanese patients
- HLA-DR3 and HLA-DQ2 are associated with carbamazepine-induced DRESS
- HLA-B*5801 is associated with allopurinol-induced DRESS
- Primary or reactivation of herpesviruses, including human herpes virus-6 (HHV-6) infection, cytomegalovirus infection, Epstein–Barr virus, and human herpes virus-7 (HHV-7), have also been implicated

## DIFFERENTIAL DIAGNOSIS

- SJS, TEN, toxic-shock syndrome, Kawasaki disease, exfoliative dermatitis, acute generalized exanthematous pustulosis, viral exanthema, acute cutaneous lupus erythematosus

## CLINICAL MANIFESTATIONS

- There is no reliable standard for diagnosis. Proposed diagnostic criteria includes acute onset of exanthema with fever, suspicion of drug reaction, hospitalization, lymphadenopathy, involvement of at least one internal organ, and hematologic abnormalities, including lymphopenia, lymphocytosis, atypical lymphocytosis, eosinophilia >10%, or thrombocytopenia
- Often a prodrome of fever, pharyngitis, and malaise 2–3 days before onset of rash
- Characteristic cutaneous features include a morbilliform exanthem with accentuation on the face, upper trunk, and proximal extremities but may progress to erythroderma. Pruritus is common. Other morphologies can occur though are less common and include vesicles, atypical targetoid plaques, purpura, and sterile pustules
- Facial edema is common, especially periorbital
- Diffuse lymphadenopathy occurs in 30–60% of patients
- Associated mucosal involvement includes cheilitis and pharyngeal erythema; erosions are rare
- Desquamation develops several days to weeks after the initial eruption and may last for several weeks
- Multiple organ systems can be involved; hepatic (hepatitis), renal (tubulointerstitial nephritis), and pulmonary complications are the most common
- Shortness of breath, tachypnea, and nonproductive cough may occur; more severe pulmonary manifestations are rare but more common with minocycline-induced DRESS and may include interstitial pneumonitis and pulmonary edema
- Myocarditis and pericarditis may occur but are rare in children. Myocarditis can occur months after withdrawal of the offending medication
- Severe, atypical cases can have neurological (encephalitis, meningitis, polyneuritis) or gastrointestinal (diarrhea, pancreatitis, gastrointestinal mucosal hemorrhage) involvement
- Neurologic manifestations are rare and typically occur weeks after the onset of the rash; they are thought to be related to reactivation of HHV-6
- Autoimmune complications can be seen as a delayed sequelae, especially autoimmune thyroiditis (Graves' disease). Development of type 1 diabetes mellitus and autoimmune hemolytic anemia have also been reported
- Rash and other abnormalities typically resolve over 1–2 months after discontinuation of the offending medication
- Avoidance of the causative medication as well as any cross-reacting medications is mandatory; family members may also be at risk and should be counseled appropriately

## DIAGNOSTICS

- *CBC:* Lymphocytosis, atypical lymphocytosis, eosinophilia, and/or thrombocytopenia may be seen
- Hepatic function tests: Elevated liver transaminases, in particular alanine aminotransferase (ALT), elevated alkaline phosphatase; markedly elevated ALT and serum bilirubin with jaundice are important predictors of acute liver failure and death
- *Metabolic panel:* Elevated serum creatinine may be seen
- *Urinalysis:* Proteinuria and eosinophilic sediment may be seen
- Lactate dehydrogenase level may be elevated
- Evaluation of HHV-6, HHV-7, EBV, and/or CMV by serum PCR

- Evaluation of hepatitis A IgM antibody, hepatitis B surface antigen, hepatitis B core IgM antibody, hepatitis C viral RNA may help exclude viral hepatitis
- Consider anti-nuclear antibody (ANA) testing if systemic lupus erythematosus is being considered
- Thyroid function testing should be performed at baseline (TSH, free T4) and then approximately 6 weeks after presentation

## MANAGEMENT

- Dermatology consultation is recommended
- Consider consultation of other specialists as appropriate depending on severity of other organ involvement
- Identify and withdraw causative medication
- Fluid replacement and correction of electrolyte abnormalities
- For cases with mild, predominantly cutaneous involvement, initiation of a mid- to high-potency topical corticosteroid is appropriate
- Antihistamines may help with associated pruritus
- For cases with significant systemic involvement initiation of systemic corticosteroids such as prednisone or methylprednisolone at a dose of 1–2 mg/kg per day is recommended. Taper gradually over weeks to months after clinical examination and laboratory abnormalities have improved; rapid taper may precipitate relapse
- IVIG at a dose of 1 g/kg per dose once daily can be considered for severe cases that do not respond to corticosteroids
- Plasmapheresis and immunosuppressive drugs such as cyclophosphamide, cyclosporine, mycophenolate mofetil, and rituximab may also be considered for corticosteroid and/or IVIG-resistant cases

## ACUTE URTICARIAL HYPERSENSITIVITY

**An acute cutaneous reaction characterized by pruritic, transient annular, and polycyclic urticarial plaques that resemble erythema multiforme.**

### ETIOLOGY

- Acute urticaria results from degranulation of mast cells and basophils and release of vasoactive substances, including histamine, bradykinin, and prostaglandin D2, which cause extravasation of plasma into the dermis
- Acute urticaria may be immune-mediated, either by IgE (most medication- and food-related urticaria), cytotoxic T-cells or immune complex formation; or may be nonimmune-mediated such as occurs with complement-mediated urticaria (radiocontrast agents, bacterial and viral infections, opioids) or physical urticaria
- In children, acute urticaria usually occurs in response to medications (most commonly penicillin and related antibiotics) or infection, most commonly respiratory viruses, gastrointestinal viruses, or Streptococcal infection, although in some cases no clear etiology can be identified

### EPIDEMIOLOGY

- Acute urticaria is very common and occurs in up to 10% of children by adolescence
- Acute urticaria occurs more commonly in infants and younger children but may be seen at any age

| TABLE 6-1 | Comparison of Acute Urticarial Hypersensitivity and Erythema Multiforme |
|---|---|
| **Acute Urticarial Hypersensitivity** | **Erythema Multiforme** |
| Annular, polycyclic urticarial lesions (centers are often pale) | Targetoid lesions (dusky centers with pale rim of edema and peripheral erythema) |
| Lesions range from small to giant | Lesions are often small to medium-sized |
| Evanescent lesions (resolve within 24 hours) | Fixed lesions (lesions persist for up to 1 week) |
| Acral edema of hands, feet, and face common | Acral edema not typically seen |
| Pruritus common | Pruritus uncommon |
| Responds to antihistamines and corticosteroids | Possible response to corticosteroids; no response to antihistamines |

## DIFFERENTIAL DIAGNOSIS

- Serum sickness, serum-sickness-like reaction, erythema multiforme, arthropod bites/ papular urticarial, annular/gyrate erythema, viral exanthema, cutaneous mastocytosis, autoimmune disease, urticarial vasculitis (Table 6-1)

## CLINICAL MANIFESTATIONS

- *Primary lesions:* Generalized annular and polycyclic urticarial papules and plaques that typically are evanescent, lasting less than 24 hours. Occasionally, lesions may resolve with a residual ecchymosis or hyperpigmentation
- Angioedema of hands, feet, and face is common and resolves more slowly than urticaria
- *Dermatographism:* Stroking of the skin results in urtication at the site
- Associated symptoms may include fever and specific symptoms suggestive of associated infection but are often absent
- Progression to anaphylaxis is rare
- By definition, acute urticaria resolves within 6 weeks, but often resolves within several days

## DIAGNOSTICS

- No specific diagnostic tests are indicated unless necessary for the identification of a specific associated infection
- Skin biopsy may be performed if the diagnosis is uncertain and manifests dermal edema; dilatation of blood and lymphatic vessels, and a sparse perivascular mononuclear infiltrate with variable numbers of eosinophils and neutrophils

## MANAGEMENT

- Discontinue potential causative medications
- H1-antagonist antihistamines may be administered at regularly scheduled intervals. As acute urticaria is self-limiting, therapy is rarely needed for more than 1–2 weeks. Use of non-sedating second-generation antihistamines (loratidine, cetirizine) or third-generation antihistamines(levocetirizine, desloratadine, fexofenadine) typically better tolerated than sedating antihistamines (diphenhydramine, hydroxyzine)
- *Consider adjunct H2-antagonist antihistamines:* Cimetidine, ranitidine
- The cutaneous urticarial reaction typically responds rapidly to antihistamines; the edema may respond more slowly
- Topical corticosteroids are not indicated

- Rarely, a short course of a systemic corticosteroid may be indicated in the case of a severe, persistent reaction unresponsive to antihistamine therapy
- Treat associated infection as indicated, although will not hasten resolution of urticaria

## ERYTHEMA MULTIFORME

**An acute, self-limited, and sometimes recurrent immunologically mediated mucocutaneous eruption characterized by target lesions with an acral predilection. The oral mucous membranes are commonly affected.**

**The use of the terms erythema multiforme minor and erythema multiforme major should be avoided.**

### EPIDEMIOLOGY

- Overall incidence is reportedly 1–6 per million
- Affects older children and young adults most commonly

### ETIOLOGY

- Erythema multiforme is a hypersensitivity reaction seen in response to a plethora of inciting agents including infectious agents, medications, vaccinations, inflammatory conditions, and environmental agents. It is believed to be a cell-mediated delayed-type hypersensitivity reaction (Table 6-2)
- Infectious agents, including numerous bacterial, viral, and fungal microorganisms, appear to be the most common inciting agents, although many cases have no clearly identifiable cause
- Recurrent erythema multiforme is strongly associated with herpes simplex virus (HSV) infection and may occur a few days to a few weeks following HSV infection or recurrence
- Drug-induced EM appears to be related to impaired metabolism of the causative drug, which results in the production of reactive and/or toxic drug metabolites that may serve as haptens

### DIFFERENTIAL DIAGNOSIS

- *Exanthematous erythematous macules and papules:* Viral exanthems, urticaria, urticarial vasculitis, secondary syphilis
- *Targetoid lesions:* Annular urticaria, fixed drug eruption, annular/figurate erythema
- *Mucositis:* Herpetic gingivostomatitis, aphthous stomatitis, pemphigus vulgaris

### CLINICAL MANIFESTATIONS

- *Primary lesions:* Classic target lesions present as erythematous papules that rapidly evolve over 1–2 days to manifest a central violaceous macule, which may blister, surrounded by an intermediate ring of pallor and a peripheral erythematous rim. Pruritus or a burning sensation may be reported. Target lesions favor extremities, including hands and feet
- *Köebner phenomenon:* Lesions may present at sites of recent trauma
- Target lesions typically present over several days, then remain fixed in location and morphology for at least 1 week, after which time they slowly resolve. May resolve with post-inflammatory hyperpigmentation
- *Mucositis:* Typically mild and limited to one mucous membrane (usually the oral mucosa); rarely involves conjunctival, urogenital mucosa
- Systemic symptoms are uncommon but may include low-grade fever, cough, and rhinorrhea

**TABLE 6-2** Evaluation and Management of Cutaneous Drug Hypersensitivity

| Primary Lesion | Clinical Features | Common Causes | Management |
|---|---|---|---|
| Urticaria | Evanescent, pruritic wheals lasting <24 hours; angioedema of hands, feet, face | Penicillin-based antibiotics | Discontinue drug; start antihistamines (consider combination of H1-antihistamine and H2-antihistamine) |
| Morbilliform eruptions | Symmetrical "measles-like" exanthem with erythematous macules and papules; may be pruritic | Antibiotics (e.g., penicillins and sulfonamides) | Discontinuation of drug advised although in some patients, reaction may resolve even if drug continued; antihistamines for pruritus; topical corticosteroids |
| Erythema multiforme | Target lesions (dusky center, pale edematous rim with erythematous border) lasting >24 hours; mild mucositis (one mucous membrane, usually oral); may be mildly pruritic | Usually occurs with infections (e.g., herpes simplex) rather than drugs | Self-limited; supportive care |
| Stevens–Johnson syndrome | Atypical target lesions; mucositis (2 or more mucous membranes) | Antibiotics (e.g., penicillins, sulfonamides); anticonvulsants (e.g., phenobarbital, phenytoin, carbamazepine); *M. pneumoniae* (may present with marked mucosal involvement with limited to no cutaneous involvement) | Prompt discontinuation of drug. Early initiation of systemic corticosteroids may be of benefit but use is controversial; severe cases may respond to IVIG; supportive care |

*(continued)*

**TABLE 6-2** Evaluation and Management of Cutaneous Drug Hypersensitivity (*continued*)

| Primary Lesion | Clinical Features | Common Causes | Management |
|---|---|---|---|
| Toxic epidermal necrolysis | Extensive areas of tender, erythematous skin associated with skin sloughing and denudation; mucositis often present; patients typically ill-appearing | Antibiotics (e.g., penicillins, sulfonamides); anticonvulsants (e.g., phenobarbital, phenytoin, carbamazepine, lamotrigine) | Prompt discontinuation of drug. Early initiation of systemic steroids may be of benefit but use is controversial; severe cases may be successfully treated with IVIG; supportive care; monitor for systemic complications |
| DRESS (drug reaction with eosinophilia and systemic signs), also known as drug-induced hypersensitivity syndrome | Exanthematous eruption associated with liver toxicity, fever, lymphadenopathy, eosinophilia, atypical lymphocytosis, although not all features may be present early in course | Aromatic anticonvulsants (e.g., phenytoin, phenobarbital, carbamazepine); sulfonamide antibiotics; minocycline | Discontinuation of drug; systemic corticosteroids; supportive care; monitor for systemic complications |

## DIAGNOSTICS

- Usually a clinical diagnosis though skin biopsy may help in atypical cases. Histology demonstrates a vacuolar interface dermatitis with vacuolar changes and dyskeratotic basal keratinocytes; a mild-to-moderate superficial perivascular lymphocytic infiltrate may be seen
- HSV PCR from an oropharyngeal specimen may be performed if there is clinical suspicion for HSV-associated EM

## MANAGEMENT

- EM is a self-limited phenomenon, often requiring only supportive care
- Bland emollients or topical antibiotics may be applied to eroded areas
- Patients with mucositis and poor oral intake may require intravenous rehydration or hyperalimentation
- Antihistamines (diphenhydramine, hydroxyzine, cetirizine) may treat associated pruritus
- In patients with HSV-associated EM, treatment with acyclovir may be indicated early in the course of the rash
- Ophthalmologic consultation is recommended for ocular involvement

## VASCULAR PHENOMENA

### COMPLICATED HEMANGIOMAS

**Hemangiomas of infancy are common vascular tumors that undergo a typical growth pattern of proliferation, stabilization (plateau), and gradual involution. Most hemangiomas require no therapy beyond active nonintervention and appropriate anticipatory guidance. Complications may arise with hemangiomas occurring near vital structures, in certain anatomic locations, or in patients with multiple hemangiomas** (Table 6-3).

## EPIDEMIOLOGY

- Occur in approximately 10% of infants
- More common in female infants, preterm infants, multiple gestations, and in association with chorionic villus sampling and amniocentesis
- Most complications arise during the proliferative phase, during the first 3–6 months of life

| TABLE 6-3 | Complications Related to Hemangiomas |
|---|---|
| **Predisposing Factor** | **Complication** |
| Periocular location | Amblyopia |
| Nasal tip, ear | Cosmetic disfigurement |
| Beard distribution | Airway involvement |
| Orolabial | Ulceration |
| Large facial, segmental distribution | PHACES syndrome |
| Large pelvic and/or buttocks, segmental distribution | PELVIS/SACRAL syndrome |
| Midline prevertebral location | Spinal dysraphism |
| Perineal or perianal site | Ulceration |
| Multiple ≥6 | Visceral hemangiomatosis |
| Large hemangiomas | Mild thrombocytopenia |
| | NOT Kasabach–Merritt phenomenon |

## ETIOLOGY

- Most cases are sporadic without clear genetic predisposing factors
- Hemangiomas of infancy share many similar cellular markers with placental tissue and may have a common precursor

## DIFFERENTIAL DIAGNOSIS

- *Vascular malformations:* Venous malformation, arteriovenous malformation, lymphatic malformation, capillary malformation
- Kaposiform hemangioendothelioma
- *Rapidly involuting congenital hemangioma (RICH):* A congenital hemangioma that involutes rapidly (during the first year) and may result in cutaneous atrophy
- *Non-involuting congenital hemangioma (NICH):* A congenital hemangioma with overlying telangiectasia that does not involute
- *Vascular tumor mimics:* Lipoblastoma, fibrosarcoma, or other soft-tissue sarcomas; these are often large, congenital lesions showing rapid growth, ulceration, and fixation to underlying tissue; dermoid cyst; myofibroma

## CLINICAL MANIFESTATIONS

- Hemangiomas are often not visible at birth and typically manifest within the first 2–8 weeks of life, often as faint areas of macular erythema that rapidly increase in size
- Superficial hemangiomas have a "strawberry" appearance. Deep hemangiomas may appear soft and bluish without much superficial change. Mixed hemangiomas may have features of both superficial and deep morphology
- Hemangiomas undergo proliferation and may grow rapidly during the first 6–9 months of life; they then plateau or stabilize until approximately 1 year of age. After 1 year of age, hemangiomas undergo slow, gradual involution over 5–8 years
- Most involute significantly, but residual telangiectasia or fibrofatty tissue may remain
- Complications prompting treatment may include rapidly growing periocular hemangiomas threatening vision, symptomatic airway hemangiomas, extensive ulcerated hemangiomas with secondary infection or sepsis, symptomatic visceral hemangiomatosis resulting in congestive heart failure, PHACES syndrome, and SACRAL/PELVIS syndrome
- *PHACES syndrome:* **P**osterior fossa abnormalities, large segmental facial **H**emangioma, cerebrovascular **A**rterial anomalies, **C**oarctation of the aorta, **E**ye abnormalities, and midline **S**ternal anomalies
- *PELVIS/SACRAL syndrome:* **P**erineal/buttock segmental hemangioma, **E**xternal genitalia anomalies, **L**ipomeningocele, **V**esicorenal anomalies, **I**mperforate anus, and **S**kin tags (perianal)

## DIAGNOSTICS

- MRI of the orbits or neck, respectively, may help delineate anatomic extent of orbital or airway hemangiomas
- MRI of the brain is recommended to evaluate for associated anomalies as seen in PHACES syndrome. MRA of head and neck is also important for delineating the cerebrovascular arterial anomalies of PHACES syndrome
- MRI of the lumbosacral spine and renal ultrasound are recommended to evaluate suspected cases of PELVIS/SACRAL syndrome
- Electrocardiogram (ECG) and echocardiography are recommended when PHACES is suspected
- Skin biopsy for atypical lesions may help confirm the diagnosis of a hemangioma and exclude a diagnosis of fibrosarcoma, other vascular tumor, or vascular malformation

## MANAGEMENT

- Consultation with Dermatology is recommended for complicated hemangiomas
- Consultation with other subspecialists, including Ophthalmology, Otolaryngology, Plastic Surgery, and Cardiology, as appropriate, should be considered when complications are present or suspected
- *The following are indications for systemic treatment:* Periocular hemangiomas threatening vision; symptomatic airway involvement; ulcerated hemangiomas unresponsive to conservative management; congestive heart failure due to coarctation of the aorta or hepatic hemangiomatosis; large segmental hemangiomas such as seen in PHACES syndrome and PELVIS/SACRAL syndrome; proliferating hemangiomas with risk for significant cosmetic disfigurement
- Consider propranolol therapy 2–3 mg/kg/day divided every 8–12 hours. Propranolol is now considered as first-line therapy. Monitor for propranolol-related side effects including bradycardia, hypotension, and hypoglycemia
- Consider systemic steroid therapy (2–3 mg/kg/day of prednisone or prednisolone) if propranolol is contraindicated or as adjunctive therapy if suboptimal response to propranolol. If initiating corticosteroids consider gastrointestinal prophylaxis with ranitidine or cimetidine
- Management of ulcerated hemangiomas should include evaluation for infection; soaks with tap water, saline, or acetic acid twice daily; topical antibiotic therapy (topical mupirocin or topical metronidazole); and daily to twice-daily dressing changes with non-adherent dressing (Telfa, petrolatum gauze, or Mepilex). Consider timolol 0.5% solution applied topically twice daily or pulsed dye laser therapy
- If response to propranolol and/or corticosteroids is suboptimal, consider surgical intervention or interventional radiologic embolization of selected hemangiomas
- Patients with six or more hemangiomas are at increased risk for visceral hemangiomatosis (although visceral hemangiomas may be seen in the absence of cutaneous hemangiomas); the liver is the most common extracutaneous site although almost any organ may be involved. Hepatomegaly, splenomegaly, congestive heart failure, and hypothyroidism are potential complications. Abdominal ultrasound or MRI, MRI of the brain, MRI of the chest, and/or MRI of the spine may help delineate extent of involvement where appropriate
- Uncomplicated hemangiomas with little to no risk for complications may be managed with active nonintervention or initiation of topical timolol 0.5% solution, as appropriate

## ATOPIC DERMATITIS

**A chronic, relapsing inflammatory skin disease characterized by pruritus, erythema, scaling, oozing, and crusting. Impaired skin barrier function and abnormalities in the immune response lead to a predilection for recurrent bacterial and/or viral skin infections. Associated with other atopic diseases: asthma, allergic rhinosinoconjunctivitis, food allergy, eosinophilic gastrointestinal disorders.**

- Infectious complications, namely bacterial superinfection with *Staphylococcus aureus* and eczema herpeticum, are associated with acute flares

### EPIDEMIOLOGY

- Atopic dermatitis affects approximately 20% of the pediatric population
- Age of onset is typically within the first 2 years of life, and while many children will "outgrow" their atopic dermatitis, a small but significant minority will develop persistent and/or progressively worsening disease

- Eczema herpeticum is seen in 10–20% of patients with atopic dermatitis and is associated with early onset atopic dermatitis and more severe disease
- Bacterial colonization and superinfection with *Staphylococcus aureus* is very common, and systemic infection such as osteomyelitis and septicemia may also occur. Staphylococcal superantigens promote inflammation
- Secondary bacterial infection with *Streptococcus pyogenes* may also be seen, either alone or in combination with *Staphylococcus aureus* infection
- In addition, patients with atopic dermatitis may develop other cutaneous infections, including widespread viral infection with molluscum contagiosum, coxsackievirus, vaccinia or papilloma virus, and fungal infections with dermatophyte molds or Pityrosporum

## ETIOLOGY

- Atopic dermatitis is a complex disease in which genetic and environmental factors contribute to chronic skin inflammation; allergic sensitization to food and environmental allergens and the production of specific IgE antibodies predicts more severe, persistent disease
- Impaired skin barrier function as a result of decreased expression of proteins involved in the formation of the cornified cell envelope, including filaggrin, and dysfunction of both innate and adaptive immunity lead to increased susceptibility to microbial colonization of the skin and cutaneous infections
- Bacterial superantigens and toxins contribute to inflammation and disease flares

## DIFFERENTIAL DIAGNOSIS

- Seborrheic dermatitis, scabies, contact dermatitis, nummular dermatitis, immunodeficiency

## CLINICAL MANIFESTATIONS

- Colonization of the skin in patients with atopic dermatitis is common and must be distinguished from infection
- Acute flares of atopic dermatitis manifest as erythematous, scaling patches and plaques, often with excoriations and crusting when secondary bacterial infection is present
- Systemic symptoms such as fever or malaise may be present but are often absent unless *Streptococcus pyogenes* infection or eczema herpeticum is present or a systemic infection has developed
- Complications of secondary bacterial infection include acute post-streptococcal glomerulonephritis
- Eczema herpeticum presents acutely with the development of grouped, monomorphous round "punched out" erosions; crusting may be present. If herpes keratoconjunctivitis is present there may be associated ocular pain, tearing, erythema, blurry vision, and/or photophobia. Secondary bacterial infection is common
- Other complications of eczema herpeticum include meningitis, encephalitis, and bacterial sepsis, which have the potential for significant morbidity and mortality

## DIAGNOSTICS

- Wound culture for bacterial Gram stain and culture may be performed from any crusted area
- HSV PCR should be performed if eczema herpeticum is suspected
- Enterovirus PCR can also be performed from vesicles or from stool if suspected coxsackievirus superinfection

## MANAGEMENT

- Initiate use of topical corticosteroids of appropriate potency based on the age of the patient, the site(s) involved, and the severity. In general, topical corticosteroids should not be withheld during the treatment of bacterial superinfection and eczema herpeticum
- In cases of suspected bacterial superinfection, parenteral antibiotics should be started empirically and adjusted based on culture results. Use of recent prior skin culture results may help guide antibiotic choice. In the absence of a history of methicillin-resistant *Staphylococcus aureus* infection, use of a first- or second-generation cephalosporin for 7–10 days is recommended. For the treatment of *Streptococcus pyogenes* use of either a first- or second-generation cephalosporin or amoxicillin/clavulanate for 10 days is recommended
- In the absence of clinical features suggestive of infection, mupirocin ointment or retapamulin ointment should be applied to eroded or crusted areas to minimize bacterial colonization
- In cases of suspected eczema herpeticum, acyclovir should be started empirically. In patients with periocular involvement, Ophthalmology consultation is recommended and use of antiviral ophthalmic medications such as 1% trifluridine or 3% vidarabine considered
- Wet wraps performed 1–2 times daily as helpful for acute flares. Apply topical corticosteroids to affected areas, followed by damp gauze or pajamas; should be left in place for at least 1–2 hours. Apply bland emollients after wet wraps are removed. Use of tubular gauze such as Tubifast® (Molnlycke) simplifies the regimen
- Atopic skin care consisting of frequent application of bland emollients, limiting bathing to less than 10 minutes, and use of a gentle non-soap cleanser is recommended
- Use of a sedating antihistamine such as diphenhydramine or hydroxyzine may be helpful in reducing pruritus and facilitating sleep at bedtime and naptime
- For patients with recurrent bacterial superinfection, initiation of bleach baths or use of an antibacterial skin cleanser such as chlorhexidine 2–3 times weekly in addition to use of mupirocin ointment to any eroded or crusted skin areas may be helpful
- For patients with recurrent eczema herpeticum, initiation of oral acyclovir at prophylactic dosing may be considered

# Emergency Medicine

*Margaret Samuels-Kalow, MD, MPhil*
*Angela Ellison, MD, MSc*

## INITIAL APPROACH TO THE SICK CHILD

Emergency evaluation differs from a standard inpatient history and physical in that less background information is available about the child and evaluation and intervention steps often need to happen at the same time. Figure 7-1 outlines some of the early steps in the evaluation of the sick child, as well as interventions to consider at each stage.

## AIRWAY AND CERVICAL SPINE STABILIZATION

- Open airway with head-tilt/jaw-thrust maneuver (use jaw thrust for trauma)
- Clear debris using large bore (e.g., Yankauer) suction catheter
- Cervical spine immobilization with collar

## BREATHING/VENTILATION

- Assess breath sounds, chest rise, and respiratory rate

## CIRCULATION

- Establish IV access within 90 seconds or three IV placement attempts then consider intraosseous access (if <8 years old) or central venous access
- Consider 20 mL/kg of lactated ringers or normal saline administered as fast as possible (typically over 5 minutes) if signs of severe dehydration or shock
- Consider chest compressions if cardiopulmonary arrest

## DISABILITY (RAPID NEUROLOGIC EVALUATION) AND DEXTROSE

- Assess mental status via Glasgow Coma Score or classify as AVPU: *Alert*, Responds to *Verbal* stimuli; Responds to *Painful* stimuli; or *Unresponsive*

## EXPOSURE/DECONTAMINATION

- Fully undress patient to evaluate for hidden injury
- Maintain normothermia to decrease metabolic needs

## OBTAIN BRIEF HISTORY

- The initial history is brief, and can be recalled by the AMPLE pneumonic (Allergies, Medications, Past medical history, Last meal, Events prior to presentation)

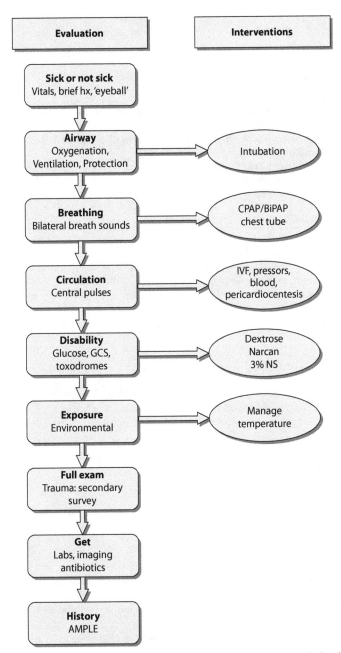

FIGURE 7-1 **Emergency evaluation and interventions.** Abbreviation: AMPLE: Allergies, Medications, Past medical history, Last meal, and Environments and events.

## BURNS

### DEFINITION

• Acute injury due to transfer of thermal energy

### EPIDEMIOLOGY

• Death from fire and burns is the third leading cause of unintentional death in children <14 years in the United States
• *Mechanisms changes with age:* Scalds, contact burns, fire, chemical, electrical radiation
  ✓ *Infants:* Bathing-related scalds, abuse
  ✓ *Toddlers:* Scalds by hot liquid spills
  ✓ *School-age:* Fire (playing with matches)
  ✓ *Adolescents:* Volatile agents and high-voltage electric lines

### PATHOPHYSIOLOGY

• *First-degree:* Redness and mild inflammatory response confined to epidermis; heals in 3–5 days without scarring
• *Second-degree:* Destruction of the epidermis and portion of the dermis; blistering; pink-red color; many weeks to heal and may need skin grafts
• *Third-degree or full-thickness:* Pale or charred color and leathery appearance; non-tender due to destruction of cutaneous nerves; most require skin grafting
• *Fourth-degree:* Full-thickness involving underlying fascia, muscle, or bone

### DIAGNOSIS

• Always evaluate airway patency/inhalational injury
  ✓ Look for soot in nares or throat
  ✓ Low threshold to intubate as airway edema will likely get worse
• Watch out for circumferential burns which may need fasciotomy
• Describe burn by degree (see Pathophysiology) + body surface area affected (Table 7-1)

### MANAGEMENT

• Analgesia
  ✓ IV opioids
    ▪ 1 mcg/kg fentanyl
    ▪ 0.1 mg/kg morphine (consider dosing in aliquots of 2 mg maximum)
  ✓ Consider covering or draping with clean sheet (decreased air exposure can decrease pain)
• Fluids
  ✓ Start with 20 cc/kg lactated ringer's bolus
  ✓ *Parkland fluid resuscitation formula:* 4 mL/kg/% body surface area
    ▪ Give half in the first 8 hours and half in the next 16 hours
    ▪ Parkland formula may underestimate evaporative loss and maintenance needs of young children
• Td (Tetanus vaccination) as needed (see below in lacerations)
• Admit or transfer to burn center
  ✓ Second degree >10% BSA or third degree burns
  ✓ Burns to hands, face, feet, genitalia, perineum
  ✓ Electrical/chemical/inhalational injury
  ✓ Circumferential burns

| TABLE 7-1 | Percent Body Surface Area by Age | | |
|---|---|---|---|
| | **Neonate (%)** | **Toddler (%)** | **Adolescent/Adult (%)** |
| Head | 18 | 15 | 9 |
| One arm | 8 | 8 | 9 |
| Front torso | 20 | 20 | 18 |
| Back | 20 | 20 | 18 |
| One leg | 13 | 15 | 18 |

✓ Previously ill children
✓ Significant associated injuries or suspected intentional injury
✓ Family inability to care for patient
- Wound care
  ✓ First and second degree burns that do not need surgical management/burn center transfer
    - Remove sloughing epidermis with gauze and sterile water
    - Do not rupture blisters
    - Cover with a topical antimicrobial agent
      ▷ Topical silver sulfadiazine cream (Silvadene)
      ▷ Bacitracin (if face or hands)
    - Daily wound dressing changes; consider pre-medication before wound care or dressing changes
    - Follow-up with burn center or with primary care provider within 2 days
- Consideration of carbon monoxide or cyanide poisoning
  ✓ Administer 100% $O_2$
  ✓ Hyperbaric oxygen if elevated CO level
    - Consult with poison control/hyperbaric oxygen service
    - *Carboxyhemoglobin levels:* Toxic=20–60%; potentially lethal=>60%
  ✓ Evaluate for neurologic symptoms or signs, signs of ischemia, or metabolic acidosis
  ✓ Cyanide antidotes if burning plastics/enclosed fire/elevated lactate
    - Cyanokit
    - Hydroxycobalamin

## CARDIAC ARREST

### DEFINITION

- Cardiopulmonary resuscitation: Attempt to restore vital functions after apparent death

### EPIDEMIOLOGY

- Ventricular fibrillation or pulseless ventricular tachycardia; only 5–15% of arrests
- 6% survival to discharge from out of hospital cardiac arrest
- 27% survival if in-hospital arrest

### PATHOPHYSIOLOGY

- Respiratory distress→respiratory failure (most common)
- Circulatory compromise→circulatory failure

## DIAGNOSIS

- Directed at identifying reversible causes
  - ✓ Hypovolemia
  - ✓ Hypoxia
  - ✓ Hydrogen (acidosis)
  - ✓ Hypoglycemia
  - ✓ Hypo- or Hyperthermia
  - ✓ Tension pneumothorax
  - ✓ Tamponade
  - ✓ Toxins
  - ✓ Thrombosis (pulmonary or cardiac)

## MANAGEMENT

- PALS algorithms (**see Appendix B**)
- *Key points:*
  - ✓ Compressions at a rate of 100 or greater
  - ✓ 4 cm depth in infants; 5 cm in children
  - ✓ Determine if rhythm shockable (defibrillate: 2 J/kg then 4 J/kg; maximum 10 J/kg or adult dose)
  - ✓ Change compressors every 2 minutes
  - ✓ Epinephrine every 3–5 minutes (0.01 mg/kg IV or IO)
- HR <60 bpm with poor perfusion is also an indication for CPR in infants and children

## DROWNING

### DEFINITION

- "Process of experiencing respiratory impairment from submersion/immersion in liquid" (WHO)
- Outcomes classified as either death, survival with morbidity, or survival with no morbidity

### EPIDEMIOLOGY

- Second leading cause of injury death in children from 1 to 14 years
- Most prevalent in toddlers/teenagers

### PATHOPHYSIOLOGY

- Hypoxemia (laryngospasm or aspiration) leads to loss of consciousness
- CNS damage begins after 4–6 minutes of hypoxemia
  - ✓ Fear/cold may trigger diving reflex which shunts blood to brain/heart
- Patients are at risk for sepsis due to breakdown of protective mucosal barriers

### DIAGNOSIS

- Usually from history
- Can have broad spectrum of clinical manifestations
- *CXR:* May reveal pulmonary edema with bilateral disseminated alveolar pattern or signs of aspiration
- Serum electrolytes
  - ✓ Seawater drowning can case intravascular volume depletion
  - ✓ Fresh water drowning may cause hyponatremia and hemolysis leading to hyperkalemia and hemoglobinuria
  - ✓ Diabetes insipidus or SIADH may occur as a result of CNS injury
  - ✓ Elevated creatinine occurs with hypoxic end organ injury
- *Arterial blood gas:* Hypoxemia and metabolic acidosis

- *ECG:* Risk for bradycardia, ventricular fibrillation, and ventricular tachycardia
- CNS imaging if CNS ischemia is suspected
- Hypoxic-ischemic injuries to kidney (elevated creatinine), liver (elevated hepatic transaminases), or pancreas (elevated amylase or lipase)

## MANAGEMENT

- Immediate management
  - ✓ Evaluate core temperature for evidence of hypothermia
  - ✓ Monitor for hypoglycemia
  - ✓ Consider continuous ECG monitoring
  - ✓ If gastrointestinal symptoms (e.g., bloody diarrhea), consider bowel rest, nasogastric suction, and gastric pH control
  - ✓ Prophylactic antibiotics are generally not recommended unless there is systemic toxicity, hemodynamic instability, or signs or symptoms of pneumonia; pipercillin-clavulanate provides broad empiric coverage if necessary
- No respiratory distress→observe for 6–12 hours
  - ✓ If normal vital signs, exam and CXR can discharge home
- If mild respiratory distress
  - ✓ *CXR:* Often normal or mild pulmonary edema
  - ✓ Monitor, supplemental oxygen as needed
  - ✓ Admit
- If significant respiratory distress
  - ✓ *CXR:* Usually abnormal
  - ✓ Monitor
  - ✓ Supplemental oxygen or intubation/PEEP as needed
  - ✓ Admit to intensive care unit

## HEAD INJURY

### DEFINITION

- *Mild:* Minimal force, no/brief LOC, normal vital signs, GCS 15
- *Moderate:* Moderate force, LOC 1–5 minutes, normal vital signs, GCS ≥13
- *Severe:* Significant force, LOC >5 minutes, abnormal vital signs, GCS ≤12

### EPIDEMIOLOGY

- Traumatic brain injury is a leading cause of death and disability in children
- However, CT scanning carries risk of radiation-induced malignancy

### PATHOPHYSIOLOGY

- *Primary brain injury:* Neuronal damage from traumatic injury
- *Secondary:* Injury to brain cells not injured by initial event
  - ✓ Hypoxia
  - ✓ Hypoperfusion
  - ✓ Metabolic derangements

### DIAGNOSIS

- For children <2 years
  - ✓ GCS =14; altered mental status; palpable skull fracture → CT
  - ✓ Occipital, parietal, temporal hematoma; LOC ≥5 seconds; severe mechanism of injury; not acting normally → CT versus ED observation
  - ✓ None of the above → CT not recommended

- Children age 2 years and older
  - ✓ GCS=14; altered mental status; signs of basilar skull fracture → CT
  - ✓ History of LOC; vomiting; severe mechanism of injury; severe headache → CT versus ED observation
  - ✓ None of the above → CT not recommended
- Severe mechanism of injury
  - ✓ Motor vehicle crash with ejection
  - ✓ Fall of >3 feet if <2 years old or 5 feet if ≥2 years old
  - ✓ Pedestrian or bicyclist without helmet struck by motorized vehicle
  - ✓ Head struck by high-impact object
- Signs of concussion
  - ✓ Headache, cognitive (e.g., feeling like in a fog), emotionally labile
  - ✓ Loss of consciousness or amnesia
  - ✓ Behavior changes such as irritability
  - ✓ Drowsiness or other sleep disturbances

## MANAGEMENT

- Elevated ICP
  - ✓ 3% NS preferred over mannitol
    - ▪ 0.1–1 mL/kg/h of 3% saline
    - ▪ 0.5–1 g/kg
  - ✓ Significant hyperventilation no longer recommended (keep $PCO_2$ 30–35)
  - ✓ Head of bed elevated 30 degrees
- Intracranial hemorrhage
  - ✓ Consider seizure prophylaxis, neurosurgical decompression
- Concussion management
  - ✓ "Brain rest" and slow return to activities
  - ✓ Follow-up exam with primary physician prior to return to play
  - ✓ Return to play guidelines available at www.cdc.gov/concussion/

## HYPOGLYCEMIA

### DEFINITION

- Infants <45 mg/dL
- Children/adolescents/adults <60 mg/dL

### EPIDEMIOLOGY

- Broad range of potential causes

### PATHOPHYSIOLOGY

- Can be primary problem or result of infection or other stress
- Differential diagnosis
  - ✓ *Ketotic:* Fasting, malabsorption, galactosemia, other inborn errors of metabolism
  - ✓ *Nonketotic:* Hyperinsulinism, adrenal insufficiency, inborn errors of metabolism
  - ✓ *Secondary causes:* Sepsis, ingestions, liver failure

### DIAGNOSIS

- Finger stick glucose
- Urine/serum ketones

| TABLE 7-2 | Rule of 50s for Glucose Correction (product of the mL/kg and the dextrose strength should equal "50") |
|---|---|
| **Age** | **Correction** |
| Infants | 5 mL/kg of D10 |
| Children | 2 mL/kg of D25 |
| Adolescents/adults | 1 mL/kg of D50 (maximum 1 ampule) |

## MANAGEMENT

- Dextrose 0.5–1.0 g/kg IV
- Need larger bore IV for higher dextrose concentrations
- Rules of 50s mnemonic for glucose correction (Table 7-2)

## HYPOTHERMIA

### DEFINITION

- Core temperature <35°C

### EPIDEMIOLOGY

- Neonates, physical disability, drug, or alcohol ingestion increase risk
- Mortality range 30–80%

### PATHOPHYSIOLOGY

- *Physiologic mechanisms to conserve heat:* Increased muscle tone, metabolism, shivering
- If fails, basal metabolic rate decreases, tissue hypoxia, and lactic acidosis
- Impaired mental status, cold-induced bronchorrhea→failure to protect airway
- *<28°C:* Increased myocardial irritability
- Can get cold-induced diuresis, DIC, decreased liver function as well

### DIAGNOSIS

- Consider with environmental exposures, trauma patients, infants, sepsis, burns
- Severe hypothermia mimics death; if hypothermia is the primary event, resuscitation should be attempted with rewarming

### MANAGEMENT

- ABCs; CPR if needed
- Correct electrolyte abnormalities
- Fluid replacement
- Warming method depends on core temperature
  - ✓ *32-35°C:* Passive rewarming, simple external rewarming
  - ✓ *<32°C:* Core rewarming, consideration of ECMO

## SEPSIS

### DEFINITION

- SIRS criteria
  - ✓ Fever
  - ✓ Leukocytosis

| TABLE 7-3 | Empiric Antibiotics in the Child with Suspected Sepsis |
|---|---|
| **Characteristics** | **Antibiotics to Consider** |
| Healthy, no central line | Vancomycin + ceftriaxone |
| Immunocompromised, recent hospitalization, chronic medical condition, central line | Vancomycin + cefepime |
| Oncology | Vancomycin + cefepime + gentamycin |
| Suspected intra-abdominal source | Piperacillin/Tazobactam or ceftriaxone plus metronidazole; consider addition of vancomycin |

✓ Tachycardia (outside of age-normal range)
✓ Tachypnea (outside of age-normal range)
- *Sepsis:* SIRS + infection
- *Severe sepsis:* Sepsis + organ dysfunction
- *Septic shock:* Cardiovascular dysfunction + sepsis
- Note that the definition includes infection + organ dysfunction; does not require hypotension because that can often be a late sign in children
- Many ill children will also present with bradycardia and/or hypothermia; consider treating as sepsis until proven otherwise

## EPIDEMIOLOGY

- Early recognition and treatment of septic shock improves outcomes
- Highest risk period is first month of life
- 10% mortality for severe sepsis

## PATHOPHYSIOLOGY

- Usually pathogenic bacteria entering into bloodstream
- Releasing toxic products (such as endotoxin) into circulation → cascade of inflammatory mediators

## DIAGNOSIS

- Flash (<1 second) or slow (>3 seconds) cap refill (measure on chest or forehead, i.e., centrally)
- Altered mental status
- Decreased or bounding pulses
- Heart rate, respiratory rate, temperature, or systolic blood pressure outside of age normal values and temperature correction
- Labs looking for end organ dysfunction, cultures looking for source

## MANAGEMENT

- IV fluids
  ✓ 20 cc/kg NS boluses repeat as needed
  ✓ After three boluses given, have vasopressors in the room
- Antibiotics (Table 7-3)
- Consider initiation of vasopressors
  ✓ Dopamine
  ✓ Epinephrine or norepinephrine

- Correct hypoglycemia, hypocalcemia
- Catecholamine resistant shock (preexisting adrenal insufficiency)
  ✓ Hydrocortisone

## TRAUMA

### DEFINITION

- *Multiple trauma:* Significant injury to two or more body areas

### EPIDEMIOLOGY

- Leading cause of death among patients <18 years
- Joint ED-surgical management of patients is the norm

### PATHOPHYSIOLOGY

- Predominant mechanism is blunt trauma
- Need to avoid triad of hypothermia, acidosis, coagulopathy

### DIAGNOSIS

- Goal is to identify life-threatening injuries (and address them)
- Primary survey
  ✓ *Airway:* Patent or not
  ✓ *Breathing:* Breath sounds present bilaterally (or not)
  ✓ *Circulation:* Central pulses
  ✓ *Disability:* GCS, moves all four extremities
  ✓ Exposure + roll (with cervical spine precautions)
- Secondary survey
  ✓ Protocolized detailed head-to-toe exam to find other injured areas
- Labs
  ✓ CBC, CMP (with LFTs), T+S, UA, consider toxicology screens
- Imaging
  ✓ Often chest and pelvic x-ray in trauma bay
  ✓ Increasing use of bedside ultrasound (FAST scan)
  ✓ Remainder determined by patient injuries

### MANAGEMENT

- Specific management for injuries identified
- Imaging of the cervical spine
  ✓ Limited data available for <8 year olds
  ✓ For >8 years of age, some suggest use of the NEXUS criteria for cervical spine imaging
    (if meet all 5 criteria below→clinically clear cervical spine without imaging)
    - No midline tenderness
    - Normal level of alertness
    - No evidence of intoxication
    - No abnormal neurologic findings
    - No painful distracting injuries

# Endocrinology

*Christine T. Ferrara, MD, PhD*
*Amanda M. Ackermann, MD, PhD*
*Andrew A. Palladino, MD*

## GLUCOSE HOMEOSTASIS

### DIABETES MELLITUS (DM)

A heterogeneous group of disorders characterized by fasting and postprandial hyperglycemia that affects 1.8 per 1000 children under 20 years of age.

#### EPIDEMIOLOGY

- *Type 1 DM*: Onset is usually in childhood, but may occur at any age; accounts for 85% of diabetes cases in children
- *Type 2 DM*: Most prevalent in obese children during puberty; more frequent in African Americans, Hispanics, Pacific Islanders, Asians, and Pima Indians; accounts for 12% of diabetes cases in children
- *Maturity Onset Diabetes of the Young (MODY)*: Autosomal dominant inheritance; onset usually between 9 and 25 years of age; accounts for 1–2% of diabetes cases in children
- *Neonatal Diabetes*: Spontaneous or inherited; onset usually <6 months of age; accounts for 1% of diabetes cases in children

#### ETIOLOGY

- *Type 1 DM*: Autoimmune-mediated destruction of β-cells in predisposed individuals (certain HLA haplotypes), trigger(s) unknown
- *Type 2 DM*: Progressive insulin secretory defect on the background of insulin resistance
- *MODY*: Genetic defects in enzymes or nuclear transcription factors involved in the regulation of insulin secretion or pancreatic islet development
- *Neonatal Diabetes*: Genetic defects in $K_{ATP}$ channel, insulin, or transcriptions factors involved in the regulation of insulin secretion or in pancreatic/islet development
- *Other*: Pancreatectomy, exocrine pancreatic disease (cystic fibrosis, hemochromatosis); other endocrinopathies (acromegaly, Cushing disease, pheochromocytoma); medications (glucocorticoids, β-blockers, phenytoin, asparaginase, cyclosporine, tacrolimus, vacor, pentamidine, diazoxide, nicotinic acid, thiazides); infections (cytomegalovirus, congenital rubella); genetic syndromes (Prader–Willi, Trisomy 21, Turner, Klinefelter)

#### PATHOPHYSIOLOGY

- Insulin deficiency and/or impaired insulin action results in the abnormal metabolism of carbohydrate, protein, and fat
- *Type 1 DM*: Destruction of pancreatic β-cells leads to absolute insulin deficiency. Lack of insulin results in excessive hepatic glucose production and impaired glucose utilization in muscle and fat leading to hyperglycemia, glycosuria, and an osmotic diuresis. Lipolysis and impaired lipid synthesis lead to elevated lipids, cholesterol, triglycerides, and free fatty acids, which are converted into ketones. Impaired utilization of glucose, excessive caloric and water losses in urine, and increasing catabolism all lead to weight loss
- *Type 2 DM*: Insulin resistance and inadequate insulin secretion result in relative insulin deficiency. Most patients have sufficient insulin to suppress lipolysis and ketogenesis

## CLINICAL MANIFESTATIONS

- *Type 1 DM*: Polyuria, polydipsia, polyphagia, weight loss, fatigue, weakness, blurred vision, increased risk of infection; frequently presents with ketosis with or without acidosis
- *Type 2 DM*: Overweight or obese; acanthosis nigricans (velvety hyperpigmented patches in skin folds of neck and axillae); may not present with polyuria, weight loss, ketosis, or diabetic ketoacidosis (DKA); may already have long-term complications at diagnosis

## DIAGNOSTICS

- *Criteria for Diagnosis of DM*: Random plasma glucose $\geq$200 mg/dL, or fasting plasma glucose $\geq$126 mg/dL, or hemoglobin A1c (HbA1c) $\geq$6.5% (all in the presence of symptoms of diabetes or on 2 separate days), or 2-hour plasma glucose $\geq$200 mg/dL during oral glucose tolerance test using a glucose load of 1.75 g/kg (up to 75 g)

### Other Tests

- Urinalysis for glucose
- HbA1c reflects average blood glucose over previous 3 months; used as an index of long-term glycemic control; $\geq$6% generally indicates diabetes; goals are: <8.5% if <6 years old, <8% if 6–12 years old, and <7.5% if >13 years old. HbA1c inaccurately reflects glycemia with certain anemias and hemoglobinopathies
- Fasting insulin and C-peptide is low in Type 1 DM, and can be low, normal, or elevated in Type 2 DM
- $\beta$-cell autoantibodies are positive in 90% of patients with Type 1 DM and are negative in most patients with Type 2 DM

## MANAGEMENT

Seek consultation from a pediatric endocrinologist. The following recommendations are general guidelines used at the authors' institution (also see DKA section).

### Long Term

- *Type 1 DM*: Daily requirement for exogenous insulin to match carbohydrate intake. Most effective insulin regimen is basal-bolus with long-acting basal insulin given once or twice daily, and short-acting bolus insulin given with meals to cover carbohydrates and to correct hyperglycemia
  - ✓ *For newly diagnosed patients, calculate the total daily dose (TDD) of insulin*: 0.4 units/kg/day for all patients, then, if necessary, adding 0.2 units/kg/day for (each) ketones, obesity, and/or puberty, which are all indicators of insulin resistance (up to 1 unit/kg/day); TDD for patients presenting in DKA should be 1 unit/kg/day
  - ✓ *Calculating basal-bolus doses*: Basal insulin dose is 50% of the TDD; carbohydrate ratio is 500/TDD (equals the grams of carbohydrate covered by 1 unit of fast acting insulin); and hyperglycemia correction factor is 1800/TDD (equals expected decrease in blood glucose (mg/dL) from 1 unit of fast acting insulin)
  - ✓ Insulin pumps deliver short-acting insulin as a continuous subcutaneous infusion plus boluses with meals (see Table 8.1)
  - ✓ An NPH/bolus or premixed insulin regimen can alternatively be used if patients are unable to adhere to basal-bolus regimen. NPH is given as 50% of the TDD with breakfast, 10% with dinner, and 10% at bedtime; 15% of the TDD is given as short-acting insulin with breakfast and another 15% with dinner
  - ✓ Premixed insulin is dosed as 70% of TDD with breakfast and 30% with dinner. Patients must adhere to a carbohydrate-restricted diet and eat at specified times. Table 8.1 outlines the pharmacokinetics of the various insulin analogs

| TABLE 8.1 | Subcutaneous Insulin Pharmacodynamics | | | |
|---|---|---|---|---|
| **Type** | **Name** | **Onset (hour)** | **Peak (hour)** | **Duration (hour)** |
| Rapid-acting[a] | Lispro (Humalog) | 0.25 | 0.75 | 3–5 |
| | Aspart (Novolog) | | | |
| | Glulisine (Apidra) | | | |
| Short-acting | Regular | 0.5 | 2–5 | 5–8 |
| Intermediate-acting | NPH | 2–4 | 6–9 | 10–12 |
| Long-acting[b] | Glargine (Lantus) | 6–10 | None | 12–24 |
| | Detemir (Levemir) | | | |
| Premixed | 70/30 | 70% NPH, 30% regular or rapid-acting | | |
| | 75/25 | 75% NPH, 25% regular or rapid-acting | | |

[a]Usually given just before meal. Also used in insulin pumps.
[b]No peak, relatively constant concentration.

- *Type 2 DM*: Weight management, increase daily physical activity, decrease sedentary activity, decrease caloric and fat intake; most require insulin or oral hypoglycemic
  - ✓ Metformin is the only oral hypoglycemic agent approved for use in children ≥10 years of age. Goal dose is 1000 mg twice daily; generally, the dose is titrated up over several weeks to avoid significant GI side effects
  - ✓ Insulin should be started in patients with HbA1c >8.5%. Generally, a premixed insulin regimen is used (70/30 or 75/25) with a TDD of 1 unit/kg/day
  - ✓ Normalize glucose, self-monitoring; normalize HgA1c, check every 3 months
- *Monitor for long-term complications:*
  - ✓ *Small vessels:* Retinopathy (regular ophthalmologic screening); nephropathy (regular screening for hypertension and microalbuminuria); peripheral neuropathy
  - ✓ *Large vessels:* Atherosclerosis (regular screening for hyperlipidemia)

## Management of Ketosis Without Acidosis (Sick-Day Rules)

- If ill or hyperglycemic (>240 mg/dL), check for presence of ketones (urine or blood)
- *Encourage oral hydration:* 1 oz/h/year of age (up to 16 oz); if glucose <200 mg/dL drink carbohydrate-containing fluids, if glucose 200–240 mg/dL, drink half carbohydrate-containing and half sugar-free fluids, if glucose >240 mg/dL drink sugar-free fluids
- If patient is not tolerating oral hydration, use IVF management similar to that used in DKA (see below)
- *Provide extra rapid-acting insulin (ketone dose):* 10% of TDD every 2 hours until ketosis resolves
- Monitor blood glucose and urine ketones every 2 hours
- Patients remaining on insulin pumps should use injections for ketone doses
- If ketones are not clearing, consider increasing ketone dose
- If signs and symptoms persist or worsen, consider DKA

## Management in Setting of Inter-current Illness Without Ketosis

- If vomiting, initiate intravenous fluids (IVFs) with dextrose, omit any standing short-acting insulin doses, give usual long-acting insulin dose, and use sliding scale insulin correction every 4 hours, or start insulin infusion (0.02–0.05 units/kg/h), and monitor serum electrolytes and glucose

- May require additional insulin (110–120% TDD) due to insulin resistance seen during illness
- *Hypoglycemic Reactions*: Due to honeymoon phase, insulin dose error, reduced oral intake, or increased activity, all patients on insulin should wear a medical alert bracelet
- Give simple carbohydrates (juice, sugar-containing soda, cake icing, or glucose tablets); recheck glucose 20 minutes later, repeat as necessary until >70 mg/dL
- If vomiting, combative, seizing, or losing consciousness, give glucagon 1 mg intramuscularly

## DIABETIC KETOACIDOSIS (DKA)

### PATHOPHYSIOLOGY

- Lack of insulin results in hyperglycemia, ketosis, and metabolic acidosis with compensatory respiratory alkalosis (rapid deep breathing, Kussmaul respirations). Ketones include acetoacetate, which is converted to acetone causing fruity breath. Glycosuria and ketonuria cause urinary water and electrolyte losses, resulting in dehydration. Dehydration, acidosis, and hyperosmolality all contribute to altered mental status. All of these symptoms can be exacerbated by concomitant trauma or infection

### DIAGNOSTICS

- *Criteria for Diagnosis of DKA*: Glucose >200 mg/dL, pH <7.3, and $HCO_3^-$ <15 mmol/L. There is associated glycosuria, ketonuria, and ketonemia

#### Other Tests

- Blood gas; electrolytes including sodium, potassium, bicarbonate, blood urea nitrogen (BUN), creatinine, glucose, calcium, magnesium, phosphorus; blood or urine ketones
- Leukocytosis and elevated serum amylase are common
- If sepsis is suspected, check blood and urine cultures

### MANAGEMENT

- Consult pediatric endocrinology. Consider admission to intensive care unit if pH <7.0, age <3 years, blood glucose >1000 mg/dL, or altered mental status. Replete intravascular volume first, then correct fluid deficit, electrolytes, and acid–base status
- *Fluids*: Replace fluid deficit, as well as ongoing maintenance requirements and ongoing losses from osmotic diuresis. Most patients are about 10–20% dehydrated. Within the first hour, give normal saline (0.9%, NS) bolus of 10–20 mL/kg; reassess and repeat as necessary to prevent hypovolemic shock. Give NS at 1–1.5 times maintenance rate for 24–48 hours
- *Electrolytes*: Monitor glucose every 1 hour, other electrolytes every 2–4 hours
  - ✓ Use a "2-bag system" to lower glucose by 50–100 mg/dL/h until in goal range 100–180 mg/dL. The 2-bag system consists of one bag of IV fluids with no dextrose and another with 10% dextrose, both with same saline and electrolyte concentrations. By varying the rate of fluid given with each bag, one can vary the dextrose infusion rate without changing electrolytes or total volume. When glucose is >300 mg/dL only use bag without dextrose unless glucose is decreasing too quickly; when glucose is 200–300 mg/dL, use each bag at half of total rate; when glucose is <200, only use bag containing 10% dextrose
  - ✓ *Potassium*: Patients are initially hyperkalemic due to acidosis; however, their total body [$K^+$] is low, and they become hypokalemic as acidosis improves and insulin and glucose are given. Potassium should be added to IV fluids when urinary output is confirmed and there is no significant hyperkalemia. Potassium should be provided as equal parts

potassium chloride and potassium phosphate: If serum [K$^+$] is <4, add 30 mEq/L KCl and 20.4 mM KPhos; if [K$^+$] is 4–5.4, add 20 mEq/L KCl and 13.6 mM KPhos. If [K$^+$] 5.5–6, add 10 mEq/L KCl and 6.8 mM KPhos. If [K$^+$] is >6.0, do not add potassium to fluids, and obtain ECG to evaluate for arrhythmia

✓ *Phosphorus:* Hyperosmolar diuresis results in phosphate loss, and hypophosphatemia can result in lactic acidosis. Phosphorus should be provided in IV fluids as KPhos

✓ *Sodium:* Hyperglycemia causes a pseudohyponatremia. Rapid changes in serum [Na$^+$] should be avoided. Corrected [Na$^+$] = serum [Na$^+$] + (1.6 × [(glucose − 100)/100])

✓ *Bicarbonate:* Metabolic acidosis corrects with insulin therapy, although it can be exacerbated by hyperchloremia in some patients treated with NS, in which case IV fluids should be changed to ½NS. Administration of bicarbonate should be avoided due to increased risk of cerebral edema

- *Insulin:* Regular insulin should be given via IV at 0.1 units/kg/h. When acidosis resolves (HCO$_3^-$ ≥15 mM or pH >7.3) and patient is tolerating oral intake, transition to subcutaneous insulin. The first dose of subcutaneous insulin should be given 15–60 minutes (15–30 minutes with rapid acting, 30–60 minutes with regular insulin) before stopping the intravenous infusion to allow sufficient time for absorption. It is optimal to convert to a subcutaneous regimen just before a meal. For patients in DKA, it is convenient, when possible, to give long-acting basal insulin while still on infusions in order to help with the transition to subcutaneous insulin. Follow sick day rules as described above until ketones are negative

- *Cerebral Edema:* Occurs in 1% of patients with DKA, but mortality rate is 40–90%. Risk factors include age <5 years, new diagnosis of diabetes, high serum osmolality, severe acidosis, and severe dehydration. Treatment includes reduced fluid rate, 3% saline 5–10 mL/kg over 30 minutes, or mannitol 10–20 g/m$^2$ (0.5–1 g/kg) IV every 2–4 hours

## HYPOGLYCEMIA

For diagnostic purposes, hypoglycemia is defined as plasma glucose <50 mg/dL. During treatment for hypoglycemia, plasma glucose of 70 mg/dL is the lowest acceptable level. Capillary and venous glucose levels are 10–15% lower than arterial glucose

### ETIOLOGY

- *Neonates:* Transient hypoglycemia on first day of life, sepsis, polycythemia, panhypopituitarism
- *Drugs:* Alcohol, salicylate, beta-blocker, calcium channel blocker
- *Ketotic Hypoglycemia:* A diagnosis of exclusion and of unknown etiology; normal fasting mechanisms, but impaired fasting tolerance. Occurs in setting of prolonged fasting or during times of illness. Typically presents at 1–5 years of age; usually resolves by 8–10 years of age
- *Hyperinsulinemia:* Infant of a diabetic mother; hyperinsulinism (congenital or perinatal stress-induced); Beckwith–Wiedemann syndrome; congenital disorders of glycosylation; factitious hyperinsulinism/surreptitious insulin administration (Münchausen syndrome, factitious disorder imposed by another [Münchausen by proxy syndrome]); sulfonylurea ingestion; insulinoma
- *Counter-regulatory Hormone Deficiency:* Growth hormone (GH) deficiency; primary or central adrenal insufficiency (see adrenal insufficiency)

#### Inborn Errors of Metabolism

- *Disorders of gluconeogenesis:* Glycogen storage disease (GSD) 1a (glucose-6-phosphatase deficiency); GSD 1b (glucose 6-phosphate transporter deficiency); fructose-1,6-diphosphatase deficiency; hereditary fructose intolerance, galactosemia

- *Disorders of glycogen storage:* GSD 0 (glycogen synthase deficiency); GSD 3 (debrancher enzyme deficiency); GSD 6 (glycogen phosphorylase deficiency); GSD 9 (phosphorylase kinase deficiency)
- Disorders of fatty acid oxidation and ketone utilization
- *Other:* Postprandial hypoglycemia (late-dumping syndrome), liver disease, Fanconi–Bickel syndrome, severe diarrhea, severe malnutrition, malabsorption, severe malaria, Jamaican vomiting sickness (from eating unripe ackee fruit of *Blighia spaida* tree), and Reye syndrome

## PATHOPHYSIOLOGY

- Normal fasting mechanisms include hepatic glycogenolysis, hepatic gluconeogenesis, adipose tissue lipolysis, fatty acid oxidation and ketogenesis, counter-regulatory hormone response, and insulin suppression. Defects in these metabolic pathways can result in hypoglycemia. Hyperinsulinism and defects in glycogenolysis result in hypoglycemia after a shorter fasting duration compared to defects in gluconeogenesis, hormone deficiencies, and fatty acid oxidation disorders

## CLINICAL MANIFESTATIONS

- Activation of the autonomic nervous system results in diaphoresis, shakiness, tachycardia, anxiety, weakness, hunger, nausea, and vomiting. Neuroglycopenia results in irritability, restlessness, headache, confusion, poor speech, poor concentration, altered level of consciousness, seizure, hypothermia, behavior and personality changes, and a sense of impending doom. Newborns may have no clinical symptoms or may exhibit cyanosis, apnea, respiratory distress, refusal to feed, or brief myoclonic jerks

## DIAGNOSTICS

- *Critical Laboratory Tests:* When blood glucose is below 50 mg/dL obtain the following labs: glucose, carbon dioxide, lactate, beta-hydroxybutyrate, free fatty acids, insulin, c-peptide, insulin-like growth factor binding protein-1, ammonia, acylcarnitine profile, free and total carnitine, GH, cortisol, urine organic acids, and urine ketones. A sulfonylurea panel should be sent if factitious hyperinsulinism is suspected
- *Glucagon Stimulation Test:* After obtaining the critical laboratory tests, when blood glucose is below 50 mg/dL, administer glucagon 1 mg IM/IV, measure glucose at 0, +10, +20, +30, and +40 minutes. If blood glucose does not rise by 20 mg/dL in 20 minutes, rescue patient with dextrose. A positive response is a rise in blood glucose by 30 mg/dL in 40 minutes

### Biochemical Profiles for the Different Causes of Hypoglycemia

- *Ketotic hypoglycemia:* Acidosis, elevated serum and urine ketones; undetectable insulin; negative glycemic response to glucagon
- *Hyperinsulinism:* Detectable insulin and/or c-peptide, low IGFBP-1; suppressed ketones, suppressed free fatty acids; positive glycemic response to glucagon; ammonia levels are elevated in hyperinsulinism/hyperammonemia (HI/HA) syndrome due to an activating mutation in glutamate dehydrogenase
- *GH deficiency:* Elevated ketones; GH <10 ng/mL; abnormal GH stimulation tests
- *ACTH/cortisol deficiency:* Elevated ketones; cortisol <18 μg/dL; abnormal stimulation tests (see Adrenal Insufficiency)
    - ✓ Abnormally low GH and cortisol values at the time of hypoglycemia have a 30% false-negative rate; the diagnosis of GH deficiency or adrenal insufficiency cannot be made based on these results alone

- *GSD 1a/b:* Lactic acidosis, hyperlipidemia, hyperuricemia, hypophosphatemia, anemia, microalbuminuria; abnormal fed glucagon stimulation test (increase in lactate with no rise in glucose); GSD 1b also has neutropenia
- *GSD 0, 3, 6, 9:* Elevated ketones, normal lactate in fasting hypoglycemic state
- *Fatty acid oxidation disorders:* Suppressed ketones, low serum carnitine, abnormal acylcarnitine profile and urine organic acids
- *Factitious hyperinsulinism due to surreptitious insulin administration:* Suppressed ketones, suppressed free fatty acids, increased insulin levels with inappropriately low c-peptide levels relative to the insulin level. With administration of sulfonylurea drugs, levels of both insulin and c-peptide will be elevated

## MANAGEMENT

- If awake and alert, give glucose orally. If impaired consciousness, give D10 or D20 2–4 mL/kg IV bolus then start continuous glucose (NG or IV). Consult a pediatric endocrinologist and/or metabolism specialist
- *Hyperinsulinism:* Glucagon 1 mg IM/IV in emergency; glucagon 1 mg/24 h continuous infusion as temporizing measure; diazoxide for perinatal stress induced hyperinsulinism and some forms of congenital hyperinsulinism (especially HI/HA syndrome); octreotide SQ/IV; pancreatectomy when warranted. Referral to a hyperinsulinism center
- *GSD:* Frequent or continuous feeds; uncooked cornstarch may extend feeding interval. For Type 1, avoid galactose, lactose, fructose, and sucrose
- *GH Deficiency:* Subcutaneous GH replacement in divided twice daily doses
- *ACTH/Cortisol Deficiency:* Glucocorticoid replacement (see Adrenal Insufficiency)
- *Postprandial Hypoglycemia (Late-Dumping Syndrome):* Acarbose (if >1 year of age); if acarbose fails, continuous feedings

## HYPOTHALAMIC-PITUITARY-ADRENAL (HPA) AXIS

### ADRENAL INSUFFICIENCY

Cortisol deficiency due to disorders of the hypothalamus, pituitary, or adrenal gland.

### ETIOLOGY

- *Primary Adrenal Insufficiency:* Autoimmune adrenalitis, autoimmune polyglandular syndromes; tuberculosis, HIV, fungal infections; Waterhouse–Friderichsen syndrome (adrenal hemorrhage associated with meningococcemia); adrenal thrombosis, infarction, or necrosis; congenital adrenal hyperplasia (CAH); adrenoleukodystrophy; triple A syndrome; primary xanthomatosis; hereditary resistance to adrenocorticotropic hormone (ACTH); metastatic carcinoma or lymphoma
- *Secondary Adrenal Insufficiency:* Long-term glucocorticoid therapy, pituitary or hypothalamic structural abnormalities, lesions or surgery, head trauma, cranial irradiation

### PATHOPHYSIOLOGY

- *Primary Adrenal Insufficiency:* Inability of the adrenal gland to produce cortisol results in elevated ACTH and melanocyte-stimulating hormone (MSH), resulting in hyperpigmentation. May also be associated with deficiency or excess of other adrenal hormones. Mineralocorticoid (aldosterone) deficiency causes hyponatremia, hyperkalemia, metabolic acidosis, dehydration, and hypotension. Androgen deficiency results in absent secondary sexual characteristics. In some forms of CAH, there are increased levels of mineralocorticoid and/or androgen due to specific enzymatic defects. Mineralocorticoid excess causes hypertension. Androgen excess results in virilization, accelerated growth, advanced bone age, increased muscle mass, acne, hirsutism, and deep voice

- *Secondary Adrenal Insufficiency*: Inability of the hypothalamus to secrete corticotropin-releasing hormone (CRH) or of the pituitary to secrete ACTH resulting in cortisol deficiency, but not mineralocorticoid deficiency

## CLINICAL MANIFESTATIONS

- Signs and symptoms of adrenal insufficiency include fatigue, apathy, listlessness, weakness, anorexia, weight loss, nausea, vomiting, diarrhea, abdominal pain, dizziness, orthostatic hypotension and tachycardia, salt craving, hyperpigmentation (in primary adrenal insufficiency), decreased axillary and pubic hair, and hypovolemia. Acute adrenal crisis is characterized by fever, confusion, hypotension, shock, and death; it is often precipitated by severe stress such as significant illness, surgery, or trauma

## DIAGNOSTICS

- *Initial Evaluation*: Hyponatremia, hyperkalemia, hypochloremia, metabolic acidosis, hypoglycemia, morning cortisol (6–8 am) <10 μg/dL or a cortisol level less than 18 μg/dL drawn in setting of acute illness
- *Diagnostic Confirmation*: Elevated ACTH, low cortisol in primary adrenal insufficiency
  ✓ *ACTH stimulation test*: ACTH normally stimulates adrenal gland production of cortisol >18 μg/dL. In primary adrenal insufficiency, there is minimal to no response to standard/high ACTH dose of 250 μg (125 μg for infants) given IV, with cortisol measured at 0, 30, 60 minutes. In secondary adrenal insufficiency, there may be some response until the adrenal glands atrophy over time, so a low ACTH dose (1 μg) is used
  ✓ *Metyrapone test*: Metyrapone inhibits 11β-hydroxylase, which converts 11-deoxycortisol to cortisol, and thereby inhibits cortisol production, leading to increased ACTH and 11-deoxycortisol if HPA axis is intact. Give metyrapone 30 mg/kg PO (maximum 3 g); measure ACTH, cortisol, and 11-deoxycortisol at 0, 120, 180, 240 minutes
  ✓ *CRH stimulation test*: Preferred test for secondary adrenal insufficiency when CRH is available. Give CRH 1 μg/kg IV and measure ACTH and cortisol at 15, 30, 60, and 90 minutes
  ✓ *Insulin-induced hypoglycemia*: Hypoglycemia stimulates counter-regulatory hormones including ACTH and cortisol. Used with caution due to risk of hypoglycemic seizure
- *Other Studies*: Plasma renin activity is elevated in patients with mineralocorticoid deficiency. Abdominal ultrasound or CT may visualize adrenal hypertrophy or hemorrhage in patients with primary adrenal insufficiency. Brain/pituitary MRI should be obtained in patients with secondary adrenal insufficiency to assess for CNS lesions

## MANAGEMENT

- If adrenal insufficiency is suspected, consult endocrinology. In patients that are stable, send studies to confirm diagnosis before starting steroids (cortisol level at a minimum). Steroid treatment will interfere with the interpretation of test results and will lead to secondary adrenal insufficiency if used long term. Patients with confirmed diagnosis should wear a medical alert bracelet
- *Fluids*: Correct hypovolemia with NS boluses as needed
- *Glucocorticoids*: Hydrocortisone is 4 times less potent than prednisone, 5 times less potent than methylprednisolone, and 25–30 times less potent than dexamethasone
  ✓ *Maintenance therapy*: Hydrocortisone 6–12 mg/m²/day PO divided TID
  ✓ *Stress dosing*: For physiologic stress (fever, vomiting, dental procedures) give hydrocortisone 50 mg/m²/day PO divided every 8 hours (or IV divided every 4 hours). For severe

stress (surgery, trauma, severe illness, or repeated emesis) give hydrocortisone 100 mg/m$^2$ IV/IM once followed by 100 mg/m$^2$/day IV divided every 4 hours

✓ *Secondary adrenal suppression:* Patients without previously diagnosed adrenal insufficiency who are treated with glucocorticoids for ≤10 days can discontinue treatment without weaning. Patients treated for >10–14 days may have HPA axis suppression, so glucocorticoids should be tapered and stress dose coverage should be provided until the HPA axis recovers (up to 12 months)

• *Mineralocorticoid Replacement*: Patients with primary adrenal insufficiency with mineralocorticoid deficiency and salt-wasting forms of CAH require fludrocortisone 0.05–0.2 mg PO daily. Some patients require NaCl replacement

## CONGENITAL ADRENAL HYPERPLASIA (CAH)

Autosomal recessive mutations of adrenal steroidogenesis enzymes result in altered glucocorticoid, mineralocorticoid, and androgen production.

### EPIDEMIOLOGY

• *21-hydroxylase deficiency:* Incidence is 1:14,000 (accounts for 90–95% of cases)
• *11β-hydroxylase deficiency:* Incidence is 1:100,000 (accounts for 5–8% of cases)
• *3β-HSD deficiency:* Accounts for <5% of cases
• *17α-hydroxylase/17,20-lyase deficiency:* Incidence is exceedingly rare (125 reported cases)
• *StAR deficiency (lipoid CAH):* Incidence is rare (<100 patients reported)

### PATHOPHYSIOLOGY

• Adrenal steroidogenic enzyme deficiency results in excess accumulation of precursors and deficiency of end products. Certain precursors and products have glucocorticoid (cortisol, corticosterone), mineralocorticoid (aldosterone, deoxycorticosterone [DOC]), and androgenic (dehydroepiandrosterone [DHEA], androstenedione, testosterone, dihydrotestosterone [DHT]) properties

### CLINICAL MANIFESTATIONS OF 21-HYDROXYLASE DEFICIENCY

• *Classic Salt-wasting CAH*: Absent 21-hydroxylase activity results in complete cortisol and aldosterone deficiency, causing salt-wasting crisis in first few days to weeks of life manifesting with lethargy, poor feeding, vomiting, diarrhea, dehydration, hyponatremia, hyperkalemia, metabolic acidosis, hypotension, shock, and death if untreated. Absence of cortisol feedback inhibition to pituitary leads to increased ACTH production, resulting in adrenal hyperplasia and accumulation of 17-hydroxyprogesterone [17OHP] and testosterone, resulting in virilization or ambiguous genitalia in females (clitoromegaly, fusion of labioscrotal folds), and accelerated skeletal maturation
• *Simple Virilizing CAH*: Decreased 21-hydroxylase activity results in virilization in females, premature puberty in males (pubic, axillary, and facial hair; phallic growth with prepubertal testes), and advanced bone age, there is no salt wasting
• *Nonclassical CAH*: Very mild 21-hydroxylase defects result in premature pubarche, mild to moderate hirsutism, menstrual irregularities, and decreased fertility in females

### DIAGNOSTICS

• *Newborn Screen*: Diagnosis of 21-hydroxylase deficiency is suggested by elevated 17OHP on newborn screen (standardized for term neonates ≥24 hours old; elevated in premature, severely ill, and normal newborns <24 hours old). Confirm 17OHP level with serum sample, do not repeat newborn screen. Diagnosis should be suspected in infants with a salt-wasting episode, ambiguous genitalia, or elevated ACTH with low cortisol

- *Diagnostic Confirmation*: Diagnosis is confirmed by standard/high-dose ACTH stimulation testing. Salt-wasting and simple virilizing CAH have significantly elevated basal and stimulated 17OHP levels with an inadequate rise in cortisol, while nonclassical CAH has normal to mildly elevated basal 17OHP level, moderately elevated stimulated 17OHP level, and a normal cortisol response
- *Other Studies*: Include electrolytes (hyponatremia, hyperkalemia in salt-wasting CAH), plasma renin activity (elevated in mineralocorticoid deficiency), measurement of baseline and ACTH-stimulated levels of other adrenal steroids (pregnenolone, progesterone, DOC, corticosterone, 18-hydroxycorticosterone, 17-hydroxypregnenolone, 11-deoxycortisol, DHEA, androstenedione, and testosterone) to distinguish from other forms of CAH and for adrenal or testicular tumors, and lastly, genetic analysis for the presumed defective enzyme

## MANAGEMENT

- If CAH is suspected, consult endocrinology (see Adrenal Insufficiency). Monitor BMP, 17OHP, androstenedione, testosterone, and plasma renin activity. If ambiguous genitalia is present, seek consultation from pediatric surgery/urology, genetics, and psychology

## CUSHING SYNDROME

Results from chronic glucocorticoid excess.

### ETIOLOGY

- *Iatrogenic*: Chronic exposure to supraphysiologic doses of glucocorticoids
- *Cushing Disease*: ACTH-secreting pituitary adenoma
- *Ectopic ACTH Syndrome*: ACTH-secreting non-pituitary tumor (neuroblastoma, pheochromocytoma, thymoma, bronchial and pancreatic carcinoma)
- *Adrenal Tumors*: Cortisol-secreting adrenal adenoma or carcinoma
- *Nodular Adrenal Hyperplasia*: Secretes both cortisol and adrenal androgens, can be associated with McCune–Albright syndrome or multiple endocrine neoplasia (MEN)

### EPIDEMIOLOGY

- Iatrogenic is the most common cause in pediatric patients. Cushing disease has a higher incidence in patients older than 7 years, whereas adrenal tumors have a higher incidence in patients younger than 7 years. Ectopic ACTH syndrome and nodular adrenal hyperplasia are rare in pediatric patients

### CLINICAL MANIFESTATIONS

- Weight gain, truncal obesity, round facies, buffalo hump, hypertension, fatigue, plethora, headache, acne, hirsutism, menstrual irregularities, precocious or delayed puberty, linear growth retardation, osteopenia, weakness, proximal muscle wasting, violaceous striae, easy bruising, psychological disturbances. Hyperpigmentation with excess ACTH

### DIAGNOSTICS

- *Cortisol*: 24-hour urinary free cortisol (>4 times the upper limit of normal), night-time salivary cortisol (>1 µg/dL at bedtime or >0.27 µg/dL at midnight), midnight plasma cortisol (>2 µg/dL)
- *Overnight Dexamethasone Suppression Test*: Dexamethasone 15 µg/kg (maximum 1 mg) PO at 10 pm, checking an 8 am plasma cortisol (>5 µg/dL is diagnostic, normal is suppression to <1.8 µg/dL)

- *Other Studies*: 8 am cortisol and ACTH, combination low-dose/high-dose dexamethasone suppression test, CRH stimulation test, inferior petrosal sinus sampling
- *Imaging*: Brain/pituitary MRI, adrenal CT or MRI, chest and/or abdomen CT or MRI

## MANAGEMENT

- Cushing disease is treated with a transsphenoidal adenomectomy. Ectopic ACTH syndrome requires surgical excision of the tumor; if tumor not resectable, consider treatment with steroidogenesis inhibitors or bilateral adrenalectomy. Adrenal tumors require unilateral adrenalectomy, whereas a bilateral adrenalectomy is indicated for nodular adrenal hyperplasia

## THYROID DISEASE

### CONGENITAL HYPOTHYROIDISM

Most common endocrine disorder (1:3500 newborns); leading cause of preventable mental retardation.

### PATHOPHYSIOLOGY

- *Thyroid Dysgenesis*: Defects in follicular cell differentiation or survival results in thyroid gland hypoplasia, complete agenesis, or ectopic location; accounts for approximately 85% of cases, and is more common in females
- *Thyroid Dyshormonogenesis*: Due to defects in thyroid hormone biosynthesis; accounts for approximately 15% of cases

### CLINICAL MANIFESTATIONS

- *Birth*: Mild phenotype, post maturity, macrosomia, large fontanels
- *Early Infancy*: Decreased tone, lethargy, poor feeding, prolonged jaundice, hoarse cry
- *Childhood*: Delayed linear growth, delayed bone age, fatigue, constipation, dry skin, cold intolerance, goiter in 2/3 of patients

### DIAGNOSTICS

- Thyroid-stimulating hormone (TSH) is elevated, and thyroxine (T4) is low. Newborn screening is now routine, preferably at 3–5 days of life; threshold TSH is 20–25 µIU/mL

### MANAGEMENT

- Levothyroxine 50 mcg/day in term normal size infants, or 10–15 µg/kg/day
- Monitor TSH (goal is lower end of normal) and T4 (goal is upper end of normal)

### CONGENITAL HYPERTHYROIDISM

Usually due to maternal Graves disease or maternal hypothyroidism.

### EPIDEMIOLOGY

- Occurs in <2% of infants of mothers with Graves disease, due to low incidence of thyrotoxicosis in pregnancy. Affects males and females equally

### PATHOPHYSIOLOGY

- Transplacental passage of maternal thyrotropin receptor stimulating antibodies (TRSAb or thyroid stimulating immunoglobulin [TSI]) leads to excessive thyroid hormone production in the offspring. Concomitant transplacental passage of thyrotropin receptor blocking antibodies (TRBAb) or thyrotropin binding inhibitory immunoglobulin (TBII) and/or antithyroid medications can affect the onset, severity, and course

## CLINICAL MANIFESTATIONS

- *Prenatal*: Fetal tachycardia, intrauterine growth retardation, goiter
- *Postnatal*: Irritability, hyperactivity, anxiety, flushing, diaphoresis, voracious appetite, decreased subcutaneous fat, goiter, exophthalmos; elevated temperature, blood pressure, heart rate, respiratory rate; advanced bone age, craniosynostosis, frontal bossing, triangular facies, microcephaly, ventriculomegaly. In severe cases, hepatosplenomegaly, jaundice, cardiac failure, and death may occur
- *Long-term Effects*: Growth retardation, intellectual and developmental impairments, secondary central hypothyroidism

## DIAGNOSTICS

- TRSAb/TSI, T4, and triiodothyronine (T3) are elevated; TSH is low

## MANAGEMENT

- Admission to a Neonatal/Newborn Intensive Care Unit with endocrinology consult
- Methimazole or propylthiouracil (PTU) (see Graves Disease for dosing)
- Saturated solution of potassium iodide (SSKI) 1 drop (48 mg iodide)/day or Lugol's solution (1–3 drops/day) accelerates decline in circulating thyroid hormone
- β-blockers if needed
- If decompensation, consider digoxin, IV fluids, corticosteroids
- Monitor TSH, T4, T3 frequently. Remission is gradual as maternal TRSAb/TSI is degraded; usually euthyroid by 3–4 months of age

## ACQUIRED HYPOTHYROIDISM

### EPIDEMIOLOGY

- Hashimoto thyroiditis or autoimmune hypothyroidism is the most common cause of acquired hypothyroidism in children. The presentation is variable as the child may be hypothyroid, euthyroid, or transiently hyperthyroid at diagnosis. Autoimmune hypothyroidism has a female predominance (2:1) and 40–50% of patients will have a positive family history of autoimmune thyroid disease. It can be associated with other autoimmune disorders, is also more common in patients with certain chromosomal disorders, such as Down syndrome and Turner syndrome

### PATHOPHYSIOLOGY

- Autoimmune hypothyroidism is the consequence of antibody-mediated (anti-thyroglobulin antibody, anti-thyroid peroxidase (TPO) antibody) destruction of thyroid tissue resulting in low thyroid hormone levels which feedback on the hypothalamus and pituitary resulting in increased levels of thyrotropin-releasing hormone (TRH) and TSH. TSH stimulation of the thyroid gland results in goiter

### CLINICAL MANIFESTATIONS

- Fatigue, cold-intolerance, constipation, non-tender goiter, bradycardia, delayed deep tendon reflexes, proximal muscle weakness, irregular menses, linear growth failure with preservation of normal weight gain

### DIAGNOSTICS

- Elevated TSH; low T4 and free T4; positive Tg and TPO antibodies. In subclinical primary hypothyroidism, there will be a mildly elevated TSH with normal T4 levels. In contrast, a child with central hypothyroidism can have a low, normal, or even elevated TSH combined with low T4 levels

## MANAGEMENT

- Thyroid hormone replacement with levothyroxine tablets, not suspension; dose recommendations based on age
  ✓ *0–3 months:* 10–15 mcg/kg/day
  ✓ *3–6 months:* 8–10 mcg/kg/day
  ✓ *6–12 months:* 6–8 mcg/kg/day
  ✓ *1–5 years:* 5–6 mcg/kg/day
  ✓ *6–12 years:* 4–5 mcg/kg/day
  ✓ *>12 years:* 2–3 mcg/kg/day
  ✓ *Adult:* 100–120 mcg/day (average adult dose)
- TSH, T4, and free T4 should be checked 6–8 weeks after initiating treatment or with dose adjustments. Thyroid function should be monitored every 6 months until growth is complete and then yearly. The goal of treatment is to keep the TSH and T4 within the normal range

## GRAVES DISEASE

### EPIDEMIOLOGY

- Graves disease is an autoimmune disease that affects the thyroid, orbital tissue, and skin. It is the most common cause of hyperthyroidism in children with peak incidence in adolescence. More common in females (5:1). Often associated with other autoimmune disorders and a family history of autoimmune thyroid disease

### PATHOPHYSIOLOGY

- TRSAb/TSI bind to and stimulate TSH receptors in the thyroid gland, resulting in excessive thyroid hormone synthesis and release, as well as follicular cell hyperplasia. These effects may be counterbalanced by TRBAb/TBII

### CLINICAL MANIFESTATIONS

- *Hyperthyroidism*: Goiter of varying degrees, exophthalmos, lid lag, tachycardia, palpitations, heat-intolerance, cardiomegaly, systolic hypertension, widened pulse pressure, tachypnea, diarrhea, tremors, proximal muscle weakness, tongue fasciculations, emotional lability, hyperactivity, difficulty concentrating, difficulty sleeping, increased appetite without change in weight or with weight loss, linear growth acceleration, bone maturation
- *Thyroid Storm*: Acute onset of hyperthermia and severe tachycardia that can progress rapidly to delirium, coma, and death

### DIAGNOSTICS

- Elevated T4, free T4, T3, free T3, thyroglobulin (Tg); low TSH; positive TRSAb/TSI; may have positive TPO or Tg antibodies and/or TRBAb/TBII

### MANAGEMENT

- *Medical Management*: Antithyroid/thionamide drugs: methimazole and PTU inhibit TPO, which oxidizes iodide into iodine so it can be incorporated into Tg tyrosine residue, thereby inhibiting thyroid hormone synthesis. PTU also inhibits 5'-deiodinase in peripheral tissues, thus inhibiting T4 to T3 conversion. Methimazole 0.25–1.0 mg/kg/day divided 1–3 times daily; PTU 5–10 mg/kg/day divided 2–3 times daily. Rare side effects of these medications include hypersensitivity reactions and agranulocytosis. PTU is only used second-line due to black box warning of liver dysfunction and death

- *β-blockers:* Propranolol is generally used for acute thyrotoxicosis. Atenolol is used for symptomatic relief of catecholamine-mediated symptoms until patient is euthyroid and is generally dosed 25–50 mg daily
- *Radioiodine (I-131) Thyroid Ablation*: Used as an alternative or adjuvant to medical or surgical therapy. Complete effects may not be seen for 2–3 months. Often results in hypothyroidism, necessitating lifelong thyroid hormone replacement. Failure rate of approximately 20%
- *Surgical Management (Total Thyroidectomy)*: Indicated if there is failure of medical therapy or concern for a coexisting carcinoma. Should be performed only after a euthyroid state has been achieved medically, in order to decrease surgical risks
- *Monitoring*: TSH, T4, T3, TRSAb/TSI (disappearance predicts remission)

## SALT AND WATER HOMEOSTASIS

### CEREBRAL SALT WASTING (CSW)

- CNS insult resulting in renal sodium loss, polyuria, hypovolemia, and hyponatremia

#### ETIOLOGY

- Head trauma, neurosurgery, CNS tumor, meningitis, hydrocephalus, stroke, brain death

#### PATHOPHYSIOLOGY

- Unclear but thought to be due to increased atrial or brain-derived natriuretic factor

#### CLINICAL MANIFESTATIONS

- Polyuria, hypovolemia, evidence of dehydration (tachycardia, poor skin turgor, dry mucous membranes), hypotension, nausea, vomiting, weakness, headache, lethargy, psychosis, coma, seizures. There is generally an associated CNS insult within past week

#### DIAGNOSTICS

- See Table 8.2. Other studies include atrial natriuretic peptide (high), anti-diuretic hormone (ADH) (normal or low), creatinine clearance (normal or low), body weight (stable or decreased)

| TABLE 8.2 | Distinguishing Features of SIADH and Cerebral Salt Wasting | |
| --- | --- | --- |
| **Feature** | **SIADH** | **CSW** |
| Serum sodium | Low | Low |
| Serum osmolality | Low | Low |
| Serum BUN and creatinine | Low | Normal or High |
| Serum aldosterone and renin | Low | Low |
| Serum uric acid | Low | Normal |
| Urine output | Low | High |
| Urine sodium[a] | High | High |
| Urine osmolality | High | High |
| Volume status | Euvolemic or Hypervolemic | Hypovolemic |
| Treatment | Fluid restriction | Volume repletion with salt and water |

[a]Generally higher in CSW compared to SIADH. Can be difficult to interpret in patients on sodium-containing IV fluids or supplements.

## MANAGEMENT

- The underlying disorder should be treated if possible. Intravascular volume should be repleted with NaCl and water (initially may need NaCl 150–450 mEq/L)
- *Acute Hyponatremia*: Correct rapidly with 3% saline 12 mL/kg over 1 hour to increase sodium by 10 mM
- *Chronic Hyponatremia*: Correct serum sodium by 0.5 mM/h or 12 mM/day; increased risk of central pontine myelinolysis if corrected too quickly
  ✓ Sodium deficit = total body water × wt in kg × (desired Na − patient Na)
- *Monitoring*: Vital signs, weight, intake/output, neuro exam, serum and urine electrolytes
- *Prognosis*: Generally resolves within 2–4 weeks; however, patients are at risk for developing other salt/water disorders (diabetes insipidus [DI], SIADH) and must be reevaluated with any change in clinical status

## SYNDROME OF INAPPROPRIATE ANTIDIURETIC HORMONE (SIADH)

Inappropriately elevated ADH (vasopressin) results in expanded intravascular volume and low serum osmolality.

### ETIOLOGY

- *CNS*: Meningitis, encephalitis, brain tumor, brain abscess, head trauma/surgery, hypoxic-ischemic encephalopathy, hydrocephalus, CNS leukemia, Guillain–Barré syndrome
- *Infections*: Pneumonia, HIV/AIDS, tuberculosis, herpes zoster, respiratory syncytial virus, aspergillosis, infantile botulism
- *Pulmonary*: Asthma, cystic fibrosis, empyema, bacterial pneumonia, abscess
- *Neoplasms*: Oat cell carcinoma; bronchial carcinoid; lymphoma; Ewing sarcoma; tumors of pancreas, duodenum, thymus, bladder, ureter
- *Drugs*: Carbamazepine, lamotrigine, chlorpropamide, vinblastine, vincristine, tricyclics
- *Other*: Post-ictal state, prolonged nausea, acute intermittent porphyria

### PATHOPHYSIOLOGY

- Inappropriate secretion of ADH by hypothalamus or ectopic secretion of ADH or ADH-like peptide stimulates renal collecting ducts to resorb water, leading to volume expansion, dilutional hyponatremia, and decreased serum osmolality. Hypo-osmolality may lead to cellular swelling and cerebral edema

### CLINICAL MANIFESTATIONS

- Anorexia, nausea, vomiting, headache, weakness, irritability, personality changes, change in mental status, seizures. In contrast to CSW, is clinically euvolemic

### DIAGNOSTICS

- See Table 8.2. Other studies include ADH (high), serum potassium (low), serum chloride (low), and body weight (stable or increased). Must rule out adrenal insufficiency, hypothyroidism, renal insufficiency, and diuretic use

### MANAGEMENT

- The underlying disorder should be treated if possible. Fluid restriction is key. Salt administration is not effective for long-term management
- *Symptomatic Hyponatremia (Seizures or Coma)*: Correct rapidly with 3% saline 1–2 mL/kg/h to increase sodium by 10 mM; increased risk of central pontine myelinolysis if chronic hyponatremia is corrected too quickly

- *Chronic Hyponatremia*: Correct serum sodium by 0.5 mM/h via fluid restriction (below)
- *Long-term Management*: Fluid restriction 1 L/m²/day (accounts for obligatory renal solute load of 500 mOsm/m²/day excreted in 500 mL/m²/day and insensible losses of 500 mL/m²/day). Demeclocycline induces nephrogenic DI and may be helpful in infants where fluid restriction will not supply enough calories for growth
- *Monitoring*: Vital signs, weight, intake/output, neurologic exam, serum and urine electrolytes and osmolality

## DIABETES INSIPIDUS (DI)

Inability to produce or respond to ADH/vasopressin results in excess urinary water loss.

### ETIOLOGY

#### Central DI

- CNS neoplasm, Sheehan syndrome (postpartum pituitary infarction), congenital midline brain lesions, head trauma (basal skull fracture, fracture of sella turcica), neurosurgery in region of hypothalamus or pituitary, intraventricular hemorrhage, brain death
- Genetic mutation in vasopressin gene (generally autosomal dominant, less commonly autosomal recessive)
- *Infiltrative disease*: Langerhans cell histiocytosis, lymphocytic hypophysitis, sarcoidosis
- *Infectious disease*: Viral encephalitis, bacterial meningitis (meningococcus, *Cryptococcus*, *Listeria*, toxoplasmosis), congenital cytomegalovirus, tuberculosis, histiocytosis, actinomycosis, Guillain–Barré syndrome
- Increased vasopressin metabolism by vasopressinase made by placenta
- DIDMOAD (diabetes insipidus, diabetes mellitus, optic atrophy, deafness)/Wolfram syndrome
- *Other*: Autoimmune diseases, drug-induced (ethanol, phenytoin, halothane), idiopathic

#### Nephrogenic DI

- *Drug-induced is most common*: Lithium, demeclocycline, foscarnet, clozapine, amphotericin, methicillin, rifampin
- X-linked mutation in vasopressin V2 receptor; accounts for 95% of congenital cases
- Autosomal recessive mutation in aquaporin 2
- *Other*: Ureteral obstruction, chronic pyelonephritis, polycystic kidney disease, medullary cystic disease, renal dysplasia, chronic renal failure, hypercalcemia, hypokalemia, sickle cell disease, Sjögren syndrome, sarcoidosis, amyloidosis, primary polydipsia (mild)

### CLINICAL MANIFESTATIONS

- Polyuria, nocturia, polydipsia (crave cold fluids, especially water), dehydration, hypernatremia, altered mental status, seizure, coma
- *Hypothalamic Tumors*: Growth failure, precocious puberty, cachexia or obesity, fever, sleep disturbance, behavioral changes, symptoms of increased intracranial pressure
- *Nephrogenic DI*: Infants exhibit irritability, poor feeding, water preference, vomiting, growth failure, and intermittent high fevers. Repeated episodes of dehydration result in brain damage, mental retardation, and abnormal behavior

### DIAGNOSTICS

- *Initial Studies*: Serum osmolality, urine osmolality, and serum sodium checked as an outpatient after the longest period of fasting the patient is known to safely tolerate. DI is unlikely if serum osmolality <270 mOsm/L or urine osmolality >600 mOsm/L. If patient does not meet criteria to rule-out or to diagnose DI (see criteria below), a water deprivation test is necessary

- *Water Deprivation Test*: Admit patient, withhold fluid, and frequently monitor serum sodium, serum osmolality, urine osmolality, urine output, urine sodium, vital signs, and body weight
  - ✓ Normal result is urine osmolality >1000 mOsm/L or >600 mOsm/L and stable
  - ✓ DI is diagnosed if serum osmolality >300 mOsm/L and urine osmolality <600 mOsm/L. Give vasopressin to determine whether central (urine output decreases and urine osmolality increases) or nephrogenic (no change in urine output or urine osmolality)
- *Other Studies*: Serum potassium, calcium, glucose, BUN; urine glucose and amino acids if suspect another cause for diuresis; MRI of pituitary and hypothalamus; ultrasound if suspect urinary tract anomaly; evaluation of anterior pituitary hormones; β-hCG for germinoma

## MANAGEMENT

### Initial Management:

- Correct free water deficit, replace ongoing excessive urinary water loss, replace vasopressin, monitor intake and output, check frequent serum sodium
- If hypotensive, give NS bolus. For fluid replacement, use enteral water when possible; otherwise, ½NS is generally preferred
  - ✓ Free water deficit = total body water × kg wt × [(current Na − desired Na)/desired Na]
  - ✓ Correct chronic hypernatremia slowly (0.5 mM/h) to avoid cerebral edema
  - ✓ Correct acute or symptomatic (seizure) hypernatremia rapidly (3–4 mM/h)
- Use IV vasopressin (Pitressin) to decrease urine output. Can be administered continuously and has a short half-life so can be titrated frequently

### Chronic Management:

- Patients with intact thirst mechanism should be allowed free access to fluids (especially in nephrogenic DI). Patients without intact thirst or unable to PO ad lib (infants, postoperative patients) should be given maintenance fluid requirement of 1 L/m²/day or 40 mL/m²/h with enteral formula or IV D5 ¼NS, in addition to replacing urine output >40 mL/m²/h or >3–5 mL/kg/h with enteral water or IV D5W
- In central DI, treatment is with desmopressin (DDAVP: a modified form of vasopressin with extended half-life) which can be administered by various routes (enteral, intranasal, subcutaneous)
- Infants with central DI can be managed with the addition of free water to formula or given between feedings; goal daily volume should be titrated in the inpatient setting and should be based on frequent serum sodium monitoring
- Patients that are without intact thirst and that are taking DDAVP should be given a fixed daily intake volume so as to avoid both hyponatremia and hypernatremia
- In nephrogenic DI, patients generally require 300–400 mL/kg/day of fluids. Salt and protein restriction minimizes renal solute load and thus diuresis; choosing foods with high ratio of calories to osmotic load in order to ensure adequate growth. Hydrochlorothiazide 1–3 mg/kg/day, alone or in combination with indomethacin (2 mg/kg/day) and/or amiloride are commonly used

## CALCIUM HOMEOSTASIS

### HYPOCALCEMIA

Serum calcium <7 mg/dL or ionized calcium <1.2 mM due to an imbalance of calcium absorption, excretion, or distribution that can be seen in a variety of disorders.

## ETIOLOGY

### Hypoparathyroidism:

- DiGeorge syndrome, surgery, hypomagnesemia, autoimmune polyglandular syndrome, parathyroid hormone (PTH) mutations, calcium sensing receptor (CaSR) activating mutations, pseudohypoparathyroidism
- *Nutritional*: Vitamin D deficiency, calcium deficiency, magnesium deficiency
- *Drugs*: Loop diuretics, chemotherapy (cisplatin, asparaginase), transfusions
- *Other*: Hyperphosphatemia, hypoalbuminemia, organic acidemias, renal insufficiency

## CLINICAL MANIFESTATIONS

- Constipation, paresthesia, Chvostek/Trousseau signs, prolonged QTc, arrhythmia, seizure

## DIAGNOSTICS

- Serum calcium, magnesium, phosphorous, BUN, creatinine, albumin, alkaline phosphatase; ionized calcium; PTH at time of hypocalcemia; 25-OH vitamin D, 1,25-(OH)$_2$ vitamin D; urine calcium, creatinine, phosphorous, magnesium, and ECG (see Table 8.3)

## MANAGEMENT

- *Acute Symptomatic Hypocalcemia*: Calcium gluconate 100 mg/kg IV bolus run over 4 hours or continuous IV calcium infusion with 1–3 mg/kg/h elemental calcium
- *Maintenance*: Oral calcium supplementation (50–75 mg/kg/day elemental calcium divided TID and administered with meals); depending on etiology, treatment may also include vitamin D, calcitriol, and/or magnesium
- *Monitoring*: Serum calcium, phosphorous, magnesium; urine calcium, creatinine, phosphorous; PTH; alkaline phosphatase; 25-OH vitamin D

| TABLE 8.3 | Laboratory Findings in Major Causes of Rickets | | | | | | | |
|---|---|---|---|---|---|---|---|---|
| Cause | Ca | Phos | PTH | 25-(OH)D | 1,25-(OH)$_2$D | Alk Phos | Urine Ca | Urine Phos |
| Calcium deficiency | ↓, NL | ↓ | ↑ | NL | ↑ | ↑ | ↓ | ↑ |
| Phosphorus deficiency | NL, ↑ | ↓ | NL, ↓ | NL | ↑ | ↑ | ↑ | ↓ |
| Vitamin D deficiency | ↓, NL | ↓ | ↑ | ↓ | ↓, NL, ↑ | ↑ | ↓ | ↑ |
| VDDR, type 1[a] | ↓, NL | ↓ | ↑ | NL | ↓ | ↑ | ↓ | ↑ |
| VDDR, type 2[b] | ↓, NL | ↓ | ↑ | NL | ↑ | ↑ | ↓ | ↑ |
| 25-hydroxylase deficiency | ↓, NL | ↓ | ↑ | ↓ | ↓ | ↑ | ↓ | ↑ |
| FHR | NL | ↓ | NL | NL | ↓, NL | ↑ | NL | ↓, NL |
| Chronic renal failure | ↓, NL | ↑ | ↑ | NL | ↓ | ↓ | ↓, NL | ↓ |

NL, normal; PTH, parathyroid hormone; VDDR, vitamin D-dependent rickets; FHR, familial hypophosphatemic rickets.
[a]Due to deficiency of 1-α hydroxylase. Also called pseudovitamin D deficient rickets.
[b]Due to mutation of the Vitamin D receptor. Also called vitamin D resistant rickets.

## HYPERCALCEMIA

- Total serum calcium $>11$ mg/dL or ionized calcium $>1.4$ mM

### ETIOLOGY

- *Transient Neonatal*: Maternal excess vitamin D intake, maternal hypocalcemia
- *Syndromes*: Williams syndrome, Bartter syndrome
- *Hyperparathyroidism*: Primary (isolated parathyroid adenoma, MEN syndrome, homozygous inactivating mutation of CaSR); secondary (renal failure, chronic hyperphosphatemia); ectopic PTH-related peptide (PTHrP) production
- *Drugs*: Thiazide diuretics, lithium, vitamin A, calcium, alkali, aminophylline
- *Other*: Excessive calcium or vitamin D intake, immobilization, neoplasia, inflammation, juvenile rheumatoid arthritis, and subcutaneous fat necrosis

### CLINICAL MANIFESTATIONS

- Constipation, abdominal pain, polyuria, renal stones, failure to thrive, confusion, bony pain, hypertension, shortened QTc, arrhythmia

### DIAGNOSTICS

- Serum calcium, magnesium, phosphorous, BUN, creatinine, albumin; ionized calcium; PTH at time of hypercalcemia, PTHrP; 25-OH vitamin D, 1,25-$(OH)_2$ vitamin D; urine calcium, creatinine, phosphorus, and ECG

### MANAGEMENT

- *Severe Symptomatic Hypercalcemia*: IV fluids, calcitonin, glucocorticoids, IV loop diuretics, bisphosphonates, surgery for parathyroid adenoma
- *Moderate Hypercalcemia and Maintenance*: Increased fluid intake, high sodium diet, limited calcium and vitamin D intake
- *Monitoring*: Serum calcium, phosphorous, magnesium; urine calcium, creatinine, phosphorous; PTH; 25-OH vitamin D

## RICKETS

- Decreased or defective bone matrix mineralization due to decreased phosphorus availability (a result of secondary hyperparathyroidism in response to hypocalcemia) for deposition of hydroxyapatite, usually involving the epiphysis and newly formed trabecular and cortical bone

### ETIOLOGY

- *Rickets of Prematurity*: 30% of affected infants have birth weight $<1000$ g

### Vitamin D Abnormalities

- *Nutritional deprivation*: Low vitamin D intake with decreased sunlight exposure; malabsorption (celiac disease, biliary obstruction, gastric resection, pancreatic-insufficient cystic fibrosis); medications that affect vitamin D metabolism (cholestyramine, phenytoin, phenobarbital)
- *Metabolic errors*: Defects in hepatic vitamin D metabolism (rare); renal 25-OH-vitamin D3-1-$\alpha$-hydroxylase deficiency (pseudovitamin D deficient rickets or vitamin D-dependent rickets [VDDR] type I); inactivating mutations in vitamin D receptor (vitamin D-resistant rickets or VDDR type 2); 25-hydroxylase deficiency

- *Calcium Deficiency*: Nutritional deprivation, hypercalciuria
- *Phosphorus Deficiency*: Nutritional deprivation: low birth weight infants, use of aluminum-containing antacids
  - ✓ *Familial hypophosphatemic rickets (FHR)*: Defective renal tubular phosphorus resorption; most common form of congenital rickets in North America; usually X-linked dominant, autosomal dominant and autosomal recessive forms are less common
  - ✓ *Kidney*: Chronic renal failure leading to renal osteodystrophy; renal tubular acidosis (primary, Fanconi syndrome, tyrosinemia type 1)
  - ✓ *Other*: Oncogenic hypophosphatemic osteomalacia, cadmium and lead excess
- *Drugs*: Aluminum, bisphosphonates, and fluoride inhibit bone mineralization
- *Hypophosphatasia*: Autosomal recessive mutations in the liver/bone/kidney alkaline phosphatase (ALPL) gene result in accumulation of pyrophosphate, which prevents formation of hydroxyapatite that is necessary for bone mineralization. Vitamin D supplementation should be avoided due to increased risk of secondary hypercalcemia

## CLINICAL MANIFESTATIONS

- Craniotabes, frontal bossing, cranial suture widening, metaphyseal flaring, rachitic rosary (enlargement of the costochondral junctions), Harrison grooves, genu varum (bow-leg) in early childhood, genu valgum (knock-knee) in late childhood, bone pain, seizures, dental abnormalities, muscle weakness, hypotonia, atelectasis, pneumonia, anemia

## DIAGNOSTICS

- Calcium, ionized calcium, phosphorus, magnesium, alkaline phosphatase, 25-OH vitamin D, 1,25-$(OH)_2$ vitamin D; urine calcium, creatinine, phosphorus; x-rays can show osteopenia with pseudofracture lines; widening, flaring, cupping, or fraying of long bone metaphyses; rachitic rosary; flaring of the lower thoracic rib cage; and rachitic changes of the iliac crest in adolescents (last to fuse). See Table 8.3

## MANAGEMENT

- *Vitamin D Deficiency*: Vitamin D2 (ergocalciferol) or D3 (cholecalciferol) 1000–5000 IU PO daily (depending on age); can also be given in larger once weekly doses; decrease to 400–1000 IU daily maintenance dose when vitamin D level and other biochemical markers have normalized; for severe vitamin D deficiency a loading dose of 25,000–50,000 IU is generally recommended
- *Elemental calcium*: 50–100 mg/kg/day prevents hypocalcemia secondary to bone matrix re-mineralization ("hungry bone" syndrome)
- *Calcitriol (1,25-$(OH)_2$ vitamin D)*: 20–100 ng/kg/day until serum calcium normalizes
- *VDDR Type 1*: Calcitriol 10–20 ng/kg/day
- *VDDR Type 2*: High doses of calcitriol (100–600 ng/kg/day) and elemental calcium (1–3 g/day) should be tried in all patients. Refractory patients may require continuous IV or intracaval elemental calcium 0.4–1.4 g/m²/day. After rickets has resolved, maintain with elemental calcium 3.5–9 g/m²/day
- *Familial Hypophosphatemic Rickets*: Elemental phosphorus 40–100 mg/kg/day divided 4–6 times/day (<3 g/day); calcitriol 20–60 ng/kg/day. If rickets recurs and/or nephrocalcinosis develops, consider adding amiloride and thiazide diuretic to increase renal tubular calcium absorption
- *Chronic Renal Disease, Renal Osteodystrophy*: Limit phosphorus intake <1200 mg/day
  - ✓ Oral elemental calcium 500–1000 mg/m²/day to decrease dietary phosphorus absorption
  - ✓ Calcitriol 10–50 ng/kg/day to maintain PTH within normal limits

✓ Occasionally requires parathyroidectomy if PTH levels do not normalize
✓ Avoid aluminum-containing medications
- *Calcium Deficiency*: Elemental calcium 25–100 mg/kg/day
- *Hypophosphatasia*: Currently no specific or effective therapy is available. Phosphate administration may heal rickets in mild cases. Vitamin D should be avoided
- *Monitoring*: Serum calcium, phosphorus, creatinine, alkaline phosphatase, PTH; urine calcium, creatinine; skeletal x-rays; renal ultrasound to evaluate for nephrocalcinosis

## TANNER STAGING

Used to define male and female pubertal development (see Table 8.4).

| TABLE 8.4 | Tanner Staging |

**Males**

| | Testes development | Penis development |
|---|---|---|
| I | Prepubertal (<4 mL) | Prepubertal |
| II | Testes enlarge (≥4 mL), scrotum reddens and changes texture | Slight enlargement |
| III | Larger | Longer |
| IV | Scrotum darkens | Larger, wider with development of glans |
| V | Adult size | Adult size |

**Female breast development**

| | |
|---|---|
| I | Prepubertal |
| II | Breast and papilla elevated as small mound with palpable subareolar bud, areolar diameter increased |
| III | Enlargement and elevation of whole breast |
| IV | Areola and papilla form secondary areolar mound |
| V | Mature breast contour, nipple projects |

**Male and female pubic hair development**

| | |
|---|---|
| I | None |
| II | Sparse, short, straight, at base of penis or medial border of labia |
| III | Darker, longer, coarser, and curlier, sparsely over pubic bones |
| IV | Coarse, curly, resembles adult hair; but spares thighs |
| V | Adult distribution with inverse triangle pattern and spread to medial thighs |

# 9 CHAPTER

# Fluids and Electrolytes

*Sonal Bhatnagar, MD*
*Lawrence Copelovitch, MD*

## BODY COMPOSITION

*Total body water (TBW):* 60% of total body weight (higher in newborns, up to 70%)
*Intracellular space:* Two-third of TBW or 40% of total body weight
*Extracellular space:* One-third of TBW or 20% of total body weight
*Interstitial space:* 75% of extracellular fluid (ECF)
*Vascular space or plasma:* 25% of ECF
*Predominant electrolytes in intracellular fluid compartment:* Potassium and magnesium
*Predominant electrolytes in ECF compartment:* Sodium, chloride, and bicarbonate

## FLUID THERAPY

### MAINTENANCE FLUID THERAPY

**Maintenance fluid requirements can be estimated by the Holliday–Segar method. Daily water requirements are calculated based on body weight and the assumption that each kilocalorie of energy metabolized results in the net consumption of 1 mL of water** (Table 9-1). **Water requirements form the basis for the estimated needs for sodium and potassium** (Table 9-2). **This method is not recommended for premature infants or term infants younger than 2 weeks of age.**

- While several studies argue strongly against the use of hypotonic maintenance fluids across all pediatric populations there are limitations in the evidence including the populations studied, study heterogeneity, and paucity of data on potential adverse events from an increased solute load
- It is equally likely that the administration of an inappropriately high **fluid administration rate** in the context of non-osmotic antidiuretic hormone release is responsible for most cases of iatrogenic hyponatremia
- The focus on tonicity of maintenance fluid without adequate study of the rate or volume clearly contributes to wide practice pattern variation
- Holliday–Segar maintenance therapy is based on the assumptions that all daily water losses occur as the result of either insensible or urine losses and that all homeostatic mechanisms are intact
- Insensible losses in the absence of conditions leading to increased fluid loss (e.g., fever, hyperventilation, prematurity and low birth weight, skin defects, burns) are usually 400–700 mL/m² body surface area (BSA) (higher in neonates, up to 1150 mL/m² BSA)

| TABLE 9-1 | Estimate of Maintenance Fluid Requirements Based on Body Weight | |
|---|---|---|
| | **Water Requirement** | |
| **Body Weight** | **Daily** | **Hourly** |
| 1st 10 kg | 100 mL/kg/day | 4 mL/kg/h |
| 2nd 10 kg | 50 mL/kg/day | 2 mL/kg/h |
| Weight above 20 kg | 20 mL/kg/day | 1 mL/kg/h |

| TABLE 9-2 | Basic Electrolyte Requirements |
|-----------|--------------------------------|
| **Electrolyte** | **Estimated Need (mEq/100 mL water)** |
| Sodium | 3 |
| Potassium | 2 |
| Chloride | 2 |

- Holliday–Segar method may not be appropriate in children with urine outputs that are abnormally high (e.g., adrenal failure, diuretic exposure) or low (e.g., hypovolemia, syndrome of inappropriate antidiuretic hormone (SIADH) secretion, renal failure, congestive heart failure, nephrotic syndrome, cirrhosis)
- Fever increases metabolic rate and therefore maintenance requirements go up (add about 10% for every °C increase > 38°C for the duration of the febrile episode)
- *Burns:* Increased needs based on percent body surface area involved
- *Oligoanuria/anuria in a euvolemic/hypervolemic child (e.g., established kidney injury):* Maintenance fluid should be prescribed by calculating insensible losses and replacing urine output every few hours
- Dextrose-containing intravenous fluids (IVFs) are used to supply a portion of the caloric needs, to prevent hypoglycemia and starvation ketosis
- Stock solutions containing 5% dextrose ($D_5$) are appropriate for most situations, but 10% dextrose ($D_{10}$) or higher is also available
- Dextrose concentrations above 12.5% are usually reserved for central catheters because the increased osmolality is irritating to peripheral veins

## MAINTENANCE ELECTROLYTE CALCULATION

- *Sodium Requirement:* 3 mEq/100 mL/day
- *Potassium Requirement:* 2 mEq/100 mL/day

**Sample Maintenance Fluid and Electrolyte Calculation:**
*Maintenance fluid, sodium, and potassium requirements for an otherwise healthy 37-kg child:*

**Water Requirement:**

| | |
|---|---|
| First 10 kg, give 100 mL/kg/day: | 10 kg × 100 mL/kg/day = 1000 mL/day |
| Second 10 kg, give 50 mL/kg/day: | 10 kg × 50 mL/kg/day = 500 mL/day |
| >20 kg give, 20 mL/kg/day: | 17 kg × 20 mL/kg/day = 340 mL/day |
| Total: | 37 kg      1840 mL/day |

OR

| | |
|---|---|
| First 10 kg, give 4 mL/kg/h: | 10 kg × 4 mL/kg/h = 40 mL/h |
| Second 10 kg, give 2 mL/kg/h: | 10 kg × 2 mL/kg/h = 20 mL/h |
| >20 kg give, 1 mL/kg/h: | 17 kg × 1 mL/kg/h = 17 mL/h |
| Total: | 37 kg      77 mL/h |

**Sodium Requirement:**

3 mEq/100 mL/day × 1840 mL/day = 55 mEq/day

$$\frac{55\,mEq\,/\,day}{1840\,mL\,/\,day} = \frac{Na^+}{1000\,mL}$$

$$Na^+ = 30\,mEq\,/\,L$$

| TABLE 9-3 | Terminology and Conversions for Stock Intravenous Solutions | | |
|---|---|---|---|
| **Stock Solution** | **Common Terminology** | **Dextrose Content (g/dL)** | **Sodium Chloride Content (mEq/L)** |
| Dextrose 5% in water | $D_5W$ | 5 | 0 |
| Dextrose 10% in water | $D_{10}W$ | 10 | 0 |
| Dextrose 5% in 0.9% NaCl | $D_5/NSS$ | 5 | 154 |
| Dextrose 5% in 0.45% NaCl | $D_5/\frac{1}{2}NSS$ | 5 | 77 |
| Dextrose 5% in 0.22% saline | D5/¼NSS | 5 | 34 |
| Dextrose 5% in 0.22% | D5/¼NSS | 5 | 34 |
| NaCl with 20 mEq KCl/L | +20 mEq KCl/L | | |
| 3% saline | "Hypertonic" saline | 0 | 513 |

NSS, 1 normal saline solution.

- *Note*: Normal saline solution (NSS) contains 0.9% NaCl or 154 mEq/L. In this case, a stock solution containing 0.22% NaCl (1/4 NSS) would provide 34 mEq NaCl/L

**Potassium Requirement:**

   2 mEq/100 mL/day × 1840 mL/day = 37 mEq/day

$$\frac{37\,mEq\,/\,day}{1840\,mL\,/\,day} = \frac{K^+}{1000\,mL}$$

$$K^+ = 20\,mEq\,/\,L$$

- The addition of 20 mEq/L of KCl would provide the approximate needs for potassium

**Therefore, an order for routine maintenance fluids for this child would be:**

   $D_5$/0.2% NaCl with 20 mEq KCl/L to run at 77 mL/h.

- It can also be written as: $D_5$/1/4 NSS + 20 mEq KCl/L @ 77 mL/h

   **Standard (Stock) Solutions for Routine Maintenance Intravenous Fluids** (Table 9-3)

   $D_5$/0.2% NS with 20 mEq KCl/L is a good choice for maintenance fluid for most routine situations. Some other helpful guidelines:

- KCl is often withheld from the IVFs until after the child's first void
- $D_{10}$ is often substituted for $D_5$ in premature infants and neonates due to their increased glucose requirements and diminished glycogen stores
- Some clinicians routinely use $D_5$/0.45% NaCl for children that weigh more than 20 kg. The increased sodium concentration is not usually problematic, but exceeds the calculated daily sodium requirement using the Holliday–Segar method
- KCl concentration in the IV solution is often reduced to 10 mEq/L to reduce irritation to the peripheral vein. This may be appropriate if additional (e.g., enteral) intake is occurring, or if it is anticipated that IV fluids alone will be used for only a limited time
- Common stock IVFs are listed in Table 9-3

## REPLACEMENT FLUID THERAPY

**Replacement therapy corrects preexisting deficits (dehydration) and ongoing losses.**

## DEHYDRATION

Consider both the extent of the dehydration and the overall balance of water and sodium that is created.

- *If pre-illness weight is available, then calculate percent dehydration:*

  % dehydration = ((Pre-illness weight − Current weight)/Pre-illness weight) × 100

- *If pre-illness weight is not available, percent dehydration can be clinically assessed:*
  - ✓ *Mild Dehydration (up to 3% in older children, 5% in infants):* Thirst, normal exam, reduced urine output
  - ✓ *Moderate Dehydration (3–6% in older children, 5–10% in infants):* Tachycardia, dry mucosa, sunken eyes, delayed capillary refill, irritable, oliguria
  - ✓ *Severe Dehydration (>6% in older children, >10% in infants):* Thready pulses, low blood pressure, anuria, cold and mottled, lethargy
- In acute dehydration (<72 hours), mainly ECF (80% of total losses) is lost. In prolonged dehydration, fluid loss is more evenly lost from both extracellular (60%) and intracellular (40%) compartments
- *Laboratory findings in dehydration:*
  - ✓ Elevation of serum creatinine and urea
  - ✓ Alteration of serum sodium, potassium, and bicarbonate
  - ✓ Increase in urine-specific gravity (except with impaired renal concentration)
  - ✓ Elevation of blood cell counts (hemoconcentration)
- *Type of dehydration*
  - ✓ *Isonatremic (serum $Na^+$ 135–145 mEq/L):* Loss of $Na^+$ and water in a balance that does not exceed the body's ability to maintain isonatremia
  - ✓ *Hyponatremic (serum $Na^+$ < 135 mEq/L):* Retention or replacement of free water in the face of $Na^+$ salt and water losses
  - ✓ *Hypernatremic (serum $Na^+$ > 145 mEq/L):* Loss of free water in excess of $Na^+$-containing fluid

## ONGOING LOSSES

- The gastrointestinal tract is a common source of ongoing losses from illness, or postoperative drainage. These ongoing losses are replaced with parenteral fluids, in volumes equivalent to the losses at a frequency that will avoid significant depletions (e.g., every 1–8 hours)
- The replacement fluid should contain electrolytes in concentrations that approximate the lost fluid. Some recommendations are listed in Table 9-4

## ORAL REHYDRATION

- Consider oral rehydration if patient is hemodynamically stable and if there is no impairment of swallowing function
- Oral rehydration solutions (ORS) are best, with concentrations of electrolytes and carbohydrates that approximate the World Health Organization/UNICEF ORS product

| TABLE 9-4 | Replacement of Ongoing Fluid Losses |
|---|---|
| **Source** | **Replacement (1 mL:1 mL)** |
| Gastric secretions | 0.45% NSS + 10 mEq KCl/L |
| Diarrhea | 0.2% NSS + 25 mEq KCl/L + 20 mEq $NaHCO_3$/L |
| Small intestine | 0.45% NSS + 20 mEq KCl/L + 20 mEq $NaHCO_3$/L |

• Small volumes (e.g., 5–10 mL) frequently (e.g., every 5–10 minutes) are initiated, and increased slowly as tolerated

## PARENTERAL REHYDRATION

*Phase I: Initial Stabilization*
• Administer 20 mL/kg IVF bolus (NSS or lactated Ringer's) and repeat as needed. This will restore intravascular volume and stabilize hemodynamics

*Phase II: After Initial Stabilization*
• IVF choice is dependent on nature/tonicity of dehydration (see below) and the degree of fluid deficit. Increased maintenance requirements (e.g., fever) may warrant further increases in the IVF rate
• Significant ongoing losses (e.g., continued vomiting and/or diarrhea) will require additional fluid replacement
• *Modifications to the rate and nature of the IVF should be guided by:*
   ✓ *Urine output:* goal = 1–2 mL/kg/h
   ✓ Weight, vital signs, clinical appearance
   ✓ *Repeat serum electrolytes:* If needed

*Phase III: Resolution*
• Trials of oral/gastric feeds usually begin with clear liquids if vomiting is present
• If vomiting is resolved, or not a factor, prompt advancement to regular diet is encouraged (including breast milk or infant formula)
• Avoid foods high in simple sugars (e.g., juices, sodas) that can worsen or prolong diarrheal symptoms
• Wean IVF rate or hold IVF for short periods to encourage oral intake

## ISONATREMIC DEHYDRATION

• Fluid lost has sodium concentration similar to blood
• Although the entire fluid deficit must be corrected sodium repletion should only be considered for fluid lost from the ECF (intracellular fluid sodium concentration is negligible)
• In acute dehydration (illness <72 hours) 80% of the fluid lost is from the ECF, in chronic dehydration (illness >72 hours) 60% of the fluid lost is from the ECF
• Don't forget that maintenance fluid should also be included in total fluid calculations
• **In general the ideal IVF solution in isonatremic dehydration will usually approximate $D_5/0.45\%$ NaCl**
• Some clinicians prefer to use $D_5/0.9\%$ NaCl in this circumstance because of the risk of hyponatremia in a subset of patients with high circulating antidiuretic hormone levels. This approach must be used cautiously in patients with acute kidney injury/oligoanuria

   Example:
   *One-year-old with 10% dehydration, with current weight 9 kg, presents with 5 days of diarrhea. Serum sodium concentration is 140 mEq/L.*
   Pre-illness weight: (Current weight (kg) × 100)/100 − % dehydration
      = (9 × 100)/100 − 10 = 900/90 = 10 kg
   Calculation of fluid deficit:
   Fluid deficit = Pre-illness weight (kg) − Current weight (kg)
   10 kg − 9 kg = 1 kg or 1 L
   Calculation of sodium deficit from ECF losses:

• Sodium deficit = Fluid deficit (L) × Percentage of fluid loss from ECF × Average ECF sodium concentration (145 mEq/L)
• Sodium deficit = 1 L × 0.6 × 145 mEq/L = 87 mEq

Calculation of maintenance fluid and sodium requirements:

- *Fluid:* $10\,kg \times 100\,mL/kg = 1000\,mL$
- *Sodium:* $1000\,mL \times 3\,mEq/100\,mL = 30\,mEq$

Total fluid and sodium requirement:

- *Fluid:* Deficit + Maintenance = $1000\,mL + 1000\,mL = 2000\,mL$
- *Sodium:* Deficit + Maintenance = $87\,mEq + 30\,mEq = 117\,mEq$

**Optimal fluid: Fluid containing 117 mEq Na/2000 mL = 58.5 mEq/L**
**Available fluid:** $D_5/0.45\%$ NaCl ($77\,mEq/L$) at a rate of $83\,mL/h$ ($2000\,mL/24\,h$)

## HYPONATREMIC DEHYDRATION

- Sodium deficit in excess of water deficit
- Start calculations as if the patient had isonatremic dehydration and then calculate the additional sodium deficit
- Sodium is freely distributed throughout the TBW (60% of the patient weight) and therefore the volume (factor) of distribution of sodium is 0.6 of the total body weight
- **In general the ideal IVF solution in hyponatremic dehydration will usually range between $D_5/0.45\%$ and $D_5/0.9\%$ NaCl**

Example:
*One-year-old with 10% dehydration, with current weight 9 kg, presents with 2 days of diarrhea. Serum sodium concentration is 123 mEq/L.*
Pre-illness weight: (Current weight × 100)/100 − % dehydration
$= (9 \times 100)/100 - 10 = 900/90 = 10\,kg$
Calculation of fluid deficit:
Fluid deficit = Pre-illness weight (kg) − Current weight (kg)
$10\,kg - 9\,kg = 1\,kg$ or $1\,L$
Calculation of sodium deficit from ECF losses (identical to isonatremic example):

- Sodium deficit = Fluid deficit (L) × Percentage of fluid loss from ECF × Average ECF sodium concentration ($145\,mEq/L$)
- Sodium deficit = $1\,L \times 0.8 \times 145\,mEq/L = 116\,mEq$

Calculation of additional sodium deficit (specific to the hyponatremic patient):
(sodium (mEq) desired − sodium (mEq) actual) × volume (L) of distribution

- *Example:* Sodium = $123\,mEq/L$, weight = $10\,kg$, assumed volume of distribution of 0.6;
Sodium deficit = $(135 - 123) \times 0.6 \times 10 = 72\,mEq$ sodium
Calculation of maintenance fluid and sodium requirements:

- *Fluid:* $10\,kg \times 100\,mL/kg = 1000\,mL$
- *Sodium:* $1000\,mL \times 3\,mEq/100\,mL = 30\,mEq$

Total fluid and sodium requirement:

- *Fluid:* Deficit + Maintenance = $1000 + 1000 = 2000\,mL$
- *Sodium:* Deficits + Maintenance = $116\,mEq + 72\,mEq + 30\,mEq = 218\,mEq$

**Optimal fluid: Fluid containing 218 mEq Na/2000 mL = 109 mEq/L**
**Available fluid:** May alternate between $D_5/0.45\%$ ($77\,mEq/L$) NaCl and D5/0.9% ($154\,mEq/L$) NaCl every 12 hours at a rate of $83\,mL/h$ ($2000\,mL/24\,h$)

## HYPERNATREMIC DEHYDRATION

- Free water deficit (FWD) in excess of salt deficit
- *Assumption:* FWD = $0.6 \times$ weight (kg) $\times$ [(actual sodium/140) − 1]

- **In general the ideal IVF solution in hypernatremic dehydration will usually range between $D_5W$ and $D_5/0.2\%$ NaCl**

  Example:
  *One-year-old with 10% dehydration, with current weight 9 kg, presents with 5 days of diarrhea. Serum sodium concentration is 155 mEq/L.*
  Pre-illness weight: (Current weight × 100)/100 − % dehydration
  $= (9 \times 100)/100 - 10 = 900/90 = 10\,kg$
  Calculation of fluid deficit:
  Fluid deficit = Pre-illness weight − Current weight
  $10\,kg - 9\,kg = 1\,kg$ or $1\,L$
  Calculation of FWD:

- FWD = $0.6 \times$ weight(kg) $\times$ [(actual sodium/140) − 1]
- *Example:* Sodium = $155\,mEq/L$, weight = $10\,kg$; FWD = $0.6 \times 10\,kg \times [(155/140) -1]/140) - 1] = 0.64\,L = 640\,mL$

  Calculation of sodium deficit from ECF losses:

- Total fluid deficit is 1000 mL, 640 mL should be replaced as free water and the remaining 360 mL should be replaced as in isonatremic dehydration
- Calculation of sodium deficit in remaining 360 mL of ECF losses:
- Sodium deficit = Fluid deficit (L) × Percentage of fluid loss from ECF × Average ECF sodium concentration (145 mEq/L)
- $0.36$ (L) $\times 0.6 \times 145\,mEq/L = 32\,mEq$

  Calculation of maintenance fluid and sodium requirements:

- *Fluid:* $10\,kg \times 100\,mL/kg = 1000\,mL$
- *Sodium:* $1000\,mL \times 3\,mEq/100\,mL = 30\,mEq$

  Total fluid and sodium requirement:

- *Fluid:* Deficit + Maintenance = 1000 + 1000 = 2000 mL
- *Sodium:* Deficit + Maintenance = 32 + 30 = 62 mEq

  **Optimal fluid: Fluid containing 62 mEq Na/2000 mL = 31 mEq/L**
  **Available fluid:** $D_5/0.2\%$ NaCl (34 mEq/L) at a rate of 83 mL/h (2000 mL/24 h)

## ELECTROLYTE ABNORMALITIES

### HYPONATREMIA

**Serum sodium concentration less than 135 mEq/L**

#### ETIOLOGY

- *Euvolemic:* SIADH, hypothyroidism, psychogenic polydipsia, dilute infant formula
- *Hypervolemic:* Congestive heart failure, nephrotic syndrome, cirrhosis, renal failure, pregnancy
- *Hypovolemic:* Vomiting, diarrhea, poor intake, third-space losses (burns, pancreatitis, trauma), renal losses (diuretics, osmotic diuresis), adrenal insufficiency

#### CLINICAL MANIFESTATIONS

- Anorexia, headache, nausea, vomiting, lethargy, muscle cramping
- *Central nervous system:* Seizures, altered mental status, decreased reflexes
- Brainstem herniation and respiratory arrest are possible

## MANAGEMENT

- Rapid correction of hyponatremia (especially if chronic hyponatremia) can lead to pontine myelinolysis. In general, correct serum sodium at a rate 0.5 mEq/L/h or less or 10–12 mEq/L in 24 hours
- *For hyponatremia with symptomatic hypovolemia:* Start with re-expansion of ECF volume with intravenous isotonic saline (e.g., NSS 20 mL/kg over 30–60 minutes; may repeat)
- *If patient has symptomatic hyponatremia (e.g., seizures):* Consider IV hypertonic saline (e.g., 2–6 mL/kg of 3% NaCl over 1 hour)
- *SIADH:* Water restriction (25–50% of daily maintenance requirement) with monitoring of serum sodium
- Definitive management requires establishing the underlying etiology. Compare urine and serum osmolality to differentiate between SIADH and water intoxication. Withhold offending medications

## IATROGENIC HYPONATREMIA IN HOSPITALIZED CHILDREN

- Hospitalized children may have various non-osmotic triggers for ADH release, including nausea, emesis, pain, stress, postoperative state, CNS disorders (e.g., meningitis, encephalitis, tumors, head injury), pulmonary diseases (e.g., pneumonia, asthma, bronchiolitis), malignancies and medications (e.g., morphine, cyclophosphamide, etc.)
- Isotonic IVFs (0.9% NaCl) are a reasonable option in children at risk for developing hyponatremia, although there is risk of hypernatremia
- Slight fluid restriction may also be considered, once the patient is euvolemic and hemodynamically stable

## HYPERNATREMIA

**Serum sodium concentration greater than 145 mEq/L.**

### ETIOLOGY

- *Hypovolemic:* Diabetes insipidus (central or nephrogenic), insensible free water losses (burns), decreased water intake, diarrhea and rehydration with inappropriately hyperosmolar formula, non-intact thirst mechanism in the context of inappropriately low free water administration
- *Hypervolemic:* Salt poisoning (sodium bicarbonate, NaCl tablets, seawater ingestion), hyperaldosteronism, Cushing's syndrome

### CLINICAL MANIFESTATIONS

- Irritability, muscle weakness, lethargy, restlessness, muscle twitching
- *CNS:* Altered mental status, seizures, coma

### MANAGEMENT

- Rapid correction of pronounced hypernatremia (especially if chronic hypernatremia) can result in life-threatening cerebral edema. In general, aim to lower serum sodium by 10–15 mEq/L per 24 hours
- If patient is severely dehydrated, start with isotonic saline bolus (e.g., NSS 20 mL/kg over 1 hour; may repeat) to restore circulation regardless of serum sodium level
- FWD should be corrected over 24–48 hours. FWD can be estimated by 4 mL FW/kg needed to reduce serum $Na^+$ by 1 mEq/L. Choose a solution that is hypotonic but that will not lower serum sodium too quickly. Remember to give maintenance fluid requirements as well
- Follow serum $Na^+$ levels frequently (e.g., every 4 hours), until stable

## HYPOKALEMIA

**Serum potassium concentration less than 3.5 mEq/L.**

### ETIOLOGY

- *Decreased intake:* Anorexia, low dietary intake, IVFs without potassium
- *Renal losses:* Medications (diuretics, amphotericin B, penicillins), renal tubular acidosis type 1, Fanconi syndrome, osmotic diuresis (e.g., diabetic ketoacidosis), mineralocorticoid excess (hyperaldosteronism, licorice abuse), Bartter syndrome, Gitelman syndrome, Liddle syndrome, hypomagnesemia
- *Extrarenal losses:* Gastrointestinal losses (diarrhea, vomiting, fistulas), sweat losses (cystic fibrosis)
- *Transcellular shift (into intracellular fluid):* Alkalosis, insulin/glucose, beta agonists, familial hypokalemic periodic paralysis

### CLINICAL MANIFESTATIONS

- *Muscle:* Weakness, paresthesias, hyporeflexia, paralysis, rhabdomyolysis
- *Renal:* Polyuria, polydipsia
- *Cardiac:* Bradycardia, prolonged QT, flattened T-wave, appearance of U-wave, AV block, premature beats, paroxysmal atrial or junctional tachycardia, ventricular arrhythmias

### MANAGEMENT

- *Determine etiology:* Electrolytes, magnesium, arterial blood gas, creatine phosphokinase, urine electrolytes (potassium, osmolarity, or creatinine)
- Obtain electrocardiogram; consider continuous ECG monitoring
- Replace potassium orally or in IVFs as potassium chloride or potassium bicarbonate (up to 40 mEq/L through peripheral IV and up to 80 mEq/L through central IV)
- For life-threatening hypokalemia, can give up to 1 mEq/kg per hour of IV potassium
- Correct underlying acid/base disorder or other etiology

## HYPERKALEMIA

**Serum potassium concentration greater than 5.5 mEq/L.**

### ETIOLOGY

- *Increased intake/production:* Excessive acute intravenous administration, hemolysis, rhabdomyolysis
- *Decreased excretion:* Renal failure, hypoaldosteronism, type IV RTA, medications (potassium-sparing diuretics, beta-blockers)
- Acidosis causing transcellular shift
- *Pseudohyperkalemia:* Hemolyzed specimen, extreme leukocytosis or thrombocytosis

### CLINICAL MANIFESTATIONS

- Paresthesias, weakness, decreased reflexes, hyporeflexia
- *Cardiac manifestations can be life-threatening:*
  - ✓ *ECG changes:* Peaked T-wave, depressed ST segment, widened P-R interval, loss of P-wave, wide QRS complex, sine wave pattern
  - ✓ *Arrhythmias:* Ventricular fibrillation, asystole

## MANAGEMENT

- Discontinue potassium intake; discontinue potassium-sparing diuretics; angiotensin converting enzymes/angiotensin receptor blockers
- Perform ECG
- *Determine etiology:* Electrolytes, arterial blood gas, creatinine phosphokinase, urinalysis, urine electrolytes (potassium, osmolarity)
- If electrocardiogram changes other than peaked T-wave or serum potassium greater than 8 mEq/L, consider the following interventions:
  ✓ Continuous ECG monitoring
  ✓ Calcium (e.g., 10% calcium gluconate 0.5 mL/kg IV over 2–5 minutes)
  ✓ Sodium bicarbonate (e.g., 2–3 mEq/kg IV over 30–60 minutes)
  ✓ Insulin (0.1–0.3 U/kg) plus glucose (1 g/kg)
  ✓ *Beta-agonist (nebulized or IV):* Controversial because may cause arrhythmia
  ✓ *Sodium polystyrene (Kayexalate):* Decreases total body potassium
  ✓ Furosemide if not in renal failure
  ✓ For renal failure or if refractory to treatment, consider dialysis

## HYPOCALCEMIA

**Serum calcium concentration less than 8.0 mg/dL (<2.0 mmol/L), or serum ionized calcium level less than 1.13 mmol/L.**

### ETIOLOGY

- *Hypoparathyroidism:* Familial, DiGeorge syndrome, idiopathic, surgical
- *Vitamin D deficiency:* Dietary deficiency, lack of sunlight, malabsorption
- *Vitamin D resistance:* Familial hypophosphatemic rickets
- *Other:* Chronic kidney disease, acute pancreatitis, magnesium deficiency, autosomal dominant hypocalcemic hypercalciuria

### CLINICAL MANIFESTATIONS

- Vomiting, muscle weakness, irritability
- *Severe:* Tetany, seizures, laryngospasm, prolonged QT interval
- *Rickets:* Craniotabes, rachitic rosary, limb deformities (genu varum and valgum), thickened wrists and ankles

### MANAGEMENT

- Management depends on underlying etiology. Initial diagnostics include:
  ✓ *Serum:* Electrolytes, calcium (total and ionized), BUN, creatinine, magnesium, phosphorus, protein, albumin, alkaline phosphatase, vitamin D levels, parathyroid hormone
  ✓ *Urine:* Calcium, phosphorus, pH, protein, glucose
  ✓ Hand/wrist x-ray
  ✓ Consider ECG
- If patient is hypoalbuminemic, correct total calcium (increase serum calcium by 0.8 mg/dL for each 1.0 g/dL that albumin is below normal) or measure ionized calcium level
- For severe symptoms, consider intravenous calcium (e.g., calcium gluconate) replacement with cardiac monitoring
- Once patient is stable, consider oral calcium replacement (e.g., calcium carbonate, calcium citrate)
- If patient is hypomagnesemic, replace magnesium (may be given IM)
- Depending on etiology, patient may need vitamin D replacement

## HYPERCALCEMIA

**Serum calcium concentration greater than 11.0 mg/dL.**

### ETIOLOGY

- Hyperparathyroidism, malignancy (bony metastases, ectopic parathyroid hormone production), immobilization, vitamin D intoxication, familial hypocalciuric hypercalcemia, hyperthyroidism, sarcoidosis, thiazide diuretics, milk-alkali syndrome, Williams syndrome, idiopathic hypercalcemia of infancy

### CLINICAL MANIFESTATIONS

- *Neurologic:* Headache, weakness, lethargy, change in mental status, coma, hyporeflexia, seizures
- *Gastrointestinal:* Constipation, nausea, vomiting, anorexia, abdominal pain
- *Renal:* Nephrocalcinosis, nephrolithiasis, polyuria, polydipsia
- *Cardiovascular:* Bradycardia, short QT interval, hypertension

### MANAGEMENT

- Attempt to identify and treat underlying etiology
- For severe hypercalcemia, consider IVFs (e.g., NSS at two to three times maintenance) followed by furosemide every 6–8 hours
- Consider bisphosphonates ± calcitonin in refractory hypercalcemia
- Steroids may be effective in specific cases (e.g., malignancy, sarcoidosis)

# Gastroenterology

*Benjamin Sahn, MD, MS*
*Petar Mamula, MD*

## ESOPHAGUS AND STOMACH

### GASTROESOPHAGEAL REFLUX DISEASE

**Gastroesophageal reflux (GER) is a physiologic process of stomach contents regurgitating into the esophagus. Gastroesophageal reflux disease (GERD) occurs when GER is accompanied by disturbing symptoms or complications such as esophagitis, respiratory disease, failure to thrive, and/or neurobehavioral manifestations.**

### EPIDEMIOLOGY

- In infants, most GER is physiologic and benign
- Functional GER occurs in more than half of all infants
- Most common esophageal disorder

### PATHOPHYSIOLOGY

- Transient lower esophageal sphincter (LES) relaxation allows gastric contents to flow retrograde up the esophagus
- Decreased gastric compliance in infants compared to adults

### CLINICAL MANIFESTATIONS

- *Functional/Simple GER:* Silent oral regurgitation, effortless spitting, or forceful vomiting; symptoms peak at 1–4 months and resolve by 12–18 months of age; usually benign
- *Complicated GER (GERD):* Significant complications develop in about 10% of untreated children
  - ✓ *Esophagitis:* Crying, irritability, food aversion, heartburn, epigastric or chest pain, odynophagia, hematemesis, anemia, and/or guaiac-positive stools
  - ✓ *Respiratory:* Laryngospasm, bronchospasm, microaspiration pneumonia
  - ✓ Failure to thrive
  - ✓ *Neurobehavioral manifestations:* Sandifer syndrome (opisthotonic posturing, head tilting, seizure-like activity); arching; excessive irritability

### DIAGNOSTICS

- With uncomplicated GER, no diagnostic tests are warranted. In infants or children with complicated GER, consider:
  - ✓ *Upper Gastrointestinal (GI) Series:* Defines anatomy; useful to exclude malrotation, pyloric stenosis, webs, atresias, or other anatomic causes; not diagnostic for reflux
  - ✓ *Scintigraphy or "Milk Scan":* Detects delayed gastric emptying and/or pulmonary aspiration; not diagnostic for reflux
  - ✓ *pH Probe:* Gold standard to quantify acid reflux; helps establish causal relationship between reflux and other symptoms

✓ *Impedance Probe:* Measures movement of air, fluid, and solids in the esophagus through electrical impedance (resistance). Can detect presence of nonacid contents and can be combined with pH probe monitoring. Particularly useful in correlating symptoms with reflux events in patient on acid suppression therapy or in postprandial period when stomach contents likely to be nonacid

✓ *Upper Endoscopy:* Allows direct visualization of the mucosa and the pathologic diagnosis of mucosal disease related to reflux; basal cell hyperplasia, papillary elongation, and an inflammatory cellular infiltrate seen in esophagitis

## MANAGEMENT

• *Conservative Therapy:* Appropriate as a component of treatment for all GER, and may be sole therapy for uncomplicated GER. These measures may mitigate GER symptoms in about 20% of affected infants

✓ Thicken formula with rice cereal (½–1 tablespoon per ounce)

✓ Hold upright during and after feeds

✓ Sleep with head elevated 30 degrees

  ▪ While prone positioning may mitigate GER symptoms, the association of sudden infant death syndrome (SIDS) with prone positioning of young infants precludes a recommendation of prone positioning as a routine strategy

✓ *Formula changes:* Allergy to cow's milk or soy-based formulas is uncommon and unlikely to present with emesis as the sole symptom. Therefore, formula changes are generally not warranted. If cow's milk protein intolerance is suspected, one may switch to a protein hydrolysate or elemental formula for a 2-week period while observing for symptom improvement

• *Medical Therapy:*

✓ *Antacid* magnesium hydroxide/aluminum hydroxide preparations (e.g., Maalox, Mylanta): 0.5 mL/kg/dose (maximum 15 mL) three times daily 10 minutes before feedings; separate from other medications by 1 hour

✓ *Acid suppression* (H2 receptor antagonists (H2RAs) [i.e., ranitidine, famotidine] and proton pump inhibitors (PPI) [i.e., omeprazole, lansoprazole, esomeprazole]) does not prevent GER but helps prevent complications. H2RAs are generally first-line therapy in infants and children <12–18 months. PPI therapy in infants is less effective at reducing symptoms than in older children based on available controlled clinical trials. Therefore, PPIs are only considered potential first-line therapy in children >18 months of age

✓ *Prokinetics:* Include metoclopramide, erythromycin, bethanechol, domperidone, and cisapride. Metoclopramide and low-dose erythromycin (3–5 mg/kg/dose) are available in the United States, but are not currently recommended for treatment of GERD based on insufficient evidence and potential for side effects. Domperidone and cisapride are available only through a clinical trial

• *Post-pyloric feedings* via feeding tube (naso-jejunal or gastro-jejunal), especially in setting of aspiration events

• *Surgical Therapy:*

✓ *Fundoplication:* Indicated for severe complicated GERD with failure of maximal medical therapy; may result in other long-term complications such as gas-bloat syndrome, chronic retching, and dumping syndrome (a cluster of symptoms resulting from rapid transit of food or formula from stomach into small intestine, including abdominal pain, nausea, vomiting, diarrhea, dizziness, flushing, fatigue, and palpitations. Symptoms are result of stretching of the intestinal wall and release of hormones leading to alterations in blood pressure and serum glucose levels.)

- Fundoplication—Surgical procedure that involves wrapping the gastric fundus around the lower esophagus. Many forms of this surgery exist based on the degree the stomach is wrapped. Efficacy in part is related to increased baseline tone of the LES and decreased transient LES relaxations
  - ▷ Increased fundoplication failure rate has been observed in early infancy and children with neurological impairment or status post esophageal atresia repair
  - ▷ Hospitalization for adverse respiratory events decreases after fundoplication surgery in children <4 years, however, no significant decrease in older children

## PEPTIC ULCER DISEASE

**Histologic inflammation and ulceration of the mucosa of the stomach and/or duodenum.**

### EPIDEMIOLOGY

- During childhood typically occurs after 8 years of age
- Accounts for 15% of abdominal pain seen in specialty practice

### ETIOLOGY

- Primary peptic ulcer disease (PUD) (typically gastritis and duodenal ulcers) tends to have a chronic relapsing and remitting course. It may be *Helicobacter pylori*-associated, non-*H. pylori*-associated, or idiopathic
- Secondary PUD (typically gastric ulcers) tends to be acute and, with therapy, recovery is usually complete. Etiologies include physiologic stress, illness, burns, sepsis, shock, head injury, trauma (e.g., retching, nasogastric tube), drugs (e.g., NSAIDs, alcohol, valproate, chemotherapy, KCl), allergic or eosinophilic gastritis, infectious, iron overdose, diabetes mellitus, Crohn's disease, Zollinger–Ellison syndrome, hyperparathyroidism, cystic fibrosis, vascular insufficiency (sickle cell disease, Henoch–Schönlein purpura), radiation gastropathy

### PATHOPHYSIOLOGY

- Imbalance between cytotoxic factors (acid, pepsin, aspirin/NSAIDs, bile acids, *H. pylori* infection) and cytoprotective factors (mucous layer, local bicarbonate secretion, mucosal blood flow)
- *Role of H. pylori:* Gram-negative rod; causes chronic active gastritis and duodenal ulcers; spread by human to human transmission; *H. pylori* infection is often acquired during childhood but uncommonly leads to PUD

### CLINICAL MANIFESTATIONS

- *Abdominal pain:* Often epigastric but may not be localized in children; may be postprandial and nocturnal
- Anorexia, weight loss, early satiety, nausea, recurrent vomiting, upper GI bleeding, anemia
- On physical exam, may note oral ulcers (e.g., Crohn's disease), wheezing (may imply GERD), abdominal tenderness
- Perform rectal exam to look for perianal disease (e.g., Crohn's disease) and occult blood in stool

### DIAGNOSTICS

- *Endoscopy:* Biopsies of the upper intestinal tract is the gold standard for diagnosis

Numerous noninvasive tests are available with variable sensitivities and specificities. Current guidelines recommend a tissue biopsy to confirm a new diagnosis, rather than relying on a noninvasive test alone. *Blood antibody tests* for *H. pylori* are NOT recommended in pediatric patients due to low sensitivity and specificity

- *Stool Antigen Test:* Useful to diagnose *H. pylori* in conjunction with endoscopic biopsy and to test for eradication of infection (4–8 weeks after treatment completion). Some tests have sensitivity >95% for detection of *H. pylori* before and after treatment. Highest yield noninvasive test available
- *Urea Breath Test:* Useful for the initial diagnosis of *H. pylori* when combined with endoscopic biopsy and to test for eradication after therapy. Has limited availability compared with stool antigen testing

## MANAGEMENT

*Acid Suppression*
- Use alone for non-*H. pylori* PUD or in conjunction with antibiotics for *H. pylori*-associated PUD
- *H2 receptor antagonist:* Ranitidine, famotidine
- *PPI:* Omeprazole, esomeprazole, lansoprazole
    IV pantoprazole 1 mg/kg/day up to 40 mg/day for inpatient treatment

*H. pylori Therapy*
- *Treatment options:* Treatment regimens 1–3 are given 7–14 days duration determined by response to therapy, medication side effects, and costs of therapy
    1. PPI + amoxicillin + clarithromycin
    2. PPI + amoxicillin + metronidazole
    3. Bismuth salts + amoxicillin + metronidazole
    4. PPI + amoxicillin for 5 days then PPI + clarithromycin + metronidazole for 5 days
        - A noninvasive test (stool antigen or urease breath test) to monitor eradication of the organism is recommended 4–8 weeks after completion of therapy

## HEPATOBILIARY SYSTEM

## ALPHA-1 ANTITRYPSIN DEFICIENCY

**An autosomal recessive disorder associated with chronic liver disease and premature pulmonary emphysema that is caused by a deficiency of the serine protease inhibitor, alpha-1 antitrypsin (Alph1-AT).**

## EPIDEMIOLOGY

- Most common inherited cause of liver disease in children
- Affects 1 in 2000 live births of white children in the United States

## PATHOPHYSIOLOGY

- Alph1-AT is predominantly produced in hepatocytes, released into the bloodstream, and functions in the lung to inhibit cleavage of connective tissue proteins
- When Alph1-AT is genetically mutated, it cannot be released from hepatocytes and becomes hepatotoxic
- Absence of Alph1-AT or abnormal function allows uninhibited cleavage of connective tissue by elastase leading to lung injury

## CLINICAL MANIFESTATIONS

- May present at any age from infancy to adulthood
- *Variable presentation:* Some allele variants cause both liver and lung disease, while others cause only lung disease
- *Liver disease (neonate to adult):* Prolonged conjugated hyperbilirubinemia in neonate, small for gestational age, acholic stools, elevated transaminases, severe bleeding episode (vitamin K deficiency from liver disease), severe liver failure, hepatomegaly, portal hypertension, varices, chronic hepatitis, cirrhosis, hepatocellular carcinoma
- *Lung disease (adult):* Emphysema
- *On physical exam:* Jaundice, hepatomegaly, splenomegaly, ascites, excoriations from pruritus

## DIAGNOSTICS

- *Serum Alph1-AT Level:* Normal is 150–350 mg/dL; may be misleading because it is an acute phase reactant and could be falsely elevated in a pro-inflammatory state. Further, a normal serum level does not equate to normal protein function
- *Pi Typing (Pi = protease inhibitor):* Defines alleles present, which indicates a normal (MM genotype) or mutant (ZZ genotype) Alph1-AT protein. Other genotypes exist, leading to variable phenotypes
- *Liver Biopsy:* Necessity for diagnosis is controversial

## MANAGEMENT

- Supportive care for liver dysfunction
- Counsel against cigarette smoking
- *Protein replacement therapy (recombinant or purified):* Only for established emphysema; does not help liver disease
- *Surgical options include:* Orthotopic liver transplantation, portocaval or splenorenal shunt, lung transplantation

## AUTOIMMUNE HEPATITIS

A chronic inflammatory liver disease of unknown etiology characterized by hypergammaglobulinemia, autoantibodies, histological findings of a portal area focused mononuclear infiltrate and interface hepatitis between the portal tract and the lobule, and clinical response to immunosuppressive therapy. There are two primary types of autoimmune hepatitis (AIH):

- *Type I:* Antinuclear antibody (ANA), anti-smooth muscle antibody (anti-SMA), and anti-F actin-positive
- *Type II:* Liver-kidney-microsomal (LKM) antibody-positive; more common in pediatrics
- Soluble liver antigen (SLA)-antibody positivity can be found in either type and is associated with more aggressive disease

## EPIDEMIOLOGY

- Relatively uncommon; may present at any age
- Female predominance (4:1)
- *About 20% of patients have at least one other autoimmune disorder:* Associations observed with autoimmune thyroiditis, nephrotic syndrome, type I diabetes mellitus, behcet disease, vitiligo, inflammatory bowel disease (IBD), and Addison's disease

## PATHOPHYSIOLOGY

- Likely autoimmune process in genetically susceptible persons
- Associated with certain HLA haplotypes (A1, B8, DR3, DR4)
- May overlap with autoimmune sclerosing cholangitis

## CLINICAL MANIFESTATIONS

- Extremely variable from asymptomatic to liver failure; may be acute or insidious and progressive
- An acute viral hepatitis syndrome is the most common presentation, characterized by fatigue, malaise, nausea, anorexia, upper abdominal discomfort, arthralgia, myalgia, oligomenorrhea, skin rashes, mild pruritus, jaundice, dark urine, pale stools
- *Physical exam should evaluate for signs of chronic liver disease:* Jaundice, cutaneous stigmata of liver disease, ascites, hepatomegaly, splenomegaly, rash, altered mental status

## DIAGNOSTICS

- ALT, AST levels are increased. Alkaline phosphatase (ALP) and GGT levels are normal or increased
- *PT, albumin:* To check liver synthetic function
- Gamma-globulin levels (high IgG, normal IgA)
- ANA; anti-SMA; anti-F actin, LKM-1; perinuclear anti-neutrophil cytoplasmic antibody (p-ANCA); rarely patients with AIH are negative for traditional antibodies (seronegative autoimmune hepatitis). The initial diagnostic evaluation should at least include ANA, anti-SMA, and LKM-1 antibodies
  - ✓ When evaluating patient for elevated aminotransferases (ALT/AST), in addition to testing for the above antibodies, additional initial evaluations to consider include antibody titers for infection (hepatitis A, B, C, EBV) and celiac disease (anti-transglutaminase Ab IgA, anti-endomysial Ab IgA), and creatine kinase (CK) to rule out muscle inflammation as source of enzyme elevation
- *Liver biopsy:* Required to confirm diagnosis and rule out other causes of chronic hepatitis. "Interface hepatitis" is the hallmark of AIH on biopsy. (Treatment may be initiated without a biopsy in the setting of acute liver failure and coagulopathy when risks of biopsy outweigh benefits)
  - ✓ The overall diagnosis is based on clinical, laboratory, and histologic findings. A scoring system for diagnosis likelihood is provided in the AASLD practice guidelines on the diagnosis and management of autoimmune hepatitis

## MANAGEMENT

- Prednisone 2 mg/kg/day, maximum 60 mg/day; gradually decrease dose over 6–8 weeks to the minimal dose required to maintain normal ALT/AST
- *Azathioprine (0.5 mg/kg/day, maximum 2 mg/kg/day):* Add if steroid alone not showing improvement
- Initial relapse after achieving remission is often treated by returning to the initial prednisone dose with addition of azathioprine for long-term maintenance therapy
- Discontinuation of therapy is considered in a subset of patients who have been treated for more than 3 years, have normal ALT/AST for 2 consecutive years, and demonstrate histological remission on liver biopsy; discontinuation of therapy just before or during puberty may be associated with higher rates of relapse; many patients require lifelong immunosuppressive therapy
- Liver transplantation for initial presentation with severe liver failure or progressive disease unresponsive to medical therapy

## BILIARY ATRESIA

**A disease of unknown etiology in which there is progressive destruction of the extrahepatic biliary tree with variable involvement of the intrahepatic biliary system.**

### EPIDEMIOLOGY

- *Incidence:* 1 in 10,000–20,000
- Slight female predominance
- 10–25% of cases associated with other congenital anomalies (see Clinical Manifestations)

### PATHOPHYSIOLOGY

- Natural history is complete obliteration of bile ducts leading to biliary cirrhosis and liver failure
- Most cases affect the entire extrahepatic biliary tree
- 10% of cases affect only the distal biliary tree
- *Untreated extrahepatic disease:* Life expectancy is 11 months

### CLINICAL MANIFESTATIONS

- Usually normal at birth
- Conjugated hyperbilirubinemia most commonly presents around 2–6 weeks of age. Approximately 10–35% will be jaundiced at birth, with the bile ductular injury occurring in the prenatal period
- *Associated anomalies:* Polysplenia, abdominal heterotaxy, intestinal malrotation, cardiovascular malformations, and anomalies of hepatic arteries/portal vein
- *On physical exam:* Jaundice/greenish hue to skin, hepatomegaly, splenomegaly, dark urine, acholic stools, ascites, edema

### DIAGNOSTICS

- *Bilirubin (total, conjugated, and unconjugated):* Conjugated fraction greater than 2 mg/dL or greater than 15% of total bilirubin
- ALT/AST (two to three times normal); GGT/ALP (markedly elevated); PT/PTT (elevated); albumin (low due to liver synthetic dysfunction)
- *Thrombocytopenia/neutropenia:* If there is hypersplenism
- *Ultrasound:* May not be diagnostic but important to rule out choledochal cyst and to detect polysplenia, heterotaxy. Absence of the gallbladder raises suspicion for biliary atresia
- *DISIDA scan (diisopropyl iminodiacetic acid labeled with 99m-technetium):* Normally after injection, this lipid-soluble, albumin-bound substance is depicted in the liver and followed by excretion into the small bowel. In biliary atresia, there is normal uptake by liver but excretion occurs into the urinary tract due to an absent/obstructed biliary tree
- *Liver biopsy:* Typically shows bile duct proliferation with cholestasis and fibrosis, but very early may not be diagnostic
- *Surgical cholangiography:* Necessary if biopsy not diagnostic and clinical suspicion remains high

### MANAGEMENT

#### Portoenterostomy (Kasai Procedure)

- Anastomosis of intrahepatic biliary tract directly to bowel at the portal plate
- 80% eventually require liver transplantation even if done early
- 70–80% success of palliation if done before 60 days of age; only 20–30% success if done after 90 days of age

- High morbidity and mortality
- Complications include cholangitis, portal hypertension/varices, malnutrition/fat-soluble vitamin deficiency

## Liver Transplantation

- Indicated for extrahepatic biliary atresia when diagnosis is delayed past time window for Kasai
- *Indicated after Kasai if:* Hepatic insufficiency, portal hypertension with recurrent variceal bleeding, irreversible failure to thrive, recurrent cholangitis, persistent cholestasis, hepato-pulmonary syndrome

## GALLBLADDER DISEASE

### DEFINITIONS

- *Cholelithiasis:* Gallstones
- *Choledocholithiasis:* Stones in common bile duct (CBD)
- *Cholecystitis:* Infected or inflamed gallbladder
- *Calculous Cholecystitis:* Infected or inflamed gallbladder that contains stones
- *Acalculous Cholecystitis:* Infected or inflamed gallbladder that does not contain stones

### EPIDEMIOLOGY

- Cholelithiasis and cholecystitis are uncommon in children and are often secondary to a predisposing condition
- More than 50% of cholecystitis in children is acalculous
- Biliary symptoms develop in only 20% of patients with gallstones

### ETIOLOGY

- *Conditions that predispose to cholelithiasis in children:* Prematurity, congenital anomaly of biliary tract, hemolytic disorders (e.g., sickle cell disease), ileal resection or disease, obesity, pregnancy, cystic fibrosis, chronic furosemide use, total parenteral nutrition (TPN), long-term ceftriaxone

### PATHOPHYSIOLOGY

#### Cholelithiasis

- Due to alteration in relative proportions of bile components
- *Cholesterol gallstones* due to bile supersaturated with cholesterol
- *Pigment gallstones:* Black pigment stones due to bile supersaturated with unconjugated bilirubin that forms complexes with free ionized calcium. Brown pigment stones involve biliary stasis and bacterial infection

#### Choledocholithiasis

- *Primary:* Stones formed in CBD
- *Secondary:* Stone migrates from gallbladder and lodges in CBD
- Causes obstructive cholestasis; may lead to pancreatitis, cholangitis

#### Cholecystitis

- *Calculous:* Obstruction of cystic duct by stone leads to acute inflammatory response of gallbladder mucosa; secondary bacterial infection may occur
- *Acalculous:* Biliary stasis (e.g., post-surgery, TPN, infectious illness) causes acute symptoms whereas functional disorders (e.g., biliary dyskinesia) cause chronic symptoms

## CLINICAL MANIFESTATIONS

- *Cholelithiasis:* 80% asymptomatic; biliary colic with right upper quadrant (RUQ) pain
- *Choledocholithiasis:* Biliary colic, obstructive jaundice, cholangitis, pancreatitis
- *Calculous Cholecystitis:* Acute presentation involves abdominal pain (RUQ or diffuse), low-grade fever, nausea, vomiting, anorexia. Chronic presentation often includes history of biliary colic or history of acute cholecystitis episode that resolved. Symptoms may be minimal
- *Acalculous Cholecystitis:* Acute presentation similar to acute calculous cholecystitis. Chronic presentation involves recurrent biliary type pain
- May be ill-appearing with abdominal tenderness, rebound, guarding, palpable gallbladder, jaundice, splenomegaly
- *Murphy's sign:* On palpation of RUQ, pain worsens with inspiration, which leads to cessation of breath

## DIAGNOSTICS

- *Bilirubin, aminotransferases, alkaline phosphatase:* May be elevated or normal
- *Leukocytosis:* Variable
- *Amylase/lipase:* May be elevated
- *Abdominal x-ray:* May show calcified stones
- *Ultrasound:* Best to detect cholelithiasis, choledocholithiasis, and acute cholecystitis
- *DISIDA scan:* No filling of gallbladder in acute cholecystitis; delayed filling in chronic cholecystitis (delayed ejection fraction with cholecystokinin [CCK] or pain with CCK stimulation suggests either chronic cholecystitis or biliary dyskinesia)
- *MRCP:* MRI of the biliary duct system. Improved resolution compared to ultrasound and may identify stones or other anomalies of the ducts missed on previous ultrasound
- *ERCP:* More invasive cholangiogram, advantage of being diagnostic and therapeutic for CBD obstruction due to stones

## MANAGEMENT

### Cholelithiasis

- Observation in asymptomatic patients

### Choledocholithiasis

- ERCP with or without sphincterotomy and biliary stent
- Elective cholecystectomy
- Surgical correction of anatomic abnormality of biliary tree, such as choledochal cyst

### Acute Cholecystitis

- Rehydration, analgesia, antibiotics, observation (usually resolves spontaneously in 2–3 days)
- *Typical antibiotic regimens:* Ampicillin-sulbactam; ampicillin-sulbactam plus gentamycin; third-generation cephalosporin plus metronidazole; ticarcillin-clavulanate; piperacillin-tazobactam; imipenem (if life-threatening)
- Elective cholecystectomy after resolution of acute illness (early or up to 2–3 months later) in uncomplicated cases
- Emergent cholecystectomy is indicated if complicated by necrosis, perforation, or empyema

### Chronic Cholecystitis

- Cholecystectomy for chronic calculous cholecystitis (in general)
- For biliary dyskinesia, cholecystectomy has variable results, with many children continuing to experience pain symptoms in the postoperative period

## GLYCOGEN STORAGE DISEASE

A family of inherited disorders affecting glycogen metabolism. Glycogen is a highly branched polymer of glucose and is stored in liver and muscle. The glycogen found in these disorders is abnormal in quantity, quality, or both.

- *Conversion of glycogen into pyruvate occurs in two parts:* Glycogenolysis from glycogen to glucose-6-phosphate and glycolysis from glucose-6-phosphate to pyruvate
- Some enzyme defects are localized in liver, others in muscles; a few are generalized

### EPIDEMIOLOGY

- Frequency (all forms) about 1/20,000 live births
- Autosomal recessive inheritance
- Types I, II, III, and IX most commonly present in early childhood; type V (McArdle disease) most common in adults

### ETIOLOGY

- More than 12 types; can be classified by organ involvement and clinical manifestations into liver and muscle glycogenoses (Table 10-1)
- *Hepatic Glycogen Storage Disease:* Type I (von Gierke disease), type III, type IV, type VI, type IX, glycogen synthetase deficiency, and glucose transporter-2 defect; typically cause hepatomegaly and fasting hypoglycemia; types III and IV are also associated with hepatic cirrhosis
- *Muscle Glycogen Storage Disease:* Divided into two groups: progressive skeletal muscle weakness, cardiomyopathy or both (type II); muscle pain, exercise intolerance, myoglobinuria and fatigue (types V, VII)

| TABLE 10-1 | Classification of Glycogen Storage Diseases | | |
|------------|---------------------------------------------|------|----------------------|
| **Type** | **Deficient Enzyme** | **Tissue** | **Main Clinical Feature** |
| Ia | Glucose-6-phosphatase "von Gierke disease" | Liver, kidney | Hypoglycemia, hepatomegaly, lactic acidosis, hyperlipidemia |
| Ib-d | Glucose-6-phosphatase-related transport | Liver | Above + neutropenia and infections (Ib) |
| II | Acid α-glucosidase "Pompe disease" | Generalized | Infant form: cardiorespiratory failureLater form: myopathy |
| III | Debranching enzyme | Liver, cardiac muscle | Hypoglycemia, hepatomegaly, myopathy |
| IV | Branching system | Liver | Hepatosplenomegaly, cirrhosis |
| V | Phosphorylase, "McArdle disease" | Muscle | Exercise intolerance |
| VI | Phosphorylase | Liver | Hepatomegaly |
| VII | Phosphofructokinase, phosphoglycerate kinase, phosphoglycerate mutase | Muscle | Exercise intolerance |
| IX | Phosphorylase b kinase | Liver | Hepatomegaly |
| O | Glycogen synthase | Liver | Hypoglycemia |

## DIAGNOSTICS

- *Hepatic glycogen storage disease*: Enzyme defects can only be detected in tissue acquired on a liver biopsy but preliminary screening can be performed with an oral glucose tolerance test or a glucagon test
- *Muscle glycogen storage disease*: Exercise test (semi-ischemic forearm test, bicycle ergometer test, or treadmill test) used to demonstrate the failure of venous lactate and pyruvate to rise and the production of uric acid, inosine, hypoxanthine, and ammonia to increase excessively; if exercise test is abnormal, myopathy should be verified by enzyme assay

## MANAGEMENT

- Prevention of hypoglycemia while avoiding storage of even more glycogen in the liver and muscle
- *Hepatic Glycogen Storage Disease:*
  - ✓ Nasogastric tube feedings at night; frequent feedings every 2–3 hours during the day using a lactose-free and sucrose-free formula
  - ✓ Uncooked cornstarch (1.75–2.5 g/kg) mixed in water, soy formula or soy milk is given every 4 hours in infants and every 6 hours in older children
  - ✓ Restrict intake of fructose and galactose
  - ✓ Supplementation with calcium and multivitamins
  - ✓ Allopurinol is used to lower the concentration of uric acid
  - ✓ Liver transplantation has been successful
- *Muscle Glycogen Storage Disease:* Muscle function may be influenced by diet (protein may compensate for increased muscle catabolism); glucose use depends on underlying condition

## WILSON DISEASE

**Autosomal recessive disease of copper metabolism that involves defective biliary copper excretion, which leads to abnormal copper accumulation in the liver, central nervous system (CNS), eyes, and kidneys.**

### EPIDEMIOLOGY

- *Prevalence:* 1:30,000

### PATHOPHYSIOLOGY

- Wilson disease gene on chromosome 13 encodes a transmembrane copper-transporting ATPase protein (ATPase 7B). Mutations result in an abnormal transporter protein, which prevents normal export of copper from hepatocytes
- Copper accumulates first in the liver and then spills over to other tissue

### CLINICAL MANIFESTATIONS

- Frequently presents in childhood but rarely before age 5 years
- *Classic triad:* Hepatic disease, neurologic disease, Kayser–Fleischer rings (brown-yellow ring around the corneo–scleral junction resulting from copper deposits)
- In children, hepatic effects precede neurologic effects and typically present in the second decade of life
- *Liver:* Acute hepatitis, chronic active hepatitis, cirrhosis, fulminant hepatic failure
- *CNS:* Basal ganglia involvement leads to dystonia, incoordination, tremor, fine motor skill difficulty, rigidity, dysarthria, and gait disturbances. Psychiatric manifestations include depression, aggressive behaviors, impulsivity, compulsivity, poor school performance, psychosis

- *Ophthalmologic:* Kayser–Fleischer rings, sunflower cataracts (cataract related to copper deposits described as brown-green deposits in anterior and posterior lens capsule)
- *Other:* Hemolytic anemia, proximal renal tubular dysfunction, bone demineralization, osteoporosis, pathologic fractures, cardiac dysrhythmias, cholelithiasis

## DIAGNOSTICS

- *Laboratory Tests:* Ceruloplasmin level less than 20 mg/dL; serum copper low or high; 24-hour urine copper greater than 100 µg/day; CBC (hemolysis); LFTs (hepatitis, cholestasis)
- *Liver Biopsy:* Gold standard; quantitation of hepatic copper, typical findings of steatosis, inflammation, +/− fibrosis
- *Head CT:* Ventricular dilatation, brain atrophy, basal ganglia abnormalities
- *Head MRI:* More sensitive than CT for specific changes

## MANAGEMENT

- *D-Penicillamine (20 mg/kg/day divided four times a day, maximum 1 g/day; start with reduced dose):* Copper chelator used as initial treatment in hepatic disease. Give 1 hour before or 2 hours after meals. Supplement with vitamin $B_6$
- *Trientine:* A copper chelator and alternative to D-penicillamine. Typical dose in range of 20 mg/kg/day in 2–3 divided doses rounded to nearest 250 mg dose
- *Zinc:* Antagonist of copper absorption used as adjunctive therapy or alternative maintenance therapy after chelation. Typical dose is 150 mg/day in larger children and adults, and 75 mg/day in smaller children. Daily dose is divided two to three times per day
- *Ammonium Tetrathiomolybdate:* Still experimental
- *Diet:* Restrict dietary sources of copper: animal liver and kidney, shellfish, chocolate, dried beans, peas, unprocessed wheat
- *Liver Transplantation:* For severe disease with fulminant hepatic failure or worsening disease unresponsive to medical therapy
- Screening of asymptomatic relatives of patients with Wilson disease

## SMALL AND LARGE INTESTINES

## CELIAC DISEASE

**An autoimmune disorder of the small intestine characterized by a permanent intolerance to wheat gluten that results in mucosal damage and malabsorption.**

## EPIDEMIOLOGY

- *Prevalence:* 1 in 300 worldwide
- More common in persons of European descent
- Associated with juvenile-onset diabetes mellitus, selective IgA deficiency, dermatitis herpetiformis, autoimmune thyroid disease, Down syndrome, Turner syndrome, and Williams syndrome
- Increased prevalence in children with first-degree relatives with celiac disease
- Increased risk of small bowel lymphoma

## PATHOPHYSIOLOGY

- Gut exposure to grain proteins in wheat, rye, barley, and oats results in an autoimmune reaction that is toxic to enterocytes and leads to a flattened mucosal lining and impaired small intestinal absorptive capacity

## CLINICAL MANIFESTATIONS

- Symptoms are variable and can present at any age
- Classically presents around age 1–3 years, but this is changing as more children are identified by increased screening practices
- Diarrhea, foul-smelling bulky greasy stools, abdominal distention and pain
- Poor growth, anorexia, malaise, muscle wasting, irritability, unexplained iron deficiency anemia
- Symptoms can be subtle with only mild diarrhea or recurrent abdominal pain or constipation complaints
- *Physical exam:* Weight loss, short stature, edema, abdominal distention, rectal prolapse, muscle wasting, dental erosion, angular stomatitis, aphthous lesions, osteopenia, rickets

## DIAGNOSTICS

- *Antibody Tests:* Anti-gliadin antibody (IgA and IgG; moderate sensitivity, low specificity), anti-endomysial IgA (sensitivity = 90–95%, specificity = 98–100%; false-negative results more common in children younger than 2 years of age), anti-tissue transglutaminase antibody (IgA anti-tTG; sensitivity = 92–98%, specificity = 96–100%)
- Antibody tests are good for initial screen but endoscopy required for definitive diagnosis
- Anti-gliadin antibodies are not used for standard screening, except in the young child less than 2 years old. Deamidated anti-gliadin antibody is more sensitive and specific than previous standard test
- May present with elevated hepatic transaminases
- *Endoscopy:* Small bowel biopsies on a *gluten-containing* diet help make diagnosis; increased epithelial lymphocytes, villous atrophy, crypt hyperplasia, infiltration of lamina propria with inflammatory cells are features consistent with celiac disease; resolution of abnormalities on gluten-free diet confirms diagnosis

## MANAGEMENT

- Permanent gluten-free diet leads to full clinical and histologic remission; gluten-free means no wheat, rye, barley, or oats; corn and rice are permitted
- Dietary counseling and careful attention to ALL food and medicinal products that may contain traces of gluten
- Multivitamin/fat-soluble vitamins
- Medical therapy for iron deficiency and rickets if present
- Very close follow-up of growth parameters and symptoms
- Periodic monitoring of dietary compliance with antibody profile; antibodies usually undetectable within 3–6 months after initiation of appropriate diet
- Screening of all immediate family members is indicated

## CONSTIPATION

**A symptom of abnormal defecation characterized by infrequent stooling, incomplete evacuation of the rectum, passage of large painful stools, involuntary soiling, or the inability to pass stool.**

### EPIDEMIOLOGY

- Occurs in more than 10% of all children
- Majority of constipation in older children is functional
- Encopresis occurs in 1–2% of all children

## ETIOLOGY

- *Anatomic:* Hirschsprung disease, imperforate anus, anal stenosis, malpositioned anus, ileal atresia, meconium ileus, colonic stricture, abdominal mass, hydrometrocolpos
- *Physiologic:* Hypothyroidism, celiac disease, lumbosacral spinal cord defect, infant botulism, muscular diseases, cystic fibrosis, diabetes, lead poisoning, post-viral "ileus," prune-belly syndrome, ascariasis, medications, excessive cow's milk ingestion, inadequate fluid intake, malnutrition, anorexia nervosa, functional constipation

## PATHOPHYSIOLOGY

- *Functional Constipation:* Cycle typically begins with voluntary withholding of stool. Stool returns from anal canal to rectum. Sensation of urge to defecate is decreased. Stool bolus becomes larger and harder, which perpetuates more withholding. Over time, rectal vault distends and normal sensation diminishes
- *Retentive Encopresis:* Involuntary soiling of liquid stool around solid stool, which results from chronic constipation
- *Grunting Baby Syndrome:* An infant with grunting, straining, and turning red while passing a *soft* stool has immature coordination of the stooling process and not true constipation

## CLINICAL MANIFESTATIONS

- *Signs of possible anatomic abnormalities:* Blood in stool, failure to thrive, emesis, abdominal distention
- *Signs of functional constipation:* Retentive posturing; infrequent passage of large, hard bowel movements; involuntary soiling
- Complaints of abdominal pain
- Stool consistency may be hard, soft, or even diarrheal
- Stool frequency can be daily or infrequent
- On physical exam, note abdominal tenderness/distention, palpable stool on abdominal palpation, anal wink, anal tone, stool in rectal vault, width of rectal vault, neurologic and back exams

## DIAGNOSTICS

- Consider laboratories depending on suspected cause

### Abdominal x-ray

- *1-view abdominal x-ray:* Most useful to diagnose fecal impaction in the rectum. Limited use in correlating colonic stool burden with degree of constipation
- *Radiopaque Sitz Marker study:* Child swallows 24 radiopaque markers in one sitting and x-ray obtained 5 days later. Location of markers aids in determining type of constipation. May be done to assess a current bowel regimen or following a bowel clean-out to assess GI transit without stool burden
  - ✓ *Slow transit:* Markers distributed throughout the colon
  - ✓ *Outlet dysfunction:* Numerous markers clustered in rectosigmoid
  - ✓ *Functional:* Less than 3 markers remaining on x-ray
- *Unprepped Contrast Enema/Rectal Biopsy:* To evaluate for Hirschsprung disease
- *L-spine MRI:* Suspected spinal cord abnormality

## MANAGEMENT

- Treat underlying medical disorders
- Surgical correction of anatomic defects
- Treatment of functional constipation may take months to years

✓ *Bowel clean-out:* Enemas, suppositories, lubricants, hyperosmolar agents
✓ *Maintenance:* Dietary fiber and fluids, hyperosmolar agents
✓ *Toilet sitting:* Twice-daily stooling attempts
✓ *Diary/journal:* Positive reinforcement
✓ Educate patient and parents. Frequent follow-up is critical to success
• *Medications used to treat constipation:*
  ✓ **Enema:** Mineral oil (rectally); sodium biphosphate (Fleets); or saline; all in children ≥2 years of age. Larger volume enemas such as polyethylene glycol enemas to relieve rectal fecal impaction may be necessary
  ✓ *Suppositories:* Glycerin, bisacodyl
  ✓ *Lubricants:* Mineral oil (orally)
  ✓ *Osmotic laxatives:* Polyethylene glycol (PEG) 3350 (Miralax), lactulose, PEG with electrolytes (Go-Lytely)
  ✓ *Stimulant laxatives:* Senna, bisacodyl, magnesium citrate, magnesium hydroxide
  ✓ *Fiber/bulk forming agents:* Benefiber, Citrucel, Metamucil, Maltsupex
• *Typical clean-out regimen:*
  ✓ Enemas to clean out rectal vault
  ✓ *Hyperosmotic and/or stimulant therapy:* May require nasogastric tube for administration. Continue until clear effluent. Monitoring serum electrolytes appropriate when using larger volumes

## GASTROINTESTINAL BLEEDING

**Loss of blood via the GI tract:**

• *Hematemesis:* Bloody emesis due to active bleeding proximal to the ligament of Treitz
• *Hematochezia:* Bright red or maroon stool due to active bleeding in the colon or brisk bleeding from a more proximal site
• *Melena:* Dark, tarry stool due to bleeding proximal to the ileocecal valve

### DIFFERENTIAL DIAGNOSIS

• Upper intestinal bleeding
  ✓ *Infant:* Swallowed maternal blood, esophagitis, gastric ulcer
  ✓ *Older child:* Esophagitis, Mallory–Weiss tear, esophageal varices, foreign body with mucosal erosion, duplication cyst, Dieulafoy lesion, gastritis, gastric ulcer, vascular malformation, duodenitis, hemobilia, swallowed blood from oral/nasal pharynx, pulmonary bleeding (hemoptysis)
• Lower intestinal bleeding
  ✓ *Infant:* Anal fissure, swallowed maternal blood, milk protein allergic colitis, infectious enterocolitis, vascular malformation, necrotizing enterocolitis, Hirschsprung disease with enterocolitis, Meckel diverticulum (>2 months), intussusception, intestinal duplication
  ✓ *Older child:* Anal fissure, perianal strep cellulitis, solitary rectal ulcer, infectious enterocolitis/*Clostridium difficile* colitis, intussusception, IBD, vascular malformations, Meckel diverticulum, polyp, intestinal duplication, Henoch–Schönlein purpura, hemolytic uremic syndrome, hemorrhoids, rectal trauma, sexual abuse

### CLINICAL MANIFESTATIONS

• Variable presentation from hemodynamically stable to shock
• Note prior use of NSAIDs, steroids, indomethacin, antibiotics

- Note history of trauma, liver disease, umbilical vein catheterization (history of umbilical vein catheterization is associated with portal vein thrombosis and development of portal hypertension predisposing to esophageal varices)
- May present with vomiting, retching, casual regurgitation of bloody fluid, abdominal pain, anorexia, fever, weight loss, sepsis, asphyxia, recent surgery, mental status changes
- Inspect mouth, nares, pharynx for trauma
- *Abdomen:* Hepatomegaly, splenomegaly, prominent abdominal vessels, right lower quadrant mass or tenderness
- *Rectal:* Blood, erythema, fissure, fistula, skin tag, polyp, hemorrhoid, rectal prolapse
- *Stool:* Blood or mucous within or surrounding stool
- *Extremities:* Capillary refill, digital clubbing, palmar erythema, purpura, or petechiae
- *Skin:* Pallor, jaundice, facial petechiae, pigmented freckles on lips/buccal mucosa, excoriations, hemangiomas, other vascular appearing lesions
- For breastfeeding infant, inspect mother's nipple (dry, cracked, bleeding nipples suggest swallowed maternal blood)

## DIAGNOSTICS

- *Stool guaiac:* False-positive results may be due to rare meat, horseradish, turnips, iron, tomatoes, fresh red cherries; false negatives may be due to vitamin C, outdated card or developing solution, storage of stool greater than 4 days
- *Nasogastric lavage:* Use normal saline at room temperature; absent blood does not exclude an upper GI source; present blood does not identify the exact origin
- *Laboratory studies:* CBC, PT/PTT, LFTs, electrolytes, type and screen
- *Stool bacterial culture and stool C. difficile toxins*
- *Abdominal x-ray:* Free air, toxic megacolon, pneumatosis, small bowel dilation
- *Air or gastrograffin contrast enema:* For suspected intussusception
- *Meckel diverticulum scan*
- *Upper GI series:* Structural abnormality, tumor, polyp, signs of IBD
- CT/MR angiography studies useful in both slower and brisk bleeding to localize lesion. CTA with oral contrast (CT Enterography) is most sensitive test if patient can tolerate oral contrast
- Tagged Red Blood Cell bleeding scan and Angiography reserved for brisk bleeding without clear localization on imaging studies
- *Endoscopy or colonoscopy:* Direct visual inspection, biopsy, culture
- *Wireless video capsule endoscopy:* For small bowel obscure GI bleeding

## MANAGEMENT

- *Initial Management of all GI Bleeding:* Identify and treat shock with IV access, isotonic fluids, oxygen, blood products
- *Non-Variceal Upper GI Bleed:* Acid reduction (ranitidine, pantoprazole); discontinue NSAIDs; endoscopic hemostasis therapy if bleed persists (bipolar electrocoagulation, heater probe, clips, injection therapy)
- *Variceal Upper GI Bleed:*
  - ✓ Fluid resuscitation; transfuse red cells to maintain hemoglobin near 10 g/dL; transfuse platelets to greater than 50,000/mm³; FFP to correct coagulopathy
  - ✓ *Octreotide (bolus 1-2 μg/kg over 2-5 minutes, then 1-2 μg/kg/h infusion):* Reduces splanchnic arterial blood flow to decrease portal pressure
  - ✓ Endoscopic band ligation, sclerotherapy
  - ✓ *Emergent surgical therapy for unresponsive severe bleeding:* Portosystemic shunt, transjugular intrahepatic portal shunt (TIPS), Blakemore–Sengstaaken tube occlusive balloon therapy, liver transplantation

- *Lower GI Bleed in an Infant:*
  - ✓ Surgical evaluation for suspected intussusception, necrotizing enterocolitis, toxic mega-colon, Hirschsprung disease
  - ✓ If otherwise healthy and has blood-streaked mucus in stool without evidence of fissure, send stool culture and consider changing to elemental formula for presumptive milk-protein allergy
  - ✓ Flexible sigmoidoscopy for persistent bloody stools despite elemental formula and negative stool culture
  - ✓ Anal fissures heal without intervention
- *Lower GI Bleed in an Older Child:*
  - ✓ Treat according to underlying cause if known
  - ✓ Treat constipation if present
  - ✓ Flexible sigmoidoscopy or colonoscopy for recurrent or persistent bleeding to detect colitis, polyps, IBD
  - ✓ Polyp removal by electrocautery
  - ✓ Meckel scan if no source identified by endoscopy
  - ✓ Surgical evaluation if severe bleed of unidentified source

## INFLAMMATORY BOWEL DISEASE

**An idiopathic chronic disease of the GI tract resulting in inflammation, tissue destruction, diarrhea, protein-losing enteropathy, GI bleeding, abdominal pain, and many extraintestinal manifestations. IBD is broadly divided into Crohn's disease, ulcerative colitis (UC), and indeterminate colitis (IC).**

### EPIDEMIOLOGY

- Family history predisposes to IBD
- 20–30% of new IBD presents in persons younger than 20 years of age
- 4% of pediatric IBD presents in children younger than 5 years of age
- More common in developed countries

### ETIOLOGY

- Interaction between environmental, gut microbiota, immunologic and genetic factors
- Dysregulation of mucosal immune system driven by normal intestinal flora

### PATHOPHYSIOLOGY

- *Crohn's Disease:*
  - ✓ May involve any segment of the GI tract, mouth to anus
  - ✓ Commonly involves small intestine and terminal ileum
  - ✓ Transmural disease with thickened nodular bowel, non-caseating granulomas, strictures, fistulas, abscesses, adhesions
  - ✓ Skip lesions, discontinuous disease
  - ✓ Perianal disease (15%)
  - ✓ Malabsorption of iron, zinc, folate, and vitamin $B_{12}$
  - ✓ Bacterial overgrowth
  - ✓ Carcinoma (increased risk over general population)
- *Ulcerative Colitis:*
  - ✓ Limited to the colon; starts in rectum and ascends continuously
    Nonspecific gastritis and/or duodenitis common

✓ Diffuse mucosal involvement/submucosal sparing
✓ Crypt abscesses; toxic megacolon (<5%)
✓ Carcinoma (significant increased risk over general population)
• *Indeterminate Colitis:*
✓ Term used when macroscopic disease is localized to colon but cannot be definitively said to be UC or CD

## CLINICAL MANIFESTATIONS

### Intestinal Manifestations:

• *Crohn's disease:* Abdominal pain, diarrhea, rectal bleeding, aphthous oral lesions, perianal fissures/tags/fistulas, abdominal abscesses, anorexia, weight loss, linear growth deceleration
• *Ulcerative colitis:* Bloody mucoid diarrhea, lower abdominal pain/tenderness, urgency to defecate, nausea/vomiting associated with defecation

### Extraintestinal Manifestations:

Occur in approximately 30% of patients with IBD, more typically after IBD diagnosis is made. A minority will manifest extraintestinal symptoms prior to intestinal-related symptoms.

• *Systemic:* Fever, malaise, anorexia, weight loss, growth delay/linear growth deceleration, delayed puberty
• *Skin:* Erythema nodosum, pyoderma gangrenosum, perianal disease
• *Joints:* Arthritis, arthralgia, clubbing, ankylosing spondylitis, sacro-ileitis
• *Eyes:* Uveitis, episcleritis, keratitis, retinal vasculitis
• *Biliary:* Sclerosing cholangitis (UC > crohn's disease), chronic active hepatitis, fatty liver, cholelithiasis
• *Bone:* Osteopenia
• *Renal:* Stones, hydronephrosis, enterovesical fistula
• *Vascular:* Thrombophlebitis, vasculitis
• *Heme:* Anemia (iron, vitamin $B_{12}$, folate deficiency, hemolysis, marrow suppression from medications, anemia of chronic disease), thrombocytosis, neutropenia
• *Oncologic:* Lymphoma, acute myelogenous leukemia, colon cancer

## DIAGNOSTICS

• Complete blood count (low hemoglobin, low mean corpuscular volume, high platelets), ESR (high), C-reactive protein (high), albumin (low), alkaline phosphatase (low), iron studies, folate, vitamin $B_{12}$ levels, electrolytes, calcium, magnesium, phosphorus
• Unique IBD-related antibody serologies are sometimes used to *aid the differentiation of crohn's disease and UC when unclear.* ASCA (anti-*Saccharomyces cerevisiae* antibody) and ANCA are most well described, although other antibodies are now available. These antibodies are generally not used as screening tests to evaluate for IBD
• *Stool guaiac:* Positive
• Stool for culture, *C. difficile* toxins A and B, ova and parasites, cryptosporidium and Giardia
• Fecal calprotectin is highly sensitive and specific for GI tract inflammation, especially colitis. Highly valuable in distinguishing between IBD and irritable bowel syndrome (IBS)
✓ When a combination of the above tests raise suspicion for IBD, the gold standard test to rule out the disease is endoscopy and colonoscopy. A radiology study (see below) may be chosen before endoscopy/colonoscopy depending on presenting symptoms (concern for obstruction, abscess, perforation)

## Radiology

There is no one perfect imaging study to evaluate the small bowel in patients with IBD. Each study has its benefits and limitations. The optimal initial study depends on the patient and his/her symptoms and course of illness.

- *Upper GI with small bowel follow-through:* Useful to evaluate for strictures. False-negatives common for superficial mucosal disease
- *Abdominal CT:* Useful to assess for complications of crohn's disease such as intra-abdominal abscess or phlegmon
- *MR Enterography:* MRI of bowel with IV and oral contrast. No ionizing radiation. Useful to assess transmural disease
- *MRI Pelvis:* Frequently used to assess perianal disease and fistulae
- *Wireless video capsule endoscopy:* Useful to assess the mucosal surface, unable to assess disease beyond bowel lumen. Risk of capsule retention at site of narrowing/stricture. A test capsule is available for those considered at higher risk
- *Bone Age:* Assess for delayed bone maturation
- *DXA Scan:* Assesses bone mineral density, which may be low in chronic inflammatory diseases such as IBD. Normal range: Z score $+2$ to $-2$. Below $Z - 2$, patients may be at risk for fracture

## Endoscopy

- Gold standard for diagnosis
- Mucosa may appear erythematous, edematous, friable, ulcerated
- Loss of normal vascular pattern
- Well-established diagnostic histology criteria—Chronic inflammation, crypt abscesses, architectural mucosal abnormalities, etc

## MANAGEMENT

### Medical

Choice of therapy for a given patient depends on many factors including disease phenotype, location of disease, severity of symptoms, growth status, age of patient, and among other factors. "Bottom up" (salicylates, steroids, antibiotics), "top down" (biologics, immunomodulators), or use of enteral therapy at time of newly diagnosed IBD may be appropriate depending on the above factors.

- *Salicylates:* Sulfasalazine, mesalamine (Pentasa, Delzicol), balsalazide (Colazal), rowasa (enemas), canasa (suppositories)
- *Antibiotics:* Metronidazole, ciprofloxacin, rifaximin, oral vancomycin
  - ✓ Antibiotics are indicated in setting of penetrating (fistulizing) luminal or perianal disease and comorbid *C. difficile* infection
  - ✓ Use in active luminal crohn's disease and UC as adjunctive therapy is patient-specific. Metronidazole and ciprofloxacin have each been shown to improve symptoms in some studies while lack significant benefit in others
- *Steroids:* Prednisone, methylprednisone, budesonide (ileal release with less systemic absorption), budesonide MMX (Multimatrix system technology; colonic release with less systemic absorption) hydrocortisone enema
- *Immunomodulators:* To reduce steroid dependency or as adjunct to infliximab
  - ✓ 6-mercaptopurine, azathioprine, methotrexate, cyclosporine, tacrolimus
- *Biologic agents:* Moderate to severe crohn's disease or UC, fibrostenotic or fistulizing crohn's disease, steroid refractory UC, other indications

✓ Infliximab (Remicade), adalimumab (Humira), certolizumab pegol (Cimzia)
✓ Obtain PPD/CXR to rule out latent TB infection before initiation
✓ Make sure vaccination series completed
- *Enteral nutritional therapy:* Nutritional-based therapy for crohn's disease, typically with delivery of semi-elemental formula via NG tube. May modulate gut microbiota to favor anti-inflammatory response. Given as 80–100% of daily caloric intake to induce remission of disease
- In acute severe UC, use of the PUCAI (pediatric UC activity index) scoring system of symptoms can guide clinical judgment regarding response to therapy and need to escalate therapy. The scoring includes abdominal pain, rectal bleeding, stool consistency, number of stools per day, nocturnal bowel movements, and activity level
  ✓ Management of an acute IBD flare that requires hospitalization often includes reevaluation of disease severity and location, with objective determination of symptoms through accurate documentation of pain pattern and stool consistency and frequency
    - Medication adherence should be inquired
    - If disease has worsen from previous baseline, escalation or change of therapy is strongly considered
- Discharge criteria following acute flare include improvement of presenting symptoms (e.g., tolerating oral intake without severe pain, minimal gross blood in stool and maintaining stable hemoglobin level, fewer diarrheal stools, gaining weight if admitted with weight loss, resolution of emesis, resolution of obstruction)

### Surgical

- Indicated in uncontrolled bleeding, bowel perforation, bowel obstruction, intractable disease, and intractable perianal disease
- *Crohn's disease:* Local resection (such as ileocecectomy), ostomy diversion, fistula management
  ✓ Incision and drainage of perirectal abscesses +/− drain placement
  ✓ Seton: A suture is placed through the fistulous tract forming a loop, to allow for continuous draining and healing from lumen to skin. Without seton, fistulous tracts tend to heal at the skin side first, and pus may be trapped creating an abscess
- *UC:* Total colectomy with ileo-anal anastomosis for medically refractory disease

## MECKEL'S DIVERTICULUM

**A true diverticulum that results from incomplete closure of the omphalomesenteric or vitelline duct. It may contain gastric or other mucosa, and occurs along the ileum usually within 100 cm of the ileocecal valve.**

### EPIDEMIOLOGY

- 2% of the population
- Has been associated with cleft palate, bicornuate uterus, and annular pancreas

### PATHOPHYSIOLOGY

- Persistence of vitelline duct; contains all three intestinal layers
- *May contain ectopic tissue:* Gastric (50%), pancreatic (5%), other
- Bleeding occurs when acid secreted by ectopic gastric mucosa causes adjacent ileal ulceration or erodes into the vitelline artery

### CLINICAL MANIFESTATIONS

- *Asymptomatic:* 95% of cases

- *Painless lower intestinal bleeding:* Most common symptom accounting for 50% of symptomatic presentations, generally in patients 2 months–2 years
- *Other manifestations:* Intestinal obstruction, intussusception, volvulus, herniation through mesenteric defect, severe right lower quadrant abdominal pain (Meckel's diverticulitis), umbilical cysts/sinuses, palpable abdominal mass

## DIAGNOSTICS

- Technetium-99m pertechnetate scintigraphic study. Test has high specificity (95–100%) but lower sensitivity (50–92%). Use of H2 receptor antagonist (ranitidine) prior to test may increase yield with a sensitivity of 62.5% with conventional study, and sensitivity of 87.5% when pretreated with ranitidine
- Tagged red blood cell scan if active bleed
- Upper GI with small bowel follow through
- Wireless video capsule endoscopy may identify isolated ileal ulcer
- Barium enema (if intussusception suspected)
- Occasionally discovered as incidental finding at laparoscopy

## MANAGEMENT

- Medically resuscitate the patient with a lower GI bleed
- Symptomatic Meckel's diverticulum should be surgically resected
- Meckel's diverticulum found incidentally during surgery performed for another reason should be resected if there is are palpable heterotopic mucosa or mass, fibrous bands to umbilicus, or surrounding inflammation

# PANCREAS

## PANCREATITIS

### DEFINITIONS

*Acute Pancreatitis:* An acute inflammatory process of the pancreas characterized by two of the following three characteristics: acute abdominal pain, elevated pancreatic enzymes at least 3× upper limit of normal, and radiologic evidence of pancreatic inflammation.
*Acute Recurrent Pancreatitis:* At least two episodes of acute pancreatitis with resolution of pain and pancreatic enzymes between episodes.
*Chronic Pancreatitis:* A condition of recurring or persisting abdominal pain, pancreatic inflammation, and progressive destruction of the pancreas that often leads to pancreatic insufficiency or failure.

### EPIDEMIOLOGY

- All ages; male = female
- Heritable forms of pancreatitis are the most common forms of chronic pancreatitis in children (cationic trypsinogen, SPINK1, CFTR gene mutations)

### ETIOLOGY

#### Acute Pancreatitis

- *Systemic Disease:* Infections; inflammatory/vascular (Henoch–Schönlein purpura, hemolytic-uremic syndrome, Kawasaki, IBD, collagen vascular); sepsis/shock; transplantation
- *Mechanical/Structural:* Trauma (blunt injury, child abuse, post-ERCP); anatomic (annular pancreas, pancreas divisum, choledochal cyst, stricture); obstruction (stones, tumor)

- *Metabolic/Toxic:* Hyperlipidemia, hypercalcemia, cystic fibrosis, severe malnutrition, refeeding, renal disease, organic acidemia, drugs/toxins
- *Idiopathic:* Up to 25% of cases
- *Chronic Pancreatitis*
- *Obstructive:* Congenital anomaly (choledochal cyst), ductal fibrosis or stricture, tumor, pseudocyst, sphincter of Oddi dysfunction, trauma, idiopathic fibrosing pancreatitis, auto-immune pancreatitis, sclerosing cholangitis
- *Calcific:* Heritable pancreatitis (cationic trypsinogen deficiency, SPINK1 and CFTR mutations), hypercalcemia, hyperlipidemia, juvenile tropical pancreatitis
- *Idiopathic:* (30%)

## PATHOPHYSIOLOGY

- *Acute Pancreatitis:* Inappropriate activation of enzymes within pancreatic parenchyma leads to inflammation and tissue destruction resulting in necrosis of peripancreatic fat, interstitial edema, and cytokine release
  ✓ Complications include hypocalcemia, hyperglycemia, GI hemorrhage, severe necrosis, pseudocyst rupture, abscess, acute tubular necrosis, gastritis, duodenitis, and pleural effusion
- *Chronic Pancreatitis:* Fibrotic parenchymal disease resulting from obstructive or calcific processes; exact mechanisms unknown
  ✓ Complications include pancreatic exocrine and endocrine insufficiency or failure
- *Hereditary Pancreatitis (cationic trypsinogen deficiency):* Autosomal dominant form of calcific chronic pancreatitis due to mutations of cationic trypsinogen, resulting in recurrent bouts of acute pancreatitis
- *Autoimmune Pancreatitis:* Associated with increased IgG levels (particularly IgG4), presence of autoantibodies, diffuse enlargement of pancreas, narrowing of main pancreatic duct, and lymphocytic infiltration of the pancreas with fibrotic changes

## CLINICAL MANIFESTATIONS

- *Acute Pancreatitis:* Severe abdominal pain of acute onset; +/− epigastric location; nausea, vomiting, anorexia. Clinical course is highly variable
  ✓ Most commonly is a self-limited process resolving over a period of 5–8 days on average in previously healthy children
  ✓ A minority may develop a systemic inflammatory response syndrome (SIRS) with hypotension, renal failure, pulmonary edema or pleural effusions, hemorrhage, and shock
- *Chronic Pancreatitis:* Recurring or persistent abdominal pain or painless; some patients have recurrent episodes of acute pancreatitis; pain diminishes as pancreas burns out (may take 10–20 years);
  ✓ Other manifestations include pancreatic exocrine or endocrine insufficiency (end-stage), steatorrhea, excessive appetite, growth failure, obstructive jaundice

## DIAGNOSTICS

- *Amylase:* Level increases early; lasts 3–5 days
- *Lipase:* More specific than amylase; typically elevated longer
- In chronic pancreatitis, enzyme levels may not be increased
- *C-reactive protein:* Peaks at 36–48 hours
- *Markers of severe disease:* Hyperglycemia, hypocalcemia, hypoxemia, hypoproteinemia, high BUN, high white blood cells, low hematocrit
- *Abdominal x-ray:* To exclude other causes of abdominal pain
- *Chest x-ray:* Evaluate for pleural effusion

- *Ultrasound:* Pancreatic inflammation, calcification, ductular dilatation, stones, pseudocyst
- *CT:* Only needed when ultrasound is technically unsatisfactory (sensitivity >90% if necrosis involves >30% of pancreas). Consider CT-guided fine-needle aspiration if diagnosis of necrosis/infection uncertain

## MANAGEMENT

- Supportive care, bed rest
- Nothing by mouth and nasogastric decompression if vomiting
- Fluid and electrolyte replacement. May need aggressive fluid resuscitation, requiring 1.5–2× maintenance intravenous fluids in early phases of disease
- Early nutrition with jejunal enteral feeds. Some evidence suggests early nasogastric feedings may be appropriate, but this remains an area of active research
- TPN reserved for patients who cannot safely tolerate enteral feedings
- Monitor acid/base status, electrolytes, renal function
- *Analgesia:* Ibuprofen, tramadol, narcotics
- *Adjuncts in chronic pancreatic pain:* Amitriptyline, nortriptyline, neurontin
- *Antibiotics:* For severe systemic illness or pancreatic necrosis (imipenem, ticarcillin-clavulanate, piperacillin-tazobactam, or ciprofloxacin + metronidazole)
- Repeat ultrasound or an alternative imaging study may be useful for patients not improving as expected to evaluate for pseudocyst, abscess, necrosis, or hemorrhage
- Attempt to identify underlying cause to help prevent recurrence
- ERCP to relieve stones or strictures
- Surgical management of complications such as symptomatic pseudocyst, abscess, necrosis, hemorrhage. Surgical correction of structural lesions is performed after acute illness resolves
- Once symptoms resolve and able to tolerate oral feedings, maintain on low-fat diet until complete recovery or indefinitely in chronic cases; consider pancreatic enzymes

---

*Medication recommendations in this chapter may be off label based on patient age or specific disease. Consult product insert for further information*

# CHAPTER 11

# Genetics

*Elizabeth Bhoj, MD, PhD*
*Rebecca Ahrens-Nicklas, MD, PhD*
*Tara L. Wenger, MD, PhD*

## GENETIC APPROACH TO EVALUATION OF COMMON PROBLEMS

### AN INFANT WITH DYSMORPHIC FEATURES OF MULTIPLE ANOMALIES

**Major anomalies are structural defects that require surgery or ongoing medical care (e.g., cleft palate, cardiac defects, hypospadias). Minor anomalies are unusual morphologic features that are of no serious medical or cosmetic consequence to the patient (e.g., single palmar crease, low-set ears, clinodactyly).**

### EPIDEMIOLOGY

- Major anomalies are detected in 3% of newborns, but up to 7% of children will have a defect identified by the age of 5 years
- Minor anomalies are found in 15% of children
- Only 1% of children have three or more anomalies, 90% of whom also have at least one major anomaly
- A child with multiple minor anomalies should be evaluated for the presence of a major anomaly

### IMPACT

- Birth defects are the second leading cause of death in the first month of life (second only to prematurity)

### ETIOLOGY

- *Chromosome rearrangements:* 5–10%
- *Single gene defects:* 10–15%
- *Environmental (nongenetic) factors:* 10%
- *Polygenic/multifactorial causes:* 35–40%
- *Unknown:* 30%

### DIAGNOSTIC CONSIDERATIONS

- *Age of parents:*
  ✓ Advanced maternal age is associated with increased rate of Trisomy 21, and other chromosomal disorders (Table 11-1)
  ✓ Advanced paternal age is associated with increased rate of de novo autosomal dominant single gene disorders
- *Multiple pregnancy losses:*
  ✓ Can indicate a balanced translocation or X-linked disorder that is lethal in males
  ✓ If available, genetic testing from these fetuses should be reviewed
- *Family history:*
  ✓ Identification of family members with similar birth defects, pregnancy losses, infertility, and whether the child resembles his or her family members

✓ Ethnicity should be elicited to determine the rarity of physical features (e.g., synophrys, hypertrophy and fusion of the eyebrows, is common in children of Middle Eastern descent, epicanthal folds are common in children of Asian descent) and to identify genetic conditions prevalent in certain ethnic groups

✓ Presence of consanguinity increases likelihood of autosomal recessive disorder in offspring

• *Medication/drug exposure during pregnancy:*

✓ Many medications (e.g., anticonvulsants, warfarin, retinoic acid) and other substances (e.g., alcohol) are associated with an increased rate of birth defects

• *Maternal medical conditions during pregnancy:*

✓ Risk due to medical condition itself (e.g., maternal diabetes associated with an increased risk of many birth defects including cardiac defects, duplicated great toe) or because of exposure to teratogenic medications (e.g., anticonvulsants, warfarin, retinoic acid)

• *Genetic screening or diagnostic testing during pregnancy:*

✓ Results of genetic screening (offered to all women) and diagnostic genetic testing (often done following abnormal screening or identification of anomalies) may not be recorded in the infant's chart, and these records should be requested

✓ Prenatal testing may have lower sensitivity than postnatal testing, and may need to be repeated

✓ Prenatal karyotypes are often limited to FISH for 13, 18, 21 and sex chromosomes. Request actual report to determine if full karyotype or limited karyotype was done, as both may be listed as "normal karyotype" in infant's chart

✓ Children with congenital heart disease may have also had FISH for 22q11.2 Deletion syndrome, which may not identify cases with duplications or smaller nested deletions, which cause a similar spectrum of defects

✓ Many prenatal microarrays do not report on copy number variants of uncertain significance during pregnancy, so consider repeating these tests after birth if clinically warranted

• *Pregnancy complications:*

✓ Some birth defects may be caused by pregnancy complications (e.g., maternal diabetes resulting in cardiac defects, oligohydramnios resulting in deformations), while some pregnancy complications may be the result of carrying an affected fetus (e.g., polyhydramnios in 22q11.2 Deletion syndrome, HELLP syndrome with fetus affected by long chain fatty acid dehydrogenase deficiency)

| TABLE 11-1 Incidence at Live Birth for Chromosomal Abnormalities | | |
|---|---|---|
| **Maternal Age at Delivery (Years)** | **Trisomy 21** | **All Chromosomal Anomalies** |
| 20 | 1/1667 | 1/526 |
| 25 | 1/1200 | 1/476 |
| 30 | 1/952 | 1/385 |
| 35 | 1/378 | 1/192 |
| 40 | 1/106 | 1/66 |
| 45 | 1/30 | 1/21 |

Reproduced with permission from Heffner LJ: Advanced maternal age—how old is too old? *N Engl J Med* 2004 Nov 4;351(19):1927-1929.

- *Medical state of infant:*
  ✓ Consider APGAR score, resuscitation, and continued support
  ✓ Determine whether appropriate exams and imaging have been done to identify other structural defects (e.g., echocardiogram, ophthalmologic exam, renal ultrasound, skeletal films)
  ✓ *For critically ill infants with suspected genetic disease:* Consider obtaining blood for DNA extraction prior to placement on ECMO, cardiopulmonary bypass, administration of whole blood, or for any critically ill infant in whom a genetic disease is suspected but not yet identified

## PHYSICAL EXAM

- Length, weight, and head circumference percentile should be corrected for gestational age, even within the "term" window and also compared to one another
- Careful identification of most severe features (e.g., Tetralogy of Fallot) along with most unusual features (e.g., epibulbar dermoids on eye exam) can help to narrow differential
- Systematic head-to-toe approach by body part (e.g., skull, hair, eyes, eyebrows, nose, ears) with focus on structure (e.g., ear placement, ear formation, presence of ear pits/folds) rather than functional organ system (e.g., cardiac exam, respiratory exam, neurologic exam) crucial for identification of minor anomalies
- Unusual features or abnormal measurements should be compared to family members (e.g., measure parental head circumferences, look at sibling photographs)

*Mimickers of Genetic Disease*
There are several recognizable syndromes that are not known to be associated with an identifiable genetic cause and typically have a low recurrence risk. As there is no specific test for these conditions, the workup in these cases primarily involves ruling out other genetic causes.

- *Decreased fetal movement (including fetal akinesia sequence):*
  ✓ Decreased fetal movement from a primary neurologic or neuromuscular cause can be associated with breech position, high arched or cleft palate, micrognathia, long fingers, abnormal skull shape, myopathic facies, and abnormal creases
- *VACTERL association:*
  ✓ *Children may have two or more of the following defects:* Vertebral anomalies (V), anal atresia (A), cardiovascular anomalies (C), tracheo-esophageal fistula (TE), renal or radial ray defects (R), and limb anomalies (L)
  ✓ Children with VACTERL have favorable cognitive outcomes and low recurrence risk
  ✓ Workup includes search for potential comorbid conditions (e.g., echocardiogram, spine imaging, limb films, renal ultrasound) and exclusion of other genetic conditions that may mimic VACTERL (e.g., genome-wide microarray to rule out aneuploidy, chromosome breakage studies to rule out Fanconi anemia in patients with involvement of radial ray)
- *Amniotic band syndrome:*
  ✓ Disruption of developing embryo or fetus by strands from amnion
  ✓ Characterized by limb or digit amputations (with normal appearing limb or digit until point where it is missing), hemangiomas, cleft lip and/or cleft palate
  ✓ Nongenetic and low risk of recurrence

- *Diabetic embryopathy:* Maternal diabetes is associated with increased rate of common birth defects as well as rare malformations, including duplicated hallux. Congenital heart disease, such as transposition of the great arteries, ventricular septal defect, and atrial septal defects are often found, as well as caudal regression, situs inversus, ureter duplex, renal agenesis, and anencephalus
  - ✓ May be associated with macrosomia or growth restriction
  - ✓ As maternal diabetes is common, genetic workup should not be limited based on presence of maternal diabetes. Diagnostic workup is focused on excluding other causes of specific malformations (e.g., microarray for congenital heart disease, sequencing of *GLI3* for duplicated hallux)
- *Moebius syndrome:*
  - ✓ Moebius syndrome is caused by palsy of the sixth and seventh cranial nerves, and is characterized by inturned eyes and limited facial movement giving an unusual facial appearance
  - ✓ Moebius has been linked to prenatal vascular insults
- *Goldenhar syndrome/hemifacial microsomia:*
  - ✓ Usually limited to underdevelopment of one or both sides of face and ear (including anotia in some), ear tags, lateral facial clefts, epibulbar dermoids, hearing loss
  - ✓ More rarely, can include life-threatening malformations of multiple organ systems (e.g., severe cardiac or skeletal anomalies)
  - ✓ Recurrence risk is low

## DIAGNOSTIC WORKUP

- First-line genetic testing will depend on level of suspicion for a specific syndrome
- Karyotype should be done for patients with suspected trisomies
- Specific gene sequencing should be done for suspected single gene disorders
- If a diagnosis is not clear from the initial exam, genome-wide microarray should be done to rule out aneuploidy
- Exome or genome sequencing may be considered for cases in which diagnosis remains elusive despite standard testing
- Metabolic workup should be considered, especially for patients with electrolyte abnormalities, involvement of multiple systems, or unexplained worsening of medical course
- Additional medical workup (e.g., ophthalmologic exam, echocardiogram, spine imaging) may help to identify comorbid conditions and narrow genetic differential

## GROWTH DISTURBANCES

**Over 1300 distinct genetic conditions with poor growth are listed in London Dysmorphology Database, of which approximately 285 have prenatal onset (London Dysmorphology Database, version 1.0.16). The majority of these syndromes have additional features, such as structural abnormalities, dysmorphic features, or developmental delay. When a genetic cause of poor or excessive growth is suspected, focused history and physical is critical to narrow differential. There are fewer genetic causes of overgrowth, but careful evaluation remains important for accurate categorization.**

## DIAGNOSTIC CONSIDERATIONS

- *Prenatal versus postnatal onset:* Birth weight, length, and head circumference should be plotted by gestational age at birth, including among term infants (37–42 weeks)
- *Degree of similarity to family member growth patterns:* Pedigree should be reviewed for recognizable inheritance pattern or size very different than relatives

- *Proportionate versus disproportionate:* Includes comparison of height, weight, and head circumference percentiles as well as individual body segment abnormalities (e.g., shortened long bones in skeletal dysplasia)
- *Symmetric versus asymmetric:* Should include comparison of limb length and girth to one another (left versus right) as well as obvious organomegaly (e.g., macroglossia) or differences in facial symmetry
- *Determine whether growth abnormality followed change in feeding patterns:* Assess for feeding difficulties or excessive eating. The presence of feeding difficulties does not preclude a genetic cause for poor growth, as some syndromes are associated with extreme feeding difficulties
- *Presence of dysmorphic features, birth defects, or intellectual disability:* When present, these features are helpful in syndrome identification
- Notable syndromes in which altered growth may be major presenting feature:

*Poor growth:*
- *Prenatal onset:* Russell–Silver syndrome (normal head circumference but short stature and low birth weight), skeletal dysplasias, chromosomal aberrations, microdeletion syndromes (e.g., Williams syndrome, 22q11.2 Deletion syndrome)
- *Postnatal onset:* Any syndrome with poor feeding or increased energy expenditure as a prominent feature

*Overgrowth:*
- *Prenatal onset:* Sotos syndrome, Weaver syndrome, Beckwith–Wiedemann syndrome, maternal diabetes
- *Postnatal onset:* Marfan syndrome

*Mixed growth pattern:*
- *Prader–Willi syndrome:* Weight gain is initially poor due to feeding difficulties, then excessive weight gain due to insatiable appetite. Very small hands and feet and short stature are usually present, sometimes requiring administration of growth hormone. Infants will also have profound hypotonia

*Asymmetric growth:*

Can be due to underdevelopment of one side, or overgrowth of the other. Identification of an abnormality on one side can be helpful in subtle cases (e.g., ear tags on smaller side of face in Goldenhar syndrome)

- *Underdevelopment of one or both sides of face:* Goldenhar syndrome, hemifacial microsomia
- *Overgrowth (asymmetry) of face or limbs:* Beckwith–Wiedemann syndrome, neurofibromatosis type I, Proteus syndrome, mosaicism (especially segmental)

## DIAGNOSTIC EVALUATION

- Karyotype, genome-wide microarray or specific gene testing may be indicated based on suspicion for individual syndromes
- Consider skeletal survey if skeletal dysplasia is suspected
- Additional medical workup including referral to Endocrinology or Gastroenterology may be necessary to rule out nongenetic etiologies while awaiting results of testing

## CARDIOMYOPATHY

**Hypertrophic Cardiomyopathy: Increased wall thickness of the left ventricle without chamber expansion, in the absence of abnormal ventricular load (i.e., not due**

**to hypertension, structural heart disease, or valve disease), with associated diastolic dysfunction.**

## EPIDEMIOLOGY

- Adult prevalence estimates of 1 in 500 adults have been reported; however, good pediatric data is lacking
- Estimated incidence in adults and children is reported to be between 0.24 and 0.47 per 100,000 per year

## GENETIC ETIOLOGIES

- *Non-syndromic:* Isolated cardiac sarcomeric gene mutations are present in at least 50% of cases where syndromic and metabolic etiologies have been excluded
- Common sites of sarcomeric gene mutations include the myosin light and heavy chains, troponins, and titin
- Usually inherited or de novo dominant mutations
- No dysmorphic features on exam
- *Syndromic:* Approximately 10% of cases are associated with a malformation syndrome

*Mutations in the RAS-MAPK pathway (Noonan, LEOPARD, and Costello syndromes):*
Due to mutations in the members of the RAS-mitogen activated protein kinase pathway, most commonly PTPN11.

- Physical features can include short stature, epicanthal folds, ptosis, hypertelorism, low posterior hairline, webbed neck, shield chest
- LEOPARD is characterized by lentigines (L), ECG abnormalities (E), ocular hypertelorism and obstructive cardiomyopathy (O), pulmonic stenosis (P), abnormalities of genitalia (A), retardation of growth (R), and deafness (D)
- Costello syndrome, due to mutations in HRAS, is associated with increased risk of malignancy and intellectual disability

*Pompe syndrome (glycogen storage disease type II):*
Due to decreased enzyme activity of acid alpha-glucosidase.

- In addition to cardiomegaly and hypertrophic cardiomyopathy, there is often hypotonia, feeding difficulties, failure to thrive, and hearing loss
- Enzyme-replacement therapy is available

## OTHER ETIOLOGIES

- *Inborn errors of metabolism:* Glycogen storage diseases, fatty acid oxidation defects, lysosomal storage diseases, mitochondrial disease
- *Neuromuscular disorders:* Friedrich's ataxia, myotonic dystrophy
- *Dilated cardiomyopathy:* Enlarged chamber volumes with normal or thinned walls and associated systolic dysfunction

## EPIDEMIOLOGY

- Annual incidence in children younger than 18 is 0.57 cases per 100,000
- Higher in boys than in girls (0.66 versus 0.47 cases per 100,000)
- Higher in African Americans than Caucasian children (0.98 versus 0.46 per 100,000)
- Higher in infants (<1 year) than in children (4.40 versus 0.34 cases per 100,000)

## GENETIC ETIOLOGIES

*Non-syndromic:* Up to 40% of dilated cardiomyopathy presents as inherited isolated cardiac disease.

- *Autosomal dominant:*
  - ✓ Extremely variable penetrance
  - ✓ Most mutations are private to individual families
  - ✓ A significant portion of nonfamilial cases are also found to have mutations
  - ✓ Unlike hypertrophic cardiomyopathy, mutations affect proteins with a variety of functions including sarcomeric, cytoskeleton, nuclear envelope, sarcolemma, calcium handling, RNA splicing, and trafficking proteins
- *Arrhythmia associated:*
  - ✓ A minority of patients may have conduction disease or supraventricular arrhythmias that may precede the diagnosis of dilated cardiomyopathy
  - ✓ Usually due to mutations in the genes encoding the nuclear envelope proteins Lamin A/C or Emerin, or the *SCN5A*-encoded cardiac sodium channel
- *Syndromic:* The vast majority of patients have isolated cardiac disease; however, a few extra-cardiac phenotypes are known
- *Dystrophinopathies:*
  - ✓ Dilated cardiomyopathy can occur in, Duchenne, and Becker muscular dystrophies due to mutations in *DMD*
  - ✓ In Duchenne, patients present with delayed milestones and progressive proximal weakness in early childhood; however, the cardiomyopathy usually presents after age 18
  - ✓ In Becker, presentation and cardiomyopathy presents later in life
- *Barth syndrome (3-methylglutaconic aciduria type 2):*
  - ✓ Due to mutations in *TAZ*, which lead to infant-onset dilated cardiomyopathy, skeletal myopathy, and neutropenia
- *Sensorineural hearing loss:*
  - ✓ Can occur in association with dilated cardiomyopathy in patients with *EYA4* mutations
  - ✓ *Initial workup:* Physical exam (with particular attention to motor exam and hearing), family history (including sudden cardiac death, arrhythmias), chest x-ray, ECHO, ECG, metabolic evaluation, genome-wide microarray, targeted gene sequencing

## STRUCTURAL CONGENITAL HEART DISEASE (CHD)

### EPIDEMIOLOGY

- CHD is the most common major congenital anomaly
- In North America estimated prevalence is 8.1 per 1000 live births
- Unlike in the past, now more than 75% of patients with CHD survive the first year, and the population of adult CHD patients is growing at a rate of almost 5% per year

### NONGENETIC ETIOLOGIES

- Causes include maternal exposures such as alcohol or antiepileptic medications, environmental exposures such as pesticides, and congenital infections such as rubella

### GENETIC ETIOLOGIES

*Syndromic due to aneuploidy:*

- Trisomy 21 (Down syndrome)
  - ✓ 40–50% of patients have CHD

✓ AV canal lesions are the prototypic finding
✓ Associated features include distinctive facial features, intellectual disability, hearing loss, thyroid disease, and short stature
- Trisomy 13 (Patau syndrome)
  ✓ 80–100% have CHD
  ✓ A wide variety of cardiac lesions can be present
  ✓ Associated features include very low survival rates, microphthalmia, polydactyly, and poor growth
- Trisomy 18 (Edwards syndrome)
  ✓ 80–100% have CHD
  ✓ A wide variety of cardiac lesions can be present
  ✓ Associated features include very low survival rates, rocker bottom feet, clenched fists, distinctive facies, and poor growth
- Monosomy X (Turner syndrome)
  ✓ 20–50% of patients have CHD
  ✓ Coarctation of the aorta is the prototypic lesion
  ✓ Associated features include short stature, webbed neck, wide-spaced nipples, and infertility

*Syndromic due to copy number variants (deletions or insertions):*

- *22q11.2 Deletion syndrome (formerly known as DiGeorge or Velocardiofacial syndrome):*
  ✓ 70–80% of patients have CHD, which is the major cause of mortality in 22q11.2 DS
  ✓ Lesions include Tetralogy of Fallot, aortic arch abnormalities, and ventricular septal defects. Cardiac defects linked to deletion of *TBX1*
  ✓ Associated features include underdevelopment of the thymus and parathyroid glands, cleft lip and/or palate, short stature, feeding difficulties, immunodeficiency, learning difficulties, and psychiatric disorders
- *Williams syndrome (7q11.23 deletion):*
  ✓ Up to 80–100% of patients have CHD
  ✓ Common lesions include supravalvar aortic stenosis, pulmonary artery stenosis, and valve abnormalities
  ✓ CHD due to deletion of *ELN*
  ✓ Associated features include distinctive facies, intellectual disability, feeding difficulties, hypercalcemia, outgoing personality, and anxiety

*Syndromic due to point mutations:*

- *Noonan and Costello syndromes:* See full description above under Cardiomyopathy, Genetic etiologies
  ✓ Both syndromes can have associated pulmonic stenosis, atrial or ventricular septal defects
- *Alagille syndrome (due to JAG1 or NOTCH2 mutations):*
  ✓ >90% of patients have CHD
  ✓ Common findings include peripheral pulmonary hypoplasia, pulmonic stenosis, and Tetralogy of Fallot
  ✓ Associated features include cholestasis with a paucity of bile ducts, eye abnormalities, and distinctive facies
- *CHARGE syndrome (due to CHD7 mutations):*
  ✓ 85% of patients have CHD
  ✓ Common lesions include pulmonic stenosis, atrial septal defects, and Tetralogy of Fallot

✓ Associated features include eye coloboma (C), heart defect (H), choanal atresia (A), retarded growth and development (R), genital hypoplasia (G), and ear and hearing abnormalities (E)

*Non-syndromic genetic etiologies:*

- Copy number variants
  ✓ About 10–15% of patients with isolated, sporadic CHD may have a rare copy number variant
- Point mutations
  ✓ Isolated CHD can be due to mutations in transcription factors and signaling molecules involved in the patterning and development of the embryonic heart. To date there have been dozens of genes identified, and this list is rapidly expanding
  ✓ *Initial workup:* Physical exam, family history, chest x-ray, echocardiogram, ECG, genome-wide microarray, targeted gene sequencing

## HYPOTONIA

**Decreased tone in any muscle or muscle group, can be divided into central hypotonia affecting the core trunk muscles, axial hypotonia affecting the limbs, or specific muscle group hypotonia, such as facial hypotonia. It may be very mild and only noticed on close testing, or so profound that respiration, swallowing, and reflexes are affected.**

### DIFFERENTIAL DIAGNOSIS

Hypotonia in an infant can be due to primary genetic cause (e.g., Trisomy 21, Prader–Willi), neurologic abnormality (e.g., lissencephaly, hypoxic-ischemic encephalopathy, myotonic dystrophy, spinal muscular atrophy), metabolic disease (e.g., Zellweger syndrome, Pompe, congenital disorder of glycosylation), or other medical issue (e.g., prematurity, sepsis, botulism).

### DIAGNOSTIC CONSIDERATIONS

*The search for a genetic cause of hypotonia, especially in a neonate, should include consideration of the following:*

- *Major malformations:* The presence of major malformations in an infant with hypotonia makes a genetic cause more likely (e.g., CHD more likely in hypotonia due to Trisomy 21 than hypotonia due to neuromuscular disease)
- *Minor dysmorphic features:* Minor dysmorphia that result from decreased fetal movement (e.g., high arched palate, long fingers, breech presentation with abnormal skull shape, abnormal creases) should be distinguished from minor dysmorphia unrelated to fetal movement (e.g., coarse facies, epicanthus)
- Prader–Willi syndrome should be considered in any infant with hypotonia and feeding difficulty. Many children with Prader-Willi will be fair compared to their family members and have very small hands and feet (less than the 3rd percentile)

### DIAGNOSTIC TESTING

- Genome-wide microarray should be done to rule out aneuploidy
- SNP microarray is preferred because it can assess loss of heterozygosity in cases where Prader–Willi is suspected
- Additional testing for Prader–Willi (methylation studies) may be indicated
- Karyotype should be done when Trisomy 21 is suspected. Additional sequencing for suspected single gene disorders can be done

- Additional nongenetic workup may include neuromuscular evaluation, electromyography, brain MRI to assess structural defects, and metabolic testing (e.g., transferrin isoelectric focusing to test for congenital disorders of glycosylation, 7-dehydrocholesterol to test for Smith–Lemli–Opitz syndrome, very long chain fatty acids to test for peroxisomal disorders)

## NOTABLE SYNDROMES LIKELY TO BE ENCOUNTERED IN AN INPATIENT SETTING

### 22q11.2 DELETION SYNDROME

**22q11.2 Deletion syndrome (22q11.2 DS), formerly known as DiGeorge syndrome and Velocardiofacial syndrome, is the most common contiguous gene deletion syndrome. Most cases affect the same about 3 Mb region encompassing approximately 45 genes.**

#### EPIDEMIOLOGY

- 1:4000 births, males and females equally affected

#### ETIOLOGY

- Approximately 90% of children with 22q11.2 DS are de novo, with 10% inherited from a parent
- There is a 50% chance of an affected parent passing the deletion to each offspring

#### CLINICAL CHARACTERISTICS

- *Cardiovascular malformations:* Most common defects include Tetralogy of Fallot, ventriculoseptal defect, interrupted aortic arch, truncus arteriosus, and vascular ring
- *Immune:* Immune deficiencies including T-cell lymphopenia, delayed IgG production, and thymic hypoplasia/aplasia
- *Palate:* Palatal defects including velopharyngeal insufficiency, cleft palate
- *Endocrine:* Endocrinologic abnormalities, including hypocalcemia
- *Neurodevelopmental:* Mild to moderate developmental delay, autism spectrum disorder (20%), psychosis (25%), and ADHD (50%)

#### DIAGNOSIS

- Genome-wide microarray or multiplex ligation-dependent probe amplification is the preferred diagnostic method for 22q11.2 DS
- The classic 22q11.2 deletion can be identified using FISH, but this technique may not identify patients with duplications or cases with atypical nested deletions

### BECKWITH–WIEDEMANN SYNDROME

**Beckwith–Wiedemann syndrome (BWS) is a disorder of imprinting that leads to somatic overgrowth and tumor predisposition, often diagnosed by the classic triad of symmetric or asymmetric gigantism, exomphalos, and macroglossia.**

#### EPIDEMIOLOGY

- Prevalence 1:14,000, with equal numbers of males and females
- No predominance in any ethnic group
- Increased risk with assisted reproduction (including in vitro fertilization and ovulation stimulating drugs)
- About 85% sporadic, 15% familial

## ETIOLOGY

- There are multiple causes of BWS, all leading to aberrant methylation at 11p15.5
- Sporadic loss of methylation at imprinting center (IC) 2 is the cause in about 50% of cases, with gain of methylation at IC1 accounting for 5% of cases
- 20% of cases are the result of paternal uniparental disomy of chromosome 11p15.5
- Another 5% are secondary to spontaneous and 40% to inherited *CDKN1C* mutations. Rarer causes include de novo and maternally derived translocations and inversions, and paternally derived duplications

## CLINICAL CHARACTERISTICS

- *Growth:* Height and weight are above the normal range early in life but final adult heights are normal (i.e., near the 50th percentile); head circumference typically remains in the 50th percentile. Hemihypertrophy can be prominent
- *Macroglossia:* May cause secondary feeding difficulties, speech problems, and obstructive sleep apnea.
- *Malignancy:* Children with BWS are at greatly increased risk (5–10%) of hepatoblastoma and Wilm's tumor, usually occurring in the first decade of life. Aggressive screening protocol including blood tests and imaging should be overseen by a pediatric oncologist
- *Hypoglycemia:* Elevated risk of hypoglycemia and hyperinsulinism
- *Other major anomalies:* Abdominal wall defects, organomegaly, renal anomalies, and cardiac malformations can also occur
- *Minor anomalies:* Common facial features include anterior earlobe creases, posterior helical pits, small midface with large mandible, facial nevus flammeus, infraorbital creases, and macroglossia; these become less striking in adulthood
- *Development:* Normal in most cases

## DIAGNOSIS

- Molecular testing is diagnostic in some cases, with slightly greater yield when an affected tissue is sampled (e.g., skin fibroblasts from the side with hypertrophy). Methylation-sensitive multiplex-ligation probe analysis, or sequencing of multiple methylation sensitive areas affected, is the standard test
- Genome-wide array (SNP rather than CGH array) should be performed rather than CGH array because SNP array can identify cases due to uniparental disomy

## NOONAN SYNDROME

**A genetic syndrome due to defect in the RAS-MAPK pathway characterized by distinctive facial features, congenital heart anomalies, and short stature.**

### EPIDEMIOLOGY

- Estimated prevalence is 1/1000–2500

### ETIOLOGY

Mutations in genes encoding RAS-MAPK pathway proteins (most commonly PTPN11) lead to overactivation of several different growth factor, cytokine, and hormone cell-signaling pathways.

### CLINICAL CHARACTERISTICS

- *Facial features:* Hypertelorism, epicanthal folds, ptosis, downslanting palpebral fissures, short broad nose, webbed neck

- *Growth:* Normal birth weight and length followed by short stature, feeding difficulties, failure to thrive, delayed puberty
- *Cardiac:* Pulmonic stenosis, hypertrophic cardiomyopathy, atrial septal defects, etc.; 25% of patients die of heart failure in the first year
- *Hematologic:* Coagulation defects, thrombocytopenia, myeloproliferative disorder
- *Other:* Hearing loss, cryptorchidism, male infertility, lymphatic abnormalities, chest deformities, widely spaced nipples, acid reflux, variable cognitive impairment

## DIAGNOSIS

- Sequencing of genes in the RAS-MAPK pathway known to cause Noonan syndrome

## PRADER–WILLI SYNDROME

**Imprinting defect due to lack of expression from paternally derived chromosome 15q11.2-q13 resulting in profound hypotonia, neonatal feeding difficulties with later hyperphagia and obesity, and developmental delay.**

### EPIDEMIOLOGY

- 1:10,000–30,000

### ETIOLOGY

- Lack of expression of paternal genes from chromosome 15q11.2-q13, either from deletion of the region of paternally chromosome 15 (70%), maternal uniparental disomy (UPD) 15 (25%), or imprinting defect (<5%.)

### CLINICAL CHARACTERISTICS

- *Hypotonia:* Neonatal hypotonia which may be profound
- *Feeding difficulty in infancy:* Poor suck and difficulty eating, often with failure to thrive as an infant
- *Hyperphagia:* After infancy period, hyperphagia predominates with resultant obesity
- *Endocrine:* Short stature, pubertal delay, and small genitalia
- *Sleep:* Sleep apnea
- *Neurodevelopment:* Developmental delay, increased rate of autism spectrum disorder, skin picking, speech articulation defects
- *Minor dysmorphic features:* Characteristic facial features of almond-shaped eyes, narrow bifrontal diameter, narrow nasal bridge, and down-turned mouth with thin upper lip; small hands and feet

### DIAGNOSIS

- Genetic testing should evaluate different mechanisms that can result in the phenotype, including methylation-sensitive PCR of 15q11.2-q13, SNP genome-wide microarray to assess for microdeletion or maternal uniparental disomy, sequencing of imprinting center for defects

## TRISOMY 21

**Also known as "Down syndrome," a genetic condition caused by an additional copy of chromosome 21, characterized by hypotonia, CHD, and intellectual disability.**

### EPIDEMIOLOGY

- 1/660 newborns, with increased risk by increasing maternal age (see Table 11.1)

## ETIOLOGY

- Caused by an additional copy of chromosome 21, by nondisjunction (94% with full Trisomy 21, 2.4% with mosaic Trisomy 21) or Robertsonian translocation (3.3%)
- Risk of recurrence low in nondisjunction (approximately 1%), high in Robertsonian translocation carriers

## CLINICAL CHARACTERISTICS

*Principle features in the neonate:* Evaluation of a neonate for Trisomy 21 should include systematic evaluation, rather than just relying on facial features. This is particularly important right after birth, when facial features may be distorted. Features seen in most neonates with Trisomy 21 include:

- Hypotonia (80%)
- Poor Moro reflex (85%)
- Hyperflexibility of the joints (80%)
- Excess skin on the back of the neck (80%)
- Flat facial profile (90%)
- Slanted palpebral fissures (80%)
- Anomalous auricles (60%)
- Dysplasia of pelvis (70%)
- Dysplasia of midphalynx of fifth finger (60%)
- Simian crease (45%)

At least four features found in 100%, and at least six features found in 89% of neonates with Trisomy 21.

*Congenital heart disease:* Cardiac defect in 40% (most often endocardial cushion defect).
*Gastrointestinal tract abnormalities:* Hirschsprung disease, duodenal atresia, tracheoesophageal fistula, omphalocele, pyloric stenosis, annular pancreas, imperforate anus.
*Endocrine:* Hypothyroidism.
*Hematologic:* Leukemia.
*Skeletal:* Atlanto-axial instability, hip dysplasia, avascular necrosis or slipped capital femoral epiphyses.
*Neurodevelopmental:* Developmental delay, hearing loss.

## DIAGNOSIS

- Standard karyotype
- Accurate identification can often be made shortly after birth by physical characteristics, but standard karyotype should be done to confirm diagnosis and determine mode of inheritance for determination of recurrence risk

## WILLIAMS SYNDROME

**Second most common contiguous gene deletion syndrome, characterized by supravalvar aortic stenosis, hypercalcemia, feeding difficulties, outgoing personality, anxiety, and developmental delay.**

## EPIDEMIOLOGY

- 1:10,000

## ETIOLOGY

- About 98% of patients have a classic 1.5–1.8 Mb deletion on chromosome 7q11.23, encompassing 26–28 genes
- 2% have a smaller deletion with a milder phenotype

## CLINICAL CHARACTERISTICS

- *Cardiac disease:* Most commonly supravalvular aortic stenosis
- *Growth:* Failure to thrive in infancy with poor growth, should use Williams syndrome specific growth charts
- *Endocrine:* Hypercalcemia
- *Musculoskeletal:* Joint laxity early in life, may develop stiffness and joint contractures
- *Neurodevelopment:* Profound intellectual disability is common, with relatively preserved language, outgoing personality, and anxiety
- *Facial features:* Delicate facial features with a low nasal bridge, described as "elfin facies"

## DIAGNOSIS

- Genome-wide microarray or MLPA is preferred for diagnosis, as FISH may miss children with atypical, nested deletions and duplications

# 12

# Hematology*

*Erin Blevins, MD, MSCE†*
*Char Witmer, MD, MSCE*

## ANEMIA

### RED BLOOD CELL (RBC) INDICES

- *Hematocrit (HCT):* Volume percentage of RBCs in blood. See Table 12-1 for age-related normal levels
- *Mean corpuscular volume (MCV):* Average RBC volume
- *Mean corpuscular hemoglobin (MCH):* Average quantity of hemoglobin per RBC
- *Mean corpuscular hemoglobin concentration (MCHC):* Grams of hemoglobin per 100 mL of packed RBCs (amount of hemoglobin per unit volume)
- *Red cell distribution width (RDW):* Index of the variation in RBC size
- *Reticulocyte count:* Percentage of young RBCs in the plasma

### DIFFERENTIAL DIAGNOSIS BASED ON MEAN CORPUSCULAR VOLUME

*Microcytic Anemia*

- Iron deficiency, thalassemia, anemia of inflammation, lead poisoning, sideroblastic anemia, copper deficiency
- *Iron deficiency versus thalassemia trait:* RBC count and RDW are often normal in thalassemia trait; in iron deficiency, low RBC count and elevated RDW; Mentzer index (MCV/RBC) serves as useful screen (<13 suggests thalassemia trait, >13 suggests iron deficiency)

*Normocytic Anemia*

- In normocytic anemia, assess the reticulocyte count. The reticulocyte index accurately reflects erythropoiesis by adjusting for the degree of anemia
- Reticulocyte index (RI) = % Reticulocyte × Patient HCT/Normal HCT
- RI is greater than 3% in compensated bleeding or hemolysis and less than 2% in anemia due to decreased RBC production; 1% is normal marrow activity without anemia
- *Reticulocytes low:* Pure RBC dysplasia (Diamond–Blackfan anemia), transient erythroblastopenia of childhood, aplastic crisis (e.g., secondary to parvovirus B19 infection), renal disease; acute bleed (without compensation), marrow infiltration (e.g., leukemia, solid tumor, or hemophagocytosis), marrow aplasia (aplastic anemia), hormone deficiencies (e.g., hypothyroidism or growth hormone deficiency), anemia of inflammation
- *Reticulocytes high:*
  - ✓ Chronic blood loss
  - ✓ *Extrinsic hemolysis:* Antibody-mediated hemolysis (e.g., auto- or drug-induced), disseminated intravascular coagulation (DIC), hemolytic-uremic syndrome (HUS),

---

*The views expressed in this presentation are those of the author and do not necessarily reflect the official policy or position of the Department of the Navy, Department of Defense, or the United States government.*
*†I am a military service member. This work was prepared as part of my official duties. Title 17, USC, §105 provides that "Copyright protection under this title is not available for any work of the U.S. Government." Title 17, USC, §101 defines a US Government work as a work prepared by a military service member or employee of the US Government as part of that person's official duties.*

| TABLE 12-1 | Normal Hemoglobin, Hematocrit, and Mean Corpuscular Volume Values by Age* | | |
|---|---|---|---|
| **Age** | **Hemoglobin (g/dL)***| **Hematocrit (%)***| **MCV (Mean −2SD)** |
| Newborn | 16.8 (13.7–20.1) | 55 (45–65) | 108 (98) |
| 2 weeks | 16.5 (13.0–20.0) | 50 (42–66) | 105 (86) |
| 3 months | 12.0  (9.5–14.5) | 36 (31–41) | 91 (74) |
| 6 months–2 years | 12.0 (10.5–14.0) | 37 (33–42) | 78 (70) |
| 7–12 years | 13.0 (11.0–16.0) | 38 (34–40) | 86 (77) |
| Women (adult) | 14.0 (12.0–16.0) | 42 (37–47) | 90 (80) |
| Men (adult) | 16.0 (14.0–18.0) | 47 (42–52) | 90 (80) |

*Mean values with ranges in parentheses. MCV, mean corpuscular volume. These data have been compiled from several sources.

thrombotic thrombocytopenic purpura (TTP), prosthetic heart valve, vitamin E deficiency, Wilson disease, liver disease, renal disease, burns

✓ *Intrinsic hemolysis:* Membrane disorders (e.g., hereditary spherocytosis), enzyme deficiencies (e.g., G6PD), hemoglobin disorders (e.g., sickle cell disease)

*Macrocytic Anemia*

- Folic acid deficiency, vitamin $B_{12}$ deficiency, normal newborn (MCV 100–125), Down syndrome, medications (e.g., valproate, trimethoprim/sulfamethoxazole, hydroxyurea, azathioprine), marrow failure (e.g., Fanconi anemia), dyserythropoietic anemia, hypothyroidism, liver disease, inborn errors of metabolism (e.g., oroticaciduria, Lesch–Nyhan)

## GLUCOSE-6-PHOSPHATE DEHYDROGENASE DEFICIENCY

**Deficiency in the major enzyme in the hexosemonophosphate shunt; results in a decrease in the oxidative protective mechanism of the RBC. An oxidative stress may cause RBC hemolysis.**

### EPIDEMIOLOGY

- X-linked inheritance; most common enzyme deficiency, affects more than 500 million people worldwide (African, Mediterranean, and Asian origins)
- African American (10–15% affected) variant is less severe than Mediterranean variant

### CLINICAL MANIFESTATIONS

- Neonatal jaundice (further discussed in management section)
- For milder forms patients are clinically and hematologically normal until they have an "oxidative challenge." Severe forms can have a baseline hemolytic anemia
- *6–24 hours after exposure to oxidative agent:* Dark urine, jaundice, pallor, tachycardia, nausea, abdominal pain
- *24–48 hours:* Low-grade fever, irritability, listlessness, splenomegaly, and hepatomegaly

### DIAGNOSTICS

- *Glucose-6-phosphate dehydrogenase (G6PD) quantitation:* G6PD concentration highest in young RBCs, so the presence of reticulocytosis can lead to overestimation of true G6PD level

*During Hemolytic Episode:*
- Normocytic, normochromic anemia with reticulocytosis
- *Smear:* Anisocytosis (reflected by increased RDW), spherocytosis, blister cells, Heinz bodies on supravital staining with methyl violet (precipitates of denatured hemoglobin)
- Elevated unconjugated bilirubin
- Urine dipstick positive bilirubin
- Direct antiglobulin test (DAT) negative (excludes autoimmune hemolysis)

## MANAGEMENT

- Avoid oxidative stressors including sulfonamides, fava beans, or antimalarial agents (table of more specifics available in most pharmacies)
- Most episodes of acute hemolysis are self-limited with hemoglobin returning to normal within 3–6 weeks
- If hemoglobin greater than 7 mg/dL and clinically stable and no hemoglobinuria, observe closely for 24–48 hours. If hemoglobin less than 7 mg/dL or between 7 and 9 mg/dL with continued brisk hemolysis (persistent hemoglobinuria), consider packed RBC transfusion (see Transfusion Medicine section)
- Management of neonatal jaundice associated with G6PD deficiency similar to approach for other causes of neonatal jaundice. Initiate prompt phototherapy if serum bilirubin greater than 15 mg/dL in first 2 days of life, or greater than 20 mg/dL during first week of life. Infants with the more severe type may require exchange transfusion to prevent kernicterus (more common in Mediterranean and Asian variants)

## HEREDITARY SPHEROCYTOSIS

**Disorder of the red blood cell membrane resulting in a decreased membrane surface area to intracellular volume ratio.**

### EPIDEMIOLOGY

- Most common in people of northern European heritage
- 75% inherited (2/3 as autosomal dominant) and 25% new mutations

### PATHOPHYSIOLOGY

- Defect or deficiency of red cell skeletal proteins (ankyrin, spectrin)
- Decreased deformability of the RBC due to membrane loss results in sequestration in the spleen and depletion of membrane lipid results in spherocytes and premature destruction of RBCs

### CLINICAL MANIFESTATIONS

- *Anemia:* Mild to severe; patients may have hyperhemolytic periods and are susceptible to an aplastic crisis from parvovirus infection
- Jaundice, splenomegaly, gallstones
- 50% of HS patients present in the newborn period with jaundice

### DIAGNOSTICS

- Normocytic hemolytic anemia with increased reticulocyte count, high RDW, and MCHC
- *Smear:* Spherocytes, anisocytosis, polychromasia
- *HS-EMA (eosin-5'-maleimide) Binding Assay:* A flow cytometry assay with improved sensitivity and specificity over the osmotic fragility test for detecting hereditary spherocytosis

## MANAGEMENT

- Daily folic acid supplementation
- *Splenectomy:* For severe cases (i.e., failure to thrive or recurrent transfusions). This stops red cell destruction in the spleen and lengthens the red cell lifespan. If possible, delay splenectomy until the patient is 5 years of age or older to decrease risk of infection
- Transfusion support if needed

## IRON-DEFICIENCY ANEMIA

**Microcytic anemia with a decreased reticulocyte count and increased RDW due to a deficiency of iron.**

### ETIOLOGY

- *Inadequate oral intake:* Excessive/exclusive cow's milk intake in toddlers or a restrictive diet
- *Inadequate iron absorption:* Loss or dysfunction of absorptive enterocytes (celiac disease, inflammatory bowel disease, bowel resection, or genetic defects in intestinal iron uptake)
- *Excessive blood loss:* Gastrointestinal blood loss (Meckel's diverticulum, gastritis, ulcer, vascular malformation, varices, inflammatory bowel disease, tumor (rare in children), parasitic infection, cow's milk induced enteropathy), hematuria, menstrual blood loss, other excessive bleeding (epistaxis), pulmonary hemosiderosis
- *Increased iron demand:* Neonatal growth, adolescent growth, pregnancy
- The most common etiology in children ages 1–3 years is dietary

### PATHOPHYSIOLOGY

- Iron is required for heme synthesis as well as other systemic enzymes (i.e., cytochromes)

### CLINICAL PRESENTATION

- Mild or moderate iron deficiency may have few overt symptoms
- Progressive pallor, irritability, difficulty sleeping, fatigue, pica (including pagophagia or ice chewing)
- History of drinking greater than 24 ounces of cow's milk a day or transition to cow's milk before 12 months is common

### DIAGNOSTICS

- CBC with reticulocyte count
- *Iron studies:* High TIBC, low transferrin, and low ferritin (first value to change with iron deficiency). Ferritin, an acute phase reactant, can be elevated in other conditions. The plasma iron level varies with recent consumption of iron and is not reliable

### MANAGEMENT

- **Iron deficiency is always secondary to an underlying cause. It is imperative that the etiology is determined in concert with iron replacement**
- *Iron:* 4–6 mg/kg/day of elemental iron in two to three divided doses (best absorption with high ascorbic acid foods/juices)
- Continue iron for 8–12 weeks after the hemoglobin (Hb) has normalized (total of 3–4 months of replacement)
- *For toddlers with excessive mild intake make dietary changes:* Limit milk intake (<24 ounces per day); only offer milk once the child has eaten a meal, stop using the bottle (if appropriate), increase intake of iron-rich foods

- *Response to therapy:* Reticulocyte count will start to increase in 2–3 days, increased in hemoglobin in 1 week, normalization in hemoglobin within 4–6 weeks, normalization of RDW after 3 months of therapy

## SICKLE CELL DISEASE

**Sickle cell disease (SCD) is a group of inherited hemoglobinopathies secondary to the production of abnormal hemoglobin complicated with an associated hemolytic anemia and vaso-occlusion. Normal adult hemoglobin (Hb A) is composed of four polypeptide globulin chains ($2\alpha 2\beta$). Sickle cell disease results from a genetic mutation in both $\beta$-globulin genes with at least one mutation resulting in HbS. Homozygous SS is the most common form of SCD and is the most severe. Additional forms of SCD include compound heterozygous states where HbS is combined with either another abnormal hemoglobin or a beta-thalassemia mutation (e.g., HbC, HbE, beta-plus ($\beta^+$) thalassemia, or beta-zero ($\beta^0$) thalassemia). Sickle cell trait, present in up to 8% of African Americans, is the heterozygous state where one gene produces normal beta globin and the other produces HbS resulting in a primarily asymptomatic carrier.**

### COMMON COMPLICATIONS OF SICKLE CELL DISEASE

*Painful Episode*

- *Definition:* Vaso-occlusive event resulting in an acute onset of pain; often involves hands and feet in infants (dactylitis)
- *Management:* Patients may be managed as outpatients with oral medications (anti-inflammatory, +/− an oral opioid) and hydration; severe pain not responsive to oral pain medications requires hospitalization, appropriate pain control includes a combination of an anti-inflammatory agent such as ibuprofen or ketorolac (IV) with an opioid, and IV hydration

*Fever*

- *Definition:* Temperature >38.5°C. Patients with SCD are more susceptible to bacterial infections because of functional asplenia. They are at highest risk for sepsis from encapsulated organisms, such as *Streptococcus pneumoniae*
- *Management:* All patients with SCD and fever need to be urgently evaluated with a physical examination, blood culture, CBC with differential and a reticulocyte count; consider a urine culture, chest x-ray (dependent on age and symptoms); administration of antibiotics (ceftriaxone or high-dose ampicillin) with observation
- To prevent bacterial infections, patients with SCD should be vaccinated (pneumococcal conjugate vaccine (PCV13) and the 23-valent pneumococcal polysaccharide vaccine) and take prophylactic penicillin VK (125 mg orally twice daily until age 3 years then 250 mg orally twice daily) from birth until at least the age of 5 years

*Splenic Sequestration*

- *Definition:* Intrasplenic trapping of RBCs
- *Clinical manifestations:* A decrease in hemoglobin with an acute enlargement of the spleen; in SCD-SS approximately 30% will have an episode by 5 years of age; often associated with acute viral/bacterial illnesses; in milder forms of SCD, such as SCD-SC or SCD-Sβ+-thalassemia, splenic sequestration can occur at an older age
- *Management:* Follow the hemoglobin and spleen size closely; if splenomegaly and anemia result in hypoxia, tachypnea, or significant tachycardia then transfuse with RBCs (5 cc/kg),

then reassess. RBC transfusion causes remobilization of sequestered blood, resulting in a higher post-transfusion hemoglobin than expected from the transfused blood alone

*Acute Chest Syndrome*

- *Definition/Clinical manifestations:* Clinical diagnosis based on the findings of fever, respiratory symptoms, and a new pulmonary infiltrate on chest x-ray (findings can lag behind the clinical symptoms). Causes include bacterial infection (*Mycoplasma pneumoniae, Chlamydia pneumoniae, Staphylococcus aureus, S. pneumoniae,* or *Haemophilus influenzae*), viral infection, fat emboli, in situ vaso-occlusion, pulmonary edema, or thromboembolism
- *Management:* Antibiotics—macrolide (erythromycin, azithromycin, or clarithromycin) and ampicillin or a third-generation cephalosporin (cefotaxime or ceftriaxone); oxygen if hypoxic; pain control; incentive spirometry; RBC transfusion (simple or exchange) for respiratory or hemodynamic instability; may require intensive care monitoring

*Aplastic Crisis*

- *Definition:* Marked anemia with reticulocytopenia, frequently secondary to parvovirus infection which causes a maturation arrest of RBC production in the bone marrow for 1–2 weeks. Patients with SCD are dependent on their high reticulocyte count to maintain their hemoglobin secondary to their shortened RBC lifespan (10–20 days in SCD-SS versus 120 days in normal patients)
- *Clinical manifestations:* Increased fatigue, pallor, fever. Reticulocytopenia begins approximately 5 days after exposure and continues for 7–10 days
- *Management:* Packed RBC transfusion may be necessary if the patient is symptomatic

*Stroke*

Children with SCD-SS and $S\beta^0$-thalassemia have a 10% risk of stroke by age of 20 years. The predominant etiology is a large-vessel vasculopathy with proliferative intimal hyperplasia.

*Clinical manifestations:* Hemiparesis, facial droop, aphasia, generalized symptoms such as mental status changes, stupor, or seizures

*Management:* Head MRI or CT Scan (if MRI is not available); obtain a CBC with retic, %S, type, and screen. Principle treatment is exchange transfusion to decrease %S. Long term: placed on a chronic RBC transfusion protocol to minimize the risk for further strokes.

*Stroke prevention* is possible through routine transcranial Doppler imaging, which measures the velocity of cerebral blood flow and detects those children who are at an increased risk for a first stroke. Children with persistently elevated transcranial Doppler measurements are placed on a chronic RBC transfusion protocol to prevent stroke.

## THALASSEMIAS

The thalassemias encompass a group of inherited disorders of hemoglobin synthesis that involve decreased or defective synthesis of one or more globin chains. Thalassemias are named after the affected globin chain, with $\alpha$ and $\beta$ thalassemia being the most common and clinically important types. When one globin chain is ineffectively produced, the unaffected chains are overproduced, causing red cell abnormalities that lead to immature red cell destruction and a subsequent microcytic, hypochromic, hemolytic anemia.

**Beta-thalassemia is usually the result of point mutations that result in impaired or decreased $\beta$-globulin production The notation $\beta^+$ indicates decreased production while $\beta^0$ indicates absent production. The various conditions produced depend on the combination of the normal ($\beta$) or abnormal ($\beta^+$ or $\beta^0$) alleles. The designation of beta thalassemia intermedia or major is a clinical designation based on severity of anemia and need for lifelong transfusions.**

- *Beta-thalassemia trait* ($\beta^+/\beta$ or $\beta^0/\beta$): Heterozygous condition (one copy), causes a mild reduction in $\beta$-chain synthesis with a resultant mild microcytic anemia
- *Beta-thalassemia intermedia* ($\beta^+/\beta^+$ or $\beta^0/\beta^+$): Homozygous condition that results in markedly reduced $\beta$-chain synthesis and moderate anemia that will occasionally require transfusion
- *Beta-thalassemia major* ($\beta^0/\beta^0$ or $\beta^0/\beta^+$): Homozygous condition with no detectable to severely reduced $\beta$-chain production resulting in a severe microcytic hypochromic anemia that requires lifelong RBC transfusions (aka Cooley's anemia)

**Alpha-thalassemia is usually due to large deletions that result in impaired $\alpha$-globulin production. There are two $\alpha$-globin genes and therefore four different forms of inherited conditions:**

- *Silent carrier:* Deficient in one $\alpha$ gene ($-/\alpha$ $\alpha/\alpha$), and there is minimal effect on hemoglobin production
- *Alpha-thalassemia trait:* Deficient in two $\alpha$ genes ($-/-$ $\alpha/\alpha$ or $-/\alpha$ $-/\alpha$)
- *Hemoglobin H ($\beta4$) disease:* Deficient in three $\alpha$ genes ($-/-$ $-/\alpha$), with tetrameric $\beta$-chain production (hemoglobin H) which results in a mild microcytic hemolytic anemia
- *Hydrops fetalis:* Deficient in all four $\alpha$ genes ($-/-$ $-/-$); not compatible with life; in utero the fetus develops hydrops fetalis

## CLINICAL MANIFESTATIONS

- *Alpha- and $\beta$-thalassemia trait:* Mild microcytic anemia, asymptomatic
- *Hb H:* Mild hemolytic anemia, jaundice, hepatosplenomegaly, gallstones
- *Beta-thalassemia intermedia:* Moderate hemolytic anemia (Hb >7 g/dL), splenomegaly, intermittent transfusion requirement
- *Beta-thalassemia major:* Massive hepatosplenomegaly, growth retardation, bony deformities including frontal bossing and maxillary prominence from extramedullary hematopoiesis (all preventable with aggressive transfusion therapy)
- If iron overload from chronic transfusions is not adequately treated with chelation therapy patients can develop cirrhosis, endocrine abnormalities, cardiac dysfunction, and skin hyperpigmentation

## DIAGNOSTICS

- Hematologic parameters vary depending on severity of condition
- *Alpha-thalassemia trait:* Mild microcytic anemia, normal levels of Hb A, A2, and F; +Hb Barts ($\gamma$-chain tetramer) on newborn screen
- *Beta-thalassemia trait:* Mild microcytic, hypochromic anemia. HbA2 level 3.5–8%; HbF level 1–5% but significant variability depending on type of mutation. Not detected on newborn screen
- *Hemoglobin H:* Moderate hypochromic, microcytic anemia (Hb 7–10 g/dL); RBC fragmentation on peripheral smear and other findings of chronic hemolysis, reticulocytosis, Hb H ($\beta4$) on electrophoresis. Newborn screen >25% hemoglobin Barts
- *Beta-thalassemia intermedia* ($\beta^+/\beta^+$ or $\beta^0/\beta^+$): Clinical designation based on having a moderate microcytic anemia, Hb >7 g/dL, that only necessitates intermittent transfusion with normal growth
- *Beta-thalassemia major* ($\beta^0/\beta^0$ or $\beta^0/\beta^+$): Clinical designation with a resultant severe anemia (Hb 3–7 g/dL); reticulocytosis; HbF 30–100%; HbA2 2–7%; MCV 50–60 fL. The newborn screen will demonstrate only hemoglobin F in patients without any beta globin production

## MANAGEMENT

- No intervention for α- or β-thalassemia trait
- Folic acid supplementation for those with Hb H
- Chronic transfusion therapy for β-thalassemia major may be required as early as 2 months, but necessary by 2 years; 10–15 mL/kg of packed RBCs required every 3–4 weeks; goal pre-transfusion hemoglobin is 9.0–10 g/dL
- Chelation therapy for chronically transfused patients with iron overload; oral/SC/IV chelators available and necessary 5–7 days per week

## TRANSIENT ERYTHROBLASTOPENIA OF CHILDHOOD (TEC)

**An acquired, self-limited anemia in a previously healthy child characterized by bone marrow erythroblastopenia, which can be severe.**

### ETIOLOGY

- Unknown; often preceded by viral illness (can be 1–2 months prior to presentation)

### EPIDEMIOLOGY

- *Age of onset:* 6 months–4 years (80% are >1 year at diagnosis)

### CLINICAL MANIFESTATIONS

- Gradually progressive pallor in an otherwise healthy child
- No organomegaly, ecchymosis, petechiae, or jaundice
- Spontaneous recovery within 1–2 months

### DIAGNOSTICS

- *Hb level:* 3–8 g/dL (normocytic and normochromic)
- Low reticulocyte count
- White blood cell and platelet counts are typically normal
- Neutropenia (ANC <1000/mm$^3$) in 10% of cases
- *Bone marrow:* Decreased RBC precursors (not required for diagnosis)

### MANAGEMENT

- Transfusions for symptomatic anemia (see Transfusion Medicine section)
- Recovery typically occurs within 1-2 months but rarely may take as long as 12 months

## BLEEDING DISORDERS

## COAGULATION STUDIES

*Activated partial thromboplastin time (aPTT):* **Measures the intrinsic clotting system, which includes factors V, VIII, IX, X, XI, XII, fibrinogen, prothrombin, and the other contact factors.**

*Prothrombin time (PT):* **Measures the extrinsic clotting system which includes factor V, VII, X, fibrinogen, and prothrombin (standardized with the International Normalized Ratio, INR).**

*Thrombin time:* **Measures the final step of the coagulation cascade with the conversion of fibrinogen to fibrin.**

*Bleeding time:* **(Rarely used due to low sensitivity) evaluates platelet plug formation.**

## HEMOPHILIA

**Bleeding disorder affecting primarily males that results from an inherited deficiency of either factor VIII (hemophilia A) or IX (hemophilia B).**

### EPIDEMIOLOGY

- *Hemophilia A:* 1 in 5000 live male births (85%)
- *Hemophilia B:* 1 in 30,000 live male births (15%)
- Both are X-linked recessive; 30% spontaneous mutation rate

### PATHOPHYSIOLOGY

- Factors VIII and IX participate in the activation of factor X
- Factor Xa converts prothrombin to thrombin, which can then cleave fibrinogen to fibrin leading to clot formation
- Deficiency of either factor VIII or IX results in impaired clot formation

### CLINICAL MANIFESTATIONS

- Hemophilia A and B are clinically indistinguishable
- *Three major classifications (bleeding is related to amount of residual factor clotting activity that is present):* less than 1% = severe; 1–5% = moderate; >5–40% = mild
- Most common cause of morbidity is bleeding into joints (hemarthrosis), especially the knees, elbows, shoulders, ankles, and hips
- Life-threatening bleeding episodes may occur in the central nervous system (CNS) or in the pharynx or retropharynx
- Other bleeding sites include the urinary tract (with or without trauma), muscle bleeds, or excessive delayed postoperative bleeding. Post-circumcision bleeding is often the initial presentation in patients without a family history of hemophilia

### DIAGNOSTICS

- Prolonged PTT, normal PT, normal bleeding time
- *Factor VIII or IX activity:* Decreased (factor IX levels are low in normal newborns making diagnosis difficult in the newborn period)
- Carrier testing and prenatal diagnosis are available. Delivery by vaginal or C-section are appropriate, but avoid instrumentation (e.g., vacuum or forceps) whenever possible

### MANAGEMENT

- Replace the missing factor; in the past these factors were derived from pooled plasma, now there are recombinant factor products
- *Factor replacement therapy:* Determined by the type and severity of the bleed. Hemostatic levels are 35–40%. For life-threatening or major bleeds or head trauma, replace 100%. The initial half-life of factor VIII concentrate is 6–8 hours, with a subsequent half-life of 8–12 hours. The initial half-life of factor IX concentrate is 4–6 hours, with a subsequent half-life of 18–24 hours
- Dose of factor VIII (units) = % desired rise in plasma factor VIII × body weight (kg) × 0.5 (may vary per patient)
- Dose of factor IX (units) = % desired rise in plasma factor IX × body weight (kg) × 1.4 (may vary depending on product or patient)

- *Desmopressin (DDAVP):* For mild hemophilia A only; patients should have a DDAVP trial prior to using therapeutically. DDAVP causes the release of stored endogenously produced factor VIII and vWF
- *Recombinant factor VIIa:* Directly activates the intrinsic pathway; can be used in patients with inhibitors
- *Aminocaproic or tranexamic acid:* Antifibrinolytic medications, useful for oral bleeding; see formulary for dosing
- Avoid medicines that negatively affect platelet function (e.g., aspirin, NSAIDs)
- *Complications:* Chronic joint destruction causing pain and limiting mobility; transfusion transmitted diseases (not reported from recombinant products); inhibitor (neutralizing antibody) formation to factor VIII or factor IX

## VITAMIN K DEFICIENCY

**Vitamin K is a fat-soluble vitamin found in green leafy vegetables, pork, soybeans, and liver. Vitamin K is required for the post-translational carboxylation of specific coagulation factors: II, VII, IX, X, and protein C and S.**

### PATHOPHYSIOLOGY

- Infants not supplemented with vitamin K after delivery may develop hemorrhagic disease of the newborn (peak incidence at 2–5 days of life); infants born to mothers who were taking anticonvulsants, phenobarbital, and phenytoin are at higher risk
- Insufficient dietary intake
- *Altered gut colonization:* Vomiting, diarrhea, malabsorption (celiac disease, cystic fibrosis, biliary atresia, gastrointestinal tract obstruction), antibiotic use
- Hepatocelluar disease
- *Drugs:* Warfarin

### DIAGNOSTICS

- PT and PTT are prolonged
- Low vitamin K-dependent factors (II, VII, IX, X, protein C and S)

### MANAGEMENT

- Vitamin K may be given orally, SC, IM, or IV; see formulary for dosing; risk of anaphylaxis with IV administration

## VON WILLEBRAND DISEASE

**Most common inherited bleeding disorder; caused by an abnormality of von Willebrand factor (vWF)**

- *Type 1:* 70–80% of cases; decreased vWF levels (normal structure)
- *Type 2A:* Decreased high-molecular-weight multimers; more severe than type 1
- *Type 2B:* Increased binding of vWF to normal platelets resulting in a mild thrombocytopenia and a decrease in high-molecular-weight multimers
- *Type 2N:* Defect of the vWF factor VIII binding region; low factor VIII levels; mild hemophilia phenotype
- *Type 2M:* Functional defect of vWF poor binding to platelets; normal multimers

- *Type 3*: Homozygous deficiency; vWF levels are undetectable with resultant low factor VIII levels due to increased clearance; severe disease; presents like hemophilia A

## EPIDEMIOLOGY

- About 1% of the population
- Autosomal dominant inheritance is most common (type 1)
- Acquired vWF deficiency may be due to neoplasms (e.g., Wilms tumor), autoimmune disorders (e.g., hypothyroidism or SLE), myeloproliferative disorders, or lymphoproliferative disorders, cardiac defects resulting in high shear stress (i.e., aortic stenosis)

## PATHOPHYSIOLOGY

- vWF is a large glycoprotein synthesized in megakaryocytes and endothelial cells
- *vWF has two roles in hemostasis:* (1) Allows platelets to adhere to damaged endothelium; (2) serves as a carrier protein for factor VIII
- DDAVP can induce the release of stored vWF from endothelial cells

## CLINICAL MANIFESTATIONS

- *Mucocutaneous bleeding:* Easy bruising, recurrent epistaxis, menorrhagia
- Postsurgical or traumatic bleeding

## DIAGNOSTICS

*Levels of vWF can fluctuate. Normal studies do not necessarily exclude vWD. When the diagnosis is strongly suspected, patients may require up to three sets of laboratory studies before excluding the diagnosis.*

- *Bleeding time (no longer performed):* Often prolonged (but can be normal)
- *PTT:* Can prolong if factor VIII is decreased (can be normal)
- *vWF antigen level:* Measures the total vWF plasma concentration
- *vWF activity (ristocetin cofactor):* Decreased in all types, except it can be normal in type 2N. Ristocetin is an antibiotic that stimulates platelet aggregation in the presence of vWF
- *Factor VIII activity:* Normal to decreased
- *vW multimers:* Helps distinguish type of von Willebrand disease (vWD)

## MANAGEMENT

- *DDAVP:* Causes endothelial release of stored vWF with a two- to fivefold increase in plasma levels; most helpful for patients with type 1 vWD; side effects include hyponatremia, facial flushing, and headache; available in IV or intranasal formulations; see formulary for dosing. Not recommended in type 2B because it can worsen thrombocytopenia
- Plasma-derived vWF concentrates (Humate P, Alphanate)

*Dosed in ristocetin units:*

1 ristocetin U/kg = About 2% increase in vWF antigen

No. of ristocetin units = (weight in kg) × (% desired) × 0.5

- *Cryoprecipitate:* Only use if concentrates are not available; not detergent treated for viruses, but lower donor exposure than FFP
- *Aminocaproic acid or tranexamic acid:* Antifibrinolytic therapy; helpful in oral bleeding and menorrhagia respectively, see formulary for dosing

## THROMBOCYTOPENIA

### DIFFERENTIAL DIAGNOSIS

#### INCREASED PLATELET DESTRUCTION

- Immune thrombocytopenia (ITP), DIC, neonatal alloimmune thrombocytopenia (NAIT), hemolytic uremic syndrome, artificial heart valves or grafts, uremia, Kasabach–Merritt syndrome (see Chapter 6), TTP, other immune-mediated thrombocytopenias (HIV, systemic lupus erythematosus)
- *Medication-induced:* Aspirin, nitrofurantoin, heparin, sympathetic blockers, clofibrate, NSAIDs, sulfonamides, penicillin, quinidine, quinine, digoxin, procainamide, methyldopa, phenytoin, valproic acid, barbiturates, gold, cimetidine, ranitidine

#### DECREASED PLATELET PRODUCTION

- *Hereditary thrombocytopenias:* Thrombocytopenia-absent radii (TAR) syndrome, amegakaryocytic thrombocytopenia, Wiskott–Aldrich syndrome, Fanconi anemia, trisomy 13, trisomy 18, inherited giant platelet disorders
- *Marrow infiltration:* Acute lymphocytic leukemia, histiocytosis, lymphomas, neuroblastoma, storage diseases, marrow failure, aplastic anemia
- *Medications:* Thiazide diuretics, chemotherapeutic agents, alcoholism, estrogen, furosemide, trimethoprim/sulfamethoxazole
- *Infection-induced:* Cytomegalovirus, Epstein–Barr virus, varicella, rubella, rubeola, mumps, parvovirus B19, tuberculosis, typhoid

#### PLATELET SEQUESTRATION

- Splenomegaly, hypothermia, burns

#### OTHER

- Pseudothrombocytopenia (clumped in collection tube); dilutional

### IMMUNE THROMBOCYTOPENIA

**An autoimmune disorder characterized by thrombocytopenia and associated mucocutaneous bleeding.**

#### EPIDEMIOLOGY

- *Frequency:* 1 case per 10,000 children per year
- *Peak age:* 5 years; range, 2–6 years; male = female
- About 80% resolve within 6 months

#### PATHOPHYSIOLOGY

- Autoantibodies (IgG) to multiple membrane glycoproteins on the surface of platelets and megakaryocytes
- Autoantibody-coated platelets are cleared by opsonization and phagocytosis primarily in the spleen, but also throughout the reticuloendothelial system

#### CLINICAL MANIFESTATIONS

- Sudden onset of widespread petechiae and/or purpura, typically days or weeks after a viral illness
- Intracranial hemorrhage is rare; incidence is 0.1–0.5%

## DIAGNOSIS

- History and physical examination
- CBC and peripheral smear
- *Bone marrow aspirate may be helpful in atypical cases. It is not routinely recommended for the diagnosis of ITP*
- ITP is a diagnosis of exclusion. Other causes of thrombocytopenia need to be considered (see Differential Diagnosis of Thrombocytopenia)

## MANAGEMENT

- There is little evidence that treatment changes the long-term outcome. Children with no to mild bleeding (skin bleeding only) may be managed with observation only regardless of the platelet count. Treatment should be considered in patients with significant bleeding symptoms (e.g., mucosal, gastrointestinal, menstrual). The goal of treatment is to obtain adequate hemostasis
- *Intravenous Immunoglobulin (IVIG):* 1 g/kg/day for 1–2 days; improves platelet count in 75% of patients within 48 hours (usually does not increase until 24 hours after first dose given); recommended for patients who are Rh negative; premedicate with acetaminophen and diphenhydramine to decrease side effects (flu-like symptoms)
- *Anti-D (WinRho):* 50–75 μg/kg; patient must be RhD(+); generally tolerated well; side effects include extravascular hemolysis (mean decreased hemoglobin of 1–2 g/dL); rare intravascular hemolysis or DIC. Should not be given to patients with anemia from bleeding or evidence of autoimmune hemolysis
- *Corticosteroids:* Multiple dosing strategies are reported. The most common is 2 mg/kg/day (maximum of 60–80 mg) for 1–2 weeks followed by a taper. Briefer higher dosing regimens are also reported
- *Chronic ITP (persistent thrombocytopenia for longer than 6 months):* Splenectomy, prednisone (intermittent use), vincristine, azathioprine, cyclosporine, cyclophosphamide, tacrolimus, rituximab, mycophenolate; new agents—thrombopoietin agonists currently being studied in pediatrics (approved for adults)

## THROMBOTIC DISORDERS

## MEDICATIONS FOR ANTICOAGULATION

### HEPARIN

- *Mechanism of action:* Complexes with natural anticoagulant antithrombin and accelerates activity; limits the expansion of thrombi by preventing fibrin formation; causes prolongation of aPTT (Table 12-2)
- *Dosage form:* Parenteral
- *Dose:*
  - ✓ *Initial bolus:* 50–75 U/kg
  - ✓ *Infusion:* younger than 1 year = 28 U/kg/h; older than 1 year = 20 U/kg/h
- *Monitoring:* Therapeutic aPTT is 60–85 seconds. Check first aPTT 4 hours after the loading dose and adjust according to Table 12-2. A therapeutic heparin anti-Xa level is 0.3–0.7 U/mL
- *Antidote:* Protamine sulfate
- *Side effects:*
  - ✓ Bleeding
  - ✓ Osteoporosis with long-term use

| TABLE 12-2 | Unfractionated Heparin Dose Adjustment Based on Activated Partial Thromboplastin Time | |
|---|---|---|
| **aPTT** | **Dose Adjustment** | **Time to Repeat aPTT** |
| <50 | 50 U/kg bolus | 4 hours after rate change |
| | ↑ Infusion rate by 10% | |
| 50–59 | ↑ Infusion rate by 10% | 4 hours after rate change |
| 60–85 | Keep rate the same | Next day |
| 86–95 | ↓ Infusion rate by 10% | 4 hours after rate change |
| 96–120 | Hold infusion for 30 minutes | 4 hours after rate change |
| | ↓ Infusion rate by 10% | |
| >120 | Hold infusion for 60 minutes | 4 hours after rate change |
| | ↓ Infusion rate by 15% | |

Adapted with permission from Michelson AD, Bovill E, Andrew M. Antithrombotic therapy in children. *Chest.* 1995 Oct;108(4 suppl): 506S–522S.

✓ *Heparin-induced thrombocytopenia (HIT):* Incidence is not clearly defined in pediatrics with a reported range of 0–2.3%. Higher risk pediatric groups include those patients undergoing cardiopulmonary bypass. HIT is characterized by symptoms appearing 5–10 days post heparin exposure with a 50% fall in the platelet count (rarely the platelet count is less than 50,000/mm$^3$) and there can be venous or arterial thrombosis. Treatment includes the removal of all heparin from the patient including avoidance of low-molecular-weight heparin. Anticoagulation should be initiated with a non-heparin anticoagulant such as a direct thrombin inhibitor (i.e., argatroban or bivalirudin)

## LOW-MOLECULAR-WEIGHT HEPARIN

• *Mechanism of action:* Accelerates antithrombin but inhibits factor Xa more than thrombin; long half-life, good bioavailability; monitor with anti-factor Xa levels
• *Dosage form:* Subcutaneous
• *Dosing (enoxaparin):*

| | **Enoxaparin Treatment** | **Enoxaparin Prophylaxis** |
|---|---|---|
| <2 months | 1.5 mg/kg every 12 hours | 0.75 mg/kg every 12 hours |
| >2 months | 1 mg/kg every 12 hours | 0.5 mg/kg every 12 hours |

• *Monitoring:* Therapeutic enoxaparin antifactor Xa level is 0.5–1 U/mL. Check anti-Xa level 4–6 hours after the second dose, and adjust as needed
• *Antidote:* Protamine causes partial reversal
• *Side effects:* Bleeding; HIT
• Use with caution in patients with renal insufficiency and avoid in renal failure

## WARFARIN (COUMADIN)

• *Mechanism of action:* Inhibits vitamin K epoxide reductase, the vitamin K regenerative enzyme; decreases the plasma concentration of vitamin K dependent factors II, VII, IX, and X along with protein C and S; causes prolongation of PT
• *Dosage form:* Oral only (no intravenous formulations)

- *Dosing:* Start while patient is therapeutic on heparin or LMWH; initially reduces protein C (shortest half-life) before other factors so initially there is a prothrombotic effect. Prolongation of PT/INR begins at 24–48 hours but takes 5–7 days for full anticoagulant effect. See formulary for dosing
- *Monitoring:* Use the INR; therapeutic range depends on clinical scenario. For patients with deep venous thrombosis, therapeutic INR is 2–3
- *Antidote:* Vitamin K, 4 Factor Prothrombin Complex Concentrate (Kcentra)
- *Side effects:* Bleeding; warfarin-related skin necrosis (result of starting warfarin without adequate anticoagulant coverage)
- Efficacy is affected by dietary intake/absorption of vitamin K as well as significant interactions with other medications. Therefore patients on warfarin should be monitored closely during illness, significant changes in the diet, or with changes in medication

## THROMBOLYTIC THERAPY

Necessary for life- or limb-threatening thrombosis and should be considered in patients with massive iliofemoral thrombosis. Options for therapy include recombinant tissue plasminogen activator (tPA) as either local or systemic therapy.
- *Mechanism of action:* Activates plasminogen to plasmin, which then degrades the fibrin clot
- *Dosing for systemic therapy:* tPA (wide variation) *low dose:* 0.03–0.06 mg/kg/h; duration depends on dose and clinical response; can be used for a relatively prolonged duration 48–86 hours. *High dose:* 0.1–0.6 mg/kg/h, reassess after 6 hours consider another 6 hours if clot not resolved

*Dosing for catheter directed tPA:* 0.5–2 mg/h

- *Monitoring:* CBC, PT, PTT, fibrinogen, and D-dimer should be checked prior to the initiation of thrombolytic therapy and every 4–8 hours while on the infusion. An elevated D-dimer and a drop in fibrinogen are indicative of a lytic state. To minimize the risk of bleeding it is important to maintain the fibrinogen >100 mg/dL and the platelet count >75,000/mm$^3$
- *Antidote:* None; if bleeding stop the drug (short half-life)
- *Side effect:* Bleeding
- *Precautions:* No IM injections; no urinary catheterization, rectal temperatures, or arterial puncture; patient should be in intensive care unit
- *Contraindications:* CNS ischemia/trauma/hemorrhage/surgery within 30 days, CNS pathology (e.g., neoplasm), seizures (within 48 hours), severe bleeding, surgery, or invasive procedure within 7–14 days, uncontrolled coagulopathy, inability to maintain a platelet count >75,000/mm$^3$ or fibrinogen >100 mg/dL, uncontrolled hypertension, serum creatinine >2 mg/dL, prematurity (gestation age <32 weeks)

## THROMBOSIS

**Complete or partial occlusion of deep veins or arteries.**

### EPIDEMIOLOGY

- Incidence of venous thromboembolism in children is 58/10,000 hospital admissions
- Usually occurs in children with acquired and/or congenital risk factors for thrombosis
- *Congenital Risk Factors:* Antithrombin deficiency, protein C deficiency, protein S deficiency, factor V Leiden (activated protein C resistance), prothrombin mutation, elevated lipoprotein(a), hyperhomocysteinemia, dysfibrinogenemia, heparin cofactor II deficiency

- *Acquired Risk Factors:* Central venous catheter (CVC, most common), antiphospholipid antibody syndrome, cancer, congenital heart disease, trauma, surgery, infection, severe dehydration, prematurity, pregnancy, nephrotic syndrome, inflammatory bowel disease, cystic fibrosis, SCD, medications (e.g., estrogen or L-asparaginase)

## PATHOPHYSIOLOGY

- Related to endothelial damage, venous stasis, or hypercoagulability and usually in combination

## CLINICAL MANIFESTATIONS

- *Extremity deep vein thrombosis (DVT):* Extremity pain, swelling, and discoloration. Consider this diagnosis in patients with a current or recent CVC in the affected extremity
- *Superior vena cava syndrome:* Swelling and plethora of the head and neck, and distended neck veins; caused by a large thrombus obstructing the superior vena cava (also associated with compression of SVC by malignancy)
- *Pulmonary embolism (PE):* Shortness of breath, pleuritic chest pain, cough, hemoptysis, fever and in the case of massive PE, hypotension and right heart failure
- *Cerebral sinovenous thrombosis:* Neonates often present with seizures, whereas older children often complain of headache, vomiting, seizures, and focal signs. They may also have papilledema and abducens nerve palsy
- *Renal vein thrombosis:* Hematuria, abdominal mass, thrombocytopenia
- *Arterial thrombosis:* Cold, pale, blue extremity with poor or absent pulses

## DIAGNOSTICS

- *Laboratory studies:* See Box 12-1
- *Doppler ultrasound:* Best for lower extremity DVT, decreased sensitivity for upper extremity DVT
- *Venography:* Helpful for upper extremity DVT if ultrasound is negative and clinical suspicion is high, requires contrast
- *Spiral CT (ventilation-perfusion scan used previously):* To evaluate for PE
- *Magnetic resonance venography of brain:* Best test for sinovenous thrombosis (can be missed on CT)


### BOX 12-1 RECOMMENDED LABORATORY EVALUATION FOR A NON-LINE ASSOCIATED OR UNPROVOKED THROMBOSIS

Complete blood cell count (CBC)
Prothrombin time (PT)
Activated partial thromboplastin time (aPTT)
Antithrombin activity
Protein C activity
Protein S activity
Factor V Leiden mutation
Prothrombin mutation
Fasting homocysteine
Lipoprotein (a)
Anticardiolipin antibody (IgG, IgM)
Anti-beta-2 glycoprotein antibody (IgG, IgM)
Dilute Russell viper venom time (or alternative test for a lupus anticoagulant)

- *CT or MR angiogram/venogram:* Helpful for proximal thrombosis or to confirm questionable findings on ultrasound

## MANAGEMENT

- *Anticoagulation:* Patients with symptomatic deep venous thrombosis should receive anticoagulation with unfractionated heparin or low-molecular-weight heparin (LMWH). Unfractionated heparin can be immediately reversed and should be used in patients who may require urgent procedures, are at high risk for bleeding, or have renal failure. Maintaining a therapeutic effect is often easier with LMWH. Length of therapy is dependent on cause of underlying thrombosis

## TRANSFUSION MEDICINE

### CRYOPRECIPITATE TRANSFUSION

#### PRODUCT

- Contains fibrinogen, FVIII, vWF, and FXIII
- One unit volume will vary, maximum is 15 mL; >150 mg/unit fibrinogen and >80 IU/unit FVIII, vWF, and FXIII

#### INDICATION

- Bleeding associated with hypofibrinogenemia
- Bleeding in patients with FVIII deficiency or vWD if factor products are not available

#### DOSAGE

- *Rule of thumb:* 1–2 units/10 kg (will result in a 60–100 mg/dL rise in fibrinogen)

### FRESH-FROZEN PLASMA TRANSFUSION

#### PRODUCT

- Contains all of the clotting factors
- FFP about 220 mL/unit; contains approximately 1 unit/mL of all coagulation factors

#### INDICATION

- To correct a factor deficiency in a coagulopathic patient with bleeding or perioperatively (DIC, vitamin K deficiency, liver disease, congenital factor deficiency, warfarin overdose)

#### DOSE

- 10–15 mL/kg, provides an approximate 10–15% factor correction with ideal recovery
- Can follow response by measuring PT/PTT and/or monitoring clinical bleeding

### PLATELET TRANSFUSION

#### PRODUCT

- *Whole blood derived* versus *single donor apheresis* platelets (single-donor product decreases the risk of antiplatelet antibodies and is preferable for patients who require multiple platelet transfusions)
- *Whole blood derived platelets:* About 50 mL/unit
- *Apheresis platelets:* 250–300 mL, equivalent to 6 units of whole blood derived platelets

## INDICATION

- Thrombocytopenic patient who is bleeding, critically ill, or requires surgical intervention. Most procedures can be done if platelet count is maintained greater than 50,000/mm³
- Given to prevent bleeding in patients with hypoproductive bone marrow (e.g., chemotherapy, aplastic anemia) when platelet count less is than 10–20,000/mm³
- Patients with platelet function defects who require surgical procedures or have active bleeding uncontrolled with local measures

## DOSE

*Whole blood derived platelets:*

- *Children less than 10 kg:* 5–10 mL/kg (increases platelet count by 50,000/mm³–100,000/mm³)
- *Patients greater than 10 kg:* 1 platelet unit/10 kg will increase by about 50,000/mm³ (maximum volume of 15 mL/kg)

*Apheresis platelets:*

   *<35 kg:* 10 mL/kg
   *>35 kg:* 1 unit/patient (with a maximum volume 15 cc/kg)
- Platelets are stored at room temperature so there is a higher risk of bacterial contamination

## RED BLOOD CELL TRANSFUSION

## PRODUCT

- Packed red blood cells (pRBCs); 180–350 mL/unit (Table 12-3)
- Patient should be typed and cross-matched prior to transfusion, but can use O-negative or O-positive blood in emergent situation (O-negative is preferable, especially in females)
- *Hematocrit varies depending on the preservative solution:* 55–65% in AS (adenine-saline) units to 70–75% in citrate-phosphate-dextrose-adenine (CPDA) units
- Leukocyte-reduced product greatly reduces risk of cytomegalovirus transmission and febrile transfusion reactions
- *Washed pRBCs:* Used for patients with IgA deficiency or a history of severe allergic transfusion reactions
- *Irradiated pRBCs:* Prevents transfusion associated graft versus host disease which is important for neonates, young infants, and immunocompromised patients

| TABLE 12-3 | Risk of Virus Transmission with Red Blood Cell Transfusion in the United States |
|---|---|
| **Virus** | **Risk of Transmission** |
| HIV I/II | 1:2,135,000 |
| Hepatitis C | 1:1,935,000 |
| Hepatitis B | 1:205,000 |
| HTLV | 1:2,993,000 |

Data from Dodd RY, Notari EP, Stramer SL: Current prevalence and incidence of infectious disease markers and estimated window-period risk in the American Red Cross blood donor population, *Transfusion.* 2002 Aug;42(8):975–979.

## INDICATION

- Treatment of symptomatic anemia (e.g., tachycardia, hypotension, hypoxia) or acute blood loss greater than 15%

## DOSE

- *Rule of thumb:* 5 cc/kg of pRBCs increases hemoglobin 1 g/dL in patients who weigh more than 70 kg: 1 unit of pRBCs increases hemoglobin by 1 g/dL
- For severe anemia in a hemodynamically compensated child, transfuse small volume, slowly (over approximately 4 hours) due to risk of precipitating heart failure; initial pRBC transfusion volume estimated as:

$$(1\,cc/kg\ of\ pRBC) \times (current\ hemoglobin)$$

## TRANSFUSION COMPLICATIONS

**Multiple reactions—Hemolytic, nonhemolytic, allergic, infectious (see Table 12-3), circulatory overload, transfusion related acute lung injury (TRALI), hypothermia, rarely electrolyte abnormalities in the setting of massive transfusion protocols (hypoglycemia or hypocalcemia or hyperkalemia). Descriptions of more common reactions are given below.**

### HEMOLYTIC TRANSFUSION REACTION

- *Acute:* Rapid destruction of red cells; usually due to blood type incompatibility (Table 12-4). Can result in fever, chills, hypotension shock, DIC, and renal failure; high mortality rate. If suspected, stop transfusion and institute supportive measures (fluids, pressors)

  *Evaluation:* Check for clinical errors, confirm patient blood type, screen for antibodies, repeat DAT on post-transfusion serum, culture donor blood for bacteria

- *Delayed:* 3–10 days after transfusion, usually in patients who had previous transfusion as a result of an antibody that was present, but undetectable at the time of the transfusion. May result in fever, fatigue, jaundice, and dark urine. Additional evaluation would include urine for hemoglobin, CBC and reticulocyte count, and markers for hemolysis

| TABLE 12-4 | Risk of Adverse Transfusion Reactions |
|---|---|
| **Hazard** | **Risk per Unit** |
| Allergic transfusion reaction | 1:50 to 1:100 |
| Febrile transfusion reaction | 1:100 |
| Sepsis (bacterial contamination) | 1:400 to 1:12,500 |
| Anaphylaxis | 1:20,000 to 1:50,000 |
| Acute hemolysis (ABO mismatch) | 1:6000 to 1:33,000 |
| Death | 1:500,000 |
| Transfusion-related acute lung injury | 1:5000 |

Data from AuBuchon JP, Kruskall MS. Transfusion safety: realigning efforts with risks. *Transfusion.* 1997 Nov-Dec; 37(11–12):1211–1216.

## FEBRILE NONHEMOLYTIC TRANSFUSION REACTION

- Temperature increase of at least 1°C in association with transfusion, with or without chills; usually due to antibody to donor WBC or plasma proteins; uncommon with leuko-reduced products. Stop transfusion and evaluate (see previous section). Consider premedication with acetaminophen

## ALLERGIC TRANSFUSION REACTION

- Reaction to donor plasma proteins; ranges from minor urticaria to anaphylaxis. Stop transfusion, treat with antihistamines (epinephrine and steroids if respiratory compromise)

# 13 Human Immunodeficiency Virus Infection

*Daniel H. Reirden, MD, AAHIVMS*

## HUMAN IMMUNODEFICIENCY VIRUS INFECTION

Human Immunodeficiency Virus (HIV) may lead to Acquired Immune Deficiency Syndrome (AIDS). Progression to AIDS is associated with opportunistic infections, cancers, and death. Advances in highly active antiretroviral treatments (HAART) have transformed HIV infection to a chronic illness with near normal life expectancy for those with access and adherence to life-long therapy. See Table 13-1 for currently approved antiretroviral drugs.

## EPIDEMIOLOGY IN THE UNITED STATES

- *Maternal to Child Transmission (MTCT):* In the United States, advances in HIV-testing, HAART use in pregnant HIV-infected women, and post-exposure prophylaxis of HIV-exposed infants have reduced MTCT to between 1% and 2%. In 2011, 53 U.S. infants were perinatally infected with HIV
- *Pediatric Infection:* There are about 3,000 children under the age of 13 years with HIV infection in the United States. This number will increase because the ban on HIV immigration to the United States was lifted, resulting in increased adoption of foreign born HIV-infected children by U.S. families and immigration of HIV-infected children and families

| TABLE 13-1 | FDA-Approved and Still Marketed Antiretroviral Medications (October 2015) |
|---|---|
| **Nucleoside/tide Reverse Transcriptase Inhibitors (NRTIs)** | **Multi-class Combination Formulations** |
| Zidovudine | Tenofovir/emtricitabine/efavirenz |
| Didanosine | Emtricitabine/tenofovir and rilpivirine |
| Stavudine | Emtricitabine/tenofovir, cobicistat, and elvitegravir |
| Lamivudine | Atazanavir and cobicistat |
| Abacavir | Darunavir and cobicistat |
| Tenofovir | **Protease Inhibitors** |
| Emtricitabine | Saquinavir |
| Zidovudine/lamivudine | Ritonavir |
| Zidovudine/lamivudine/abacavir | Indinavir |
| Abacavir/lamivudine | Nelfinavir |
| Tenofovir/emtricitabine | Atazanavir |
| **Non-Nucleoside Reverse Transcriptase Inhibitors (NNRTIs)** | Fosamprenavir |
| | Tipranavir |
| Nevirapine | Darunavir |
| Delavirdine | Lopinavir/ritonavir |
| Efavirenz | **Integrase Strand Transfer Inhibitor** |
| Etravirine | Raltegravir |
| Rilpivarine | Doultegravir |
| **Fusion Inhibitors** | Elvitegravir |
| Enfuviritide | **CCR5 Inhibitor** |
| | Maraviroc |

- *Adolescent and Young Adult Infection:*
  - ✓ *Perinatally Acquired Infection:* With changes to the HIV immigration laws in 2010 and improvements in antiviral therapies leading to prolonged life expectancies, the number of HIV-infected adolescents is increasing
  - ✓ *Behaviorally Acquired Infection:* The Centers for Disease Control and Prevention (CDC) classifies modes of transmission as: male-to-male (men who have sex with men, MSM) sexual contact; injection drug use (IDU); MSM and IDU; heterosexual contact; or other. The incidence of HIV infection has remained stable or decreased except in MSM
    - ▪ 60% of youth who tested HIV-positive are previously unaware of their diagnosis

## DIFFERENTIAL DIAGNOSIS

- *Infancy and childhood:*
  - ✓ Congenital immunodeficiencies; congenital infections, infections, such as *Mycobacterium tuberculosis*; malignancies; malnutrition; or other causes of failure to thrive, such as inflammatory bowel disease, celiac disease, or cystic fibrosis
- *Adolescents and young adults:*
  - ✓ *Acute infection:* Any viral syndrome such as influenza, mononucleosis (EBV, CMV); primary HSV; bacterial or viral meningitis; arbovirus infections; gastrointestinal infections; malignancy; rheumatologic disease, such as idiopathic rheumatoid arthritis; primary or secondary syphilis
  - ✓ *Advanced infection:* Differential will vary depending on presentation, some examples are included below:
    - ▪ *Infectious:* Pneumonia (bacterial, viral, fungal, parasitic); meningitis (bacterial, viral, fungal); sepsis, chronic fatigue syndrome; syphilis, tuberculosis , chronic vaginal candidal infection
    - ▪ *Wasting:* Malignancy, anorexia nervosa, inflammatory bowel disease, celiac disease, or cystic fibrosis
    - ▪ *Malignancy:* Burkitt's lymphoma, Kaposi sarcoma, cervical dysplasia or cancer

## PATHOPHYSIOLOGY

- *Perinatally Acquired Infection:*
  - ✓ *Intrauterine:* Virus crosses the placenta to infect an unborn infant. Providing HAART therapy to HIV-infected pregnant women reduces the viral load and reduces the chance of intrauterine infection
  - ✓ *Intrapartum:* Passage through the birth canal exposes the infant to the virus from genital secretions and blood. Having therapeutic levels of antiretrovirals in the infants system is analogous to pre-exposure prophylaxis. Post-exposure prophylaxis is provided to protect the infant from maternal blood exposure during birth and the possibility of acquisition of HIV by swallowing fluids during the delivery
  - ✓ *Breast-Feeding:* An additional 10–20% of maternal to child HIV transmission may occur through breast-feeding. HIV-infected women in the United States are advised to avoid breast-feeding as there is ready access to infant formulas
- *Behaviorally Acquired infection:* The virus is introduced into the bloodstream directly (e.g., intravenous drug use) or from transmucosal exposure (e.g., sexual exposure). The virus attaches to a CD4+ cell by using both the CD4 receptor and a CCR5 co-receptor. The virus is inserted into the CD4+ lymphocyte and the viral RNA is transcribed to proviral DNA though the use of virally supplied reverse transcriptase enzyme. This proviral DNA is then transported to the host cell nucleus where it is integrated into the host cell DNA through

the use of an integrase enzyme. When activated, the host DNA will make HIV proviral RNA that is transported into the cytoplasm where protease enzymes assemble the RNA into a viral capsule, which is then transported to the cell wall where an infectious HIV virus can bud from the host cell. Without treatment intervention, this generally results in the steady decline of CD4+ T lymphocytes over a period of years. Additional immune dysfunction is caused by B-cell dysregulation

## CLINICAL MANIFESTATIONS

Clinical manifestations vary by age at time of presentation.

- *Infancy and childhood:*
  - ✓ HIV-infected infants have a high risk of pneumonia due to *Pneumocystis jiroveci* (PCP) during the first 6 months of life
  - ✓ 30–80% will present with some abnormal physical finding by age 1 year, especially lymphadenopathy; hepatosplenomegaly; recurrent oropharyngeal candidal infections after age 1; pneumonias; recurrent bacterial infections; or failure to thrive
- *Adolescents and young adults:*
  - ✓ *Acute HIV Infection:* Consider acute HIV infection in any sexually active adolescent or young adult with fever of unknown origin or sexually transmitted infection, particularly syphilis
  - ✓ *Latent HIV Infection:* Due to the long duration of asymptomatic latency, infected persons may have no symptoms and may not be aware of their HIV infection
  - ✓ *Advanced HIV Infection:* Varied clinical manifestations include the pneumonia (recurrent bacterial, *Pneumocystis jiroveci, M. tuberculosis*); meningitis (toxoplasmosis, cryptococcal); fever of unknown origin (e.g., *Mycobacterium avium* intercellulare (MAI), CMV, HSV); candidiasis (oropharyngeal, vaginal, or esophageal); diarrheal illness (e.g., microsporidium, cryptosporidium, isospora, CMV, MAI), malignancy (e.g., Burkitt's lymphoma, cervical cancer, Kaposi sarcoma), and renal failure (from HIV nephropathy)

## DIAGNOSTICS

Western Blot is no longer the gold standard for confirming HIV infection (see algorithm in Figure 13-1).

- *Maternal–Child Transmission:*
  - ✓ Women whose HIV status is unknown or undocumented should have a rapid HIV test or ELISA/EIA during delivery
  - ✓ Most infants will tests positive on ELISA or EIA testing due to the passage of maternal IgG antibodies across the placenta. These antibodies may remain present in the infant until age 18 months
  - ✓ Quantitative HIV RNA viral load testing (≥5000 copies sensitivity 100% at birth, 1, 3, and 6 months of age), or qualitative HIV DNA (same sensitivities as RNA viral load testing), are used to confirm the presence or absence of HIV transmission from HIV-infected mothers. Infants are tested as follows:
    - ▪ Testing at birth in high-risk infants is recommended
    - ▪ *PCR should be performed at:*
      - ▹ 14–21 days of life
      - ▹ 1–2 months of life
      - ▹ 4–6 months of life
    - ▪ If any PCR test is positive, a second test should be performed as soon as possible on a separate specimen

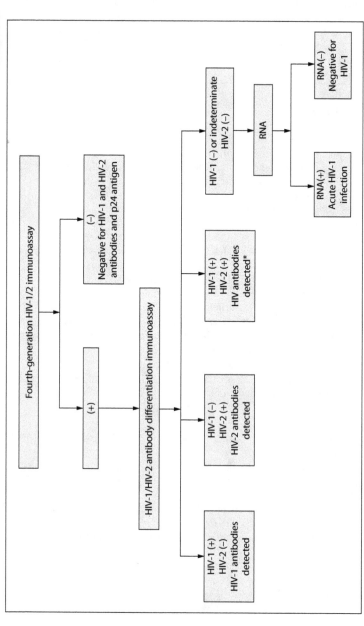

**Abbreviation:** HIV = human immunodeficiency virus.

* Additional testing required to rule out dual infection with HIV-1 and HIV-2.

**FIGURE 13-1 HIV testing algorithm 2013.** Centers for Disease Control and Prevention. Detection of acute HIV infection in two evaluations of a new HIV diagnostic testing algorithm—United States, 2011–2013. *MMWR.* 2013;62:491. Reproduced with permission from Centers for Disease Control and Prevention. Detection of Acute HIV Infection in Two Evaluations of a New HIV Diagnostic Testing Algorithm —United States, 2011– 2013 *MMWR Morb Mortal Wkly Rep.* 2013 Jun 21;62(24):489–494

✓ *Confirmation of negative HIV status in non-breast-fed infants:* Two negative PCR-based tests, one obtained at ≥1 month of age and one obtained at ≥4 months of age, or two negative HIV antibody tests obtained at ≥6 months of age
- Weaker evidence (grade BIII) supports HIV negative status if HIV-negative by antibody testing at 12–18 months of age
- *Suspected Acute HIV Infection:*
✓ Due to the lag in the development of HIV antibodies, HIV ELISA and EIA testing can provide false-negative results
✓ *Quantitative HIV-RNA testing is the recommended test of choice:* ≥10,000 copies/mL are diagnostic of acute HIV infection with a sensitivity of close to 100%; specificity = 98%
- *Latent HIV Infection:*
✓ See Figure 13-1 for current testing algorithm; FDA has two approved fourth-generation tests that both require blood or plasma
✓ Both the Centers for Disease Control and Prevention (CDC) and the United States Preventative Services Task Force (USPSTF) recommend routine HIV testing in all sexually active individuals at least once in their lifetime; repeat testing should be performed in those with other risk factors

## MANAGEMENT

- *Infants and children:*
✓ *Intrapartum Antiretroviral Therapy/Prophylaxis:*
- All HIV-infected pregnant women should be treated with HAART without respect to their viral load;
- For pregnant women on HAART and not optimally suppressed, HIV genotype testing should be considered prior to modifying HAART;
- For HIV-infected pregnant women in the United States naïve to treatment, genotyping should be done, but medications can be initiated prior to receiving the results. General recommendations are:
  ▷ 2 Nucleoside/tide (NRTIs) should be part of any regimen. There has been extensive experience with zidovudine (AZT) and lamuvidine (3TC) in pregnancy and it remains the recommended backbone of HAART triple therapy. AZT has a high placental transfer rate
  ▷ Protease Inhibitors are recommended in addition to the dual NRTI backbone. Examples:
    ○ Atazanavir (ATV) boosted with ritonavir. May require increased dosing in second and third trimester based on drug levels
    ○ Lopinavir (LPV) boosted with ritonavir. May require increased dosing in second and third trimester based on drug levels
- Continuous infusion of zidovudine should be administered to those women who have HIV RNA levels >400 copies/mL (or unknown viral load) near delivery. Dosing is 2 mg/kg IV over first hour followed by continuous infusion of 1 mg/kg/h until delivery
- If the HIV RNA viral load is >1000 copies/mL near time of delivery a scheduled cesarean section should take place at 38 weeks gestation. For those women with HIV RNA viral loads <1000 copies/mL, vaginal delivery is acceptable
- The infant should receive oral zidovudine as soon as possible after birth and continue this for 6 weeks. High-risk infants (those born to HIV-infected women who have not received HAART before labor or during delivery) should receive combination therapy: zidovudine for 6 weeks along with 3 doses of nelfinavir (at birth, 48 hours later, and then 96 hours after the second dose)
  ▷ For infants >35 weeks gestation the dose of zidovudine is 4 mg/kg per dose orally twice daily
- Breast-feeding is not recommended for infants born in the United States to HIV-infected women

- HIV-Infected Children
  - ✓ HIV-infected infants <12 months of age be treated regardless of CD4 count or percentage or viral load
  - ✓ HAART is recommended for all children >1 year of age with minimal or no symptoms; deferral, though rare, may occur in special circumstances based on age and CD4 count and percentage
  - ✓ In children <5 years old, the CD4 percentage is generally preferred to stage immune status due to age-related variability in absolute CD4 counts
  - ✓ Immunologic monitoring including CD4 count, percentage, and viral load should be performed every 3–4 months. See Table 13-2 for disease classification status in children
  - ✓ Initiation of HAART in Antiretroviral Naïve Children
    - ▪ Treatment should generally include two NRTIs, plus either a NNRTI or PI
    - ▪ HIV genotyping for viral resistance should be performed prior to initiation of HAART
    - ▪ Initial recommended regimens vary by age. The preferred regimens are:
      - ▷ *Children aged birth to 3 months:* Zidovudine plus NNRTI or PI
      - ▷ *Children aged ≥ 14 days and <3 years:* two NRTIs plus lopinavir/ritonavir
      - ▷ *Children aged ≥ 3 years and <6 years:* two NRTIs and lopinavir/ritonavir
      - ▷ *Children >= 6years:*
        - ○ two NRTIs plus atazanvir and low dose boosted ritonavir
        - ○ two NRTIs plus lopinavir/ritonavir
- Adolescents and Young Adults
  - ✓ HAART is recommended for all HIV-infected individuals to reduce disease progression and likelihood of transmission to others
  - ✓ Patients and providers may elect to delay treatment based on individual circumstances
  - ✓ HIV genotyping should occur prior to starting HAART. If necessary, treatment may begin pending results and then modified if resistance to a particular drug is discovered
  - ✓ HLA B*5701 testing should be done in anyone for whom treatment with abacavir is being considered
  - ✓ An antiretroviral combination generally consists of two NRTIs in combination with a third active antiviral medication from one of three drug classes: an integrase strand transfer inhibitor, a NNRTI, or a protease inhibitor with a pharmokinetic enhancer (ritonavir or cobicistat). The 2015 *Guidelines for the Use of Antiretroviral Agents in HIV-1 Infected Adults and Adolescents* recommend as preferred initial HAART regimens in treatment-naïve individuals include:
    - ▪ Preferred Dual NRTI backbone
      - ▷ Tenofovir** + emtricitabine or lamivudine (Caution with tenofovir use in those with renal insufficiency and prior to Tanner Stage 4)
      - ▷ Abacavir*** + emtricitabine or lamuvidine (Only for those without a positive mutation at HLA-B57*01)
    - ▪ PI-Based Regimen
      - ▷ Darunavir + ritonavir + tenofovir + emtricitabine (Caution with tenofovir use in those with renal insufficiency)
    - ▪ Integrase Strand Transfer Inhibitor-Based Regimens
      - ▷ Dolutegravir + abacavir + lamivudine (Only for those without a positive mutation at HLA-B57*01)
      - ▷ Dolutregravir + tenofovir + emtricitabine (Caution with tenofovir use in those with renal insufficiency and prior to Tanner Stage 4)
      - ▷ Elvitegravir + cobicistat + tenofovir + emtricitabine (Only for use in those with pre-treatment creatinine clearances > 70mL/min)
  - ✓ Alternate regimens may be appropriate in some situations
  - ✓ Common side effects of HAART medications are given in Table 13-3

**TABLE 13-2** 1994 Revised HIV Pediatric Classification System: Clinical Categories

Category 1: Not Symptomatic

Children who have no signs or symptoms considered to be the result of HIV infection or who have only one of the conditions listed in Category 2.

Category 2: Mildly Symptomatic

Children with two or more of the following conditions but none of the conditions listed in Categories 3 and 4:

- Lymphadenopathy ($\geq$0.5 cm at more than two sites; bilateral = one site)
- Hepatomegaly
- Splenomegaly
- Dermatitis
- Parotitis
- Recurrent or persistent upper respiratory infection, sinusitis, or otitis media

Category 3: Moderately Symptomatic

Children who have symptomatic conditions, other than those listed for Category 2 or Category 4, that are attributed to HIV infection. Examples of conditions in Clinical Category 3 include, but are not limited to, the following:

- Anemia (<8 g/dL), neutropenia (<1000 cells/mm³), or thrombocytopenia (<100,000 cells/mm³) persisting $\geq$30 days
- Bacterial meningitis, pneumonia, or sepsis (single episode)
- Candidiasis, oropharyngeal (i.e., thrush) persisting for >2 months in children aged >6 months
- Cardiomyopathy
- Cytomegalovirus infection with onset before age 1 month
- Diarrhea, recurrent or chronic
- Hepatitis
- Herpes simplex virus (HSV) stomatitis, recurrent (i.e., more than two episodes within 1 year)
- HSV bronchitis, pneumonitis, or esophagitis with onset before age 1 month
- Herpes zoster (i.e., shingles) involving at least two distinct episodes or more than one dermatome
- Leiomyosarcoma
- Lymphoid interstitial pneumonia (LIP) or pulmonary lymphoid hyperplasia complex
- Nephropathy
- Nocardiosis
- Fever lasting >1 month
- Toxoplasmosis with onset before age 1 month
- Varicella, disseminated (i.e., complicated chickenpox)

Category 4: Severely Symptomatic

Children who have any condition listed in the 1987 surveillance case definition for AIDS (below), with the exception of LIP, which is a Category 3 condition:

- Serious bacterial infections, multiple or recurrent (i.e., any combination of at least two culture-confirmed infections within a 2-year period), of the following types: septicemia, pneumonia, meningitis, bone or joint infection, or abscess of an internal organ or body cavity (excluding otitis media, superficial skin or mucosal abscesses, and indwelling catheter-related infections)

*(continued)*

**TABLE 13-2** *(continued)*

- Candidiasis, esophageal or pulmonary (bronchi, trachea, lungs)
- Coccidioidomycosis, disseminated (at site other than or in addition to lungs or cervical or hilar lymph nodes)
- Cryptococcosis, extrapulmonary
- Cryptosporidiosis or isosporiasis with diarrhea persisting >1 month
- Cytomegalovirus disease with onset of symptoms at age >1 month (at a site other than liver, spleen, or lymph nodes)
- Encephalopathy(at least one of the following progressive findings present for at least 2 months in the absence of a concurrent illness other than HIV infection that could explain the findings): (a) failure to attain or loss of developmental milestones or loss of intellectual ability, verified by standard developmental scale or neuropsychological tests; (b) impaired brain growth or acquired microcephaly demonstrated by head circumference measurements or brain atrophy demonstrated by computerized tomography or magnetic resonance imaging (serial imaging is required for children aged <2 years); (c) acquired symmetric motor deficit manifested by two or more of the following: paresis, pathologic reflexes, ataxia, or gait disturbance
- Herpes simplex virus infection causing a mucocutaneous ulcer that persists for >1 month or bronchitis, pneumonitis, or esophagitis for any duration affecting a child aged >1 month
- Histoplasmosis, disseminated (at a site other than or in addition to lungs or cervical or hilar lymph nodes)
- Kaposi sarcoma
- Lymphoma, primary, in brain
- Lymphoma, small, non-cleaved cell (Burkitt), or immunoblastic or large cell lymphoma of B-cell or unknown immunologic phenotype
- *Mycobacterium tuberculosis*, disseminated or extrapulmonary
- Mycobacterium, other species or unidentified species, disseminated (at a site other than or in addition to lungs, skin, or cervical or hilar lymph nodes)
- *Mycobacterium avium* complex or *Mycobacterium kansasii*, disseminated (at site other than or in addition to lungs, skin, or cervical or hilar lymph nodes)
- *Pneumocystis jiroveci* pneumonia
- Progressive multifocal leukoencephalopathy
- Salmonella (nontyphoid) septicemia, recurrent
- Toxoplasmosis of the brain with onset at age >1 month
- Wasting syndrome in the absence of a concurrent illness other than HIV infection that could explain the following findings: (a) persistent weight loss >10% of baseline; OR (b) downward crossing of at least two of the following percentile lines on the weight-for-age chart (such as 95th, 75th, 50th, 25th, 5th) in a child ≥1 year of age; OR (c) <5th percentile on weight-for-height chart on two consecutive measurements, ≥30 days apart PLUS (1) chronic diarrhea (i.e., ≥2 loose stools per day for >30 days), OR (2) documented fever (for ≥30 days, intermittent or constant)

Adapted with permission from Centers for Disease Control and Prevention. 1994 Revised classification system for human immunodeficiency virus infection in children less than 13 years of age. *MMWR*, 1994. 43 (No. RR-12): p. 1–10.

| TABLE 13-3 Common Side Effects of HIV Medicine Classes | |
| --- | --- |
| **Medication** | **Common Side Effects** |
| **Nucleoside/tide Reverse Transcriptase Inhibitors (NRTIs)** | Anemia |
| | Thrombocytopenia |
| | Pancreatitis |
| | Hepatotoxicity |
| | Lipoatrophy |
| | Hypersensitivity reaction (abacavir) |
| **Non-Nucleoside Reverse Transcriptase Inhibitors (NNRTIs)** | Rash |
| | Psychiatric effects (efavirenz) |
| | • Abnormal dreaming |
| | • Insomnia |
| | • Depression |
| | • Anxiety |
| | Hepatotoxicity |
| | Hypersensitivity reaction (nevirapine) |
| | Teratogenic (efavirenz) |
| **Protease Inhibitors (PIs)** | Gastrointestinal symptoms (nausea, diarrhea) |
| | Dyslipidemia |
| | Hyperglycemia |
| | Hyperbilirubinemia (atazanavir) |
| | Hepatotoxicity |
| **Integrase Strand Transfer Inhibitor-Based Regimens (INSTIs)** | Nausea, diarrhea, flatulence |
| | Elevations in amylase and liver function tests |
| | Headache |
| | Dizziness, abnormal dreams |
| | Pruritus, rash |
| | Fatigue, muscle pain |
| **Fusion Inhibitors** | Injection site reactions |

## PRIMARY PROPHYLAXIS OF OPPORTUNISTIC INFECTIONS

- *Mycobacterium avium* complex (MAC)
  - ✓ *Children ≤1 year of age:* <750 CD4 cells
  - ✓ *Children 1–2 years of age:* <500 CD4 cells
  - ✓ *Children 2–5 years of age:* <75 CD4 cells
  - ✓ *Children ≥6 years of age:* <50 CD4 cells
  - ✓ Azithromycin or clarithromycin may be used

- *Pneumocystis jiroveci* pneumonia (PCP): Chemoprophylaxis is based on a combination of age and CD4 count or percentage:
  - ✓ *Children ≤1 year of age:* All HIV-infected infants
  - ✓ *Children 1–5 years of age:* CD4 count <500 cells/mm³ or CD4 <15%
  - ✓ *Children ≥6 years of age:* CD4 count <200 cells/mm³ or CD4 <15%
  - ✓ Trimethoprim-sulfamethoxazole (TMP-SMX) is the drug of choice for primary prophylaxis
- *Toxoplasma gondii*
  - ✓ Data less well established in children than in adolescents or adults
  - ✓ CD4 <15% and seropositivity for IgG antibodies to *Toxoplasma gondii* warrant primary prophylaxis
  - ✓ TMP-SMX is the drug of choice for primary prophylaxis
- *Vaccine Preventable Diseases:*
  - ✓ Follow recommendations of the Advisory Committee on Immunization Practices. Available at: http://www.cdc.gov/mmwr/pdf/other/su6201.pdf. Accessed on October 19, 2013
  - ✓ In general, live vaccines should be avoided in HIV-infected infants with severe immuno-suppression. Varicella and measles-mumps-rubella (MMR) may be given to those with HIV disease classifications of 1 or 2 (see Table 13-2)
  - ✓ *Vaccines against encapsulated organisms can reduce risk of disease burden in HIV-infected children:*
    - ▪ *Meningococcal vaccination (MCV-4):* 2 doses given soon after age 2 years separated by 8 weeks
    - ▪ Polysaccharide pneumococcal vaccination (PCV-23) should be given after 2 doses of protein-conjugate vaccination after age 2 years and then repeated in 3–5 years
  - ✓ *Hepatitis B vaccine:*
    - ▪ Immunogenicity is reduced in children with HIV infection. Titers should be checked after the 3-dose vaccine series and if <10 mIU/mL, a repeat of the 3-dose vaccine is recommended

## MANAGEMENT OF OPPORTUNISTIC INFECTIONS (OI) AND INFLAMMATORY SYNDROMES

**Opportunistic infections remain an important cause of morbidity and mortality. Risk factors include undiagnosed HIV infection; lack of proper prophylaxis of OI; virologic and immunologic failure while on HAART; and, suboptimal adherence to HAART.**

- *Differential Diagnosis:*
  - ✓ Distinguishing between OI and infections that non-immunocompromised individuals may also acquire can be difficult. Immune Reconstitution Inflammatory Syndrome (IRIS), a paradoxical systemic inflammatory reaction to either an active infection or a latent infection, can present weeks to months after the initiation of HAART. Its presentation is similar to an infectious illness, but it is purely inflammatory in nature
  - ✓ A good rule of thumb is to always consider common infections that can present in any child without HIV infection, then consider the OIs, oncologic processes, and IRIS
  - ✓ See Table 13-4 for diagnosis and treatment of OIs in infants and children
  - ✓ See Table 13-5 for diagnosis and treatment of OIs in adolescents and young adults

**TABLE 13-4** Opportunistic Infections in HIV-Infected Infants and Children

| Etiology | Clinical Presentation | Laboratory/Radiological Findings | Preferred Treatment |
|---|---|---|---|
| **Bacterial Infections** | | | |
| *Bartonella*, ssp. *henselae* and *quintana* | FUO, bacillary angiomatosis, endocarditis, osteomyelitis, splenitis | CD4 count <100 cells/mm³ <br> Elevated antibody titer to organism <br> Histopathology or PCR | Doxycycline 2–4 mg/kg orally per day for 3–4 months. |
| **Mycobacterial Infections** | | | |
| *Mycobacterium tuberculosis* | <u>Pulmonary:</u> Cough, fever, failure to thrive, weight loss <br><br> <u>Extrapulmonary:</u> Most common sites in children are lymph nodes or CNS. However, blood (miliary), cardiac, joint, bone, skin, kidney, eye, and abdomen can be initial sites. | • + Mantoux PPD ≥5 mm <br> • + Interferon-gamma release assay (IGRA): Caution in those <5 years of age <br> • Sputum sample with acid fast bacilli (AFB) <br> • Gastric aspiration (early morning) <br> • Tissue sampling <br> • Chest x-ray | Disseminated disease may progress quickly in infants; prompt initiation of treatment should be considered. Caution with drug–drug interactions with HAART. 4 drug regimen recommended: <br><br> • Ethambutol 20 mg/kg daily dose (max 2.5 g) <br> • Isoniazid 10–15 mg/kg daily dose (max 300 mg) <br> • Pyrazinamide 30–40 mg/kg daily dose (max 2 g) <br> • Rifampin 10–20 mg/kg daily dose (max 600 mg) |

*(continued)*

**TABLE 13-4**  (continued)

| Etiology | Clinical Presentation | Laboratory/Radiological Findings | Preferred Treatment |
|---|---|---|---|
| *Mycobacterium avium intracellulare* (MAI) | • Pulmonary: Less common presentation in children<br><br>• Disseminated: More common in children. Rare in first year of life. Symptoms include: fever, night sweats, weight loss, abdominal pain, diarrhea, lymphadenitis | • CD4 counts <50 copies/mm$^3$ or CD4 % ≤15–25% depending on age, with the lower % for younger children<br><br>• + Blood culture or culture from site. May use culture of normally sterile site (e.g., bone marrow)<br><br>• + AFB stain of blood, sputum, or stool (confirm with culture or PCR testing)<br><br>• Perform susceptibility testing to azithromycin and clarithromycin | Two drug combination therapy for 12 months.<br><br>Preferred regimen:<br><br>• Clarithromycin 7.5–15 mg/kg orally twice daily (max 500 mg per dose) +<br>• Ethambutol 15–25 mg/kg once daily (max 2.5 g/day)<br>• Severe disease add rifabutin 10–20 mg/kg once daily (max 300 mg daily)<br><br>Alternate regimen:<br><br>• Azithromycin 10–12 mg/kg once daily (max 500 mg daily) may be substituted for clarithromycin<br><br>Secondary prophylaxis is needed after treatment completion. |
| **Viral Infections** | | | |
| Cytomegalovirus (CMV): End organ disease typically occurs in those with profound immunosuppression (CD4 counts <50 cell/mm$^3$). | • Retinitis: Most common presentation; may be unilateral: floaters, central or peripheral visual loss.<br><br>• Other sites: GI, liver, kidney, sinuses, or CNS<br><br>• Symptoms often nonspecific: Fever, weight loss, odynophagia | • CMV can be isolated in cell culture from blood leukocytes, urine, or tissue<br><br>• Positive blood buffy-coat culture<br><br>• DNA PCR of blood, fluid, or tissue<br><br>• Ophthalmoscopic exam | Symptomatic congenital infection:<br><br>• Ganciclovir 6 mg/kg IV every 12 hours for 6 weeks<br><br>Disseminated disease and retinitis:<br><br>• Ganciclovir 5–7.5 mg/kg IV every 12 hours for 14–21 days<br><br>• Followed by 5 mg/kg IV per day for 5–7 days per week for chronic suppression |

| | | |
|---|---|---|

Cytomegalovirus (continued)

CNS disease: Also followed by chronic suppression:

- Ganciclovir 5–7.5 mg/kg IV every 12 hours; PLUS
- Foscarnet 60 mg/kg IV every 8 hours until symptoms improved
- Poor prognosis in pre-HAART era.
- HAART has increased survival time and is the only treatment that has demonstrated benefit.

Jackson Canyon (JC) virus: The causative agent of Progressive Multifocal Leukodystrophy (PML); causes demyelinating disease of the CNS. Rare in children.

Usually insidious in onset. May present with focal neurologic deficits, cognitive dysfunction, visual disturbances, paralysis, ataxia, or aphasia.

- PML is generally associated with profound immunosuppression, i.e., CD4% <15.
- MRI of white matter will reveal:
- Deceased signal on T1 images
- Increased signal on T2 and FLAIR sequences
- Presence of JC virus in CNS by PCR in conjunction with MRI findings
- Brain biopsy is gold standard with specificity of 100%, but carries significant risk.

## Fungal Infections

Aspergillosis: Most common spp. causing infection are A. fumingatus, followed by A. flavus

- Invasive pulmonary aspergillosis is the most common: Fever, cough, dyspnea, pleuritic pain
- Other sites: Tracheobronchitis, CNS, skin, and sinuses

- Profound immunosuppression (CD4% <15) associated with higher risk
- Blood cultures generally not helpful
- CXR or CT scan for pulmonary involvement
- Biopsy for fungal culture of suspected site

Invasive pulmonary aspergillosis:

- Voriconizole 6–8 mg/kg IV every 12 hours for 2 doses followed by 7 mg/kg either IV or orally twice daily for 12 weeks

*(continued)*

TABLE 13-4 (continued)

| Etiology | Clinical Presentation | Laboratory/Radiological Findings | Preferred Treatment |
|---|---|---|---|
| *Candida* Infections | • Oral thrush and diaper dermatitis occur in a majority of HIV-infected children; primarily caused by *C. albicans*.<br><br>• Esophageal candidiasis presents with odynophagia, retrosternal pain, and children can present with nausea, vomiting, and weight loss.<br><br>• Disseminated candidiasis: Blood infections are generally caused by non-*albicans* species of *Candida*. | Oral thrush:<br>• Potassium hydroxide preparation of samples will show budding yeast cells.<br>• Culture may need to be done in refractory cases or failure of treatment.<br><br>Esophageal thrush:<br>• Barium swallow will demonstrate a classic cobblestone appearance<br>• Refractory causes may require endoscopy to rule out other causes.<br><br>Disseminated candidiasis:<br>• Blood cultures (1–2 days for growth and 1–2 days for speciation)<br>• Beta-D-glucan assays (limited validation in children)<br>• PCR, but can currently only identify to the *Candida* species level.<br>• Consider ultrasound to identify liver and kidney dissemination<br>• Ophthalmology exam to detect eye involvement. | Oral thrush:<br>• Fluconazole 3–6 mg/kg orally once daily (max 400 mg/dose) for 7–14 days.<br><br>Esophageal thrush:<br>• Fluconazole 6 mg/kg orally once daily on day 1 followed by 3–6 mg/kg orally once daily (max 400 mg/dose) for 14–21 days.<br>• Itraconazole cyclodextrin oral solution 5 mg/kg once daily for 14–21 days.<br><br>Disseminated candidiasis:<br>• Amphotericin B 0.5–1.5 mg/kg IV once daily<br>• Treat for at least 2–3 weeks after the last positive blood culture.<br>• Longer treatment may be needed for some sites (e.g., CNS, lung) |

**Coccidioidomycosis:** Etiology is attributed to two species, *C. immitis* and *C. posadasii*. *C. immitis* is confined to California while *C. posadasii* is more widely distributed throughout the Southwest, Mexico, and Latin America.

Pulmonary:
- Fever, malaise, cough and chest pain.
- Hemoptysis is less common

Meningitis:
- Headache, change in mental status, focal deficits, vomiting often occur. Hydrocephalus is common.

Disseminated disease:
- Generalized lymphadenopathy
- Skin nodules or ulcers
- Peritonitis
- Liver involvement

- Tissue histology that shows spherules containing endospores are diagnostic
- Blood cultures and CSF cultures are rarely positive
- Sputum cultures often positive
- Serologic assays, such as complement fixation assays of IgG and IgM may be helpful; however may be falsely negative in severely immunocompromised children.
- Clinical symptoms are nonspecific so consider evaluation in those with travel to endemic areas.

Pulmonary or disseminated non-meningeal disease:
- Amphotericin B 0.5–1 mg/kg IV once daily until clinical improvement (min of several weeks).

Meningeal infection:
- Fluconazole 5–6 mg/kg IV or orally twice daily (max 800 mg/day).

**Cryptococcosis:** Generally caused by *Cryptococcus neoformans*. Infections are rare in children, particularly in the post-HAART era.

Generally occurs in profoundly immunocompromised individuals.

Meningoencephalitis:
- Insidious onset
- Fever, headaches, possibly nuchal rigidity

Disseminated cryptococcosis:
- Cutaneous lesions that resemble molluscum contagiosum
- Nodules
- Ulcers

- Cryptococcal antigen in serum, CSF, or other body fluid is the recommended test.
- CSF analysis:
  - High opening pressure
  - India-ink stained wet mount of CSF (no longer performed in some centers)
- Culture of blood, CSF, and sputum

CNS disease:
Acute therapy (2-week induction) is followed by consolidation therapy.
- Amphotericin B 0.7–1 mg/kg IV daily; PLUS
- Flucytosine 100 mg/kg orally divided 4 times daily

Consolidation therapy:
- Fluconazole 12 mg/kg on day 1, followed by 6-12 mg/kg (max 800 mg daily) either IV or orally for minimum of 8 weeks.

*(continued)*

**TABLE 13-4** *(continued)*

| Etiology | Clinical Presentation | Laboratory/Radiological Findings | Preferred Treatment |
|---|---|---|---|
| Cryptococcosis (continued) | Pulmonary:<br>Rare in children, but may include fever, dry cough, x-ray with focal or diffuse infiltrates. | | Localized diseased (not CNS):<br>• Fluconazole 12 mg/kg on day 1, followed by 6–12 mg/kg (max 800 mg daily) either IV or orally. Treatment duration varies<br><br>Disseminated disease (no CNS):<br>Amphotericin B 0.7–1 mg/kg IV daily (+/− flucytosine) |
| Histoplasmosis: Etiology is inhalation of microconidia of *Histoplasmosis capsulatum*. Most highly endemic in the Ohio and Mississippi river valleys. It is been rare in children in both the pre and post-HAART eras. | Progressive disseminated histoplasmosis: Most common presentation in HIV-infected children.<br>• Prolonged fever<br>• Failure to thrive<br>• Splenomegaly<br>• Cough<br>• Lymphadenopathy<br>• Ulcerative cutaneous lesions | • Culture is often invasive and slow to grow organism<br>• EIA probes can detect infection in serum, sputum, and CSF<br>• CSF can also be tested for histoplasmal antigen. | Disseminated disease:<br>• Itraconazole oral solution. Loading dose of 2–5 mg/kg (max 200 mg) orally for days 1–3, followed by 2–5 mg/kg (max 200 mg) per dose twice daily for 12 months. (Urine antigen should be checked for relapse) |
| Pneumocystis Pneumonia (PCP): Etiology is *Pneumocystis jiroveci*. The organisms are found worldwide in lungs of humans. | Pneumonia:<br>• Remains a common AIDS defining illness<br>• Highest incidence in 1st year of life (3–6 months peak age)<br>• Fever<br>• Cough (nonproductive)<br>• Tachypnea | • CD4 counts are generally <200 cells/mm³ or % <15%.<br>• Hypoxia is hallmark<br>• LDH is nonspecific, but often elevated<br>• Chest x-ray classically shows bilateral diffuse interstitial infiltrates described as "ground glass" in appearance. But, can be normal. | Trimethoprim-Sulfamethoxazole (TMP-SMX) TMP 15–20 mg/kg/day IV or orally divided every 8 hours.<br>• Duration of treatment is 21 days followed by suppressive therapy.<br>• In severe disease, corticosteroids may reduce morbidity and mortality |

Pneumocystis Pneumonia (continued)

- Dyspnea

- Stains of sputum (obtained through induced mechanism, bronchoaveolar lavage) include silver stain, toluidine blue, and Wright stain may be used
- Direct fluorescent antibody stains may also be use.

## Parasitic Infections

Cryptosporidiosis/Microsporidiosis:

Cryptosporidium spp. are ubiquitous protozoal parasites. Microspora spp. are intracellular spore forming protozoa.

Cryptosporidiosis:
- Non-bloody watery diarrhea
- Abdominal cramping
- Fever
- Vomiting
- Can invade biliary duct causing acalculous cholecystitis or sclerosing cholengitis

Microsporidiosis:
- Diarrheal illness, non-bloody
- Hepatitis
- Peritonitis
- Myositis
- Keratoconjunctivitis
- Cholangitis

Cryptosporidiosis:
- EIA is preferred
- Cannot be cultured
Microsporidiosis:
- Trichrome stain

Cryptosporidiosis:
- Effective HAART treatment
Microsporidiosis:
- Effective HAART treatment
- Albendazole 7.5 mg/kg (max 400 mg/dose) orally twice daily may be used for disseminated, but not ocular infection for microsporidia other than *E. bienuesi*.

(continued)

TABLE 13-4 (continued)

| Etiology | Clinical Presentation | Laboratory/Radiological Findings | Preferred Treatment |
|---|---|---|---|
| Toxoplasmosis: Etiology is *Toxoplasma gondii*. Infection can occur congenitally or through exposure later in life. In pre-HAART era, CNS toxoplasmosis was rare in children. | CNS disease: <br> • Focal encephalitis <br> • Headache <br> • Fever <br><br> With progression: <br> • Seizures <br> • Coma <br><br> Non-CNS presentations are rare in those with HIV/AIDS. | | Congenital toxoplasmosis: <br> • Pyrimethamine: Loading dose, 2 mg/kg orally once daily for 2 days, then 1 mg/kg orally once daily for 2–6 months, then 1 mg/kg orally 3 times weekly; PLUS <br> • Leucovorin (folinic acid), 10 mg orally or IM with each dose of pyrimethamine; PLUS <br> • Sulfadiazine, 50 mg/kg orally twice daily <br> • Treatment duration: 12 months <br><br> Acquired toxoplasmosis, acute induction therapy (followed by chronic suppressive therapy): <br> • Pyrimethamine: Loading dose, 2 mg/kg (max 50 mg) orally once daily for 3 days, then 1 mg/kg body weight (max 25 mg) orally once daily; PLUS <br> • Sulfadiazine, 25–50 mg/kg (max 1.0–1.5 g/dose) orally per dose 4 times daily; PLUS <br> • Leucovorin, 10–25 mg orally daily <br> • Followed by chronic suppressive therapy <br> • Treatment duration (followed by chronic suppressive therapy): ≥6 weeks (longer if clinical or radiologic disease is extensive or response is incomplete at 6 weeks). |

| Etiology | Clinical Presentation | Laboratory/Radiological Findings | Preferred Treatment |
|---|---|---|---|
| **Bacterial Infections** | | | |
| *Bartonella*, ssp. *henselae* and *quintana* | FUO, bacillary angiomatosis, endocarditis, osteomyelitis, splenitis | CD4 count <100 cells/mm³<br><br>Elevated antibody titer to organism<br><br>Histopathology or PCR | Bacillary angiomatosis, peliosis, bacteremia, and osteomyelitis:<br>• Doxycycline 100 mg orally per day for 3 months.<br><br>Endocarditis:<br>• Doxycycline 100 mg IV every 12 hours; PLUS<br>• Gentamycin 1 mg/kg IV every 8 hours for 2 weeks, then<br>• Doxycycline 100 mg by mouth twice daily for 3 months. |
| Syphilis: Etiology is the spirochete *Treponema pallidum*. While not necessarily an opportunistic infection, there has been a resurgence in the United States in recent years. | • HIV coinfection can alter the clinical presentation in every stage.<br>• Primary syphilis: Painless chancre at the site of inoculation.<br>• Secondary syphilis: Almost any rash, adenopathy, malaise, headache.<br>• Latent syphilis:<br>  ∘ Early: Absence of symptoms, but + RPR and treponemal-specific confirmatory assay within 12 months of a previously negative RPR<br>  ∘ Late/Unknown duration: Asymptomatic and + RPR and treponemal specific confirmatory assay over 12 months beyond a previously negative RPR | • Dark-field microscopy, where available, can detect treponemes in primary syphilis.<br>• Non-treponemal specific screening tests:<br>  ∘ Venereal Disease Research Laboratory (VDRL)<br>  ∘ Rapid plasma regain (RPR)<br>  ∘ Enzyme-linked Assays (EIA)<br>  ∘ RPR allows for the assessment of titer levels<br>• Treponemal specific confirmatory tests:<br>  ∘ FTA-ABS: Generally remains positive after one episode of syphilis | Primary, secondary, and early-latent syphilis:<br>• Penicillin-G 2.4 million units IM × 1<br><br>Late-latent or syphilis of unknown duration:<br>• Penicillin-G 2.4 million units IM weekly × 3 weeks<br><br>Neurosyphilis:<br>• Penicillin-G 24 million units IV per day divided every 4 hours for 14 days |

(continued)

**TABLE 13-5** (continued)

| Etiology | Clinical Presentation | Laboratory/Radiological Findings | Preferred Treatment |
|---|---|---|---|
| Syphilis (continued) | • Neurosyphilis:<br><br>◦ Can occur at any stage of syphilis and manifest in varied clinical presentations, such as cranial nerve dysfunction, stroke, meningitis, acute or chronic change in mental status, loss of vibration sense, and auditory or ophthalmic abnormalities. It is important to note that asymptomatic neurosyphilis may be more common in HIV-infected individuals | | |

**Mycobacterial Infections**

| Etiology | Clinical Presentation | Laboratory/Radiological Findings | Preferred Treatment |
|---|---|---|---|
| *Mycobacterium tuberculosis* | Pulmonary: Cough, fever, night sweats, weight loss<br><br>Extrapulmonary: Blood (miliary), cardiac, joint, bone, skin, kidney, CNS, eye, and abdomen can be initial sites and increasing immunosuppression increases likelihood of extrapulmonary presentation. | • + Mantoux PPD $\geq$5 mm<br>• + Interferon-gamma release assay (IGRA)<br>• Sputum sample with acid fast bacilli (AFB)<br>• Tissue sampling<br>• Chest x-ray | Disseminated disease may progress quickly in infants; prompt initiation of treatment should be considered. Caution with drug–drug interactions with HAART. Four-drug regimen recommended:<br>• Ethambutol: Weight-based dosing for 50 kg person, 800 mg daily<br>• Isoniazid: 300 mg daily<br>• Pyrazinamide: Weight-based dosing for 50 kg person, 1000 mg daily<br>• Rifampin: 600 mg daily dose (Note interactions with HAART) |
| *Mycobacterium avium intracellulare* (MAI): Decreased incidence in post-HAART ear. | • In patients with AIDS who are not on ART, MAC disease typically is a disseminated, multi-organ infection. | • CD4 counts <50 copies/mm$^3$<br>• + Blood culture or culture from site. May use culture of normally sterile site, e.g, bone marrow or lymph node | Two-drug combination therapy is needed. With:<br>• Clarithromycin 500 mg orally twice daily+ |

MAI (continued)

- Early symptoms may be minimal and can precede detectable mycobacteremia by several weeks.
- Symptoms include fever, night sweats, weight loss, fatigue, diarrhea, and abdominal pain.

- + AFB stain of blood, sputum, or stool (confirmation needs to be made with culture or PCR testing)
- Susceptibility testing to azithromycin and clarithromycin is recommended

- Ethambutol 15 mg/kg orally daily, or
- Azithromycin 500–600 mg + ethambutol 15 mg/kg orally daily if drug interaction or intolerance precludes the use of clarithromycin

Duration:

- At least 12 months of therapy, can discontinue if no signs and symptoms of MAC disease and sustained (>6 months) CD4 count > 100 cells/μL in response to ART.

## Viral Infections

Cytomegalovirus (CMV): Acquisition of infection is common.

- More common with CD4 count <50 cells/mm$^3$
- Retinitis is the most common manifestation of the disease. Usually unilateral, but can be bilateral: floaters, scotomata, or peripheral visual loss is common.
- Extra-ocular disease: Can affect GI, lung, liver, kidney, sinuses, or CNS
- Symptoms often nonspecific: Fever, weight loss, odynophagia, or profuse bloody diarrhea.
- Pneumonitis is very uncommon

- More common at CD4 <50 cells/mm$^3$
- CMV can be isolated in cell culture from blood leukocytes, urine, or tissue
- Positive blood buffy-coat culture
- DNA PCR of blood, fluid, or tissue

CMV retinitis:

*Induction therapy: For immediate sight-threatening lesions (adjacent to the optic nerve or fovea):*

- Intravitreal injections of ganciclovir (2 mg) or foscarnet (2.4 mg) for 1–4 doses over a period of 7–10 days to achieve high intraocular concentration faster; PLUS

*Preferred systemic induction therapy:*

Valganciclovir 900 mg orally twice daily for 14–21 days

*For peripheral lesions:*

- Valganciclovir 900 mg orally twice daily for 14–21 days

Chronic maintenance (secondary prophylaxis):

- Valganciclovir 900 mg orally daily

*(continued)*

**TABLE 13-5** (continued)

| Etiology | Clinical Presentation | Laboratory/Radiological Findings | Preferred Treatment |
|---|---|---|---|
| Cytomegalovirus (continued) | | | CMV esophagitis or colitis:<br>• Ganciclovir 5 mg/kg IV every 12 hours; may switch to valganciclovir 900 mg orally twice daily once the patient can tolerate oral therapy<br>• Duration: 21–42 days or until symptoms have resolved<br>• Maintenance therapy is usually not necessary, but should be considered after relapses.<br>Histologically confirmed CMV pneumonia:<br>• Experience for treating CMV pneumonitis in HIV patients is limited.<br>• Use of IV ganciclovir or IV foscarnet is reasonable (doses same as for CMV retinitis)<br>CMV neurological disease:<br>*Note: Treatment should be initiated promptly.*<br>• Ganciclovir 5 mg/kg IV every 12 hours + (foscarnet 90 mg/kg IV every 12 hours or 60 mg/kg IV every 8 hours) to stabilize disease and maximize response, continue until symptomatic improvement and resolution of neurologic symptoms.<br>The optimal duration of therapy and the role of oral valganciclovir have not been established for pulmonary or CNS CMV. |

Jackson Canyon (JC) virus: The causative agent of Progressive Multifocal Leukodystrophy (PML); causes a demyelinating disease of the CNS.

Usually insidious in onset. May present with focal neurologic deficits, cognitive dysfunction, visual disturbances, paralysis, ataxia, or aphasia.

- PML is generally associated with profound immunosuppression, i.e., CD4 count <100–200 cells/mm³.
- MRI of white matter will reveal:
  - Decreased signal on T1 images
  - Increased signal on T2 and FLAIR sequences
- Presence of JC virus in CNS by PCR in conjunction with MRI findings
- Brain biopsy is gold standard with specificity of 100%, but carries significant risk.

- Poor prognosis in pre-HAART era.
- HAART has increased survival time and is the only treatment that has demonstrated benefit.

## Fungal Infections

Aspergillosis: Rare in the post-HAART era, but significantly lethal in pre-HAART era. Most common spp. causing infection are *A. fumingatus*, followed by *A. flavus*

- Invasive pulmonary aspergillosis is the most common presentation: Fever, cough, dyspnea, pleuritic pain, necrotizing pneumonia
- Other presentations include: Tracheobronchitis, CNS disease, skin, sinus disease

- Profound immunosuppression (<100 CD4 cells/mm³) associated with higher risk
- Blood cultures generally not helpful
- CXR or CT scan for pulmonary involvement
- Fungal histology/culture of suspected site
- BAL galactomannan is very specific

Invasive pulmonary aspergillosis:
- Voriconizole 6–8 mg/kg IV every 12 hours for 2 doses followed by 7 mg/kg either IV or orally twice daily for 12 weeks

*Candida* Mucocutaneous Infections: *Candida* ssp. are the most common fungal infections in HIV-infected adolescents and young adults.

Oral thrush: Primarily caused by *C. albicans*. Oral thrush characteristically presents white patches with underlying inflamed mucosa when the patch is removed. Other presentations are possible.

Oral thrush:
- May be made clinically
- Potassium hydroxide preparation of samples will show budding yeast cells.

Oral thrush:
- Fluconazole 100 mg orally daily for 7–14 days.

(continued)

| TABLE 13-5 (continued) | | | |
|---|---|---|---|
| **Etiology** | **Clinical Presentation** | **Laboratory/Radiological Findings** | **Preferred Treatment** |
| Candida Mucocutaneous Infections (continued) | • Esophageal candidiasis presents with odynophagia, retrosternal pain.<br>• Vulvovaginal candidiasis: Presents similarly to HIV-uninfected women with a white, cottage-cheese-like vaginal discharge and vaginal itching. | • Culture may need to be done in refractory cases or failure of treatment.<br><br>Esophageal thrush:<br>• Barium swallow will demonstrate a classic cobblestone appearance<br>• Refractory causes may require endoscopy to rule out other causes.<br><br>Vulvovaginal candidiasis:<br>• May be made clinically<br>• Potassium hydroxide preparation of samples will show budding yeast cells and hyphae. | Esophageal thrush:<br>• Fluconazole 100 mg orally once daily for 14–21 days.<br>• Itraconazole oral solution 200 mg once daily for 14–21 days. |
| Coccidioidomycosis:<br>Etiology is attributed to two species, *C. immitis* and *C. posadasii*. *C. immitis* is confined to California while *C. posadasii* is more widely distributed throughout the Southwest, Mexico, and Latin America. | Pulmonary:<br>• Fever, malaise, and chest pain.<br>• Cough and hemoptysis is a rare presentation<br>Meningitis:<br>• Headache, change in mental status, focal deficits, vomiting often occur. Hydrocephalus is common<br>Disseminated disease:<br>• Generalized lymphadenopathy<br>• Skin nodules or ulcers<br>• Peritonitis<br>• Liver involvement | • Tissue histology that shows spherules containing endospores are diagnostic<br>• Blood cultures and CSF cultures are rarely positive<br>• Sputum cultures often positive.<br>• A coccidioidomycosis-specific antigen is available for urine and serum and is useful in making the diagnosis | Mild disease (e.g., focal pneumonia):<br>• Fluconazole 400 mg orally daily<br>Severe, non-CNS infection, or disseminated disease:<br>• Liposomal amphotericin B 4–6 mg/kg IV daily until clinical improvement and then switch to an azole.<br>Meningeal infection:<br>• Fluconazole 400–800 mg IV or orally daily.<br>Chronic suppressive therapy:<br>• Fluconazole 400 mg orally daily |

| | | |
|---|---|---|
| Cryptococcosis: Generally caused by *Cryptococcus neoformans*, but occasionally by *C. gattii* (in Australia, subtropical regions, and the Pacific Northwest). | Generally occurs in profoundly immunocomprised individuals.<br><br>**Meningoencephalitis:**<br>• Insidious onset<br>• Fever, headaches, possibly nuchal rigidity<br><br>Disseminated cryptococcosis:<br>• Cutaneous lesions that resemble molluscum contagiosum<br>• Nodules<br>• Ulcers<br><br>**Pulmonary:**<br>• May include fever, dry cough, x-ray with focal or diffuse infiltrates.<br>• Mimics PCP | • Cryptococcal antigen in serum, CSF, or other body fluid is effective for rapid diagnosis<br>• CSF analysis:<br> ○ High opening pressure (≥25 cm H$_2$O)<br> ○ India-ink stained **wet mount** of CSF<br>• Culture of blood, CSF, and sputum | CNS disease:<br>Acute therapy (2-week induction) is followed by consolidation therapy.<br>• Liposomal amphotericin B 3–4 mg/kg IV daily; PLUS<br>• Flucytosine 100 mg/kg orally divided 4 times daily (renal dosing needed)<br>Consolidation therapy: For minimum of 8 weeks followed by maintenance therapy.<br>• Fluconazole 400 mg daily either IV or orally<br>Maintenance therapy:<br>• Fluconazole 200 mg orally daily for at least 12 months.<br><br>Non-CNS, extrapulmonary, and diffuse pulmonary disease:<br>• Treat the same as meningitis above.<br>Non-CNS with mild to moderate symptoms and focal pulmonary infiltrates:<br>• Fluconazole 400 mg orally daily for 12 months. |
| Histoplasmosis:<br>Etiology is inhalation of microconidia of *Histoplasmosis capsulatum*. Most highly endemic in the Ohio and Mississippi river valleys, Puerto Rico, and Latin America. | Progressive disseminated histoplasmosis:<br>• Prolonged fever<br>• Hepatosplenomegaly<br>• Fatigue<br>• Cough<br>• Weight Loss | • Histoplasma antigen in blood or urine is sensitive for rapid diagnosis of acute pulmonary disease and disseminated disease<br>• Culture is often invasive and slow to grow organism<br>• EIA probes can detect infection in serum, sputum, and CSF | Moderately severe to severe disseminated disease:<br>*Induction therapy (for at least 2 weeks or until clinically improved):*<br>• Liposomal amphotericin B 3 mg/kg IV daily<br>*Maintenance therapy:*<br>• Itraconazole 200 mg orally three times daily for 3 days, then 200 mg orally twice daily. |

*(continued)*

213

**TABLE 13-5** (continued)

| Etiology | Clinical Presentation | Laboratory/Radiological Findings | Preferred Treatment |
|---|---|---|---|
| Histoplasmosis (continued) | CNS disease:<br>• Fever<br>• Headache<br>• Focal deficits<br>GI disease:<br>• Diarrhea<br>• Abdominal pain<br>• Weight loss<br>Pulmonary disease:<br>• Cough<br>• Fever<br>• Pleuritic chest pain | • CSF can also be tested for histoplasmal antigen. | Less severe disseminated disease:<br>*Induction and maintenance therapy:*<br>• Itraconazole 200 mg orally thrice daily for 3 days, then 200 mg orally twice daily for at least 12 months<br>Meningitis:<br>*Induction therapy (4–6 weeks):*<br>• Liposomal amphotericin B 5 mg/kg/day IV daily<br>*Maintenance therapy:*<br>Itraconazole 200 mg orally twice daily for ≥1 year and until resolution of abnormal CSF findings |
| Pneumocystis Pneumonia (PCP): Etiology is *Pneumocystis jiroveci.* The organisms are found worldwide in lungs of humans. | Pneumonia:<br>• Often subacute onset<br>• Fever<br>• Cough (nonproductive)<br>• Tachypnea<br>• Dyspnea | • CD4 counts are generally <200 cells/mm³ or % <14%.<br>• Hypoxia is hallmark<br>• LDH is nonspecific, but often elevated<br>• Chest x-ray classically shows bilateral diffuse interstitial infiltrates described as "ground glass" in appearance. But, can be normal.<br>• Stains of sputum (obtained through induced mechanism, bronchoaveolar lavage) include silver stain, toluidine blue, and Wright stain may be used<br>• Direct fluorescent antibody stains may also be used. | • Trimethoprim-Sulfamethoxazole (TMP-SMX) TMP 15–20 mg/kg/day IV or orally divided every 8 hours.<br>• Duration of treatment is 21 days followed by suppressive therapy.<br>• In severe disease, corticosteroids reduce morbidity and mortality |

## Parasitic Infections

Cryptosporidiosis/
Microsporidiosis:
*Cryptosporidium* spp.
are ubiquitous protozoal
parasites. *Microspora*
spp. are intracellular
spore-forming protozoa.

Cryptosporidiosis:
- Non-bloody watery diarrhea
- Abdominal cramping
- Fever
- Vomiting
- Can invade biliary duct causing acalculous cholecystitis or sclerosing cholengitis

Microsporidiosis:
- Diarrheal illness, non-bloody
- Hepatitis
- Peritonitis
- Myositis
- Keratoconjunctivitis
- Cholangitis

Cryptosporidiosis:
- EIA is preferred
- Cannot be cultured

Microsporidiosis:
- Trichrome stain

Cryptosporidiosis:
- Effective HAART treatment

Microsporidiosis:
- Effective HAART treatment
- Albendazole 7.5 mg/kg (max 400 mg/dose) orally twice daily may be used for disseminated, but not ocular infection for microsporidia other than *E. bienuesi*.

Toxoplasmosis: Etiology
is *Toxoplasma gondii*.
Prevalence of serum
antibodies varies
through the United
States and the world.
Disease is primarily due
to reactivation of latent
cysts.

CNS disease: The most common clinical presentation.
- Focal encephalitis
- Headache
- Fever

With progression:
- Seizures
- Coma

Non-CNS presentations are rare in those with HIV/AIDS.

- CT or MRI with contrast will show ring-enhancing lesions in the gray matter of the cortex or basal ganglia. Edema is often present.
- IgG antibodies are uniformly present.
- Stereotactic CT-guided brain biopsy is the only definitive diagnostic tool.
- Detection of *Toxoplasma gondii* by PCR in CSF is very specific, but has low sensitivity.

Treatment of acute infection:
- Pyrimethamine 200 mg orally 1 time, followed by weight-based therapy.
- If <60 kg, pyrimethamine 50 mg orally once daily + sulfadiazine 1000 mg orally every 6 hours + leucovorin 10–25 mg orally once daily
- If ≥60 kg, pyrimethamine 75 mg orally once daily + sulfadiazine 1500 mg orally every 6 hours + leucovorin 10–25 mg orally once daily

*(continued)*

215

**TABLE 13-5** *(continued)*

| Etiology | Clinical Presentation | Laboratory/Radiological Findings | Preferred Treatment |
|---|---|---|---|
| Toxoplasmosis (continued) | | | • Leucovorin dose can be increased to 50 mg daily or twice daily. <br><br> Duration for acute therapy: <br><br> • At least 6 weeks longer duration if clinical or radiologic disease is extensive or response is incomplete at 6 weeks. <br><br> Chronic maintenance therapy: <br><br> • Pyrimethamine 25–50 mg orally daily + sulfadiazine 2000–4000 mg orally daily (in 2–4 divided doses) + leucovorin 10–25 mg orally daily. This should be continued for at least 6 months after CD4 counts have exceeded 200 cells/mm³ before consideration of stopping secondary prophylaxis. |

## POST-EXPOSURE PROPHYLAXIS

- *Occupational (PEP):* Guidelines available from the 2013 "Updated US Public Health Service Guidelines for the Management of Occupational Exposures to Human Immunodeficiency Virus and Recommendations for Post-exposure Prophylaxis"
  - ✓ Risk of HIV transmission following a percutaneous exposure is about 0.3%. Higher HIV viral loads in infected persons, a larger, hollow-bore needle, or an arterial source increase risk of transmission
  - ✓ HIV testing the source patient is preferred when possible
  - ✓ Initiate PEP as soon as possible, preferably within hours. If the source patient is later found to be HIV-negative PEP can be discontinued
  - ✓ Baseline HIV, syphilis, and Hepatitis C testing should be offered to the exposed individual
  - ✓ *Three drug regimens are now recommended in all exposures in which PEP is being recommended:*
    - The preferred regimen is Raltegravir 400 mg by twice daily, plus Tenofovir DF 300 mg + emtricitabine 200 mg orally daily (available in a combination pill)
    - Treatment duration is 4 weeks
  - ✓ Follow-up should occur at 72 hours, 6 weeks, 12 weeks, and 6 months after exposure
  - ✓ Local expert guidance should be sought or PEP guidance is also available at PEPline at www.nccc.ucsf.edu/about_nccc/pepline or by phone at 888-448-4911
- *Nonoccupational Post-exposure Prophylaxis (nPEP):*
  - ✓ Defined as nonoccupational exposure to blood, genital secretions, or other potentially infectious body fluids
  - ✓ If treatment is chosen, it should be started ≤72 hours after exposure
  - ✓ Table 13-6 shows relative risk of HIV transmission per exposure type
  - ✓ Figure 13-2 shows the Center for Disease Control's algorithm for determining the need for nPEP

| TABLE 13-6 Estimated Per-Act Risk for Acquisition of HIV, by Exposure Route | |
|---|---|
| **Exposure Route** | **Risk Per 10,000 Exposures to an Infected Source** |
| Blood transfusion | 9000 |
| Needle-sharing injection-drug use | 67 |
| Receptive anal intercourse | 50 |
| Percutaneous needle stick | 30 |
| Receptive penile–vaginal intercourse* | 10 |
| Insertive anal intercourse* | 6.5 |
| Insertive penile–vaginal intercourse* | 5 |
| Receptive oral intercourse* | 1 |
| Insertive oral intercourse* | 0.5 |

*Estimates of risk for transmission from sexual exposures assume no condom use.
Reproduced with permission of Smith DK, Grohskopf LA, Black RJ, et al: Antiretroviral postexposure prophylaxis after sexual, injection-drug use, or other nonoccupational exposure to HIV in the United States: recommendations from the U.S. Department of Health and Human Services, *MMWR Recomm Rep* 2005 Jan 21;54(RR-2):1–20

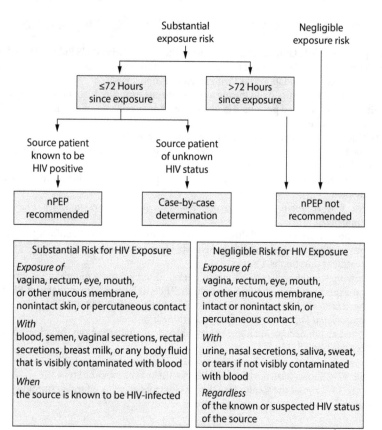

**FIGURE 13-2 Algorithm for evaluation and treatment of possible nonoccupational HIV exposures.** Reproduced with permission of Smith DK, Grohskopf LA, Black RJ, et al: Antiretroviral postexposure prophylaxis after sexual, injection-drug use, or other nonoccupational exposure to HIV in the United States: recommendations from the U.S. Department of Health and Human Services, *MMWR Recomm Rep* 2005 Jan 21;54(RR-2):1–20

# 14     Immunology

*Gita Ram, MD*
*Soma Jyonouchi, MD*

## APPROACH TO PRIMARY IMMUNODEFICIENCY

**Warning Signs for Immune Deficiency. Consider immune deficiency when two or more of the following are present (data from Jeffrey Modell Foundation).**

- Recurrent otitis (≥8 episodes), sinusitis (≥2 episodes), or pneumonia (≥2 episodes) in 1 year (from Jeffrey Modell Foundation)
- Two or more invasive infections (meningitis, sepsis, osteomyelitis, etc.)
- Recurrent deep skin or organ abscesses
- Infections with unusual or opportunistic organisms
- Failure to thrive
- Persistent thrush in mouth or elsewhere on skin after 1 year of age
- Need for intravenous antibiotics to clear common infections
- Family history of immunodeficiency

## MAJOR CATEGORIES

The major categories of primary immune deficiencies reflect the various arms of the immune system (Tables 14-1 and 14-2).

| TABLE 14-1   Classification of Primary Immune Deficiencies | |
| --- | --- |
| **Category** | **Select Conditions** |
| **B cell disorders** | • X-linked agammaglobulinemia (XLA) |
| | • Common variable immune deficiency (CVID) |
| | • Transient Hypogammaglobulinemia of Infancy (THI) |
| | • IgA deficiency |
| **Combined B and T cell disorders** | • Severe combined immune deficiency (SCID) |
| | • 22q11.2 deletion syndrome |
| | • Wiskott–Aldrich syndrome |
| | • Ataxia-Telangiectasia |
| **Phagocyte disorders** | • Chronic granulomatous disease (CGD) |
| | • Leukocyte adhesion deficiency (LAD) |
| | • Severe congenital neutropenia (SCN) |
| | • Hyper IgE syndrome |

| TABLE 14-2 | Features and Diagnostic Approach for Primary Immune Deficiencies | |
|---|---|---|
| | **General Features** | **Diagnostic Approach** |
| **B cell (antibody/ humoral) disorders** | • Usually present after 3–6 months of age after maternal antibodies decrease; exception is common variable immunodeficiency (CVID), which can present at any age including adulthood. | *Quantitative measures:*<br><br>• Serum immunoglobulin levels (IgG, IgA, IgM), flow cytometry<br>• B cell enumeration<br><br>*Functional measures:* |
| | • Predisposition for infections of the upper and lower respiratory tract with encapsulated bacteria (*Streptococcus pneumoniae* and *Haemophilus influenzae*). *Mycoplasma* spp. and *Ureaplasma* spp. infections can cause pneumonia and destructive septic arthritis. Enterovirus infections (*polio, coxsackie, echo virus*) can cause chronic diarrhea, meningitis, or fatal disseminated infections in patients with X-linked agammaglobulinemia. | • IgG responses to vaccinations— pneumococcal serotype-specific antibodies after pneumococcal conjugate (Prevnar) or polysaccharide (Pneumovax) vaccination, tetanus and diphtheria antibodies after DTaP vaccination |
| | • The cornerstone of therapy is immunoglobulin replacement therapy to reduce the frequency of infections. | |
| **T cell and combined (T and B cell) disorders** | • Present at birth or in early infancy<br>• Failure to thrive, chronic diarrhea<br>• Develop prolonged and severe respiratory viral infections<br>• Predisposition for fungal infections and opportunistic infections such as *Pneumocystis jiroveci* (formerly *Pneumocystis carinii*)<br>• Association with autoimmune diseases<br>• Severe combined immune deficiency (SCID) is characterized by a complete absence of T cells and is fatal in the first year of life without bone marrow transplantation.<br>• Milder forms of T cell deficiencies include 22q11.2 deletion syndrome and ataxia-telangiectasia. | *Quantitative measures:*<br><br>• Absolute lymphocyte count (ALC) on CBC with differential (80% of the ALC is comprised of T cells)<br>• Flow cytometry for T cell subset enumeration<br>• Many states now have a TREC assay newborn screen—this test result is near zero for patients with SCID<br><br>*Functional measures:*<br><br>• Mitogen proliferation assay |

| TABLE 14-2 | *(continued)* | |
|---|---|---|
| | **General Features** | **Diagnostic Approach** |
| **Phagocyte disorders** | • Present in early childhood<br>• Predisposition to skin infections, pneumonia, lymphadenitis, and osteomyelitis from catalase-positive organisms *Staphylococcus aureus, Burkholderia cepacia, Nocardia asteroides, Serratia marcescens, Aspergillus fumigatus*<br>• Poor wound healing, delayed separation of the umbilical cord, and omphalitis | *Quantitative measures:*<br>• Absolute neutrophil count (ANC) on CBC with differential<br>*Functional measures:*<br>• Neutrophil oxidative burst (DHR assay) |
| **Complement disorders** | • Extremely rare<br>• Early complement component defects: predisposition for bacterial respiratory tract infections and immune complex disease (systemic lupus erythematosus)<br>• Terminal complement component defects: predisposition for recurrent meningococcal disease | • CH50 is typically near zero for affected patients |

## SPECIFIC IMMUNODEFICIENCIES

### X-LINKED AGAMMAGLOBULINEMIA (XLA)

**A defect of B cell maturation, resulting in B cell and antibody deficiencies with recurrent bacterial infections.**

#### EPIDEMIOLOGY

• Approximately 1/100,000–200,000

#### ETIOLOGY

• *Btk* (Bruton tyrosine kinase) gene, on Xp22

#### PATHOPHYSIOLOGY

• Btk is required for B cell maturation after the pre-B stage. As a result, patients with XLA have arrest of B cell development in the bone marrow at the pro-B to pre-B stage. Mature B cells and plasma cells do not develop, causing a deficiency of all antibody isotypes
• Btk is also expressed in myeloid stem cells so patients may also present with neutropenia

#### DIFFERENTIAL DIAGNOSIS

• *Primary immunodeficiencies:* Autosomal recessive agammaglobulinemia (BLNK deficiency, Igα and Igβ deficiency, μ heavy-chain deficiency, and λ5 deficiency), CVID, hyper

IgM syndrome, WHIM syndrome, transient hypogammaglobulinemia of infancy, GATA2 deficiency, dyskeratosis congenita

- *Immunoglobulin loss:* Nephrotic syndrome, severe burns, intestinal lymphangiectasia, severe enteropathy
- *Prematurity:* Maternal IgG is transferred to the fetus during third trimester

## CLINICAL MANIFESTATIONS

- Bacterial respiratory tract infections such as sinusitis, otitis, pneumonia, and bronchitis with encapsulated organisms (*Streptococcus pneumoniae, Haemophilus influenzae*) are very common
- Patients do not have difficulty with common viral respiratory infections
  - ✓ There is, however, an increased susceptibility to enterovirus infections (e.g., poliovirus, coxsackievirus, echovirus) which can cause chronic diarrhea, meningitis, or fatal disseminated infection
- Profound neutropenia is found in 10% of XLA patients at initial presentation (usually in the setting of acute infections). The neutropenia typically resolves after the infectious episode is treated. Sepsis, especially with *Pseudomonas aeruginosa* and *Staphylococcus aureus*, can occur during episodes of neutropenia
- Absence of lymphoid tissue (tonsils, adenoids, lymph nodes) is a classic finding

## DIAGNOSTICS

- Low levels of IgG, IgA, and IgM antibodies in children beyond the first 6 months of life
  - ✓ IgG subclass evaluation is not necessary
  - ✓ T cell studies are not warranted if the clinical picture is highly suggestive of immunoglobulin deficiency
- Peripheral B lymphocyte counts are typically <1%
- Neutropenia can be seen during acute infectious episodes
- Absence of detectable Btk protein (by flow cytometry or western blotting) and genetic testing confirms the diagnosis

## MANAGEMENT

- IVIG replacement (400–500 mg/kg every 3–4 weeks) is the cornerstone of therapy and helps to prevent serious infectious complications. IVIG provides passive immunity to common pathogens such as tetanus, diphtheria, pneumococcus, and hepatitis B

## COMMON VARIABLE IMMUNODEFICIENCY (CVID)

**A heterogeneous group of disorders characterized by decreased antibody production and recurrent bacterial infections. Approximately 25% of patients also suffer from autoimmune complications.**

## EPIDEMIOLOGY

- 1/10,000–1/100,000 children affected
- Onset can occur at any age, but there are two peaks of presentation, the first and third decades of life

## ETIOLOGY

- The exact genetic cause of most CVID cases remains unknown. This is likely a heterogeneous disorder with a common clinical phenotype. In recent years, a number of monogenic causes of CVID have been identified in a minority of patients, but this disorder is likely polygenic in most patients

## DIFFERENTIAL DIAGNOSIS

- *Primary immunodeficiencies:* XLA and autosomal recessive agammaglobulinemia, hyper IgM syndrome, WHIM syndrome, transient hypogammaglobulinemia of infancy, combined immunodeficiencies, X-linked lymphoproliferative disease
- *Immunoglobulin loss:* Nephrotic syndrome, severe burns, intestinal lymphangiectasia, and severe enteropathy
- *Drug-induced:* Antimalarial agents, captopril, carbamazepine, glucocorticoids, rituximab, phenytoin, sulfasalazine
- *Malignancy:* Chronic lymphocytic leukemia, thymoma, non-Hodgkin's lymphoma, B cell malignancy

## PATHOPHYSIOLOGY

- Defects in B cell differentiation or B cell co-stimulatory signaling result in impaired immunoglobulin production

## CLINICAL MANIFESTATIONS

- >90% of patients suffer from recurrent infections of the sinopulmonary tract (sinusitis and pneumonia)
- Autoimmune diseases are common (25%) and include autoimmune hemolytic anemia and immune thrombocytopenic purpura. Autoimmune complications can precede the onset of infections
- Patients are also at greater risk for developing certain malignancies including lymphoma (incidence, 8%) and gastric carcinoma (incidence, 2%)
- Gastrointestinal diseases, including inflammatory bowel disease and malabsorption are common; chronic infectious diarrhea (often *Giardia lamblia* or *Campylobacter jejuni*) can also occur
- Non-caseating granulomas of lungs, liver, and spleen can occur

## DIAGNOSTICS

- Two of three immunoglobulin isotypes (IgG, IgA, IgM) are 2 SD below age-appropriate normal levels
- Poor antibody response to vaccine antigens at least 4 weeks postvaccination
- T and B cell enumeration by flow cytometry. A CD4 lymphopenia may be present in some patients. B cell numbers are typically normal but may be low in some patients. Patients with low or absent switched memory B cells appear to be at greatest risk for bronchiectasis and autoimmune complications

## MANAGEMENT

- IVIG replacement every 3–4 weeks
- Prophylactic antibiotics can be considered as adjunctive therapy in patients with recurrent infections. The type of prophylaxis should be directed at the site of infection and offending pathogens (e.g., amoxicillin 20 mg/kg/day or azithromycin 10 mg/kg/week)
- Routine screening for autoimmune and infectious complications
  - ✓ CBC to monitor for autoimmune cytopenias (e.g., ITP hemolytic anemia)
  - ✓ Other testing should be guided by clinical symptoms
  - ✓ Routine or screening imaging studies are not recommended for detection of malignancy in the absence of suggestive signs or symptoms

## TRANSIENT HYPOGAMMAGLOBULINEMIA OF INFANCY

**A prolongation of the physiologic nadir of immunoglobulin production which typically occurs between 3 and 6 months of life.**

### EPIDEMIOLOGY

• Approximately .061 per 1000 live births

### ETIOLOGY

• A maturational delay in endogenous IgG production

### DIFFERENTIAL DIAGNOSIS

• *Primary immunodeficiencies:* XLA and autosomal recessive agammaglobulinemia, CVID, hyper IgM syndrome, WHIM syndrome (warts, hypogammaglobulinemia, infections, and myelokathexis), combined immunodeficiencies, X-linked lymphoproliferative disease
• *Immunoglobulin loss:* Nephrotic syndrome, severe burns, intestinal lymphangiectasia, and severe enteropathy
• *Drug-induced:* Antimalarial agents, captopril, carbamazepine, glucocorticoids, rituximab, phenytoin, sulfasalazine
• *Malignancy:* Chronic lymphocytic leukemia, thymoma, non-Hodgkin's lymphoma, B cell malignancy
• *Prematurity:* Maternal IgG is transferred to the fetus during third trimester

### PATHOPHYSIOLOGY

• Transplacental transfer begins during the second trimester of pregnancy and peaks during the third trimester; IgG measured in the infant at birth is almost entirely maternal. Maternal IgG gradually declines and a physiologic nadir is reached around 6 months of age, when the infant's endogenous IgG production begins to develop
• Transient hypogammaglobulinemia is a delay in endogenous IgG production leading to prolonged hypogammaglobulinemia

### CLINICAL MANIFESTATIONS

• Low IgG levels
• Normal vaccine antigen responses
• Many patients are asymptomatic and identified incidentally, but some may present with recurrent bacterial sinopulmonary infections
• Spontaneous improvement in IgG levels usually occurs by 18 months of age, but some may not have full recovery until 5 years of age
  ✓ 67% normalize by 24 months of age
  ✓ 100% normalize by 5 years of age

### DIAGNOSTICS

• Low IgG levels with decreased or normal IgM and IgA levels
• Normal or low normal vaccine responses (in contrast to CVID patients who have low IgG and absent vaccine response). If vaccine antibody levels are low, patients should be revaccinated and have levels rechecked 4–6 weeks later
• Absolute T, B, and NK cells are normal
• Transient hypogammaglobulinemia remains a diagnosis of exclusion and the absence of other primary immunodeficiencies (XLA, HIGM, CVID) must be documented

## MANAGEMENT

- No therapy is needed if patients are asymptomatic. Immunoglobulin levels and vaccine antibody responses should be rechecked every 6–12 months until resolution of hypogammaglobulinemia can be documented
- Antibiotic prophylaxis (e.g., amoxicillin 20 mg/kg divided twice daily) can be considered for those with recurrent sinopulmonary infections
- IVIG is typically not indicated for transient hypogammaglobulinemia of infancy unless patients continue to suffer from severe infections despite antibiotic prophylaxis. IVIG therapy should be stopped within 1–2 years to assess endogenous antibody levels and vaccine responses

## IgA DEFICIENCY

**The most common immunodeficiency, characterized by isolated undetectable serum IgA.**

### EPIDEMIOLOGY

- The most common immunodeficiency, manifesting in 1/200–1/1000 among Caucasians

### ETIOLOGY

- A selective deficiency in IgA production secondary to a B cell maturational defect

### DIFFERENTIAL DIAGNOSIS

- *Primary immunodeficiencies:* CVID, XLA, hyper IgM deficiency
- *Maturational delay:* Younger patients under the age of 4 years may have low IgA levels due to immaturity of the humoral immune system

### PATHOPHYSIOLOGY

- The IgA is the predominant immunoglobulin found in mucosal surfaces
- IgA is normally concentrated in mucosal secretions (pulmonary secretions, saliva, tears, breast milk, GI secretions); its concentration in the serum is relatively low
- In IgA deficiency, a maturational defect in B cells leads to expression of immature IgA on the cell surface with co-expression of IgM and IgD. Development into IgA-secreting plasma cells is impaired

### CLINICAL MANIFESTATIONS

- Most (85%) patients with selective IgA deficiency are asymptomatic and do not require treatment or regular follow-up
- A minority of patients, particularly those with concurrent IgG subclass deficiency, may present with sinopulmonary infections with encapsulated bacteria
- Autoimmune disorders (ITP, autoimmune hemolytic anemia, SLE, vitiligo), gastrointestinal disorders (giardiasis, inflammatory bowel disease), and atopic diseases (asthma, allergic rhinitis, atopic dermatitis, food allergy) are also increased in patients with IgA deficiency
- Very rarely, anaphylactic transfusion reactions to IgA containing blood products may occur
- Selective IgA deficiency may progress to CVID. Thus, patients who are symptomatic with sinopulmonary infections should be followed longitudinally to determine if CVID develops

### DIAGNOSTICS

- Undetectable IgA levels, with normal IgG and IgM levels
- Normal antibody responses to vaccines

## MANAGEMENT

- No treatment is required for asymptomatic patients who do not suffer from increased infections
- If patient suffers from recurrent infections, prophylactic antibiotics can be considered. These should be tailored to the pathogens and sites of repeated infections (e.g., amoxicillin 20 mg/kg/day, azithromycin 10 mg/kg/week)
- Patients with selective IgA deficiency are not candidates for IVIG

## SEVERE COMBINED IMMUNODEFICIENCY (SCID)

**A heterogeneous group of disorders characterized by profound T cell dysfunction resulting in severe infections and death within the first year of life without stem cell transplantation.**

### EPIDEMIOLOGY

- Incidence between 1/50,000 and 1/70,000 live births
- Increased incidence in males (X-linked SCID is the most common form)

### ETIOLOGY

- Although there are many different causes of SCID (more than 30 have been described to date), the unifying feature shared by all types is a complete absence of T cell development. Although some mutations allow for B cell development to occur, B cell function is invariably impaired due to the absence of T cell co-stimulatory signaling
- Classification of the different types of SCID based on the pattern of lymphocyte subpopulation depression is a useful strategy for determining the underlying genetic defect
  - ✓ **T−B+NK+SCID:** IL-7 receptor deficiency, CD3 deficiencies, CD45 deficiency
  - ✓ **T−B+NK−SCID:** IL-2 receptor gamma deficiency (X-linked SCID), ADA deficiency
  - ✓ **T−B−NK+SCID:** Rag1/2 deficiency, Artemis deficiency
  - ✓ **T−B−NK−SCID:** Adenosine deaminase (ADA) deficiency, purine nucleotide phosphorylase (PNP) deficiency, adenylate kinase 2 deficiency (reticular dysgenesis)

### DIFFERENTIAL DIAGNOSIS

- *Primary immunodeficiencies:* Wiskott–Aldrich syndrome, 22q deletion syndrome, MHC class I or II deficiency, cartilage hair hypoplasia
- HIV infection

### PATHOPHYSIOLOGY

- The unifying feature shared by all types of SCID is a complete absence of T cell development. Some mutations allow for B cell development to occur, but B cell function is invariably impaired due to the absence of T cell co-stimulatory signaling
  - ✓ In common gamma chain receptor SCID, the gamma chain forms the functional signaling unit of the IL-2, IL-4, IL-7, IL-9, IL-15, and IL-21 receptors, thus affecting T and NK cell development
  - ✓ In ADA deficiency SCID, accumulation metabolites that are toxic to all types of lymphocytes results in a T−B−NK−SCID phenotype

### CLINICAL MANIFESTATIONS

- SCID patients present during early infancy with pneumonia, diarrhea, otitis, sepsis, or skin infections. Recalcitrant oral candidiasis, *Pneumocystis jiroveci* lung infections, and severe viral respiratory infections are common

- Lymphoid tissue, including the thymus, is often decreased or absent
- Failure to thrive secondary to recurrent infections
- Patients can develop severe infections after receiving live virus vaccines (rotavirus, BCG, MMR, Varicella)
- Graft-versus-host (GVHD) reactions from engrafted maternal T cells can result in severe cutaneous, gastrointestinal, and hematologic disease. Lymphadenopathy and hepatospleno-megaly can also occur

## DIAGNOSTICS

- Newborn screening for SCID is now available in a number of states and is based on measuring T cell receptor excision circles (TRECs) which are by-products of T cell development. Patients with SCID typically have undetectable TREC values
- A CBC with differential typically reveals a low absolute lymphocyte count ($<3000/mm^3$) but a normal CBC does not exclude SCID as a possibility
- Flow cytometry to enumerate T, B, and NK cells (T cell numbers are markedly reduced. B and NK cell numbers vary depending on the type of SCID)
- Immunoglobulin levels are markedly reduced (although IgG can be normal in young infants due to maternally transferred immunoglobulin)
- T cell proliferation in response to mitogens usually reveals poor T cell function
- Thymic tissue is typically absent on chest x-ray
- HIV DNA PCR to exclude HIV infection

## MANAGEMENT

- Isolation—Minimize sick contacts
  ✓ Contact and respiratory precautions should immediately be instituted. Hospitalization is often necessary
- Trimethoprim-sulfamethoxazole (TMP-SMX) prophylaxis to prevent *Pneumocystis jiroveci* infections
- IVIG replacement therapy (400–600 mg/kg once monthly to maintain IgG levels greater than 800 mg/dL)
- Avoid all live virus vaccinations (rotavirus, BCG, varicella, MMR)
- All blood products must be irradiated, CMV-negative, and leukocyte reduced. Patients can develop GVHD from retained leukocytes and CMV infections from blood products
- Breastfeeding should be avoided to prevent transmission of CMV
- HLA-typing for the patient and any siblings for bone marrow transplantation. There is a 95% success rate (i.e., survival $>10$ years) for bone marrow transplantation performed within the first 3 months of life

## 22q11.2 DELETION SYNDROME

**A genetic disorder characterized by cardiac defects, hypocalcemia, developmental delay, facial dysmorphology, and variable T cell defects.**

- DiGeorge syndrome, velocardiofacial syndrome, and similar syndromes involve deletions within the 22q region, but wide heterogeneity of the phenotype results from differing amounts of chromosomal loss

## EPIDEMIOLOGY

- 1/3000–1/4000 live births
- Found in 8% of children with cleft palates and 1% of children with congenital heart disease

## ETIOLOGY

- The most common deletion which causes this syndrome includes a region containing more than 35 genes. *TBX1* gene has emerged as one of the most likely causes of the clinical phenotype
- Chromosome 10p deletions and CHD7 mutations (CHARGE syndrome) can result in a similar clinical phenotype

## DIFFERENTIAL DIAGNOSIS

- *Primary immunodeficiencies:* Other T cell and combined immunodeficiencies
- *Genetic syndromes:* CHARGE syndrome, chromosome 10p deletions
- HIV infection

## PATHOPHYSIOLOGY

- Impaired embryogenesis of the 3rd and 4th pharyngeal arches results in thymic hypoplasia (which impairs T cell development), parathyroid hypoplasia (which results in hypocalcemia), conotruncal heart defects, and facial dysmorphology

## CLINICAL MANIFESTATIONS

- Low T cell numbers are present in 80% of patients with 22q11.2 deletion syndrome. The decrease in T cell numbers is typically mild to moderate but with preservation of T cell function
- A severe form of this syndrome resulting from complete thymic aplasia (resulting in near total absence of T cells) occurs in approximately 1% of patients. Patients with this condition require a thymic transplant in order to survive
- Patients typically have normal B cell numbers and immunoglobulin levels
- Tetany and seizures from hypocalcemia is present in 10–30% of neonatal patients. The hypocalcemia is self-limiting; most children do not require calcium supplementation beyond 1 year
- 80–90% of patients have congenital heart disease. Most commonly—interrupted aortic arch, right arch, ventricular septal defect, aberrant right subclavian and internal carotid arteries, tetralogy of Fallot, and truncus arteriosus
- Speech delay, nonverbal learning disorders, and mild mental retardation (40–50%)
- Paranoid schizophrenia and depression in adolescence
- Autoimmune diseases occur in 9%. Most commonly—juvenile idiopathic arthritis, immune thrombocytopenic purpura, and autoimmune hemolytic anemia
- *Characteristic facial features:* Low set, cupped or folded ears, small mouth, short philtrum, hypertelorism, high-arched or cleft palate, micrognathia

## DIAGNOSTICS

- Patients with heart disease, characteristic facial features, and hypocalcemia should immediately be screened for a 22q11.2 deletion
- Chromosome 22q11 deletions via FISH
- Genome Wide Array—This is fast becoming the preferred method for diagnosis because it has the ability to identify atypical deletions and other chromosomal abnormalities such as 10p deletions and CHD7 deletions
- Serum calcium levels (including ionized calcium)
- Parathyroid hormone level (frequency depends on initial levels as some patients never develop hypocalcemia)
- Echocardiography, ECG, and chest x-ray to identify conotruncal or other cardiovascular abnormalities in all infants with a high degree of clinical suspicion

- Flow cytometry for T cell and B cell subsets (along with CBC)
  - ✓ Low T cell numbers may result from thymic hypoplasia
  - ✓ T cell numbers may be normal if the thymus is well-developed
- Immunoglobulin levels and antibody responses to vaccinations
  - ✓ Low IgG levels and poor specific antibody response to pneumococcal, diphtheria, and tetanus occur in 5% of patients

## MANAGEMENT

- Live viral vaccines are generally given to patients who have a CD8 T cell count >300 cells/mm³ and normal specific antibody responses to non-live viral vaccine antigens
- Thymic transplant is indicated for patients with complete thymic aplasia resulting in complete absence of T cells and severe immunodeficiency
- Antibody deficiency can be present in rare patients who would therefore require IVIG therapy
- Calcium supplementation if necessary

## WISKOTT–ALDRICH SYNDROME (WAS)

**A combined T and B cell immunodeficiency associated with thrombocytopenia (small platelets), eczema, susceptibility to opportunistic infections, and increased risk for B cell lymphoma.**

### EPIDEMIOLOGY

- WAS occurs in 1/250,000 live male births
- Case reports of heterozygotic females due to inactivation of the unaffected X-chromosome

### ETIOLOGY

- Defect in the *WAS* gene (Xp11.23)

### DIFFERENTIAL DIAGNOSIS

- *Primary immunodeficiencies:* Severe T cell and combined immunodeficiencies (SCID)
- HIV infection
- Immune thrombocytopenia purpura (ITP); ITP typically has normal to large platelet size
- Inherited thrombocytopenias (May–Hegglin, Fechter syndrome, Bernard–Soulier, Sebastian syndrome, gray platelet syndrome, Montreal platelet syndrome); these typically have giant platelets

### PATHOPHYSIOLOGY

- WASP protein functions to enhance actin polymerization and branching allowing cells to rearrange their actin cytoskeleton. Cytoskeletal rearrangement is vital for a number of key functions in immune cells such as endocytosis, exocytosis, chemotaxis, and formation of the immunologic synapse

### CLINICAL MANIFESTATIONS

- 30% have classic triad of thrombocytopenia, eczema, and chronic sinopulmonary infections
- Recurrent otitis media, sinusitis, and pneumonia. Other infections include sepsis, meningitis, severe viral infections, and opportunistic infections (including *Pneumocystis jiroveci*)
- Infants often present with petechiae and bleeding (e.g., bloody diarrhea, epistaxis, or prolonged bleeding after circumcision), especially if platelet counts are less than 10,000/mm³

- Mild to severe eczema develops in a majority of patients with WAS. The eczema is often complicated by superinfection with bacterial and viral (e.g., HSV) pathogens
- Malignancies develop in 13% of patients and occur during adolescence or adulthood (most commonly EBV-positive B cell lymphoma and leukemia)
- Autoimmune disease (e.g., autoimmune cytopenia, vasculitis, colitis) occurs in 40% of patients

## DIAGNOSTICS

- Thrombocytopenia (typically <70,000/mm$^3$) with small platelets (mean platelet volume, 3.8–5.0 fL)
- T cell lymphopenia and reduced lymphocyte proliferation to mitogens
- Normal IgG, reduced IgM, and increased IgA and IgE levels
- Assess antibody responses to protein and polysaccharide vaccine antigens as these can be decreased
  ✓ Diphtheria and tetanus (DTaP if age <2 years)
  ✓ Pneumococcus (13-valent conjugate pneumococcal vaccine if age <2 years and 23-valent polysaccharide pneumococcal vaccine if age >2 years)
- Reduced WASP protein expression (by flow cytometry or western blot). Protein expression can be normal in some patients
- Genetic testing for mutations in the *WAS* gene can confirm the diagnosis

## MANAGEMENT

- WAS patients with antibody deficiency benefit from IVIG replacement therapy (400–600 mg/kg once each month)
- *Pneumocystis jiroveci* prophylaxis with TMP-SMX
- While splenectomy may improve thrombocytopenia, the risk of future invasive bacterial infections increases significantly. Therefore, splenectomy is not recommended
- Patients with severe disease who have an HLA-identical donor are good candidates for bone marrow transplantation. This therapy can cure both the immunological and hematological abnormalities seen in patients. Five-year survival following fully matched transplantation is 90% (survival for haploidentical transplants is approximately 50%). Outcomes are significantly better when transplant occurs before 5 years of age

## ATAXIA-TELANGIECTASIA

**Combined T and B cell immunodeficiency with neurocutaneous findings and a predisposition for malignancy.**

### EPIDEMIOLOGY

- Incidence between 1/100,000 and 1/300,000, equal across races

### ETIOLOGY

- Ataxia-telangiectasia mutated (ATM) protein (gene on chromosome 11q22.3)
- Autosomal recessive inheritance

### PATHOPHYSIOLOGY

- ATM protein functions to detect double-stranded DNA breaks and to initiate cell cycle checkpoint arrest—This delay in cell cycle progression allows for the repair of DNA damage

## DIFFERENTIAL DIAGNOSIS

- *Other DNA breakage syndromes:* Nijmegen breakage syndrome, Bloom syndrome
- Other T cell or combined immunodeficiencies

## CLINICAL MANIFESTATIONS

- Although walking develops normally by 1 year of life, progressive ataxia develops, and patients are generally wheelchair bound after 10 years of age. Other neurologic abnormalities include oculomotor apraxia, dysarthria, and choreoathetosis
- The onset of ataxia precedes the development of cutaneous telangiectasias which are present by 3–5 years of age
  ✓ Telangiectasias typically develop on the bulbar conjunctiva, ear pinna, and nose
- Patients suffer from recurrent sinopulmonary infections at high frequency, but opportunistic infections are rare. Aspiration pneumonia secondary to dysfunctional swallowing is common
- There is an increased risk of malignancy in patients with ataxia-telangiectasia; approximately one-third of patients develop non-Hodgkin's lymphoma, leukemia, or solid malignancies
- Diminished large-fiber sensation

## DIAGNOSTICS

- Definitive diagnosis is established by identification of mutations in the *ATM* gene
- Elevated serum alpha-fetoprotein (AFP) after 1 year of age; AFP can normally be elevated in infants
- Brain MRI may reveal cerebellar atrophy in older children with ataxia-telangiectasia
- B cell abnormalities include low immunoglobulin levels and low antibody responses to vaccinations
- T cell abnormalities include low T cell numbers via T cell enumeration and reduced T cell function via T cell proliferation in response to mitogens

## MANAGEMENT

- IVIG supplementation for hypogammaglobulinemia (400–600 mg/kg once monthly with a goal IgG level >800 mg/dL)
- x-rays and ionizing radiation should be avoided to minimize the risk of future malignancies

## CHRONIC GRANULOMATOUS DISEASE (CGD)

**A phagocyte immune deficiency resulting from impaired activation of key proteolytic enzymes in the neutrophil phagosome.**

## EPIDEMIOLOGY

- Prevalence varies by mutation (e.g., genes for gp91, a component of the NADPH oxidase complex, have mutations as follows: CYBB 1/250,000; CYBA 1/2,000,000)
- 65–70% X-linked inheritance; remainder autosomal recessive

## ETIOLOGY

- Mutations affecting the NADPH oxidase complex

## DIFFERENTIAL DIAGNOSIS

- *Primary immunodeficiency:* Hyper IgE syndrome, leukocyte adhesion deficiency, severe congenital neutropenia

## PATHOPHYSIOLOGY

CGD is caused by defects in the NADPH oxidase system, which consists of six proteins (two membrane bound and four cytosolic). Upon cellular activation, the cytosolic components assemble with the membrane bound components to form the active complex.

Oxygen and NADPH+H are reduced by NADPH oxidase to produce NADP+ and super-oxide radical. This stimulates an influx of potassium cations into the cell which then activates the release of neutrophil proteases (neutrophil elastase and cathepsin G).

## CLINICAL MANIFESTATIONS

- *Patients present within the first few years of life with severe deep-seated infections:* Pneumonia (79%), skin or visceral abscesses (68%), lymphadenitis (53%), and osteomyelitis (25%)
- *Patients are susceptible to catalase positive organisms: Staphylococcus aureus, Serratia marcescens, Burkholderia cepacia, Nocardia* spp., and *Aspergillus fumigatus*
- Inflammatory bowel disease resulting in malabsorption may occur, particularly in X-linked CGD. Obstructive GI tract and urinary tract granulomas are problematic complications

## DIAGNOSTICS

- Flow cytometry for dihydrorhodamine 123 (DHR) dye conversion to rhodamine 123 is more sensitive and specific than the historically used nitroblue tetrazolium (NBT) test. It can be used to detect carrier status and can differentiate X-linked CGD from other forms in a majority of cases

## MANAGEMENT

- Long-term prophylaxis with TMP-SMX and itraconazole to reduce severe bacterial and fungal infections
- Interferon-gamma prophylaxis has also been shown to reduce the frequency of infectious complications
  - ✓ Side effects such as fever and flu-like symptoms limit use of this medication
- Bone marrow transplantation (BMT) is a viable curative therapy
  - ✓ BMT should be considered as soon as possible for patients with X-linked CGD and those with autosomal recessive CGD with severe symptoms
  - ✓ CGD patients with autosomal recessive CGD with little or no reactive oxygen intermediate (ROI) production have greatly reduced long-term survival compared with patients with residual production of ROI

## LEUKOCYTE ADHESION DEFICIENCY (LAD)

**An autosomal recessive phagocyte immunodeficiency resulting from a defect in neutrophil migration leading to recurrent bacterial infections (neutrophil number and function are normal).**

### EPIDEMIOLOGY

- Extremely rare with less than 400 cases of LAD 1 reported in the United States
- LAD 2 reported primarily in Middle East

### ETIOLOGY

- *LAD 1:* Deficiency or defect in the common beta chain of the beta 2-integrin family CD18
- *LAD 2:* Mutations in the gene encoding GDP-fucose transporter 1 (FUCT1)
- *LAD 3:* Mutations in the gene for KINDLIN3, which is a protein involved in integrin activation

## DIFFERENTIAL DIAGNOSIS

- *Primary immunodeficiencies:* Severe congenital neutropenia, cyclic neutropenia, CGD, hyper IgE syndrome
- Leukemoid reaction

## PATHOPHYSIOLOGY

- Patients with LAD have normal absolute neutrophil counts and normal neutrophil function. However, their neutrophils are unable to adhere to the endothelium of vessels and migrate to sites of active infection or inflammation
  - ✓ LAD 1: Defective firm adhesion of neutrophils to endothelium
  - ✓ LAD 2: Defective leukocyte rolling but intact firm adhesion
  - ✓ LAD 3: Normal integrin expression and structure but impaired integrin activation (and thus binding)

## CLINICAL MANIFESTATIONS

- *LAD 1*—This is the most common form of LAD and is characterized by markedly elevated WBC count (50,000–100,000/µL) even in the absence of infection, delayed separation of the umbilical cord with omphalitis, recurrent bacterial skin infections, impaired wound healing and pus formation, and pneumonia with staphylococcus and gram negative bacilli. Patients with severe forms of LAD 1 often die during infancy without bone marrow transplantation
- *LAD 2*—This is characterized by a milder phenotype than LAD 1. Patients develop mild leukocytosis (10,000–40,000/µL) and have reduced (but not absent) pus formation. Bacterial skin and lung infections are typically not life-threatening. Patients have severe mental, growth, and motor retardation as well as microcephaly
- *LAD 3*—The clinical phenotype is identical to patients with LAD 1

## DIAGNOSTICS

- Marked leukocytosis in the absence of infection
- Decreased or absent expression of CD18 via flow cytometry in LAD 1 (normal in LAD 2 and LAD 3)
- Absence of CD15a on leukocytes on LAD 2 (flow cytometry)
- Gene sequencing—ITGB2 (LAD 1), SLC35C1 (LAD 2), or KINDLIN 3 (LAD 3)

## MANAGEMENT

- *LAD 1:* Bone marrow transplantation should be a consideration for patients with severe forms of LAD 1. BMT has a success rate of 80% when a matched donor is available and 50% in cases of haploidentical transplants
- *LAD 2:* Aggressive treatment of infections and prophylactic antibiotics. Fucose supplementation as early as possible to help prevent psychomotor retardation
- *LAD 3:* As with LAD 1, early intervention with bone marrow transplantation is a consideration

## SEVERE CONGENITAL NEUTROPENIA (SCN)

**A heterogeneous group of immunodeficiencies characterized by persistent severe neutropenia and severe recurrent bacterial infections.**

## EPIDEMIOLOGY

- The exact prevalence of SCN is difficult to determine but there appears to be at least 6 cases per million inhabitants

## ETIOLOGY

- SCN is a genetically heterogeneous disease with autosomal dominant (ELANE and GFI-1), autosomal recessive (HAX1), and X-linked (WAS) forms of inheritance reported
  - ✓ An underlying genetic defect has not been elucidated in up to 40% of patients

## DIFFERENTIAL DIAGNOSIS

- *Primary immunodeficiencies:* X-linked hyper IgM syndrome, XLA, WHIM syndrome, reticular dysgenesis, cyclic neutropenia, Chediak–Higashi syndrome, Shwachman–Diamond syndrome, Griscelli syndrome type 2, Hermansky–Pudlak type 2, dyskeratosis, congenital, Fanconi pancytopenia
- *Metabolic diseases associated with neutropenia:* Glycogen-storage disease type 1b, propionic acidemia; methylmalonic acidemia
- *Infection:* HIV, parvovirus, hepatitis viruses, malaria
- *Immune-mediated:* Autoimmune neutropenia, Felty syndrome
- *Nutrition:* Vitamin $B_{12}$, transcobalamin II, copper, or folate deficiency
- *Hematologic diseases:* Aplastic anemia, myelodysplastic syndromes
- *Drug-induced:* Chloramphenicol, penicillin, sulfonamides, aspirin, acetaminophen, phenylbutazone, barbiturates, benzodiazepines, chlorpromazine, phenothiazines, levamisole

## PATHOPHYSIOLOGY

Pathophysiology varies depending on the genetic mutation causing the disease.

- *ELANE (AD):* ELANE (also known as ELA2) encodes for the protein neutrophil elastase (a serine protease synthesized during the early stages of primary granule production in promyelocytes). Heterozygous mutations in this gene account for 50–60% of autosomal dominant SCN cases. Mutations in ELANE are also known to cause cyclic neutropenia
- *HAX1 (AR):* Mutations in the *HAX1* gene cause a form of autosomal recessive neutropenia. HAX1 appears to be critical for maintaining the inner mitochondrial membrane potential and protecting against neutrophil apoptosis
- *WAS (XL):* Missense mutations in the cdc42 binding site of the *WAS* gene can result in X-linked neutropenia without other clinical findings associated with WAS (eczema, thrombocytopenia, and T cell immunodeficiency)
- *GFI-1 (AD):* Heterozygous mutations in the growth factor-independent 1 (*GFI-1*) gene cause a rare autosomal dominant form of SCN. GFI-1 is a transcription factor which regulates key genes for neutrophil differentiation

## CLINICAL MANIFESTATIONS

- Typically present during the first year of life with neutropenia (ANC $<500/mm^3$) leading to recurrent, occasionally life-threatening, bacterial infections
- *Staphylococcus aureus* is the most common cause of infectious complications, including cellulitis, skin abscesses, omphalitis, oral ulcers, and pneumonia
- Neurologic disorders including developmental delay and epilepsy have been associated with patients with SCN due to HAX1 mutations
- Increased risk of developing myelodysplastic syndrome and acute myeloid leukemia
- Patients with cyclic neutropenia have a milder clinical course

## DIAGNOSTICS

- CBC with differential 2 times per week for 6 weeks to diagnose or exclude cyclic neutropenia
- Anti-neutrophil antibody levels

- Bone marrow examination typically reveals arrest of neutrophil development at the pro-myelocyte stage
- Genetic testing should be performed to confirm the diagnosis of SCN

## MANAGEMENT

- Recombinant G-CSF therapy is the cornerstone of therapy for patients with SCN. This therapy increases the neutrophil count and decreases the number of serious infections. Patients who require higher doses of G-CSF (>8 μg/kg/day) are at markedly increased risk for death from infections and malignancy; thus these patients are strong candidates for early bone marrow transplantation

## HYPER-IgE SYNDROME (STAT3 DEFICIENCY)

**A primary immunodeficiency characterized by invasive bacterial skin and lung infections, dermatitis, elevated IgE levels, and musculoskeletal abnormalities.**

### EPIDEMIOLOGY

- Incidence unknown, but rare; equal incidence in males and females, and across races

### ETIOLOGY

- Autosomal dominant mutations in the *STAT3* gene

### DIFFERENTIAL DIAGNOSIS OF ELEVATED IgE

- *Primary immunodeficiencies:* Omenn syndrome (an SCID variant characterized by eryth-roderma, lymphadenopathy, and hepatosplenomegaly), WAS, Netherton syndrome, IPEX syndrome, DOCK8 deficiency
- *Infections:* HIV, malaria, parasitic infections
- Atopy, eczema, allergic bronchopulmonary aspergillosis

### PATHOPHYSIOLOGY

- Mutations in STAT3 impair differentiation and function of IL-17 secreting (Th17) cells. IL-17 secreted by Th17 cells stimulate granulopoiesis through induction of G-CSF, recruit neutrophils to the site of infection through induction of IL-8, and stimulate production of antimicrobial peptides such as β-defensins

### CLINICAL MANIFESTATIONS

- Eczematous rash in infancy or early childhood
- Retained primary teeth (60–70%) often requiring dental extraction
- Recurrent bacterial infections, including upper and lower respiratory tract infection (90%). Pneumatoceles following pneumonias are common. Organisms include *Staphylococcus aureus, Haemophilus influenzae, Pseudomonas aeruginosa,* and *Aspergillus fumigatus*
- Skin infections are common, including abscesses (hot and cold)
- Mucocutaneous fungal infections including thrush, esophageal candidiasis, and onycho-mycosis in 80% of patients
- Pathologic fractures following minor trauma (60–70%)
- *Characteristic facial features:* Coarse facies—wide nose, deep-set eyes, prominent chin and forehead. High arched palate

### DIAGNOSTICS

- Elevated IgE greater than 2000 IU/mL (100%), although this can fluctuate
- Elevated eosinophil count greater than 2 SD above normal (93% of patients)

- *Dental x-rays:* Delayed development and retained primary teeth
- Abnormal neutrophil chemotaxis assay
- Antibody responses to pneumococcus, diphtheria, and tetanus should be assessed as some patients have impaired antibody responses to vaccine antigens
- Low Th17 cell numbers
- Genetic testing to identify mutations in the *STAT3* gene can confirm the diagnosis

## MANAGEMENT

- Anti-staphylococcal antibiotic prophylaxis (usually TMP-SMX at a dose of 2.5 mg/kg/day of the trimethoprim component)
- IVIG for patients with impaired antibody immunity

Katie Chiotos, MD
Lori Handy, MD, MSCE
Salwa Sulieman, DO
Jeffrey S. Gerber, MD, PhD

## SYNDROMES AND COMPLEXES

### BITE WOUND INFECTIONS

**Infections usually localized to site of bite. Rare sequelae include meningitis, brain abscess, endocarditis, and septic arthritis.**

### EPIDEMIOLOGY

- Infection follows 10–15% of dog bites and approximately 50% of cat bites
- Greatest rate of infection after bites to the hands (28–63%)
  ✓ Other common sites: Face/head/neck (6–16%), arm/leg (10–32%), trunk (2–10%)

### ETIOLOGY

- Usually polymicrobial; derived from oral flora of biting animal
- Cat and dog bite infections: *Pasteurella canis* (dog), *Pasteurella multocida* (cat), Streptococci, *Staphylococcus aureus*, *Moraxella* spp, *Neisseria* spp, and anaerobes
- Human bites: *Staphylococcus aureus*, viridans group Streptococci, *Streptococcus pyogenes*, *Eikenella corrodens*, *Streptococcus intermedius*, *Capnocytophaga* spp, *Neisseria* spp, *Haemophilus* spp
- Horse/sheep bite: *Actinobacillus* spp, *Streptococcus equisimilis*
- Marine settings/fish bite: *Halomonas venusta*, *Vibrio* spp, *Aeromonas hydrophila*, *Plesiomonas shigelloides*, *Pseudomonas* spp, *Mycobacterium marinum*
- Monkey bite: B virus

### PATHOPHYSIOLOGY

- Infection follows direct inoculation of bacteria into tissues
- Hematogenous dissemination may occur

### CLINICAL MANIFESTATIONS

- Note wound type (puncture, laceration, avulsion), edema, erythema, tenderness, drainage, depth of penetration, bruising, deformity, involvement of underlying structure, sensation, regional lymphadenopathy
- Look for signs of systemic infection (e.g., fever, hypotension)
- Animal: Record type of animal, health of animal, provoked or unprovoked attack; observe for signs of rabies if applicable
- Patient: History of asplenia (increased risk of *Capnocytophaga* spp); immunosuppression or other illnesses; last tetanus immunization

### DIAGNOSTICS

- Gram stain and culture of wound if time from injury greater than 8 hours or if signs and symptoms of infection exist

- Blood culture if fever present
- Radiographs indicated for penetrating injuries overlying bones or joints, suspected foreign body, or fracture

## MANAGEMENT

### Immediate Management

- Examine for foreign body, irrigate with copious amounts of normal saline, debride devitalized tissue
- Suturing is controversial. Leave wound open if greater than 8 hours old or a puncture wound; primary wound closure for injuries to face and when cosmetic outcome is important
- Indications for operative exploration and debridement: Extensive tissue damage; involvement of metacarpophalangeal joint from clenched fist injury; cranial bites by large animals

### Tetanus Prophylaxis

- Clean minor wounds: Administer tetanus toxoid if >10 years since last tetanus-containing vaccine dose, if vaccine history is unknown, or if <3 doses received
- Puncture or severe wounds: If <3 doses received, administer tetanus toxoid and tetanus immunoglobulin. If patient has completed primary immunization but it has been ≥5 years since last tetanus-containing vaccine dose, administer tetanus toxoid

### Rabies Post-Exposure Prophylaxis

- Prophylaxis:
  - ✓ Active: Four doses of rabies vaccine on days 0, 3, 7, 14 (five doses for immunocompromised hosts)
  - ✓ Passive: Rabies immune globulin (RIG) given on day 0 with the first dose of vaccine, infiltrate wound with as much as possible; give remainder IM
- Dogs, cats, ferrets: If animal is healthy and available for 10 days of observation, prophylaxis (immunization) only if animal develops signs of rabies; if animal suspected or determined to be rabid, administer both immunization and RIG; if unknown, consult public health officials
- Bats, skunks, raccoons, foxes, woodchucks, and most other carnivores: Regarded as rabid unless geographic area is known to be free of rabies or proven negative via laboratory tests; patients require rabies immunization and RIG
- Livestock, rodents, and lagomorphs: Typically not high risk, but consult local public health officials

### Antibiotic Management

- See Table 15-1

## BRONCHIOLITIS

**Acute lower respiratory tract infection that causes inflammation of the bronchioles and results in distal airway obstruction frequently accompanied by wheezing**

## EPIDEMIOLOGY

- Children usually younger than 2 years of age
- One-third of children develop bronchiolitis in the first 2 years of life; approximately 10% of these children will be hospitalized
- All geographic areas; winter to early spring

| TABLE 15-1 | Antibiotic Management of Bite Wounds | | |
|---|---|---|---|
| **Source** | **Most common Organisms** | **Antibiotic** | **Comments** |
| **Dog, cat** | *Pasteurella* spp, *Staphylococcus aureus*, streptococci, anaerobes, *Capnocytophaga* spp, *Moraxella* spp, *Corynebacterium* spp, *Neisseria* spp | Orally: Amoxicillin-clavulanate<br>IV: Ampicillin-sulbactam<br>*Alternative if PCN-allergic:*<br>Trimethoprim-sulfamethoxazole PLUS<br>Clindamycin | • Consider MRSA coverage for severe wounds or refractory infections<br>• 3–5 days for prophylaxis; treatment of infected wounds typically 7–10 days depending upon source control and wound severity |
| **Human** | *Streptococci, Staphylococcus aureus, Eikenella corrodens, Haemophilus* spp, anaerobes | Orally: Amoxicillin-clavulanate<br>IV: Ampicillin-sulbactam<br>*Alternative if PCN-allergic:*<br>Trimethoprim-sulfamethoxazole PLUS<br>Clindamycin | |

Adapted with permission from the Committee on Infectious Diseases; Kimberlin DW, Brady MT, Jackson MA, Long SS: Red Book: 2015 *Report of the Committee on Infectious Disease. American Academy of Pediatrics.*

• Risk factors for severe illness: Age less than 3 months, gestational age less than 34 weeks, ill or toxic appearance, respiratory rate >70 per minute, pulse oximetry <94%, cardiac or pulmonary disease, immunodeficiency

## ETIOLOGY

• Infectious agents: Respiratory syncytial virus (RSV; 50–80% of cases); parainfluenza viruses types 1, 2, and 3; adenovirus; influenza virus; rhinovirus; coronaviruses; *Mycoplasma pneumoniae*; human metapneumovirus. Patients may have coinfections

## PATHOPHYSIOLOGY

• Necrosis of airway epithelium and ciliated lining causes mucosal inflammation. Lymphocytic infiltration of peribronchial and peribronchiolar epithelium causes edema of submucosa and adventitia
• Impaired mucociliary clearance leads to obstruction of smaller caliber distal airways without significant alveolar involvement causing partial or total obstruction to airflow
• Varying degrees of obstruction lead to rapidly changing clinical signs and symptoms
• Epithelial regeneration lags behind clinical recovery

## CLINICAL MANIFESTATIONS

• Incubation period of causal pathogens ranges from 2 to 8 days. Acute illness ranges from 3 to 7 days. Recovery is gradual over 1–3 weeks
• Signs and symptoms: Rhinorrhea (profuse), cough, low-grade fever, lethargy, increased work of breathing, tachypnea, wheezing, cyanosis, apnea (especially in age less than

3 months), and retractions (suprasternal, subcostal, intercostal, and, with severe illness, supraclavicular)
- Auscultation: Prolonged expiratory phase, wheezing, rales, rhonchi

## DIAGNOSTICS

- Diagnostic testing is typically not indicated for routine bronchiolitis
- Chest x-ray (if performed) demonstrates hyperinflation, patchy atelectasis, peribronchial cuffing; CXR is not typically required
- Rapid viral identification from nasopharyngeal aspirate may be useful for cohorting hospitalized patients but has little impact on management; routine viral testing is not necessary
- Consider arterial blood gas and serum electrolytes if there is concern for impending respiratory failure

## MANAGEMENT

- Respiratory support:
  - ✓ Supplemental oxygen should be initiated in previously healthy infants only if oxygen saturation values fall persistently below 90%, and should be discontinued if oxygen saturation is greater than 90% while feeding well with minimal respiratory distress
  - ✓ Discontinue use of pulse oximetry or transition to intermittent pulse oximetry during the convalescent stage of illness (e.g., if oxygen saturation >90% in room air for >2–4 hours)
  - ✓ High flow nasal cannula decreases intubation rate, respiratory rate, and ICU length of stay
  - ✓ Mechanical ventilation should be considered for infants with signs of respiratory failure, shock, or persistent apnea
- Pharmacologic interventions:
  - ✓ Nebulized beta-2 adrenergic agonists (albuterol, levalbuterol) are not *routinely* indicated. For moderate to severely ill infants, consider trial doses with assessment of clinical response. May have more benefit in those with asthma history or ventilated patients. Potential exists for paradoxical effects and increased airway resistance
  - ✓ Nebulized alpha/beta adrenergic agonists (racemic epinephrine) are not *routinely* indicated. In moderately ill infants, consider trial doses with assessment of clinical response
  - ✓ Heliox has been shown to reduce respiratory distress in first hour after administration, but studies have not yet demonstrated reduction in need for mechanical ventilation or length of ICU admission
  - ✓ Treatment with hypertonic (3%) saline may reduce length of stay; further trials needed to determine quantify magnitude of benefit and optimal delivery methods and treatment duration
    - Most common regimen is either 1.5 mg racemic epinephrine mixed with 4 mL of 3% saline or 1–2.5 mg albuterol mixed with 4 mL 3% saline; administered every 2–8 hours until discharged
  - ✓ Corticosteroids not *routinely* indicated; studies do *not* show consistent clinical improvement with either systemic or inhaled formulations; infants with strong family history of asthma *and* a previous episode of wheezing might benefit from early systemic steroid administration, though data are conflicting
  - ✓ Antivirals (ribavarin) not *routinely* indicated and virtually never used; consider for high-risk patients (e.g., complex congenital heart disease)
- Suctioning: Lapses in suctioning >4 hours associated with increased length of stay
- Chest physiotherapy has not been shown to reduce the length of disease, improve clinical scores, or reduce hospital stay

- Infants with extreme tachypnea are at risk of aspiration; consider nothing-by-mouth status, IV hydration, and consider nasogastric tube for enteral feeds
- Infection prevention and control: Viruses causing bronchiolitis are transmitted primarily by direct contact with secretions and/or fomites. Appropriate hand hygiene is paramount. Contact precautions and patient cohorting are indicated
- Palivizumab (humanized monoclonal RSV antibody) prophylaxis:
  - ✓ Recommended during the first year of life to infants born before 29 weeks, 0 days' gestation and to infants with hemodynamically significant heart or chronic lung disease of prematurity
  - ✓ The recommended dose is 15 mg/kg/dose for a maximum of 5 monthly doses during RSV season
  - ✓ The AAP guidelines provide additional guidance on eligibility for administration (*Pediatrics* 2014;134:e1474–e1502)
  - ✓ Palivizumab does not interfere with response to vaccines

## CENTRAL-LINE ASSOCIATED BLOODSTREAM INFECTION

**Bacteria or yeast cultured in the presence of a central venous catheter (CVC).**

### EPIDEMIOLOGY

- Risk with nontunneled is greater than tunneled which is greater than totally implantable catheter
  - ✓ Tunneled = Hickman, Broviac, Groshong, and Quinton catheters
  - ✓ Totally implantable = Portacath, permacath (hemodialysis)
- Lower risk with silver chelated collagen cuff, antibiotic impregnated catheter (e.g., minocycline + rifampin, chlorhexidine + silver sulfadiazine), and chlorhexidine preparation compared to betadine preparation

### ETIOLOGY

- Coagulase-negative staphylococci, *Staphylococcus aureus*, *Enterococcus*, *Pseudomonas aeruginosa*, and other gram-negative bacilli, *Candida* spp, rapid-growing mycobacteria (e.g., *M. chelonae, M. fortuitum, M. abscessus*)

### PATHOPHYSIOLOGY

- Migration of skin organisms into catheter
- Contamination of catheter hub by health care worker hands or environmental sources
- Hematogenous seeding of catheter from another focus of infection or translocated bacteria from the gastrointestinal tract

### CLINICAL MANIFESTATIONS

- Fever alone
- Fever, hypotension, tachycardia, tachypnea (septic shock)
- Abscess or cellulitis at catheter insertion site
- Complications include sepsis, bacterial endocarditis, mycotic aneurysms, disseminated candidiasis (endophthalmitis, endocarditis, or hepatosplenic or renal candidiasis)

### DIAGNOSTICS

- Blood cultures from the catheter *and* periphery are preferred. The following criteria implicate CVC as source of infection:
  - ✓ *Quantitative blood cultures:* (1) CVC culture yields a colony count at least fivefold *higher* than peripheral blood culture; (2) 15 or more CFU from catheter tip by *semiquantitative*

culture (colony counts directly from agar plate); or (3) 100 or more CFU from catheter tip by *quantitative* culture

✓ *Differential time to positivity*: Positive result from CVC culture at least 2 hours earlier than from peripheral culture with similar culture volume. Compared to quantitative blood culture methods, differential time to positivity has sensitivity = 80–90% and specificity = 75–94%

• Consider echocardiogram if:
  ✓ Culture grows *Staphylococcus aureus* or HACEK organism
  ✓ Culture positive greater than 3 days despite appropriate therapy
  ✓ New murmur develops

• Rapid-growing mycobacteria grow in conventional blood culture bottles. Isolation of MAI requires special AFB isolator blood culture tubes (check with Microbiology Laboratory)

• If culture grows *Candida* spp, risk of dissemination to at least one organ is about 17%, including dissemination to the eye (3%), central nervous system (12%), abdomen (8-23%), and heart (8%). Obtain ophthalmologic exam and consider imaging the brain and abdomen as well as an echocardiogram

## MANAGEMENT

• Empiric regimens may vary depending on regional antibiotic susceptibility patterns. Guiding principles include coverage for skin flora, which may include MRSA and nosocomial Gram-negative organisms if patient is ill or frequently hospitalized. If the patient is already on antimicrobial therapy, empiric antibiotics should be broader than the current regimen (**Figure 15-1**)

• Fever alone in presence of a central catheter:
  ✓ Vancomycin and cefepime for inpatients; ceftriaxone if stable for home while awaiting blood culture results

• Shock in presence of a central catheter:
  ✓ Add an aminoglycoside (to vancomycin and cefepime) for additional gram-negative coverage
  ✓ Consider antifungal coverage if the patient is immunocompromised, has been on prolonged antibiotics, or is on TPN

• Reasons to discontinue the central catheter: (1) Rapid clinical deterioration; (2) cellulitis or abscess at or along catheter site; (3) persistently positive blood culture results despite appropriate therapy; (4) endocarditis/septic thrombophlebitis; (5) organism is known to be difficult to clear such as *Bacillus, Burkholderia, Candida, Staphylococcus aureus, Stenotrophomonas,* and *Mycobacteria*

• Treatment duration is individualized by organism, clinical course, CVC status (salvage or removal), and clearance of bacteremia

• General recommendations include:
  ✓ *Candida* spp: Minimum 14 days (line removal recommended)
  ✓ *Staphylococcus aureus:* Minimum 14 days (line removal recommended)
  ✓ Coagulase-negative staphylococci: 10 days if line remains in place, 3 days if line removed
  ✓ Enterococcus and viridans streptococci: 7 days
  ✓ Gram-negative organisms: 10 days (line removal preferred)

• Antibiotic or ethanol locks can be considered as part of salvage therapy and for CVC maintenance (prevention) for patients with recurrent CVC infection

**FIGURE 15-1 Antimicrobial spectra of commonly used antibacterial agents.**

| | PENICILLIN | AMPICILLIN | OXACILLIN | AMP-SULB | TICAR-CLAV | PIP-TAZO | CEFAZOLIN | CEFUROX | CEFOXITIN | CEFTRIAX | CEFTAZIDIME | CEFEPIME | IMIPENEM | MEROPENEM | DOXYCYCLINE | CLINDAMYCIN | AMINOGLYC | CIPRO | LEVO | AZITHRO | TMP-SMX | VANCO | LINEZOLID | METRO |
|---|---|---|---|---|---|---|---|---|---|---|---|---|---|---|---|---|---|---|---|---|---|---|---|---|
| **Gram +** | | | | | | | | | | | | | | | | | | | | | | | | |
| Strep. Grp. A/B | + | + | + | + | + | + | + | + | + | + | + | + | + | + | + | + | − | +/− | + | +/− | − | + | + | − |
| Streptococcus pneumoniae | + | + | + | + | + | + | + | + | + | + | + | + | + | + | + | + | − | +/− | + | +/− | + | + | + | − |
| E. faecalis | + | + | − | + | +/− | + | − | − | − | − | − | − | + | +/− | − | − | s | +/− | + | − | − | + | + | − |
| E. faecium | +/− | +/− | − | +/− | +/− | +/− | − | − | − | − | − | − | +/− | − | − | − | s | − | − | − | − | +/− | + | − |
| Staphylococcus aureus | − | − | + | + | + | + | + | + | + | + | − | + | + | + | + | + | + | + | + | − | + | + | + | − |
| MRSA | − | − | − | − | − | − | − | − | − | − | − | − | − | − | + | + | s | +/− | +/− | − | + | + | + | − |
| Listeria | + | + | − | + | | | − | − | − | − | − | − | + | + | + | | s | + | + | + | + | + | + | − |
| **Gram −** | | | | | | | | | | | | | | | | | | | | | | | | |
| H. influenzae | − | +/− | − | + | + | + | + | + | + | + | + | + | + | + | + | − | + | + | + | + | +/− | − | +/− | − |
| N. Meningitidis | + | + | − | + | + | + | − | + | +/− | + | +/− | + | + | + | + | − | − | + | + | + | + | − | − | − |
| E. coli | − | +/− | − | + | + | + | + | + | + | + | + | + | + | + | +/− | − | + | + | + | − | +/− | − | − | − |
| Klebsiella | − | − | − | + | + | + | + | + | + | + | + | + | + | + | − | − | + | + | + | − | +/− | − | − | − |
| Enterobacter | − | − | − | − | + | + | − | +/− | − | + | + | + | + | + | − | − | + | + | + | − | | − | − | − |
| Serratia | − | − | − | − | + | + | − | +/− | − | + | + | + | + | + | − | − | + | + | + | − | +/− | − | − | − |
| Pseudomonas | − | − | − | − | + | + | − | − | − | − | + | + | + | + | − | − | + | + | +/− | − | − | − | − | − |
| **Anaerobes** | | | | | | | | | | | | | | | | | | | | | | | | |
| Oral anaerobes | + | + | − | + | + | + | − | − | + | − | − | − | + | + | + | + | − | − | + | − | − | − | + | + |
| Gut anaerobes (B. fragilis) | − | − | − | + | + | + | − | − | + | − | − | − | + | + | − | + | − | − | − | − | − | − | +/− | + |

Results may vary; consult local clinical microbiology laboratory for most relevant data. S = synergy when used in combination with cell wall active agent; empty cells = no data.

243

## CELLULITIS/ABSCESS

**A primary, superficial skin infection.**

### ETIOLOGY

• Immunocompetent children: *S. pyogenes* (predominant with simple cellulitis), *Staphylococcus aureus* (predominant with purulence/abscess formation). Consider *S. agalactiae* in neonates
• Immunocompromised children: Also *Pseudomonas* spp, Enterobacteriaceae, *Cryptococcus neoformans*, anaerobes

### PATHOPHYSIOLOGY

• Acute infection of the skin involving the dermis and subcutaneous tissues, most commonly following local trauma (e.g., abrasions)
• Hematogenous dissemination is less common since introduction of *Haemophilus influenzae* type B vaccine, but is still seen with *Streptococcus pneumoniae*

### CLINICAL MANIFESTATIONS

• Constitutional symptoms including fever, chills, malaise
• Skin edema, warmth, erythema, tenderness, or fluctuance
• Red, lymphangitic streaks
• Regional lymphadenopathy
• Break in skin may be found on exam

### DIAGNOSTICS

• Culture of aspirate, skin biopsy, and blood cultures collectively yield causal organism in 25% of cases; blood cultures positive in <1% of uncomplicated cellulitis and roughly 12% of complicated infections
• Blood cultures should be performed in young patients or those who are systemically ill
• Drain areas of fluctuance (especially in areas of high methicillin-resistant *Staphylococcus aureus* [MRSA] prevalence)

### MANAGEMENT

• Well-appearing children can be treated as outpatients: Cephalexin or amoxicillin-clavulanate can be used for simple cellulitis and for purulent cellulitis/abscess formation in regions with low MRSA prevalence; trimethoprim-sulfamethoxazole (TMP-SMX) or clindamycin for purulent cellulitis/abscess formation in areas of high MRSA prevalence
• Incision and drainage of abscesses is paramount and might obviate antimicrobial therapy for simple abscesses
• An increased risk of treatment failure requiring drainage, hospitalization, or change in antibiotics has been noted with TMP-SMX compared to β-lactams in children with non-drained, non-cultured skin and soft tissue infections. Additional factors associated with treatment failure include treatment in the emergency department, presence or history of fever, and presence of either induration or small abscess
• Ill-appearing patients with high fever, rapid progression, or lymphangitis require hospitalization and IV antibiotics. Consider oxacillin, cefazolin, or clindamycin. Critically ill patients require coverage with vancomycin due to possible MRSA resistance to clindamycin. (*Refer to section on MRSA*)
• Duration of therapy depends on clinical response and adequate drainage; typically 5–7 days

## COMMUNITY-ACQUIRED PNEUMONIA

**Infection of lung parenchyma.**

### EPIDEMIOLOGY/ETIOLOGY

- Viruses account for up to 35% of childhood community-acquired pneumonia (CAP), but almost 80% of CAP in children <2 years
- Neonates: Group B *Streptococcus*, enteric gram-negative rods, cytomegalovirus (CMV), herpes simplex virus (HSV), *L. monocytogenes*
- One to 3 months: RSV; parainfluenza viruses; *Streptococcus pneumoniae*; *C. trachomatis*; *Bordetella pertussis*
- Three months to 5 years: RSV; parainfluenza viruses; influenza; adenovirus; *Streptococcus pneumoniae*; *Haemophilus influenzae*; *Staphylococcus aureus*; *Mycoplasma pneumoniae*
- Five to 15 years: *Streptococcus pneumoniae*, *M. pneumoniae*, *C. pneumoniae*, influenza
- Clinically significant pleural effusions:
  - ✓ Common: *Streptococcus pneumoniae* and *Staphylococcus aureus*
  - ✓ Less common: *S. pyogenes*, *M. tuberculosis*
- Aspiration pneumonia: Enteric gram-negative rods, oral anaerobes; frequently polymicrobial

### PATHOPHYSIOLOGY

- Absent systemic or secretory immunity to an organism
- Impaired lower respiratory tract defenses
- Direct inhalation or hematogenous seeding of organism

### CLINICAL MANIFESTATIONS

- Fever, cough, tachypnea (most sensitive indicator)
- Hypoxia, nasal flaring, grunting, retractions
- Dyspnea, chest or abdominal pain, malaise
- Crackles, decreased breath sounds, egophony, whispered pectoriloquy
- Wheezing suggests a viral or atypical bacterial cause

### DIAGNOSTICS

- Chest x-ray findings suggest etiology but may lag behind clinical symptoms:
  - ✓ Lobar or segmental abnormality, pleural effusion: Bacterial infection
  - ✓ Bilateral, diffuse infiltrates: Viral, *M. pneumoniae*, *Legionella pneumophila*
  - ✓ Hilar adenopathy: *M. tuberculosis*, endemic fungi (e.g., *Histoplasma capsulatum*, *Coccidioides immitis*), *M. pneumoniae*; Epstein–Barr virus
  - ✓ Pneumatocele: *Staphylococcus aureus*, gram-negative rods, occasionally Streptococcus pneumoniae

#### Laboratory Studies

- Blood culture result positive in 10–25% with pleural effusion; 3–7% of hospitalized children with pneumonia; less than 2% of outpatients with pneumonia
- Pleural fluid:
  - ✓ Transudate: pH greater than 7.2; LDH less than 1000 U/L; white blood cell (WBC) count less than 1000/mm$^3$; no bacteria on Gram stain; glucose greater than 40 mg/dL; pleural/serum LDH ratio less than 0.5

✓ Exudate: pH less than 7.1; LDH greater than 1000 U/L; WBC count greater than 10,000/mm³; bacteria present on Gram stain; glucose less than 40 mg/dL; pleural/serum LDH greater than 0.5

✓ Send acid-fast culture and stains if concerned for *M. tuberculosis*

### Diagnosis of Specific Agents

- Viral pathogens: Nasopharyngeal aspirate PCR, antigen detection, or culture
- *M. pneumoniae* and *C. pneumoniae*: PCR (rapid, accurate); serology (time-consuming); cold agglutinins (poor sensitivity)
- Tuberculosis: Tuberculin skin test (PPD); culture and acid-fast smear of sputum, bronchoalveolar lavage, or gastric aspirates

## MANAGEMENT

- Specific treatment ultimately depends on cause
- Antibiotic selection depends on clinical presentation: See Table 15-2
- Possible causes of persistent fever despite antibiotics include development of effusion/empyema, viral or mycoplasmal cause, necrotizing pneumonia, or, less likely, resistant bacteria
- Chest ultrasound is preferred imaging modality to quantify and characterize pleural effusions identified on chest x-ray
  ✓ Small: <10 mm on lateral decubitus film or opacifies less than ¼ of hemithorax; fluid drainage not required
  ✓ Moderate: >10 mm but opacifies less than ½ of hemithorax; drainage required if patient has respiratory compromise or if suggestive of empyema
  ✓ Large: Opacifies greater than ½ of hemithorax: drainage should be performed
  ✓ If exudative/simple fluid, requires chest tube +/− fibrinolysis
  ✓ If loculated/complex fluid, may warrant video-assisted thoracoscopy (VATS) or chest tube with fibrinolysis; open decortication not usually necessary but may be used in cases of treatment failure despite chest tube or VATS
- Complications: Empyema, lung abscess, necrotizing pneumonia

## CROUP

**Upper airway obstruction due to virus-induced inflammation that may involve the larynx, infraglottic tissues, and trachea (laryngotracheitis) leading to inspiratory stridor, barking cough, and hoarseness**

## EPIDEMIOLOGY

- Usually between ages 6 months and 3 years (peak at 18 months), though can occur up until age 6
- Epidemics begin in late fall and peak in early winter

## ETIOLOGY

- Common: Parainfluenza viruses (>65% of cases)
- Less common: RSV, influenza virus A and B, adenovirus, coxsackieviruses, and measles
- Bacterial croup (laryngotracheobronchitis and laryngotracheobronchopnemonitis) is due to secondary bacterial infection from organisms such as *Staphylococcus aureus*, group A *Streptococcus*, *Streptococcus pneumoniae*, *Haemophilus influenza*, and *Moraxella catarrhalis*

## PATHOPHYSIOLOGY

- Viral infection of the nasopharynx spreads to respiratory epithelium
- Infection causes diffuse inflammation of the trachea and vocal cords

**TABLE 15-2**    Empiric Therapy for Community-Acquired Pneumonia (CAP) in Children >3 Months of Age

| Pneumonia Category | First-Line Therapy[1] | β-Lactam Allergy[2] | Target Pathogen(s) | Comments |
|---|---|---|---|---|
| **Mild (Outpatient)** | Amoxicillin | Clindamycin OR Levofloxacin | Streptococcus pneumoniae | • **High-dose amoxicillin** active against most Streptococcus pneumoniae<br>• **Clindamycin** active against about 90% of Streptococcus pneumoniae<br>• **Levofloxacin** active against >95% of Streptococcus pneumoniae<br>• **Orally cephalosporins** inferior to high-dose amoxicillin for Streptococcus pneumoniae<br>• **Azithromycin** resistance in up to 40% of Streptococcus pneumoniae |
| **Moderate (Inpatient)** | Ampicillin | Clindamycin OR Levofloxacin | Streptococcus pneumoniae | • **High-dose** ampicillin active against most Streptococcus pneumoniae<br>• **Ceftriaxone** for incompletely immunized patients or treatment failure[4] with outpatient amoxicillin |
| **Complicated[3] (Inpatient)** | Clindamycin AND Ceftriaxone | Clindamycin AND Levofloxacin | Streptococcus pneumoniae, Streptococcus pyogenes, Staphylococcus aureus | Consult Infectious Diseases and Surgery for pneumonia with mod–large effusion/empyema to consider alternate etiologies and evaluate for drainage |
| **Severe (ICU)** | Vancomycin AND Ceftriaxone | Vancomycin AND Levofloxacin | Streptococcus pneumoniae, S. pyogenes, Staphylococcus aureus | Consult Infectious Diseases and Surgery for pneumonia with mod–large effusion/empyema to consider alternate etiologies and evaluate for drainage |

[1]For **typical,** presumed bacterial community-acquired pneumonia.

[2]Defined by urticaria or anaphylaxis.

[3]Includes pneumonia with moderate–large parapneumonic effusion

[4]After >48 hours of therapy with high dose amoxicillin in a patient tolerating a PO regimen

**Atypical pneumonia** (often characterized by non-lobar, patchy, or interstitial pattern on CXR; insidious onset; low-grade fever, malaise, H/A, cough; minimal auscultatory findings relative to CXR) is often caused by respiratory viruses, but may be caused by atypical bacterial pathogens including **Mycoplasma pneumoniae.** Most atypical pneumonia is mild and self-limited; however, for disease requiring hospitalization, consider PCR testing for respiratory viruses and **M. pneumoniae.** For confirmed **M. pneumoniae,** or for presumed infection in the presence of severe pneumonia, include **azithromycin OR levofloxacin.**

- Inflammation of the subglottic trachea (narrowest part of child's upper airway) leads to dramatic airflow restriction
- Bacterial croup is due to inflammatory cell infiltrate, ulceration, formation of pseudomembranes and microabscesses

## CLINICAL MANIFESTATIONS

- Initial rhinorrhea, pharyngitis, and low-grade fevers
- Upper airway obstruction 8–12 hours later
- Signs of obstruction include "barking" cough, hoarseness, inspiratory stridor, accessory muscle use, and hypoxia. Dysphagia is not typical
- Fever, tachypnea, restlessness, coryza
- Children with bacterial infections are toxic

## DIAGNOSTICS

- Diagnosis is made on clinical grounds
- Neck x-rays are not required but can support the initial diagnosis
- Only 50% of cases demonstrate abnormal neck x-ray findings. Antero-posterior view: narrowed air column in subglottic area (steeple sign). Lateral view: overdistention of the hypopharynx
- In severe cases, or with concern for bacterial superinfection, a nasal wash specimen or tracheal secretions can be used for direct identification of organisms

## MANAGEMENT

- Cool mist tent or vaporizer is not recommended as it may increase patient anxiety leading to worsening respiratory distress
- Corticosteroids: Proven benefit for moderate to severe croup; decreases subglottic edema beginning 6–8 hours after dose. Consider dexamethasone (0.6 mg/kg orally or intramuscularly for one dose, maximum 10 mg) or nebulized budesonide (2–4 mg) for one dose; no current evidence to suggest longer courses provide additional benefit
- Nebulized racemic epinephrine (2.25%): Consider for hypoxia or severe croup. Adrenergic effects induce vasoconstriction leading to decreased subglottic edema. Onset occurs in less than 10 minutes. Duration of effect is less than 2 hours; requires 3- to 4-hour observation before discharge. Repeated treatments may decrease need for intubation in ill patients
- Criteria for discharge include: No stridor at rest; normal air entry, color, and level of consciousness
- Heliox therapy (70% helium, 30% oxygen mixture) for severe distress: Helium improves laminar gas flow in edematous airway and decreases the mechanical work of respiratory muscles. Heliox may be effective only if the supplemental oxygen requirement is less than 30%, but larger studies are needed
- Patients with superimposed bacterial laryngotracheobronchitis or laryngotracheobronchopneumonia often require endotracheal intubation and should receive antimicrobials targeting the most common organisms

## ENCEPHALITIS

**Inflammation of the brain parenchyma.**

### EPIDEMIOLOGY

- Most frequently observed in summer and early fall when enteroviruses and arboviruses are most prevalent

- Reported incidence is between 3.5 and 16/100,000. Epidemiological studies are difficult to perform due to lack of standard case definitions
- Commonly associated with meningitis (meningoencephalitis)

## ETIOLOGY

- Viruses most commonly implicated: Arboviruses (West Nile, St. Louis, Eastern and Western equine, Venezuelan equine, California, Powassan, and Colorado tick fever), enteroviruses, herpes simplex 1 and 2, human herpesvirus 6 and 7, varicella zoster, influenza A and B, parainfluenza 1–3, mumps, measles, RSV, rotavirus, adenovirus, Epstein–Barr, rabies, Nipah virus, CMV, parvovirus, lymphocytic choreomeningitis virus, Japanese encephalitis virus
- Bacteria: *Haemophilus influenzae*, *Neisseria meningitidis*, *Streptococcus pneumoniae*, *Mycobacterium tuberculosis*, *Bartonella henselae*
- Other infections: *Mycoplasma pneumoniae*, Rocky Mountain spotted fever, ehrlichia, *Cryptococcus neoformans*, *Coccidioides immitis*, *Histoplasma*, parasites, and helminthes
- Postinfectious diseases: Guillain–Barré, Miller–Fisher, acute cerebellar ataxia, ADEM
- Other: Metabolic disorder, seizure disorder, toxin ingestion, mass lesion, subarachnoid hemorrhage, acute demyelinating disorder, acute confusional migraine, vasculitis, NMDA receptor antibodies

## PATHOPHYSIOLOGY

- Most commonly occurs by hematogenous spread to the brain following viremia or bacteremia
- May occur as a result of retrograde movement through the peripheral nerves (e.g., HSV and rabies)
- Pathogenesis can include direct viral cytopathology and/or a parainfectious or postinfectious inflammatory response

## CLINICAL MANIFESTATIONS

- Common: Acute febrile illness, headache, altered mentation
- Other: Behavioral or personality changes, generalized or focal seizures, hemiparesis, ataxia, movement disorders
- Neurologic abnormalities are based on areas of the brain affected; altered level of consciousness, cranial nerve palsies, ataxia, weakness
- If meningitis: Nuchal rigidity, Kernig and Brudzinski signs (see Meningitis section)

## DIAGNOSTICS

- Clinical diagnosis is based on fever and altered mental status
  Diagnostics: See Table 15-3

- Detailed vaccination, travel, and exposure history should guide additional diagnostics
- Laboratory or imaging features may be suggestive of more unusual causes and consultation with infectious diseases expert and neurologist can guide additional testing

## MANAGEMENT

- If associated with meningitis suggestive of bacterial disease then begin appropriate empiric antibiotics (see Meningitis section) after obtaining CSF culture
- HSV encephalitis: In neonates, acyclovir 60 mg/kg/day divided every 8 hours (older children, 1500 mg/m$^2$/day divided three times daily). Acyclovir may also be indicated in VZV infections—consult with an infectious disease specialist

| TABLE 15-3 | Diagnostic Approach for Encephalitis |
| --- | --- |

## Routine Studies

*Cerebrospinal fluid (CSF)*

Opening pressure, white blood cell count + differential, red blood cell count, protein, glucose

Gram stain and bacterial culture

Herpes simplex virus PCR

Varicella zoster virus PCR

Enterovirus PCR

Cryptococcal antigen and/or India Ink staining

Oligoclonal bands and IgG index

VDRL

*Serum*

Blood culture

CBC with differential

Chemistry panel

Liver function tests

Toxicology screen

HIV serology

Treponemal testing

Hold acute and collect convalescent serum 10–14 days later for paired antibody testing

*Imaging/Neurophysiology*

Neuroimaging (MRI preferred to CT if available)

Chest imaging if respiratory symptoms present

EEG

## Conditional Studies

*Immunocompromised Patients*

CSF cytomegalovirus PCR

CSF human herpesvirus 6/7 PCR

CSF HIV PCR

CSF Epstein–Barr virus PCR

CSF JC virus PCR

CSF *Toxoplasma gondii* PCR with serum serology

CSF acid-fast bacilli culture and smear

CSF fungal culture

CSF and serum West Nile virus serologies plus additional regional arboviruses

CSF and serum PCR for arboviruses

Serum *Coccidioides immitis* complement fixation antibodies

Urine *Histoplasma capsulatum* antigen

*Season and Exposure*

Summer/Fall: Serum and CSF IgG and IgM for arboviruses specific to geographic location; serum serology of tick-borne diseases

Cat exposure: Serum Bartonella antibody, ophthalmologic evaluation

Tick exposure: Serum serology of tick-borne diseases endemic to region

Animal bite/bat exposure: Rabies testing in concert with regional health department

Swimming/diving in fresh water or sinus irrigation: CSF wet mount and PCR for *Naegleria fowleri*

PCR, polymerase chain reaction.

- Most patients with other viral encephalitides require only supportive care
- Physical, occupational, and speech therapy are important in children with severe disease and long-term complications
- Complications: Cerebral edema, long-term neurologic dysfunction, seizure disorder, death

## FEVER IN NEONATES AND YOUNG INFANTS

**Temperature 38.0°C or greater in neonate (age 0–28 days) or young infant (age 29–56 days)**

### EPIDEMIOLOGY

- Serious bacterial infection (SBI) occurs in 9–13% of febrile neonates, including urinary tract infections (4–8%), bloodstream infections (2%), pneumonia (1%), and meningitis (0.5–1%). Additional sources of infection to consider, guided by history and physical exam, include osteomyelitis, gastroenteritis, and skin/soft tissue infections

### ETIOLOGY

- Urinary tract infections: *E. coli*, *Klebsiella*, and *Enterobacter* spp, group B *Streptococcus* (GBS), *Enterococcus*
- Bloodstream infections: GBS, *E. coli*, *Klebsiella*, and *Enterobacter* spp; *Listeria monocytogenes*; coagulase-negative staphylococci (catheter-associated infection); *Staphylococcus aureus*; enteroviruses; HSV
- Pneumonia: GBS; *E. coli*, *Klebsiella*, and *Enterobacter* spp; *L. monocytogenes*; *Chlamydia trachomatis*; respiratory viruses; CMV
- Meningitis: GBS; *E. coli*, *Klebsiella*, and *Enterobacter* spp; *L. monocytogenes*; enteroviruses; HSV (see Neonatal HSV section)

### PATHOPHYSIOLOGY

- Degree of neonatal immune compromise is inversely related to gestational age and birth weight
- High risk of systemic dissemination from any bacterial infection
- Labor and delivery expose neonates to unique pathogens

## CLINICAL MANIFESTATIONS

- Important history: Maternal fever or infection, birth history, ill contacts, level of activity, irritability, feeding, lethargy, vomiting, bowel habits, urine output, jaundice, respiratory distress, fever, or rashes
- Medical history should include immunization status, existing medical conditions (e.g., HIV, asplenia), prematurity
- Neurologic: Bulging fontanelle, lethargy, irritability, hypotonia, hypertonia, weak suck or cry
- Respiratory: Tachypnea, grunting, nasal flaring, retractions, hypoxemia, apnea, cyanosis
- Cardiovascular: Tachycardia, bradycardia, hypotension, delayed capillary refill, diminished pulses
- Gastrointestinal: Abdominal tenderness, distended or firm abdomen, diminished bowel sounds, periumbilical ecchymoses or erythema, discharge from umbilical stump
- Skin: Jaundice, mottled skin, petechiae
- Skeletal: Focal bone tenderness

## DIAGNOSTICS AND MANAGEMENT

- Specific protocol may vary by hospital. The Philadelphia protocol is described subsequently
- All infants 56 days old or younger undergo complete evaluation due to inability to rely on physical exam: CBC with differential; blood culture; urinalysis with Gram stain and cell count; urine culture; CSF cell count, glucose, protein and culture; chest x-ray (if respiratory signs)
- Hospitalize all neonates (age 0–28 days) to administer empiric intravenous antibiotic therapy until either an organism is identified or all culture results are negative for 48 hours or longer: Ampicillin + gentamycin OR ampicillin + cefotaxime. Diagnosis of UTI in neonates does not obviate lumbar puncture, as the rate of coexisting meningitis may occur
- In young infants (age 29–56 days), the Philadelphia protocol identifies those at low risk for bacterial disease who may not require empiric antibiotic therapy. Criteria to identify low-risk infants (29–56 days) are:
  ✓ Exam: Well appearance and normal exam
  ✓ CBC: Less than 15,000 WBC/mm³; band to neutrophil ratio less than 0.2
  ✓ Spun urinalysis: Less than 10 WBC/hpf; no bacteria on Gram stain
  ✓ CSF: Less than 8 WBC/mm³; no bacteria on Gram stain
  ✓ Chest x-ray (if performed): No evidence of discrete infiltrate
- If *ALL* results meet low-risk criteria and follow-up within 24 hours by a physician can be ensured, then consider outpatient management without antibiotics for those age 29–56 days. If any results are abnormal, admit to the hospital and treat empirically with intravenous antibiotics as for neonates (may use cefotaxime alone). If culture results are negative after 48 hours and suspicion for SBI no longer exists, then discharge. If any culture result is positive, alter therapy appropriately
- Infants 29–60 days who test positive for RSV are at lower risk for an SBI than those who test negative; although a clinically important rate of urinary tract infections have been documented (requiring evaluation of blood and urine), lumbar puncture may be deferred in some cases
- Consider viral PCR testing for enterovirus, parechovirus, and HSV from the serum and cerebrospinal fluid when testing is readily available

## FEVER OF UNKNOWN ORIGIN

**Fever (documented temperature 38.3°C or greater) for 14 days or longer with cause not apparent after physical exam and initial screening laboratory tests**

### EPIDEMIOLOGY

- Infection (28–52%), collagen vascular disease (6–20%), malignancy (3–16%)
- Resolution of fever without diagnosis in 20–40%
- *Differential Diagnosis:* See Table 15-4

### PATIENT HISTORY/DIAGNOSTIC CONSIDERATIONS

- Constitutional: Fever onset and height, method used to take temperature, weight loss, night sweats, chills, anorexia
- History: Travel, animal exposure, exposure to unpasteurized dairy products, tick bite, blood transfusion, trauma, fractures or puncture wounds, congenital or acquired heart disease, immune deficiency, foreign body ingestion, CVC, medications

| TABLE 15-4 | Differential Diagnosis of Fever of Unknown Origin | | |
|---|---|---|---|
| **Common Infectious Causes** | **Less Common Infectious Causes** | **Rare Infectious Causes** | **Noninfectious Causes** |
| Systemic viral syndrome | Tuberculosis | Q fever | Collagen vascular diseases |
| Respiratory tract infection | Cat-scratch disease | Brucellosis | Juvenile rheumatoid arthritis |
| Osteomyelitis | Infectious mononucleosis | Tularemia | Systemic lupus erythematosus |
| Urinary tract infection | Lyme disease | Leptospirosis | Dermatomyositis |
| CNS infection | Rickettsial diseases | Intra-abdominal abscess | Scleroderma |
| Enteritis | Malaria | Toxoplasmosis | Vasculitis |
| | Periodontal abscess | Syphilis | Malignancy |
| | Endocarditis | Endemic fungi (e.g., histoplasmosis) | Kawasaki syndrome |
| | HIV | Psittacosis | Inflammatory bowel disease |
| | Viral hepatitis | Chronic meningococcemia | Munchausen syndrome by proxy |
| | Acute rheumatic fever | | Factitious fever |
| | | | Periodic fever syndrome |
| | | | Central fever |
| | | | Dysautonomia |
| | | | Hyperthyroidism |
| | | | Drug fever |

- Family stressor (Munchausen by proxy, pseudofevers)
- Perform repeated and thorough physical exams searching for findings that suggest specific cause

## MANAGEMENT

### *Initial Studies* (Select Tests Based on History *and* Exam)

- Blood:
  - ✓ Blood culture, CBC, CRP, ESR, hepatic function panel
  - ✓ Serology for HIV, EBV, CMV, cat-scratch, Lyme, and streptococcal enzyme titers (ASO, anti-DNase B)
  - ✓ Antinuclear antibodies
- Urine: Urinalysis and culture
- Stool: Hemoccult testing, culture (bacterial/viral), ova and parasite exam
- Radiologic: Chest radiograph
- Miscellaneous: Tuberculin skin test, throat culture, rapid viral antigen testing of nasopharyngeal aspirate

### Additional Studies to Consider

- Blood:
  - ✓ Repeat blood culture
  - ✓ Serology for toxoplasmosis, hepatitis A, B, and C, tularemia, brucellosis, leptospirosis, Rocky Mountain spotted fever, ehrlichiosis, and Q fever
- Stool: *C. difficile* toxins A and B
- Radiologic: Radiographs of involved bones if tenderness or edema on exam, sinus CT, gastrointestinal barium study with small bowel follow-through (if symptoms suggest inflammatory bowel disease), abdominal ultrasound, bone scan, or gallium scan, MRI of pelvis, spine, or specific extremity, echocardiogram
- Miscellaneous: Ophthalmologic exam, bone marrow biopsy (if abnormal CBC or suspected malignancy), lumbar puncture, evaluation for immune deficiency

## GASTROENTERITIS

**Infection of the gastrointestinal tract usually associated with vomiting and diarrhea**

### EPIDEMIOLOGY

- Infectious cases due to viruses (75–90%), bacteria (10–20%), or parasites (up to 5%)

### ETIOLOGY

- See Table 15-5

### PATHOPHYSIOLOGY

- *Osmotic/Malabsorptive:* Intestinal epithelial damage leads to malabsorption and osmotic diarrhea (e.g., *Giardia*)
- *Inflammatory:* Exudation of mucus, blood, and protein into the luminal space exacerbates water and electrolyte loss (e.g., *Shigella*, STEC)
- *Secretory/Toxigenic:* Toxin release results in active secretion of water into the luminal space (e.g., cholera toxin, rotavirus)

### CLINICAL MANIFESTATIONS

- See Table 15-5

TABLE 15-5  Clinical Features of Common Gastrointestinal Pathogens

| Pathogen | Clinical Manifestations | Epidemiologic Clues | Diagnosis | Management |
|---|---|---|---|---|
| **Viral** | | | | |
| Rotavirus | Watery diarrhea associated with fever and vomiting | Children <5, peaks in spring | Antigen detection via EIA, PCR | Supportive once infected; prevention by universal rotavirus vaccination |
| Norovirus | Sudden onset of vomiting, watery diarrhea, abdominal pain, and fever | Outbreaks in daycares, cruise ships; most common cause of food-borne disease outbreaks | PCR, stool antigen or antibody EIA available in research/reference labs | Supportive |
| Sapovirus, adenovirus (40/41), and astrovirus | Milder illness than norovirus or rotavirus characterized by watery diarrhea, less commonly associated with vomiting or fever | Primarily in children <4 | Commercial assays available for sapovirus; EIA for adenovirus available | Supportive |
| **Bacterial** | | | | |
| *Bacillus cereus* | Nausea, abdominal cramps, can be predominantly vomiting (preformed toxin ingestion) or predominantly diarrhea (spore ingestion) | Food borne; preformed toxin most commonly in fried rice, spores in contaminated meat or vegetables | Organism or toxin can be detected in *food* | Supportive |
| *Campylobacter jejuni* | Bloody diarrhea with severe abdominal pain, fever, occasionally bacteremia; immune-mediated manifestations including Guillain–Barré syndrome, Miller–Fisher syndrome, and reactive arthritis can occur following infection | Ingestion of improperly cooked poultry, unpasteurized milk, untreated water; exposure to young animals (i.e., new pets); travel to dairy farms | Culture using selective media; commercially available EIA | Generally supportive, but azithromycin × 3 days or erythromycin × 5 days can shorten duration of illness and organism shedding when given early in illness |

(continued)

**TABLE 15-5** (continued)

| Pathogen | Clinical Manifestations | Epidemiologic Clues | Diagnosis | Management |
|---|---|---|---|---|
| *Clostridium difficile* | See section on *C. difficile* | | | |
| *Escherichia coli* | | | | |
| Shiga-toxin producing (STEC) | Hemorrhagic colitis with bloody diarrhea appearing 3–4 days after onset of symptoms, may cause HUS | Undercooked beef, contaminated greens, unpasteurized milk, petting zoos, person–person | Culture on sorbitol containing selective media, EIA for Shiga toxin production; monitor CBC, BUN, and creatinine for development of HUS | Supportive; antibiotic therapy in patients with STEC is associated with increased risk of developing HUS in some studies but no increased risk or benefit found on meta-analysis of trials, so antibiotic therapy not currently recommended |
| Enteropathogenic (EPEC) | Watery diarrhea | Exclusively in children <2 and in resource-limited countries | Clinical/epidemiological; cannot distinguish from normal flora | Supportive |
| Enterotoxigenic (ETEC) | Watery diarrhea, abdominal cramping; "traveler's diarrhea" | Resource-limited settings (and travelers to these settings) | Clinical/epidemiological; cultures cannot distinguish from normal flora | Azithromycin or ciprofloxacin × 3 days |
| Enteroinvasive (EIEC) | Fever, watery or bloody diarrhea | All age groups, occasionally food borne | Clinical/epidemiological; cultures cannot distinguish from normal flora | Supportive |
| Enteroaggregative (EAEC) | Mild watery diarrhea, may be chronic | All age groups | Clinical/epidemiological; cultures cannot distinguish | Supportive |

| Non-typhoidal Salmonella | Diarrhea, abdominal cramps, and fever; can be complicated by bacteremia, osteomyelitis, brain abscesses, and meningitis | Undercooked poultry or beef, dairy products, contaminated water, contact with reptiles; most common in children <4 | Stool culture | Only indicated for those at high risk of invasive disease: Children <3 months, chronic GI disease, HIV, or other immunocompromising condition. Amoxicillin or TMP-SMX for susceptible strains; otherwise fluoroquinolones, azithromycin, or ceftriaxone |
|---|---|---|---|---|
| *Salmonella typhii* | Initially fever, malaise, myalgias, abdominal pain, constipation or bloody diarrhea, then hepatosplenomegaly and rose spots by the second week of illness; associated with bacteremia and sometimes meningitis | Humans are the only hosts, most common in resource-limited settings and travelers to those settings | Blood culture, bile culture, or bone marrow aspirate; stool cultures are often negative | Empiric treatment with ceftriaxone with definitive therapy determined based on sensitivities and continued × 10–14 days; azithromycin, ampicillin, TMP-SMX, and fluoroquinolones all active against susceptible strains. |
| *Shigella* | Varies from watery stools without constitutional symptoms to bloody stools associated with high fever, abdominal pain, and tenesmus; can be complicated by pseudomembranous colitis, toxic megacolon, and HUS (Shiga toxin producing *S. dysenteriae*). Generalized seizures and postinfectious reactive arthritis have been associated | Low inoculum required for infection, often associated with childcare outbreaks | Stool culture | Indicated for severe illness, dysentery, or underlying immunosuppressive conditions. Amoxicillin or TMP-SMX can be given for susceptible strains for 5 days; otherwise azithromycin × 3 days, ceftriaxone × 5 days, or fluoroquinolone × 3 days pending susceptibility testing |

(*continued*)

**TABLE 15-5** (continued)

| Pathogen | Clinical Manifestations | Epidemiologic Clues | Diagnosis | Management |
|---|---|---|---|---|
| *Vibrio cholerae* | Painless, watery diarrhea leading to significant electrolyte imbalances | More common in the developing world; most cases in the United States are associated with consuming raw or undercooked shellfish | Stool cultures; must request selective media. Serologic testing also available but require acute and convalescent serums | Indicated for moderate to severe illness. Single dose doxycycline or azithromycin or tetracycline for 3 days for susceptible strains; otherwise ciprofloxacin, ofloxacin, or TMP-SMX |
| *Yersinia enterocolitica* | Fever and bloody diarrhea in young children; pseudoappendicitis syndrome resulting from mesenteric adenitis with fever, abdominal pain, and tenderness and leukocytosis in older children; may cause bacteremia or distant foci of infection uncommonly. | Principal reservoir is swine; infection results from contaminated and incompletely cooked pork, unpasteurized milk, well water, chitterlings, and tofu. Uncommon in the United States. | Stool culture; must request selective media | Indicated only for immunocompromised hosts with gastrointestinal infection; generally sensitive to TMP-SMX, aminoglycosides, cefotaxime, fluoroquinolones, tetracycline, doxycycline, and chloramphenicol. Extraintestinal foci of infection or bacteremia should always be treated. |
| *Yersinia pseudo-tuberculosis* | Fever, rash, diarrhea, and pseudoappendicitis; extraintestinal manifestations include sterile pleural and joint effusions and erythema nodosum; mimics Kawasaki disease. | Reservoirs include ungulates, rodents, rabbits, and birds; outbreaks linked to contaminated fresh fruit | Stool culture; must request selective media | Same as *Yersinia enterocolitica* above. |

**Parasites**

| | Clinical features | Epidemiology | Diagnosis | Treatment |
|---|---|---|---|---|
| Cryptosporidiosis | Frequent, watery diarrhea occasionally associated with fever, fatigue, abdominal pain, vomiting, and anorexia. Immunocompromised patients may have chronic diarrhea associated with weight loss and malnutrition. | Contaminated drinking and recreational water, more common in the summer. Livestock and petting zoos. Daycare outbreaks due to person–person transmission. | Direct immunofluorescent antibody, EIA, and rapid immune chromatographic tests available. Can detect oocysts on stool ova and parasite testing, but requires special specimen preparation and staining. | No specific therapy for immunocompetent hosts. HIV+ or otherwise immunocompromised hosts, nitazoxanide. Alternatives include paromomycin or combination of paromomycin + azithromycin. TMP-SMX × 7–10 days, longer in HIV+ patients |
| Cyclosporiasis | Watery diarrhea with anorexia, nausea, vomiting, abdominal pain, fatigue, and weight loss. Symptoms can be relapsing. | Endemic in resource-limited settings, linked to imported fresh produce and recent travel. | Stool examination for ova and parasites, may need repeated examinations. | TMP-SMX × 7–10 days, longer in HIV+ patients |
| Giardia lamblia | Acute illness with watery diarrhea or more chronic illness with foul smelling stools, flatulence, and anorexia. Postinfectious lactose intolerance occurs in 20–40% | Daycare outbreaks, camping trips, outbreaks from contaminated water supplies. | Stool EIA or DFA testing preferred; stool examination for ova and parasites, may need repeated examinations. | Tinidazole (single dose), metronidazole (5–10 days), nitazoxanide (3 days). |
| Entamoeba histolytica | Spectrum of disease from asymptomatic excretion of cysts to mild, noninvasive disease to intestinal amebiasis (most common) characterized by gradual onset of bloody diarrhea, lower abdominal pain, tenesmus, and weight loss; complications include toxic megacolon, fulminant colitis, and bowel perforation. Extraintestinal manifestations include most commonly liver abscesses | Resource-limited countries | Stool ova and parasite examination; serologic testing | For asymptomatic cyst excretion: Iodoquinol, paromomycin, diloxanide. For intestinal amebiasis or extra-intestinal disease: Metronidazole or tinidazole, followed by iodoquinol or paromomycin. |

PCR, polymerase chain reaction; EIA, enzyme immunoassay; HUS, hemolytic uremic syndrome; TMP-SMX, trimethoprim-sulfamethoxazole.

259

## DIAGNOSTICS

- See Table 15-5
- CBC may show excessive band forms (*Shigella*) or evidence of hemolysis (in Shiga toxin producing strains of *E. coli* and *Shigella*)
- Serum electrolytes not routinely indicated unless there are signs of severe dehydration or as part of evaluation for hemolytic uremic syndrome (HUS)
- Fecal occult blood and WBC testing rarely affect clinical management
- Stool cultures are generally low yield and should be reserved for cases of dysentery, suspected STEC, recent foreign travel, immunocompromised hosts with fevers, or when a diagnosis is needed for public health reasons. Stool cultures and ova and parasite testing are particularly low yield in patients hospitalized for >3 days and are not recommended in this population

## MANAGEMENT

- See Table 15-5 for indications for antibiotic therapy
- Oral rehydration is the preferred therapy in cases of mild to moderate dehydration given its low failure rate (3.6%). Small but frequent oral challenges can be given with assessments in response
- Consider a single dose of ondansetron, which enhances success of oral rehydration therapy and decreases need for admission and IV hydration by 50%
- Severe dehydration can be life-threatening. Isotonic IV fluids (0.9% saline or lactated Ringer's) are recommended. IV boluses (20 mL/kg) can be given initially for resuscitation and transitioned to maintenance/replacement fluids and, ultimately, oral rehydration solutions (see Fluids and Electrolytes, Chapter 9)

## INFECTIOUS MONONUCLEOSIS

**Clinical syndrome characterized by fever, exudative pharyngitis, lymphadenopathy, hepatosplenomegaly, and malaise. Caused by Epstein-Barr virus (EBV). However, infections caused by CMV, *Toxoplasma gondii*, adenovirus, or acute HIV infection can have a similar presentation.**

## EPIDEMIOLOGY

- Spread by close personal contact usually via saliva, but can also be transmitted through blood products and sexual contact
- Incubation period is 30–50 days
- Virus can be excreted in oral secretions for over 6 months following infection
- Often causes asymptomatic infection in early childhood. Approximately 90% of US adults have been infected

## PATHOPHYSIOLOGY

- EBV infects oropharyngeal lymphoid tissue B cells, which disseminate to involve the entire lymphoreticular system
- Following infection, the virus remains latent within memory B cells and can later reactivate at times of immune suppression

## CLINICAL MANIFESTATIONS

- EBV can cause a wide spectrum of disease, including asymptomatic infection (most common presentation in young children), infectious mononucleosis (most commonly in adolescents), and lymphoproliferative disease in immunocompromised hosts

- A 3–5 day prodrome of malaise, fatigue, headache, and low-grade fevers may precede clinical infection
- Classic presentation includes triad of high fever, exudative pharyngitis, and generalized lymphadenopathy, most commonly involving the cervical chain
- Other common findings include severe fatigue, malaise, splenomegaly (more common with EBV than CMV), hepatomegaly (10–35%), generalized maculopapular or morbilliform rash (can be triggered by amoxicillin or ampicillin use), and abdominal pain (especially in young children)
- Rare findings and complications include splenic rupture, pneumonia, myocarditis, pancreatitis, mesenteric adenitis, myositis, acute renal failure, glomerulonephritis, Guillain–Barré syndrome, meningoencephalitis, transverse myelitis, peripheral neuritis, optic neuritis, and hemophagocytic syndrome
- Rash
  ✓ Can be pruritic or maculopapular and is typically generalized
  ✓ Occurs in 3–15% of patients without antibiotic exposure and in 23% following antibiotic exposure, most commonly with β-lactams
  ✓ May occur 5–10 days after the antibiotic exposure
  ✓ Rechallenge with a β-lactam does not cause rash
- Fever can occasionally persist for over 2 weeks

## DIAGNOSTICS

- Laboratory findings:
  ✓ Hematologic abnormalities include lymphocyte predominant leukocytosis with >10% atypical lymphocytes, mild thrombocytopenia (platelet count *rarely* <100,000/mm$^3$), and hemolytic anemia (<1% of cases)
  ✓ Mild elevation of hepatic transaminases (50–65% of patients)
- Heterophile antibody tests (including "monospot"):
  ✓ False negatives may occur in children younger than 4 years of age (up to 50% with EBV will have a false-negative monospot)
  ✓ False positives may also occur with leukemia, lymphoma, systemic lupus erythematosus, and serum sickness
  ✓ Most useful for rapid diagnosis in older children, where testing is 85% sensitive and over 90% specific by the second week of illness. Becomes undetectable over 3–6 months
- Specific EBV serologies are reliable in all ages, including with negative heterophile antibody tests
  ✓ *Acute infection:* Elevated viral capsid antigen (VCA) IgM and IgG; EBV nuclear antigen (EBNA) IgG negative
  ✓ *Recent infection:* VCA IgM negative (disappears 4–8 weeks after infection); VCA IgG positive; EBNA negative
  ✓ *Past infection:* VCA IgM negative; VCA IgG and EBNA positive (appears 1–6 months after infection)
  ✓ *Note:* Early antigen assays are unreliable so are not useful for diagnosis
- EBV PCR is most useful in evaluation of immunocompromised patients with suspected EBV infection

## MANAGEMENT

- Supportive care for fever and pharyngitis
- Corticosteroids reserved for patients with impending airway obstruction, which is rare (e.g., prednisone 1 mg/kg/day for 7 days followed by a taper)

- Acyclovir, ganciclovir, and foscarnet demonstrate in vitro activity against EBV but have *not* been shown to improve clinical outcomes in previously healthy children
- Avoid contact sports until full clinical recovery and spleen is not palpable (generally 6–8 weeks)
- Reduction of immunosuppressive therapy for patients with EBV-associated post-transplant lymphoproliferative disorders

## LYMPHADENITIS AND LYMPHADENOPATHY

**Lymphadenopathy is defined as enlargement (>10 mm) of a single lymph node (isolated), a contiguous group of lymph nodes (regional), or noncontiguous groups of lymph nodes (generalized). Lymphadenitis is inflammation within a lymph node or group of lymph nodes, usually the result of infection. The condition may be acute, subacute, or chronic.**

### ETIOLOGY

- Depends on location and clinical presentation
- Bacterial (usually involving cervical chain):
  - ✓ Commonly due to group A beta-hemolytic streptococci and *Staphylococcus aureus*
  - ✓ Less commonly due to anaerobes (dental source), cat-scratch disease, and nontuberculous mycobacteria
  - ✓ Rarely tularemia or diphtheria
- Parasitic: Toxoplasmosis, leishmaniasis
- Fungal: Histoplasmosis, coccidioidomycosis, blastomycosis, cryptococcosis
- Viral: EBV, CMV, adenovirus, HIV, rubella, measles, mumps, HSV, VZV, HHV6, HHV7, hepatitis B, parvovirus B19, dengue
- Other: Oncologic process; Kikuchi–Fujimoto disease (a typically benign, self-limited condition characterized by painful cervical lymphadenopathy and necrosis noted on pathology); Rosai–Dorfman (benign histiocytic proliferation leading to lymphadenopathy, most commonly of the cervical chain)

### PATHOPHYSIOLOGY

- Pyogenic lymphadenitis: Organisms enter lymph nodes and cause proliferation of lymphoid cells in response to antigenic stimuli; also can cause microabscesses and suppuration; may also occur secondary to lymphatic drainage of a localized infected site
- Generalized lymphadenopathy: Organisms may enter lymphatics after hematogenous spread from a systemic infection and cause more generalized proliferation of lymphoid tissue

### CLINICAL MANIFESTATIONS

- Most important to distinguish lymphadenitis from lymphadenopathy and define whether there is local or generalized involvement
- Lymphadenitis: Localized involvement; affected nodes are tender with overlying warmth or erythema. Fluctuance suggests abscess formation
- Torticollis (cervical node involvement); dysphagia, drooling, and dyspnea (retropharyngeal node); cough, stridor, dyspnea (mediastinal node); abdominal pain (mesenteric adenitis); limp (inguinal node)
- Concerning for malignancy if very rapid increase in node size; confluent and matted shape; firm rubbery consistency; lack of tenderness; fixation to surrounding soft tissue structures

- Overlying violaceous discoloration of skin with draining sinus is characteristic of mycobacterial adenitis, but can also occasionally occur with *Staphylococcus aureus*
- Specific sites:
  - ✓ Preauricular: Adenovirus, tularemia, *B. henselae* (causes Parinaud oculoglandular syndrome; see cat-scratch disease)
  - ✓ Postauricular: Scalp infections, HHV6, HHV7, rubella, parvovirus B19
  - ✓ Occipital: Tinea capitis (kerion), scalp infection (cellulitis), or superinfection of eczema or seborrheic dermatitis, rubella, toxoplasma
  - ✓ Supraclavicular: Left-sided "Virchow's node" associated with abdominal source (consider malignancy); right-sided associated with thoracic source (e.g., histoplasmosis, tuberculosis)
  - ✓ Axillary: Cat-scratch disease, BCG vaccination
  - ✓ Inguinal: Sexually transmitted infections including chancroid and lymphogranuloma venereum, *Yersinia pestis*
  - ✓ Generalized: CMV, EBV, toxoplasmosis, HIV, syphilis, endemic mycoses, noninfectious autoimmune or oncologic processes

## DIAGNOSTICS

- Radiologic evaluation is not necessary in most mild to moderate cases of lymphadenitis and rarely in cases of lymphadenopathy
- Ultrasonography preferred to identify drainable abscesses complicating lymphadenitis; CT scan rarely necessary
- Consider needle aspiration or incisional drainage of lymph node if (1) poor response to IV antibiotics; (2) fluctuance or evidence of extension into neck by radiologic studies. Send specimen for bacterial Gram stain and culture, mycobacterial culture and acid-fast smear, and surgical pathology. Fungal culture may be helpful in certain clinical scenarios
- Depending on clinical situation, consider cat-scratch serology or PCR of nodal aspirate, PPD (5–10 mm may be seen with non-tuberculous mycobacteria; usually greater than 15 mm with tuberculosis) and viral serologies or PCRs

## MANAGEMENT

- Empiric antibiotics for suspected bacterial adenitis:
  - ✓ Oral: Clindamycin, amoxicillin-clavulanate, cephalexin
  - ✓ IV: Clindamycin, ampicillin-sulbactam, cefazolin; rarely require vancomycin
  - ✓ If not improving on above therapy, consider repeat imaging to identify a drainable collection and/or biopsy
  - ✓ Average duration of therapy is 10 days
- Special situations (also see Cat-Scratch Disease section)
  - ✓ Non-tuberculous mycobacteria: Standard therapy requires surgical resection of all visibly affected nodes; incisional drainage not recommended since it may lead to a draining sinus tract. Medical management alone with clarithromycin, ethambutol, or rifampin is seldom successful
  - ✓ *M. tuberculosis*: Isoniazid, rifampin, and pyrazinamide + ethambutol or streptomycin and infectious diseases consultation to evaluate for extent of disease

## MASTOIDITIS

**Acute mastoiditis: Mastoid air cell infection resulting from an extension of acute otitis media (OM)**

**Chronic mastoiditis: Low grade but persistent mastoid air cell infection resulting from chronic suppurative OM or, less commonly, inadequately treated acute mastoiditis**

## ETIOLOGY

- Acute mastoiditis:
  - ✓ Common: *Streptococcus pneumoniae, S. pyogenes, Staphylococcus aureus*
  - ✓ Less common: *Haemophilus influenzae, Pseudomonas aeruginosa*, other enteric gram-negative bacilli, anaerobes, *M. tuberculosis*
- Chronic mastoiditis: *Pseudomonas aeruginosa, Staphylococcus aureus, Streptococcus pneumoniae*

## PATHOPHYSIOLOGY

- Mastoid is a series of interconnected air cells located on posterior process of temporal bone, which is connected to the middle ear by a thin channel
- Purulent material from middle ear under pressure invades mastoid air cells and can cause destruction of the bony septa within the mastoid (coalescent mastoiditis) or abscess formation
- Complications arise due to extension of infection into adjacent structures:
  - ✓ Anterior: Facial nerve palsy, labyrinthitis due to invasion of the auditory canal, jugular vein, internal carotid
  - ✓ Posterior: Occipital osteomyelitis
  - ✓ Medial: Petrositis, intracranial complications including meningitis, subdural empyema, epidural abscess, or sinus venous thrombosis
    - ▪ Petrositis may manifest as Gradenigo syndrome, the triad of pain behind the eye, ear discharge, and abducens nerve palsy
  - ✓ Inferior: Abscess of deep neck musculature
  - ✓ Lateral: Subperiosteal abscess within the lateral cortex of the mastoid

## CLINICAL MANIFESTATIONS

- Acute mastoiditis:
  - ✓ Fever, ear pain, tinnitus, postauricular swelling, tenderness, and erythema
  - ✓ Tympanic membrane often bulging, immobile, and opaque, or has ruptured with otorrhea present
  - ✓ May have a history of recent OM (days–weeks)
  - ✓ Pinna deviated outward and downward (infant) or upward (older child)
- Chronic mastoiditis:
  - ✓ Persistent posterior auricular swelling, history of recurrent OM or effusion, chronic otorrhea, hearing loss, and ear pain

## DIAGNOSTICS

- Usually clinical
- Culture from tympanocentesis or drainage procedure useful to guide therapy
- Associated lab findings can include elevated peripheral WBC count, ESR, and CRP
- Temporal bone CT with IV contrast is imaging modality of choice; destruction of bony septa, mastoid air cell coalescence, or rim enhancing fluid collections all suggest mastoiditis, whereas fluid-filled air cells are often seen in uncomplicated OM
- Head CT with contrast (or MRI) may reveal associated intracranial complications

## MANAGEMENT

### Medical

- Acute: Ampicillin-sulbactam or cefotaxime $+/-$ vancomycin depending on severity of illness; may switch to oral antibiotics once patient improves (amoxicillin-clavulanate; levofloxacin; or clindamycin) for a total duration of 3–4 weeks
- Chronic: Piperacillin-tazobactam or ticarcillin-clavulanate $+/-$ vancomycin
- Modify antibiotics based on culture results

### Surgical

- ENT consultation: Myringotomy $+/-$ tympanostomy tubes
- Mastoidectomy if (1) no improvement within 48 hours of myringotomy; (2) subperiosteal abscess, facial nerve palsy, or intracranial extension

### Follow-up

- Audiology exam

## MENINGITIS

**Inflammation of the meninges, which manifests as increased CSF white blood cells**

### EPIDEMIOLOGY

- Viral meningitis most common during late summer and early fall during enteroviral season
- Neonatal bacterial meningitis occurs in 80 cases per 100,000 live births with group B *Streptococcus* accounting for the majority of infections
- Incidence of bacterial meningitis is 6.9/100,000 in children 2–23 months of age and <0.5/100,000 in children 2–17 years of age

### ETIOLOGY

- Bacteria
  - ✓ Neonates (0–1 month): Group B *Streptococcus, E. coli, Listeria monocytogenes, Streptococcus pneumoniae*, enteric gram-negative bacilli
  - ✓ Infants (1 month–1 year): *Streptococcus pneumoniae*, group B *Streptococcus, Neisseria meningitidis, Haemophilus influenzae*
  - ✓ Children older than 1 year: *Streptococcus pneumoniae, Neisseria meningitidis, Haemophilus influenzae*. Incidence of *Streptococcus pneumoniae* is increasing, but studies are under way to track serotype replacement since the introduction of pneumococcal 13-valent vaccine
  - ✓ Other bacterial causes: *Borrelia burgdorferi, M. tuberculosis, Staphylococcus aureus, Treponema pallidum*
- Viruses: Enteroviruses, HSV 1 and 2, varicella zoster, adenovirus, parainfluenza, mumps, measles, influenza A and B, lymphocytic choriomeningitis virus, arboviruses, HIV
- Fungi: *Blastomyces dermatitidis, Coccidioides immitis, Cryptococcus neoformans, Candida* species, *Histoplasma capsulatum*

### PATHOPHYSIOLOGY

- Bacteria and viruses gain entry into the bloodstream through mucosal surfaces. After entry into the blood, the organism invades the meninges and replicates, inducing an inflammatory response

## CLINICAL MANIFESTATIONS

- Neonates and infants: Fever, lethargy, poor feeding, and/or irritability. On exam: bulging fontanelle, nuchal rigidity, inconsolable irritability. In neonates, fever alone should prompt an evaluation for meningitis
- Toddlers and children: Fever, severe headache, chills, photophobia, neck stiffness, seizures, and vomiting. On exam: nuchal rigidity, photophobia, presence of Kernig and/or Brudzinski signs
- Kernig sign: While legs are flexed 90 degrees at the hip, extension of the lower legs cannot be accomplished beyond 135 degrees
- Brudzinski sign: Passive neck flexion elicits involuntary hip flexion
- Complications: Circulatory collapse, focal neurologic findings (paralysis, facial nerve palsy, visual field defects, hearing loss), seizures, hydrocephalus, brain abscess, subdural effusions, syndrome of inappropriate diuretic hormone release

## DIAGNOSTICS

- Laboratory studies: Blood culture, CBC with differential, chemistry panel, liver function tests (especially if suspecting HSV)
- The Bacterial Meningitis Score can be used to predict children at very low risk of bacterial meningitis (see Table 15-6); when all 5 predictors are absent, outpatient management can be considered if the patient appears well and has scheduled clinical follow-up (negative predictive value >99% for absence of bacterial meningitis if all 5 predictors are absent)
- CSF studies (Table 15-7): Cell count with differential, protein, glucose, Gram stain and culture, enterovirus PCR during summer and fall, HSV PCR if consistent with clinical picture
- Radiology:
  ✓ CT scan if evidence of increased intracranial pressure or focal neurologic exam to identify masses, infarcts, and cerebral edema that may put patient at risk for cerebral herniation during lumbar puncture or to aid with prognosis
  ✓ Imaging also indicated for *Citrobacter* and *Cronobacter* infections due to high rate of abscess formation

## MANAGEMENT

- Empiric therapy in patients with suspected bacterial meningitis:
  ✓ Neonate (0–1 month): Ampicillin and cefotaxime IV, dosed for CNS penetration. Begin acyclovir in infants <21 days of age and those who are ill appearing or with other stigmata of HSV disease while awaiting HSV testing results
  ✓ All other children: Vancomycin IV and ceftriaxone or cefotaxime, dosed for CNS penetration

| TABLE 15-6 | Bacterial Meningitis Score |
|---|---|
| **Bacterial Meningitis Score Predictors Criteria*** | |
| CSF Gram stain | Positive result |
| CSF ANC | ≥1000 cells/mm³ |
| CSF protein | ≥80 mg/dL |
| Peripheral blood ANC | ≥10,000 cells/mm³ |
| Seizure | Onset at or prior to time ≥of presentation |

*Bacterial meningitis is unlikely if none of these 5 predictors are present.
ANC, absolute neutrophil count; CSF, cerebrospinal fluid.

| TABLE 15-7 | Typical Cerebrospinal Fluid Profiles | | | |
| --- | --- | --- | --- | --- |
| | WBC (cells/mm³) | WBC Differential | Protein (mg/dL) | Glucose (mg/dL) |
| Normal neonate (0–28 days) | 0–19 | | <115 | 2/3 of serum |
| Normal infant (29–56 days) | 0–9 | | <89 | 2/3 of serum |
| Normal children/ Adolescents | 0–10 | | 5–40 | 2/3 of serum |
| Viral meningitis | <1000 | Lymphocyte predominant* | Normal or <100 | 2/3 of serum |
| Bacterial meningitis | >1000 | Neutrophil predominant | >100–150 | <40 |
| Lyme meningitis | <500 | Lymphocyte predominant | <100 | 2/3 of serum |
| TB meningitis | <300 | Lymphocyte predominant | >200–300 | <40 |

*Neutrophil predominance can be seen in early viral meningitis.

- If CSF culture results remain negative for 48 hours, the antibiotics can be discontinued. However, if antibiotics are administered prior to lumbar puncture, an empiric treatment course of antibiotics should be considered, which can be done in consultation with an infectious diseases specialist
- Duration of therapy varies by organism and patient course. Typically: *N. meningitidis*, 5–7 days; *Streptococcus pneumoniae*, 10 days; group B *Streptococcus*, 14 days
- Audiology exam indicated during follow-up

## NEONATAL CONJUNCTIVITIS

**Conjunctivitis occurring in infants less than 4 weeks of age**

### EPIDEMIOLOGY

- Historically, *C. trachomatis* and *N. gonorrhoeae* most common pathogens. Frequency related to rates of maternal genital infection; however, there is increasing incidence of non sexually transmitted bacterial pathogens
- *Chlamydia trachomatis* acquisition in 50% of infants born vaginally to infected mothers; after acquisition, risk of conjunctivitis is 25–50%

### ETIOLOGY

- Infectious (common): *C. trachomatis*, *N. gonorrhoeae*. Other organisms include *Staphylococcus aureus, Streptococcus pneumoniae, group A and B streptococci, Haemophilus influenzae* (nontypeable), *Pseudomonas aeruginosa* (hospitalized preterm infants)
- Chemical: Silver nitrate, erythromycin, foreign body

### PATHOPHYSIOLOGY

- Infection: Can be acquired in utero, transvaginally, or after birth
- Incubation: *N. gonorrhoeae*, 2–7 days; *C. trachomatis*, 5–14 days

## CLINICAL MANIFESTATIONS

- Conjunctival injection, edema of eyelids, chemosis (swelling)
- Eye discharge may be serosanguineous or purulent
- *C. trachomatis* pneumonia develops in 11–20% of exposed infants at 3–12 weeks of age (afebrile, nasal congestion, diffuse infiltrates, rales)
- *N. gonorrhoeae* may rapidly progress to corneal ulceration and perforation resulting in blindness
- *Pseudomonas aeruginosa* may cause systemic infection

## DIAGNOSTICS

- Culture and Gram stain of the discharge; *N. gonorrhoeae* appears as intracellular gram-negative diplococci on Gram stain
- *Chlamydia trachomatis* can be identified by nucleic acid amplification test (NAAT) on conjunctival or nasopharyngeal (pneumonia) swab. Culture or detection of intracytoplasmic inclusions on Giemsa-stained conjunctival epithelial cells also diagnostic

## MANAGEMENT

- Prevention: Perinatal ocular prophylaxis with topical 0.5% erythromycin, 1% silver nitrate, or 1% tetracycline ointment reduces risk of conjunctivitis; all active against *N. gonorrheae*, but do not prevent transmission of *C. trachomatis*
- *Chlamydia trachomatis* (conjunctivitis or pneumonia)
  - ✓ Oral erythromycin for 14 days (50 mg/kg/day in four doses) has 80% efficacy. Alternate regimens include oral azithromycin (single dose or for 3 days) or sulfonamides
  - ✓ Newborns born to untreated mothers with chlamydia require close observation (without treatment) because efficacy of prophylactic oral erythromycin is unknown
- *Neisseria gonorrhoeae*
  - ✓ Hospitalization, consider evaluation (blood and CSF cultures) to exclude disseminated infection
  - ✓ Ceftriaxone: 25–50 mg/kg single dose IV or IM (maximum 125 mg) for infected infants and for those born to an infected, untreated mother. Cefotaxime if hyperbilirubinemia is present
  - ✓ Saline eye irrigations hourly initially and then every 2–3 hours until resolution of discharge

## OSTEOMYELITIS

**Inflammation of bone, usually secondary to bacterial infection**

### EPIDEMIOLOGY

- 50% of cases occur in children <5 years of age
- Boys are affected more often than girls (except in first year of life)

### ETIOLOGY

- *Staphylococcus aureus* is most common with increasing rates of MRSA
- Other organisms: *Streptococcus pneumoniae* (less common due to widespread vaccination); *Streptococcus pyogenes*; *Kingella kingae*; enteric Gram-negative rods and group B *Streptococcus* (neonates); *Neisseria gonorrhoeae* (adolescents); coagulase-negative staphylococci (prosthetic material-related); anaerobes (complicated sinusitis, superinfection of

fracture site); *Salmonella* (sickle hemoglobinopathies); *Pseudomonas aeruginosa* (puncture wound through sneaker)

## PATHOPHYSIOLOGY

- Hematogenous spread (most common) or extension of contiguous skin/muscle structure infection
- In neonates, infection often extends to joint space via transphyseal capillaries, which recede by 18 months of age

## CLINICAL MANIFESTATIONS

- Most frequently occurs in long bones (in order of decreasing frequency): Femur, tibia, hands and feet, humerus, pelvis, fibula
- 75% of cases have single bone involvement
- Fever, occasionally anorexia, malaise, vomiting, irritability
- Pain and reluctance to use affected extremity ("pseudoparalysis")
- Focal swelling, point tenderness, warmth, and erythema (usually over metaphysis)
- Tenderness out of proportion to soft tissue findings
- Range of motion intact, limited only by pain/muscle spasm
- Neurologic deficits in vertebral osteomyelitis
- In neonates, the entire limb may have swelling, edema, and discoloration

## DIAGNOSTICS

- Leukocytosis (often but not always)
- C-reactive protein (CRP): Elevated in more than 95% (may be normal in chronic osteomyelitis)
- Erythrocyte sedimentation rate (ESR): Elevated in 90%
- Blood culture results: Positive in 35–50%
- Bone aspirate: Culture of bone, blood, and/or joint fluid positive in 50–80%
- Plain radiographs: Low sensitivity for diagnosing early osteomyelitis; 10–20 days after onset, may detect lytic lesions, periosteal elevation, and new bone formation
- Radionuclide bone scanning: Useful in early diagnosis (sensitivity 80–100%)
  ✓ Helpful if multiple sites suspected or poorly localizable pain
- MRI: Best sensitivity (92–100%)
  ✓ Differentiates cellulitis from osteomyelitis
  ✓ Use of contrast allows for better differentiation of bone and soft tissue edema caused by osteomyelitis

## MANAGEMENT

### Medical

- Empiric therapy: Oxacillin, cefazolin, or clindamycin (if high prevalence of MRSA). If patient severely ill, consider vancomycin
- CRP typically begins to decline 2–3 days after initiation of antibiotics (normal within 7–10 days). ESR begins to decline approximately 5–7 days after initiation of antibiotics (normal within 3–4 weeks)
- Early transition to oral therapy, often prior to discharge is the preferred strategy. Treatment failure rates between children treated with early conversion to oral therapy are not significantly different than those treated with prolonged courses of intravenous antibiotics
- Oral therapy with either a targeted agent or empiric clindamycin (dose 30–40 mg/kg/day) or cephalexin (dose 150 mg/kg/day) may be considered. Discuss with infectious diseases specialist
- Duration of therapy: Normalization of CRP, resolution of signs/symptoms of infection, and minimum 3 weeks of therapy (typical duration 3–6 weeks)

## Surgical

- Considerations for surgery: (1) Subperiosteal abscess; (2) bacteremia persisting beyond 48–72 hours of treatment; (3) continued fever, pain, swelling after 72 hours of therapy; (4) development of sinus tract

## OTITIS MEDIA

**Classification of otitis media (inflammation of mucosal lining of middle ear):**

**Acute otitis media (AOM): Purulent fluid in the middle ear with acute signs and symptoms of local or systemic illness**
**Otitis media with effusion (OME): Asymptomatic middle ear effusion**
**Chronic suppurative otitis media (CSOM): Purulent drainage through perforated tympanic membrane for more than 6 weeks**

### EPIDEMIOLOGY

- 90% of children have at least one episode of AOM by 2 years of age; incidence peaks between 6 and 18 months of age

### ETIOLOGY

- AOM: *Streptococcus pneumoniae* (35–48%); nontypeable *Haemophilus influenzae* (20–29%); *Moraxella catarrhalis* (12–23%)
  - ✓ Less common pathogens include group A *Streptococcus* and *Staphylococcus aureus*
  - ✓ After initiation of PCV7 in 2000 and PCV13 in 2010, non-vaccine serotypes of *Streptococcus pneumoniae* and nontypeable *Haemophilus influenza* have emerged as the predominant bacterial pathogens
- Viral pathogens responsible for 10–40% of middle ear effusions in AOM, including RSV, parainfluenza, influenza, and adenovirus
- CSOM is usually polymicrobial: *Pseudomonas* spp; *Staphylococcus aureus*

### PATHOPHYSIOLOGY

- AOM: Transient (e.g., upper respiratory tract infection) or chronic eustachian tube dysfunction causes negative middle ear pressure
- Middle ear fluid accumulates with subsequent bacterial superinfection

### CLINICAL MANIFESTATIONS

- Abrupt onset of fever and ear pain (holding, tugging, rubbing of the ear in a nonverbal child)
- Middle ear effusion: Bulging tympanic membrane, impaired membrane mobility by pneumatic otoscopy, or air-fluid level behind membrane
- Middle ear inflammation: Tympanic membrane with red or yellow color; otalgia

### DIAGNOSTICS

- Diagnosis made by physical exam with pneumatic otoscopy
- Tympanocentesis considered for: (1) Relief of severe pain; (2) confirmation of pathogens in neonates, immunocompromised, or after failed antibiotic therapy; (3) part of treatment for acute mastoiditis
- Tympanometry confirms middle ear effusion when pneumatic otoscopy cannot be performed

## MANAGEMENT

**Based upon the American Academy of Pediatrics Guideline for the Diagnosis and Management of AOM**

### Initial Management of Acute Otitis Media

- Pain control: Acetaminophen or ibuprofen; in children >5 years, consider topical benzocaine (e.g., auralgan, americaine otic)
- For ages 6 months–2 years:
  - ✓ Otorrhea or bilateral AOM—Treat with antibiotics
  - ✓ Unilateral or bilateral AOM with severe symptoms (toxic appearing child, persistent otalgia >48 hours, fever >39°C, or uncertain follow up)—treat with antibiotics
  - ✓ Unilateral AOM without otorrhea—Consider initial observation without antibiotics if non-severe illness or uncertain diagnosis and then treat if no improvement within 48–72 hours. *If observation option exercised, must ensure mechanism for communication with physician, reevaluation, and obtaining medication if necessary*
- For ages >2 years:
  - ✓ Same as above except consider initial observation of patients with bilateral AOM without otorrhea

### Antibiotic Options for Acute Otitis Media

- First-line, *non-severe* symptoms (if decision made to treat and/or the patient has not received amoxicillin in the last 30 days): High-dose amoxicillin, 80–90 mg/kg/day in two divided doses
  - ✓ Alternate agents for penicillin allergy: Cefdinir, cefuroxime, cefpodoxime, azithromycin, clarithromycin, or clindamycin
- First-line, *severe* symptoms (or the patient has received amoxicillin in the last 30 days): Amoxicillin-clavulanate using 90 mg/kg/day of amoxicillin component with 6.4 mg/kg/day of clavulanate in two divided doses
  - ✓ Alternate agent for penicillin allergy: Ceftriaxone (1–3 days)
- Clinically defined treatment failure (no improvement within 48–72 hours): Amoxicillin-clavulanate using 90 mg/kg/day of amoxicillin component (if previously on amoxicillin); otherwise use ceftriaxone (3 days) or clindamycin +/− tympanocentesis
- Duration of therapy: 5–7 days if child >6 years of age and with mild to moderate symptoms; 7 days if child 2–6 years of age with uncomplicated AOM; 10 days in child <2 years of age or with underlying medical conditions, recurrent AOM, or tympanic membrane perforation

### Additional Considerations

- Persistence of middle ear effusion after AOM: 60–70% at 2 weeks, 40% at 1 month, and 10–25% at 3 months
- Recurrent AOM (three episodes in 6 months or four episodes in 1 year, with one episode in the preceding 6 months): Prophylactic antibiotics not indicated
- Indications for tympanostomy tubes: (1) Chronic OME and associated conductive hearing loss greater than 15 dB; (2) tympanic membrane retraction with ossicular erosion or cholesteatoma formation
- OME:
  - ✓ First 3 months: observe
  - ✓ After 3 months (chronic): Tympanostomy tubes if bilateral effusions and hearing loss greater than 15 dB. Antibiotics and corticosteroids not indicated because effusion rapidly re-accumulates upon cessation

- CSOM: 7–14 days of ototopical antibiotics (ciprofloxacin, ofloxacin, neomycin, polymyxin B)
  ✓ Consider oral agents as for AOM
- Complications: Middle ear (e.g., conductive hearing loss, cholesteatoma); temporal bone (e.g., mastoiditis, petrositis; see Mastoiditis topic); inner ear (e.g., labyrinthitis); intracranial (e.g., subdural abscess, lateral sinus thrombosis, meningitis)

## PERIORBITAL/PRESEPTAL AND ORBITAL CELLULITIS

**Periorbital or preseptal cellulitis: Infections anterior to orbital septum**
**Orbital cellulitis: Infections posterior to the orbital septum**

### EPIDEMIOLOGY

- Preseptal cellulitis: Usually in children under 5 years of age
- Orbital cellulitis: Mean age is 12 years; more common in boys

### ETIOLOGY

**Preseptal Cellulitis**

- Infection after local trauma: *Staphylococcus aureus*, *S. pyogenes*
- Hematogenous seeding: Usually *Streptococcus pneumoniae* (since introduction of *Haemophilus influenzae* type B vaccine)
- Soft tissue swelling in periorbital area due to compression of ophthalmic veins secondary to sinusitis (not true cellulitis): *Streptococcus pneumoniae*, *Moraxella catarrhalis*, nontypeable *Haemophilus influenzae*

**Orbital Cellulitis**

- Usually extension of sinusitis into orbit
- Often polymicrobial; most commonly *Streptococcus pneumoniae*, *S. pyogenes*, *Staphylococcus aureus*, and anaerobic bacteria of the upper respiratory tract

### CLINICAL MANIFESTATIONS

- Fever
- Eyelid edema and erythema (>95% unilateral)

**Preseptal Cellulitis**

- Evidence of local trauma
- Normal visual acuity, pupillary responses, intraocular pressure, and extraocular movements
- No pain with eye movement

**Orbital Cellulitis**

- Proptosis
- Impaired or painful extraocular eye movements
- Loss of visual acuity or pupillary responses

### DIAGNOSTICS

- Obtain CBC and blood culture for suspected or confirmed orbital cellulitis, periorbital cellulitis with fever, or toxic appearance
- Perform a lumbar puncture if signs or symptoms of meningitis
- CT scan of orbits and sinuses is recommended if: (1) Orbital involvement confirmed by exam; (2) orbital involvement is suspected or cannot be excluded by exam; (3) progression of disease despite parenteral antibiotic treatment

## MANAGEMENT

### Preseptal Cellulitis

- Oral antibiotics if mild infection and child nontoxic
  - ✓ First-line: Amoxicillin-clavulanate; consider clindamycin in areas of high MRSA prevalence
- Intravenous antibiotics if ill appearing or failed oral treatment
  - ✓ First-line: Ampicillin-sulbactam; consider clindamycin or vancomycin in areas of high MRSA prevalence
- Alternate: Clindamycin, ceftriaxone, vancomycin
- Total duration: 10 days; may be completed orally if clinical improvement is documented

### Orbital Cellulitis

- Requires intravenous antibiotics initially:
  - ✓ First-line: Ampicillin/sulbactam
  - ✓ Alternate: Clindamycin, vancomycin, ceftriaxone
  - ✓ Total duration approximately 14 days, depending on clinical improvement and surgical drainage (if necessary)
- If no clinical improvement is noted in 36–48 hours or if symptoms progress: Repeat CT scan and consider surgical drainage
- Surgical drainage for large, well-defined abscess on initial or repeat CT scan; complete ophthalmoplegia; significant visual impairment

## RETROPHARYNGEAL AND PERITONSILLAR ABSCESS

**Peritonsillar abscess: Purulent collection in the tonsillar fossa**
**Retropharyngeal abscess: Deep neck abscess involving the potential space between the posterior pharyngeal wall and the alar division of the deep cervical fascia**

### EPIDEMIOLOGY

#### Peritonsillar Abscess

- Typically occurs in older children/adolescents (mean age 11 years) as a complication of streptococcal pharyngitis; 15% complicate EBV infection
  - ✓ Increasing incidence likely due to community acquired (CA)-MRSA

#### Retropharyngeal Abscess

- Typically occurs in young children (<5 years) and complicates pharyngitis. In older children and adolescents, it often complicates penetrating injury to the posterior pharynx

### ETIOLOGY

#### Peritonsillar Abscess

- Common: *S. pyogenes*
- Less common: *Staphylococcus aureus*, anaerobes (*Fusobacterium, Peptostreptococcus, Bacteroides*), *Haemophilus influenzae*

#### Retropharyngeal Abscess (Usually Polymicrobial)

- Common: *S. pyogenes, Staphylococcus aureus*, viridans group streptococci
- Less common: Oral anaerobes (*Fusobacterium, Peptostreptococcus, Bacteroides* spp), *Eikenella corrodens, Haemophilus influenzae, Streptococcus pneumoniae*

## PATHOPHYSIOLOGY

• Peritonsillar abscess begins with pharyngitis or cellulitis and progresses to abscess

### Retropharyngeal Abscess

• Retropharyngeal space:
  ✓ Limited posteriorly by the alar division of deep cervical fascia and anteriorly by the posterior pharyngeal wall
  ✓ Divided by a midline raphe into two lateral compartments with each half containing lymph nodes
• Infection of the nasopharynx spreads to retropharyngeal space by lymphatic routes; lymph node inflammation followed by necrosis leads to abscess
• Retropharyngeal abscess is unlikely in older children due to regression of lymph nodes
• Complications: Extension to carotid sheath (carotid artery, internal jugular vein, vagus nerve) or posteriorly (atlantoaxial dislocation); spontaneous rupture may cause aspiration, asphyxiation, empyema, or mediastinitis

## CLINICAL MANIFESTATIONS

### Peritonsillar Abscess

• Adolescent with fever, sore throat, unilateral pain, drooling, dysphagia, and "hot potato" (muffled) voice
• Trismus in two thirds
• Oropharynx: Displacement of uvula away from affected side, palpable peritonsillar fluctuance, +/− tonsillar exudate
• Ipsilateral cervical adenopathy

### Retropharyngeal Abscess

• Fever, decreased oral intake, sore throat
• Drooling, dysphagia, odynophagia
• Neck stiffness or pain with neck extension
• Torticollis, trismus, stridor, and dyspnea are less common (<5%)

## DIAGNOSTICS

• Leukocytosis with neutrophil predominance (CBC not routinely recommended)
• Rapid streptococcal antigen test by throat swab
• Lateral neck x-ray in retropharyngeal abscess: Retropharyngeal space wider than one-half of the C2 vertebrae or greater than 7 mm (false negative rate of 14%)
• Neck CT with contrast: In peritonsillar abscess, assesses extent of infection; in suspected retropharyngeal abscess, distinguishes cellulitis from abscess (false-negative rate of 10%)

## MANAGEMENT

### Peritonsillar Abscess

• Incision and drainage with 18-gauge needle confirms diagnosis and provides immediate relief
• Empiric therapy: Ampicillin-sulbactam/amoxicillin-clavulanate, or clindamycin
• Duration of therapy: 7–10 days

### Retropharyngeal Abscess

• Emergency: Secure airway (if necessary); obtain IV access; order nothing by mouth (NPO)
• Early detection (no mature abscess) may obviate surgery

- Most cases of mature abscess require surgical drainage
  - ✓ Transoral approach limits exposure of vessels; used to drain abscesses medial to great vessels
  - ✓ Transcervical (i.e., external) approach limits aspiration risk; used to drain abscesses lateral to great vessels or if there is a large lateral component
- Antibiotics: Ampicillin-sulbactam. Alternate: ceftriaxone + clindamycin. Use IV antibiotics initially, and switch to oral antibiotics when symptoms have improved to complete 10- to 14-day course. Longer courses may be necessary for undrained collections

## SEPSIS

**Systemic inflammatory response syndrome (SIRS) in response to a suspected or documented infection with or without organ system dysfunction (severe sepsis) or cardiovascular dysfunction unresponsive to fluid resuscitation (septic shock).**

### ETIOLOGY/EPIDEMIOLOGY

- Neonatal: Group B *Streptococcus*, enteric gram-negative bacilli, less commonly *Listeria monocytogenes*; *Staphylococcus aureus*, *Candida* spp, coagulase-negative *Staphylococci*, other gram negatives in hospitalized neonates, especially those with CVCs
- Community acquired, non-immunocompromised host: *Streptococcus pneumoniae*, *Neisseria meningitidis*, *Streptococcus pyogenes*, enteric gram negatives, *Staphylococcus aureus*, rickettsial disease
- Immunocompromised host: Enteric gram negatives, *Staphylococcus aureus*, coagulase-negative *Staphylococcus*, viridans group *Streptococci*, fungi
- Central venous catheter: See "catheter related blood stream infection" section
- As many as 50–75% of children with sepsis will have no confirmed cause
- Figure 15-2 shows the laboratory classification of commonly isolated bacteria

### PATHOPHYSIOLOGY

- Activation of the immune response by pathogen leads to leukocyte mobilization, upregulation of pro-inflammatory cytokines, complement activation, and activation of coagulation
- These processes lead to capillary injury, vasodilation, microvascular thromboses and subsequent cardiac and other end-organ dysfunction

### CLINICAL MANIFESTATIONS

- Sepsis is defined as signs of systemic inflammation related to suspected or documented infection, including:
  - ✓ Temperature >38.5 or <36°C
  - ✓ Tachycardia >2 standard deviations above normal for age
  - ✓ Tachypnea >2 standard deviations above normal for age
  - ✓ Leukocytosis or leukopenia for age, or >10% bands
- Evidence of organ system dysfunction, including altered mental status, increased work of breathing, tachypnea, hypoxia, tachycardia, poor perfusion, hypotension, petechiae or purpura

### DIAGNOSTICS

- Complete blood count, electrolytes, liver function tests, dextrose stick, PT, PTT, fibrinogen, lactate, and co-oximetry (if patient has a CVC) can help assess end-organ function and adequacy of perfusion
- Type and screen
- Consider random cortisol level

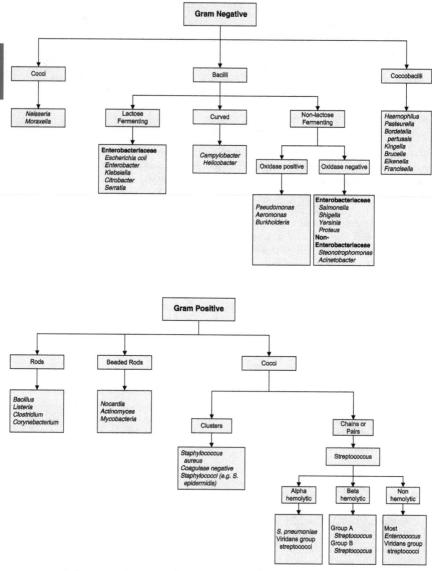

FIGURE 15-2 **Laboratory features of common organisms.**

- Cultures of all potential sources of infection *before* antibiotics (if doing so does not delay antibiotic administration); blood culture should be obtained in all cases of sepsis (prefer cultures from both peripheral blood and central line, if present), as well as urine culture, CSF Gram stain and culture, respiratory Gram stain and culture, and wound Gram stain and culture of any identifiable soft tissue abscesses, as clinically indicated

- Consider viral testing for HSV and/or enterovirus from serum, as well as influenza, adenovirus, and/or RSV from respiratory secretions
- Chest x-ray, imaging of possible foci of infection as clinically indicated

## MANAGEMENT

- Immediate establishment of intravenous or intraosseus access (preferably at least two access points in severely ill patients)
- Rapidly administer 20 mL/kg bolus, repeated as needed, with goal of 60 mL/kg within the first 1 hour
- If not responsive to 60 mL/kg fluid resuscitation, consider initiation of inotropes
- Administer antibiotics within 1 hour of diagnosis of sepsis
  - ✓ Neonate: Ampicillin and cefotaxime +/− acyclovir
  - ✓ Infants and children, community acquired: Vancomycin and cefotaxime or ceftriaxone
  - ✓ Immunocompromised, hospitalized, or CVC: Vancomycin and an antipseudomonal beta-lactam *plus* second gram-negative agent (aminoglycoside or ciprofloxacin)
  - ✓ Intra-abdominal source: Add metronidazole
  - ✓ Toxin-mediated process: Add clindamycin
  - ✓ Suspected rickettsial illness (Rocky Mountain spotted fever, ehrlichiosis): Add doxycycline
  - ✓ High risk for fungal infection (neutropenia, prior broad spectrum antibiotics, TPN dependent): Consider adding echinocandin (caspofungin, micafungin) or amphotericin
  - ✓ If type I hypersensitivity to penicillin: Aztreonam in place of cephalosporins
  - ✓ Modify above recommendations based on sensitivity profile of prior isolates and local resistance patterns
- Source control as soon as feasible (drainage of soft tissue abscesses, debridement of necrotic tissues, removal of infected CVCs)

## SEPTIC ARTHRITIS

**Microbial invasion of the joint space**

### EPIDEMIOLOGY

- Peak incidence in children <3 years of age

### ETIOLOGY

- Most common across all age groups: *Staphylococcus aureus*
- Neonates: *Staphylococcus aureus*, group B *Streptococcus*, enteric gram-negative rods
- School age: *Staphylococcus aureus*, *Kingella kingae*, *S. pyogenes*, *Streptococcus pneumoniae*, *Haemophilus influenzae*
- Older children: *Staphylococcus aureus*, *S. pyogenes*, *Borrelia burgdorferi*, *N. gonorrhoeae*
- Less common causes: *N. meningitidis*, *Pseudomonas* spp, *Candida* spp, Brucella spp, tuberculous and non-tuberculous mycobacteria, *Nocardia asteroids*, *Borrelia burgdorferi* (Lyme disease—seen in endemic areas)

### PATHOPHYSIOLOGY

- Mechanism: (1) Hematogenous dissemination; (2) contiguous extension (10–16% of cases); (3) direct inoculation
- Risk factors: Joint instrumentation, diabetes, immunodeficiency, skin or soft tissue infection, hemoglobinopathy, IV drug use

## CLINICAL MANIFESTATIONS

- Fever, malaise, poor appetite, irritability (infants)
- Frequency of joint involvement (in order of decreasing frequency): Knee, hip, ankle, elbow, shoulder, other
- Severe joint pain, decreased mobility, refusal to walk
- Joint swelling, erythema, warmth, exquisite tenderness, decreased range of motion
- Septic hip held flexed and externally rotated
- 90% of cases are monoarticular
- Dermatitis-arthritis syndrome, sexually transmitted diseases (*N. gonorrhoeae*)
- History of erythema migrans (EM) rash, significant swelling, minimal pain (Lyme)

## DIAGNOSTICS

- CBC: 70% with elevated WBC
- CRP: Elevated at presentation in 95%
  - ✓ CRP >2 mg/dL has been shown to be the strongest independent risk factor
- ESR: Elevated at presentation in 90%
- Blood culture results: Positive in 40%
- Joint fluid aspiration for cell count (Table 15-8)
- Joint fluid culture results: Positive in 50–60%; yield increased if joint fluid inoculated directly into blood culture bottle (especially for detection of *K. kingae*)
- Low synovial fluid glucose concentration (<40 mg/dL) suggests infection but this criterion has a sensitivity of only 50%
- If Lyme disease exposure: Lyme serology +/− Lyme joint fluid PCR (useful in antibiotic-refractory disease)
- Joint radiographs: Important to exclude other causes of joint pain; not diagnostic for septic arthritis but may reveal distortion of fat pad, soft tissue swelling, joint space widening, and focal source of osteomyelitis
- Ultrasound: Preferred initial study to identify excess joint space fluid
- MRI: Highly sensitive in early detection of joint fluid; detects involvement of adjacent bone or soft tissue

## MANAGEMENT (THIS IS A MEDICAL EMERGENCY)

### Surgical

- Hip or shoulder: Prompt surgical drainage, joint space irrigation
- Knee, ankle, or wrist: Needle aspiration; consider joint space irrigation if unable to perform adequate drainage
- Open surgical drainage of joints other than hip and shoulder is usually not required

| TABLE 15-8 | Typical Synovial Fluid Findings |
| --- | --- |
| **Diagnosis** | **Typical WBC per mm³** |
| Normal | <150 |
| Bacterial arthritis | >50,000 |
| Lyme arthritis | Typical: 40,000–80,000* |
| Reactive arthritis | <15,000 |

*Range: 200–140,000; WBC, white blood cell.

## Medical

- Empiric antibiotic therapy
  - ✓ Neonate: Intravenous oxacillin (or clindamycin or vancomyicin if MRSA common) + gentamycin (or cefotaxime)
  - ✓ Older children: Intravenous clindamycin or vancomycin, switch to oxacillin or cefazolin if methicillin-sensitive *Staphylococcus aureus* (MSSA) is isolated
  - ✓ Consider both oxacillin + vancomycin if hip or shoulder involved
  - ✓ Add cefotaxime/ceftriaxone if risk factors for gram-negative rods
  - ✓ Consider *Kingella kingae* as a cause in pre-school age children and those with poor response to clindamycin
  - ✓ Consider doxycycline (children >8 years old) or amoxicillin (children <8 years old) if concern for Lyme disease
  - ✓ Specific antibiotic therapy based on culture results
- Oral versus intravenous antibiotics
  - ✓ Oral therapy can be substituted for IV therapy after infection is adequately controlled if an oral antibiotic appropriately covers the organism and follow up is ensured
  - ✓ For severe infections involving any joint space (especially the hip or shoulder): IV therapy may need to be extended
- Duration:
  - ✓ Three to 4 weeks for *Staphylococcus aureus* or enteric gram-negative rods
  - ✓ In general, 2–3 weeks is sufficient for most other organisms (must be individualized based on patient's course)
- Response to therapy: ESR peaks at end of first week and normalizes at 3–4 weeks. CRP peaks by day 2–3, and normalizes by day 7–9

## SINUSITIS

**Inflammation of paranasal sinuses secondary to allergic, bacterial, fungal, or viral etiology. Bacterial sinusitis is classified clinically by the duration and severity of symptoms:**

- Acute bacterial sinusitis: Symptoms for less than 30 days
- Subacute sinusitis: Symptoms for 30–90 days
- Chronic sinusitis: Symptoms for greater than 90 days

### EPIDEMIOLOGY

- Complicates 5–10% of upper respiratory infections
- Peak prevalence in the winter months

### ETIOLOGY

- Acute and subacute bacterial sinusitis:
  - ✓ *Streptococcus pneumoniae; Haemophilus influenzae; Moraxella catarrhalis*
  - ✓ Less commonly: Group A *Streptococcus*, group C *Streptococcus*, viridans group streptococci, anaerobes, *Eikenella* spp
- Chronic sinusitis:
  - ✓ Aerobic bacteria found in acute sinusitis, *Staphylococcus aureus*, anaerobes

### PATHOPHYSIOLOGY

- Ciliary dysfunction and increased secretions lead to sinus obstruction
- Contamination of usually sterile sinuses with nasopharyngeal bacteria

- Recurrent bacterial sinusitis should prompt investigation for underlying predisposition (e.g., allergic rhinitis, cystic fibrosis, dysmotile cilia, and HIV)

## CLINICAL MANIFESTATIONS

- Acute sinusitis:
  - ✓ Persistent illness: Nasal discharge of any quality or daytime cough or both, lasting more than 10 days without improvement
  - ✓ Worsening course: Worsening or new onset of nasal discharge, daytime cough, or fever after initial improvement
  - ✓ Severe onset: Concurrent fever (temperature of 102.2°C or greater) and purulent nasal discharge for at least 3 consecutive days
- Chronic sinusitis: Respiratory symptoms for longer than 90 days; nasal discharge of any quality; headache; fever uncommon
- On physical exam: Periorbital edema; mucopurulent discharge in nose or posterior pharynx; erythematous or boggy and pale nasal mucosa; tenderness to palpation and/or percussion over paranasal sinuses; malodorous breath

### Complications

- Orbital complications: Orbital abscess, orbital cellulitis, optic neuritis
- Intracranial complications: Epidural or subdural empyema, cavernous or sagittal sinus thrombosis, meningitis, brain abscess, osteomyelitis; require neurosurgical and infectious diseases consultation

## DIAGNOSTICS

- Diagnosis usually based on clinical findings
- Confirmatory imaging not indicated in cases of uncomplicated sinusitis
- Imaging indicated if: (1) Complicated sinusitis; (2) numerous recurrences; (3) protracted or unresponsive course; (4) anticipated surgical drainage
  - ✓ Contrast-enhanced CT better than MRI to assess suspected suppurative complications

## MANAGEMENT

### Medical

- Persistent illness: Either prescribe antibiotic therapy OR offer additional observation for 3 days
- Worsening course or severe onset: Antibiotic therapy indicated
- First-line therapy: Amoxicillin or amoxicillin-clavulanate
  - ✓ High-dose amoxicillin (90 mg/kg/day) should be used in areas of high prevalence of penicillin-resistant *Streptococcus pneumoniae* (>10%)
  - ✓ High-dose amoxicillin with clavulanate should be used in children that attend daycare, age <2 years, or have had antibiotic use within the last 4 weeks
- Consider alternate agent if (1) allergy to penicillin; (2) failure to improve on amoxicillin or amoxicillin-clavulanate after 3 days; (3) moderate to severe illness; (4) protracted symptoms (>30 days)
- Alternate agents: Ceftriaxone, cefdinir, cefuroxime, cefpodoxime
  - ✓ Agents not recommended as empiric therapy due to high rates of resistance: Macrolides, TMP/SMX
- Duration: 10 days
- Empiric therapy for complicated sinusitis (e.g., subdural extension): Vancomcyin + third-generation cephalosporin + metronidazole

### Sinus Aspiration

- Indications: (1) Failure to respond to multiple course of antibiotics; (2) severe facial pain; (3) orbital or intracranial complications; (4) evaluation of an immunocompromised host

## TOXIC SHOCK SYNDROME

**An acute streptococcal or staphylococcal exotoxin-mediated infection resulting in fever, diffuse erythroderma, hypotension, and impairment of three or more organ systems**

### EPIDEMIOLOGY

- 90% of cases in 1980s occurred in context of superabsorbent tampon use. Now <50% of cases are associated with tampon use. Other associations include foreign body placement, primary *Staphylococcus aureus* infection, postoperative wound infection, and mucous membrane or skin disruption
- *Streptococcus pyogenes*-associated toxic shock syndrome (TSS) is associated with varicella infection, diabetes mellitus, and HIV infection

### ETIOLOGY

- *Staphylococcus aureus* strains producing one or more of the following exotoxins: TSST-1, enterotoxin A, B, C, or D
- *S. pyogenes* strains producing streptococcal pyrogenic exotoxins A, B, or C, mitogenic factor, or streptococcal superantigen

### PATHOPHYSIOLOGY

- TSST-1 and other exotoxins act as superantigens by crosslinking MHC II and TCR, bypassing normal MHC-mediated antigen presentation. T cell activation causes massive cytokine release
- Exotoxins cause perivascular infiltrates, decreased peripheral resistance, and interstitial edema resulting in intravascular volume depletion, hypotension, and shock
- Activation of the coagulation cascade and thrombolytic enzymes induce microangiopathic hemolytic anemia and DIC

### CLINICAL MANIFESTATIONS

- Fever, rash, hypotension, arthritis with multi-organ involvement and clinical illness out of proportion to degree of local infection
- Diffuse erythroderma or blanching macular erythema that desquamates 1–2 weeks later

### DIAGNOSTICS

- Elevated creatinine
- Platelets less than $100,000/mm^3$ or signs of DIC
- Elevated alanine aminotransferase, aspartate aminotransferase, or total bilirubin
- Blood, throat, and CSF cultures are usually negative; blood cultures may be positive in *Staphylococcus aureus*-related TSS
- Diagnosis of Staphylococcal TSS requires: Fever >38.9°C, diffuse macular erythrodermic rash (with subsequent desquamation), hypotension, and multisystem organ involvement (>3 organ systems)
- Diagnosis of Streptococcal TSS requires: Isolation of *S. pyogenes* from a sterile or non-sterile site, hypotension, and multisystem organ involvement (>2 organ systems)

## MANAGEMENT

- Anticipate shock and multisystem organ failure
- Remove or drain any loculated source of infection
- Empiric IV antibiotics: Beta-lactamase resistant antistaphylococcal antibiotic (e.g., oxacillin, vancomycin) plus a protein-synthesis inhibitor (clindamycin), which provides (1) a mechanism of bacterial growth inhibition not dependent on replication (to address stationary phase *Staphylococcus aureus/S. pyogenes*) and (2) suppression of toxin production. Consider adding Gram-negative coverage until diagnosis is more certain
  - ✓ For *S. pyogenes* cases, switch to penicillin + clindamycin
  - ✓ For methicillin sensitive *Staphylococcus aureus* cases, continue with an appropriate beta-lactam antibiotic (based on susceptibility testing) and clindamycin
  - ✓ For methicillin resistant *Staphylococcus aureus* cases, continue with vancomycin and clindamycin
  - ✓ Total antibiotic course of 10–14 days may include high-dose oral therapy when the patient is no longer critically ill
- IVIG may be considered as adjunctive therapy for patients with an inaccessible focus of infection or those with continued deterioration following fluid and vasopressor support (dose: 400 mg/kg once); however, its effectiveness for treatment of TSS has not been established in randomized clinical trials

## URINARY TRACT INFECTION

**Infection of lower (cystitis) or upper (pyelonephritis) urinary tract**

### EPIDEMIOLOGY

- About 5% prevalence in young febrile children without a source
- Age and gender influence prevalence:
  - ✓ Incidence (in order of decreasing frequency): Neonates, infants, school-aged
  - ✓ Neonates: Boys affected more often than girls; uncircumcised boys at higher risk
  - ✓ Age older than 1 year: Girls affected more often than boys

### ETIOLOGY

- *E. coli* (70–90% of urinary tract infections [UTIs])
- Other organisms include: *Klebsiella*, *Proteus* spp (boys >1 year); *Pseudomonas aeruginosa*; *Enterococcus* spp; *Staphylococcus saprophyticus* (female adolescents); group B streptococci (neonates); *Staphylococcus aureus* (suggests hematogenous seeding from additional site of infection, e.g., osteomyelitis, endocarditis, renal abscess)

### PATHOPHYSIOLOGY

- Host factors: Inability to empty bladder completely (e.g., neurogenic bladder, posterior urethral valves, indwelling catheter); vesicoureteral reflux (20–30% of children with UTI)

### CLINICAL MANIFESTATIONS

- Neonates and Infants: Fever or temperature instability; poor feeding; vomiting; jaundice; decreased activity
- Children 2–5 years of age: Fever; abdominal pain; bedwetting or incontinence in previously toilet-trained child; foul-smelling urine
- Children older than 5 years: Fever; vomiting; abdominal pain; dysuria; frequency; urgency; bedwetting or incontinence in previously toilet-trained child; suprapubic or costovertebral angle tenderness

- Risk factors (general): History of UTI, renal disease, undiagnosed febrile episodes, sexual activity, genitourinary trauma
- Risk factors for girls: White race, age <12 months, temperature >39°C, fever >2 days, absence of other source of infection
  ✓ No more than 1 present: <1% probability of UTI, no more than 2 present: <2% probability of UTI
- Risk factors for boys: Nonblack race, temperature >39°C, fever >24 hours, absence of another source of infection
  ✓ No more than 2 present and uncircumcised: <1% probability of UTI, no more than 3 present and circumcised: <2% probability of UTI

## DIAGNOSTICS

### Laboratory Screening

- Urinalysis (on centrifuged urine):
  ✓ With positive leukocyte esterase, positive nitrites, or 5 or more WBCs per high-power field, sensitivity of 99.8% and specificity of 70%. Thus, urinalysis is a useful screening test but cannot replace culture for diagnosis

### Laboratory Confirmation

- Midstream clean catch method preferred in toilet trained children (Table 15-9)
- Straight catherization recommended in children unable to provide clean catch specimen
- Suprapubic aspiration unsuccessful in 10% of attempts
- Urine bag specimens are *not* appropriate for culture
- To establish the diagnosis of UTI, urinalysis must show pyuria and/or bacteriuria AND >50,000 CFU/mL on urine culture; bacteriuria in the absence of pyuria should raise suspicion for asymptomatic bacteriuria or contaminated culture

## MANAGEMENT

### Medical

- Febrile UTI or suspected pyelonephritis *outpatient* therapy:
  ✓ Oral therapy acceptable for uncomplicated pyelonephritis
  ✓ Children must be older than 1 month of age, well-hydrated, and tolerating oral medications; 7–14 days of treatment; empiric therapy (oral): Cephalexin, cefdinir, cefixime, amoxicillin-clavulanate, TMP-SMX (depending on local resistance rates); children <1 month may also be candidates for oral therapy, depending on response to initial intravenous therapy

| TABLE 15-9 | Interpretation of Urine Culture Results | |
| --- | --- | --- |
| **Method** | **Probable** | **Possible** |
| Suprapubic | ≥100 CFU/mL | Any growth |
| | One pathogen | One pathogen |
| Catheterization | ≥50,000 CFU/mL | ≥10,000 CFU/mL |
| | One pathogen | One pathogen |
| Clean catch | ≥100,000 CFU/mL | ≥50,000 CFU/mL |
| | One pathogen | One pathogen |
| | Two cultures | One culture |

CFU, colony-forming unit.

283

- Febrile UTI or suspected pyelonephritis *inpatient* therapy:
  - ✓ Hospitalization and initial intravenous therapy for those with moderate dehydration, ill appearance, significant emesis, underlying urologic abnormalities, poor compliance, and failure of outpatient therapy
  - ✓ Seven to 14 days of treatment; empiric therapy (intravenous): Ampicillin + gentamycin, ceftriaxone/cefotaxime, ciprofloxacin; may switch to oral therapy when patient clinically improved
- No benefit to routine repeat urine cultures after initiation of therapy. Consider repeat cultures if fever or symptoms persist >72 hours
- Consider antimicrobial prophylaxis for children with severe (grade V) VUR

### Imaging

- Ultrasound of urinary tract identifies: Hydronephrosis, dilatation of distal ureters, hypertrophy of bladder wall, presence of ureteroceles
  - ✓ Recommended by AAP for: (1) All children younger than 2 years of age with first UTI; (2) if clinical improvement is slower than anticipated with appropriate treatment
- Voiding cystourethrogram (VCUG) identifies: Vesicoureteral reflux (VUR), posterior urethral valves, bladder abnormalities
  - ✓ VCUG should not be performed routinely after the first febrile UTI. Recommended by AAP for children with renal ultrasounds suggestive of VUR or >1 documented UTI

## SPECIFIC PATHOGENS

### CAT-SCRATCH DISEASE

**A subacute, self-limited regional lymphadenitis syndrome caused by cutaneous inoculation with *Bartonella henselae* (a fastidious pleomorphic gram-negative rod) through cat scratches or bites. Rarer causes include *Afipia felis* and *Bartonella clarridgeiae*.**

### EPIDEMIOLOGY

- Broad geographic distribution; peaks in fall and early winter
- Cats are the natural reservoir, with anywhere from 13 to 90% seroprevalence
- 90% of cases have a history of recent contact with healthy cats, especially cats younger than 1 year of age or cats with fleas
- The most common cause of chronic, unilateral regional lymphadenitis in US children

### CLINICAL MANIFESTATIONS

- Primary cutaneous inoculation lesion (papules at site of inoculation) often precedes lymphadenopathy by 1–2 weeks
- Unilateral subacute tender lymphadenopathy in axillary, cervical, submandibular, periauricular, supraclavicular, epitrochlear, femoral, or inguinal locations; 1–5 cm in size, up to 30% suppurate. Incubation time from cat scratch to appearance of lymphadenopathy is 5–50 days (median 12 days)
- Constitutional symptoms in up to 30% of patients (fever, malaise, fatigue)
- *Parinaud's oculoglandular syndrome:* Conjunctival granuloma with ipsilateral preauricular lymphadenitis
- Encephalopathy may develop 1–6 weeks after primary disease and is associated with seizures and rarely coma with recovery in several weeks. Head CT is typically normal. CSF shows slight mononuclear pleocytosis. EEG is abnormal
- Fever: Up to 5% of cases of fever of unknown origin due to cat-scratch disease (CSD)

- Granulomatous hepatitis or splenitis
- Rare manifestations: Osteomyelitis, endocarditis, thrombocytopenic purpura, bacillary angiomatosis in immunocompromised hosts (HIV)

## DIAGNOSTICS

- *Serology by indirect fluorescence assay:* IgG titers <1:64 = no current infection; >1:64 but <1:256 = possible infection, repeat in 10–14 days; >1:256 = current or recent infection
- *PCR* (blood, CSF, or tissue biopsy specimens): Useful to diagnose rare *B. henselae* manifestations
- *Histopathology:* Warthin–Starry silver stain may demonstrate pleomorphic bacilli in chains (not routinely necessary)
- *Culture:* Difficult to isolate organism from tissue or blood
- *CT scan:* May reveal multiple hypodense liver or spleen lesions

## MANAGEMENT

- Routine antibiotic use for cat-scratch adenitis is controversial because spontaneous resolution typically occurs within 1–4 months. Azithromycin, clarithromycin, rifampin, or ciprofloxacin may hasten initial decrease in lymph node volume
- Consider needle aspiration of painful suppurative nodes for symptomatic relief. Surgical excision is not typically required
- No controlled trials of therapy exist for less common sites of infection (e.g., hepato-splenic CSD, osteomyelitis, bacillary angiomatosis). Consider parenteral gentamycin or azithromycin. Transition to oral therapy when patient is improved. Duration of therapy is unclear

## CLOSTRIDIUM DIFFICILE INFECTION

***Clostridium difficile* is an anaerobic spore-forming bacterium that causes diarrhea and colitis.**

### EPIDEMIOLOGY

- Up to 70% of infants and 1–3% of adults are asymptomatic carriers
- Predisposing factors: Hospitalization, prolonged antibiotics, abdominal surgery, inflammatory bowel disease, immune deficiency

### PATHOPHYSIOLOGY

- Disturbance of normal colonic flora, usually as a result of antibiotic exposure, allows *C. difficile* to flourish
- Spores produce toxins (A and B) that cause mucosal damage

### CLINICAL MANIFESTATIONS

- Spectrum of mild diarrhea to severe pseudomembranous colitis to toxic megacolon
- Fever and crampy abdominal pain may accompany foul-smelling, watery stools
- Pseudomembranous colitis characterized by diarrhea with blood or mucous, abdominal pain, fever, and systemic toxicity
- Toxic megacolon, intestinal perforation, and death are more common in neutropenic patients or in patients with inflammatory bowel disease

### DIAGNOSTICS

- Stool studies:
  ✓ *C. difficile* toxins A and B by enzyme immunoassay (relatively low sensitivity)

✓ Two-step testing: Enzyme immunoassay for glutamine dehydrogenase (highly sensitive) with confirmatory toxin testing (to increase specificity)
✓ Nucleic acid amplification techniques (excellent sensitivity and specificity)
✓ Test of cure *not* recommended
- CBC: Leukocytosis, possibly anemia if stool is bloody
- Consider endoscopy when diagnosis is unclear; findings include classic pseudomembrane with a white or yellow plaque along hyperemic and inflamed colonic mucosa. Mucosa may be friable and erythematous without pseudomembrane

## MANAGEMENT

### Initial Medical Management

- Discontinue offending antibiotics when possible
- Treat any dehydration, anemia
- Surgical consultation if toxic megacolon is present
- Mild to moderate infection: Metronidazole orally/IV (orally preferred) 30 mg/kg/day (maximum 2 g/day) divided four times daily for 10–14 days
- Severe disease (ICU patient, pseudomembranous colitis, underlying intestinal tract disease): Vancomycin orally (IV not effective) 40 mg/kg/day divided four times daily for 10–14 days (maximum 2 g/day)

### Management of Relapse

- Up to 25% relapse within 4 weeks of stopping therapy due to reinfection, persistent spores, chronic antibiotics, or a predisposing underlying disease
- Initial relapse: Repeat metronidazole course
- Second relapse: Vancomycin
- Fidaxomicin, a non-absorbed macrolide antibiotic approved for treatment of *C. difficile* in adult patients, is associated with lower rate of recurrence compared to oral vancomycin

### Management of Chronic Relapsing C. difficile

- Prolonged oral vancomycin in a tapered or pulsed regimen; investigational therapies include nitazoxanide, tinidazole, fecal transplants, and immune globulin therapy

## HEPATITIS A

**Hepatitis A virus (HAV) is the predominant form of viral hepatitis and is typically an acute, self-limited illness.**

## EPIDEMIOLOGY

- Fecal–oral transmission, rarely bloodborne
- Since introduction of HAV vaccine in 1995, decrease in both sporadic cases and outbreaks

## PATHOPHYSIOLOGY

- Viral shedding in stool approximately 3 weeks before onset of symptoms
- HAV replicates in hepatocytes and is released into the bloodstream, causing viremia

## CLINICAL MANIFESTATIONS

- Spectrum of disease varies greatly, ranging from asymptomatic infection to fulminant hepatitis; risk of symptomatic disease increases with age, with most infants and children under 6 experiencing no or mild symptoms

- Fever, malaise, nausea, emesis, anorexia, abdominal pain, and diarrhea during prodrome
- Jaundice, dark urine, acholic stool, and hepatomegaly are more common in older children and adults, occurring in 40–70% of infections in this age group

## DIAGNOSTICS

- Elevation of ALT, AST, GGT, bilirubin, and alkaline phosphatase; ALT and AST elevation most prominent, peaking day 3–10 of illness
- Anti-HAV IgM and total anti-HAV antibody detected by immunoassay
- Anti-HAV IgM detectable 5–10 days before onset of symptoms and suggests acute infection, whereas total anti-HAV could reflect past infection or immunization

## MANAGEMENT

- Supportive: No specific antiviral therapy is available
- Prevention: Routine hepatitis A vaccination, pre- and post-exposure vaccination, and pre- and post-exposure IVIG in certain circumstances

## HEPATITIS B

**Hepatitis B virus (HBV) causes both acute and chronic liver disease, including cirrhosis and hepatocellular carcinoma.**

## EPIDEMIOLOGY

- Transmitted by perinatal, percutaneous, and sexual exposures as well as by close person–person contact
- Breast-feeding does not increase the risk of transmission and babies who have received hepatitis B vaccination and hepatitis B immune globulin (HBIG) can safely breast-feed
- Risk of vertical transmission without post-exposure prophylaxis: 70–90% if mother is HBsAg and HBeAg positive; 5–20% if mother is HBsAg positive but HBeAg negative

## PATHOPHYSIOLOGY

- Cytotoxic T cells attack HBV-infected hepatocytes, causing inflammation and necrosis
- Extrahepatic manifestations (e.g., rash, arthritis) are thought to be immune mediated

## CLINICAL MANIFESTATIONS

- Severity of acute illness increases with age and ranges from asymptomatic seroconversion (most common in perinatal acquisition) to acute hepatitis with jaundice (occurs in 5–15% of children age 1–5 and 33–50% of older children and adults) to fulminant fatal hepatitis (can occur at any age but is uncommon [<1%])
- Risk of chronic infection is *inversely* related to the age at infection; chronic infection occurs in 90% of infants infected perinatally, 25–50% of children infected at age 1–5, and 5–10% of older children and adults
- Incubation period ranges from 50 to 180 days
- Acute infection: 1–2 weeks of malaise and anorexia followed by nausea, vomiting, abdominal pain, jaundice, hepatomegaly, and splenomegaly
- Chronic infection (defined as presence of HBsAg in serum >6 months after acute infection): Often asymptomatic but can progress to cirrhosis and hepatocellular carcinoma years after infection

- Extrahepatic manifestations include arthritis, arthralgias, rash (urticarial, macular, papular acrodermatitis), membranoproliferative glomerulonephritis, and polyarteritis nodosa

## DIAGNOSTICS

- See Table 15-10
- In perinatally exposed infants, testing for HBsAb and HBsAg should be done at 9–18 months of age to avoid detection of maternal antibody or HBIG; IgM anti-Hbc is unreliable for diagnosis of perinatal infection
- HBeAg is a marker of viral replication and infectivity
- HBV DNA PCR test is useful to follow response to therapy

## MANAGEMENT

### Prevention

- Universal immunization of infants, children, adolescents, and high-risk adults
- Mother with positive HBsAg: Administer HBIG 0.5 cc IM and first dose of recombinant HBV vaccine (at different sites) within 12 hours of birth. This combination prevents perinatal transmission in 95% of exposed infants
- Mother with unknown HBV status: Administer first HBV vaccine to infant within 12 hours of birth regardless of weight and gestational age and test mother immediately
  ✓ If infant is <2000 g, administer HBIG within 12 hours of life if HBV status is still unknown
  ✓ If infant is term and >2000 g, can await mother's HBsAg testing and administer HBIG to infant as soon as possible but within 7 days

### Medical

- Acute HBV infection: No specific therapy
- Chronic HBV infection: Treatment initiation based on ALT levels, age, liver biopsy findings, comorbidities, and family history. Approved therapies for children include interferon alfa-2b, lamivudine, adefovir, and entecavir
- Children with chronic HBV infection should be screened periodically for sequelae such as hepatocellular carcinoma
  ✓ HBeAg and HBeAb, serum ALT, HBV DNA, and AFP should be evaluated at the time of chronic hepatitis B diagnosis
  ✓ If ALT and AFP levels are normal and the patient is HBeAg positive, they are at low risk of progression to hepatocellular carcinoma and AFP and ALT levels should be repeated every 6–12 months with HBeAg/HBeAb repeated yearly
  ✓ If ALT or AFP levels are elevated, or the patient has elevated HBV DNA (>2000 IU/mL) with negative HBeAg, consultation with a pediatric liver specialist is recommended to determine the appropriate interval for lab follow up as well as ultrasound imaging
  ✓ Patients with a family history of hepatocellular carcinoma or cirrhosis should also be referred to a pediatric liver specialist

| TABLE 15-10 | Serology During Four Stages of HBV Infection | | | |
| --- | --- | --- | --- | --- |
| **Test** | **Acute Disease** | **Window Phase** | **Complete Recovery** | **Chronic Carrier** |
| HBsAg | Positive | Negative | Negative | Positive |
| HBsAb | Negative | Negative | Positive | Negative |
| HBcAb | Positive (IgM) | Positive (IgM) | Positive (IgG) | Positive (IgG) |

HB, hepatitis B; sAg, surface antigen; sAb, surface antibody; cAb, core antibody; Ig, immunoglobulin.

## HEPATITIS C

**Hepatitis C virus (HCV) causes acute and chronic liver disease, which can lead to cirrhosis and hepatocellular carcinoma.**

### EPIDEMIOLOGY

- Transmitted through blood and blood product transfusions, intravenous drug use, accidental needle stick injuries, sexual contact, and vertically from mother to infant
- Estimated 5% vertical transmission rate with higher rates observed in cases of HIV coinfection, prolonged rupture of membranes, and higher viremia
- *Not* transmitted through breast milk
- Incubation period: 6–7 weeks (range 2 weeks–6 months)

### PATHOPHYSIOLOGY

- Hepatocyte death due to immune attack by cytotoxic T cells on infected hepatocytes

### CLINICAL MANIFESTATIONS

- Acute HCV infection only develops in 20-30% of cases, symptoms include anorexia, nausea, jaundice, dark urine, and right upper quadrant abdominal pain
- *Chronic infection:* Develops in approximately 80% of perinatally infected children and less commonly in children infected postnatally
- Less than 5% go on to develop cirrhosis
- Fulminant hepatic failure is exceedingly rare

### DIAGNOSTICS

- Anti-HCV IgG appears 8–10 weeks after infection, but can be delayed up to 6 months. Serologic testing is 97% sensitive and 99% specific, but does not distinguish between acute and chronic infection and no IgM assay is currently available
- HCV RNA appears within 1–2 weeks of infection and indicates current infection. Most useful in screening perinatally exposed infants, to identify anti-HCV positive individuals with current infection, to diagnose early infection, and to monitor response to therapy. A single negative test is not conclusive because viral RNA may be only intermittently detectable
- For neonates born to HCV positive mothers, can either test for anti-HCV IgG after 18 months of age or by HCV PCR if earlier diagnosis is desired

### MANAGEMENT

- Decision to proceed with therapy depends primarily on liver biopsy findings
- Acute infection: Adult studies suggest that treatment in the acute phase may lead to higher sustained virologic response than treatment in the chronic phase; pediatric studies are in progress
- Chronic infection: Peginterferon alfa-2b in combination with ribavirin is approved for children >3 years old but is associated with significant adverse events including flu-like symptoms, hematologic abnormalities, thyroid abnormalities, ischemic retinopathy, uveitis, and growth disturbance. Direct acting antiviral drugs, including telaprevir or boceprevir, are being used successfully in adult patients; pediatric studies are in progress

## LYME DISEASE

**Tick-borne illness caused by the spirochete *Borrelia burgdorferi***

## EPIDEMIOLOGY

- Geographic regions: Northeast, upper Midwest, West Coast
- In endemic areas: Incidence of 20–100 cases/100,000
- Seasonal occurrence: April–October
- Incidence highest among children 5–14 years old

## ETIOLOGY

- *Borrelia burgdorferi* is transmitted by the bite of infected tick vectors: *Ixodes pacificus* (West Coat), *Ixodes scapularis* (East and Midwest)

## PATHOPHYSIOLOGY

- Initial infection site: Skin
- Tick must stay on skin >36 hours for transmission
- Once disseminated into bloodstream, *B. burgdorferi* adheres to multiple cell types and persists in tissue unless treated
- Cytokines amplify inflammatory response and cause local tissue damage

## CLINICAL MANIFESTATIONS

- Three stages: Early localized, early disseminated, late disseminated disease
- *Early localized:* EM (erythematous annular lesion with central clearing, usually >5 cm); fever, malaise, headache, myalgias, and arthralgias
- *Early disseminated (3–5 weeks after tick bite):* Multiple EM lesions, cranial nerve palsies (especially VII, usually last 2–8 weeks and then resolves), fatigue, myalgia, headache, occasionally meningitis or carditis (AV block)
- *Late disseminated disease (months to years after tick bite):* Mono-articular arthritis of a large joint (knee in >90%); CNS involvement (chronic demyelinating encephalitis, polyneuritis, memory problems) rare in children
- Jarisch–Herxheimer reaction: Transient fever, headache, myalgias after therapy is started

## DIAGNOSTICS

- Two-test approach: EIA (sensitive but not specific) and, if EIA is positive, Western blot (necessary to confirm infection)
- IgM peaks at 3–6 weeks; IgG peaks weeks to months after the bite
- Antibodies to *B. burgdorferi* usually often not detectable in patients with early localized EM rash, so at this stage can empirically treat without testing
- False-positive EIA tests may be secondary to other spirochetal infections (syphilis, leptospirosis), systemic lupus erythematosus, EBV, varicella
- Lumbar puncture to confirm lymphocytic meningitis of early disseminated disease; typically reveals 10–150 WBC/mm$^3$ and less than 10% segmented neutrophils, elevated protein, normal glucose. PCR has poor sensitivity in CNS
- ECG: Detect heart block in patients with disseminated Lyme
- Joint aspiration: WBC typically 25,000–80,000/mm$^3$ (but range from 200 to 140,000/mm$^3$) and positive Lyme PCR of joint fluid
- *No* proven utility of blood PCR or urine PCR or antigen tests

## MANAGEMENT

- Early localized: 14–21 days of amoxicillin (<8 years) or doxycycline (≥8 years)
- Early disseminated (multiple EM lesions) and arthritis: Oral amoxicillin or doxycycline (21–28 days); cefuroxime (preferred) or erythromycin may be used in young children with

penicillin allergy. If arthritis unresponsive after 2 months or there is a recurrence, consider a second course of oral therapy (4 weeks) or initiate IV therapy (2–4 weeks)
- Arthritis unresponsive to oral therapy, meningitis, and carditis: IV ceftriaxone for 21–28 days. For carditis, if degree of heart block is mild (e.g., first or second degree and asymptomatic) may switch to oral therapy. For meningitis, may consider oral therapy with doxycycline for 14 days

## MALARIA

**Intraerythrocytic parasitic infection caused by *Plasmodium* species (*P. vivax*, *P. ovale*, *P. malariae*, *P. knowlesi*, and *P. falciparum*)**

### EPIDEMIOLOGY

- Endemic throughout tropical areas; view countries with malaria risk at CDC website (www.cdc.gov/travel)

### PATHOPHYSIOLOGY

- Transmission is primarily through the bite of an infected *Anopheles* species mosquito. Uncommon modes of transmission include transplacental and bloodborne (e.g., transfusion, needle stick)
- Sporozoites from mosquito infect hepatocytes, differentiate to merozoites, and infect RBCs
- Periodic RBC lysis releases merozoites to infect other RBCs
- *P. vivax* and *P. ovale* have a dormant hepatic phase that can cause late relapse if not properly treated

### CLINICAL MANIFESTATIONS

- Characteristic high fever that may have a cyclical pattern (every 48–72 hours, depending on species) or may occur daily, especially with *P. falciparum*
- Chills, headache, sweats, malaise, myalgias, nausea, vomiting, diarrhea, arthralgias, abdominal or back pain
- Pallor, jaundice, hepatosplenomegaly, anemia, and thrombocytopenia
- *P. falciparum* may lead to severe disease including:
  - ✓ Cerebral malaria: Altered mentation, seizures, increased ICP, and progression to coma and death
  - ✓ Severe hemolysis ("black water fever"), acute tubular necrosis, adrenal insufficiency, hypoglycemia, shock, respiratory failure
- *P. vivax* and *P. ovale*:
  - ✓ Relapse due to latent intra-hepatic stage as long as 3–5 years after infection
  - ✓ Hypersplenism, which may lead to splenic rupture
- *P. malariae*:
  - ✓ Nephrotic syndrome, chronic asymptomatic parasitemia
- *P. knowlesi*:
  - ✓ Found in southeast Asia and can cause severe disease and death due to hyperparasitemia

### DIAGNOSTICS

- Giemsa-stained thick and thin peripheral blood smears, which detect organisms (thick) and allow determination of species and percent parasitemia (thin)
- Multiple smears (every 12 hours) over 48–72 hours may be necessary if the first is negative and clinical suspicion is high, or to monitor response to therapy
  - ✓ Parasitemia >2% suggests *P. falciparum*

- Rapid antigen test is most sensitive for *P. falciparum* (90–95%), but significantly less sensitive for remaining species, so should be followed by thick and thin blood smears
- Other findings: Anemia, leukopenia, thrombocytopenia, hypoglycemia, proteinuria, hematuria, elevated hepatic transaminases, and indirect bilirubin (hemolysis)

## MANAGEMENT

- Treatment regimen depends on:
  - ✓ *Infecting species*: *P. falciparum and P. knowlesi* cause more rapidly progressive infections than other species and require rapid initiation of treatment. *P. vivax* and *P. ovale* require additional therapy (primaquine phosphate) to eradicate dormant hypnozoites in the liver
  - ✓ *Likelihood of chloroquine resistance*: Depends on (1) the region of the world where infection was acquired and (2) whether or not chemoprophylaxis was taken (consider resistance of infecting *Plasmodium* species to chemoprophylactic regimen)
  - ✓ *Presence of severe illness*: Parasitemia greater than 5%, signs of cerebral malaria or other end-organ involvement, shock, hemoglobin <7, acidosis, or hypoglycemia requires parenteral therapy with quinine, quinidine, or artesunate
- If disease is uncomplicated, outpatient therapy is often reasonable, but consider admission for suspected or confirmed *P. falciparum* because of the potential for rapid clinical deterioration, particularly in nonimmune hosts
- Supportive care includes monitoring for hypoglycemia, anemia, fluid and electrolyte disturbances, and renal failure
- Consider exchange transfusion for parasitemia greater than 10% or severe complications at lower parasitemia (e.g., cerebral malaria, renal failure)
- Parasitemia should decrease over first 48–72 hours to 25% of initial parasitemia
- Refer to 2012 Redbook, CDC website (www.cdc.gov/malaria), or CDC malaria hotline (770-488-7788) for specific drug regimens based on patient age, severity of illness, region where infection was acquired, and clinical response

## METHICILLIN-RESISTANT *STAPHYLOCOCCUS AUREUS* (MRSA)

*Staphylococcus aureus*, a Gram positive coccus, is the most commonly isolated human bacterial pathogen and causes both superficial and invasive infections. Methicillin-resistant *Staphylococcus aureus* (MRSA) isolates are resistant to all available penicillins and other β-lactam antimicrobial drugs.

### EPIDEMIOLOGY

- Both MSSA and MRSA are major causes of hospital-acquired infections
- MRSA has emerged as a significant cause of community-acquired infection (CA-MRSA) in both children and adults; most commonly as cutaneous abscesses but also as severe, invasive infections (e.g., pneumonia, bone/joint infections)
- Hospital-acquired MRSA infections are decreasing with better infection control practices, but the incidence of CA-MRSA infection remains high

### PATHOPHYSIOLOGY

- *Staphylococcus aureus* infections are due to direct tissue invasion causing inflammation, hematogenous dissemination, or toxin release leading to tissue necrosis
- MRSA strains almost universally carry the mecA gene, which affords β-lactam resistance
- CA-MRSA both colonizes more body sites and displays a higher attack rate (colonization to infection) than MSSA
- Transmission is via direct contact

## CLINICAL MANIFESTATIONS

- Skin and soft tissue infections: Impetigo, abscess, cellulitis, wound infection, ocular infection, pyomyositis
- Bone/joint infections: Osteomyelitis, pyogenic arthritis, diskitis
- Respiratory tract infections: Pneumonia, lung abscess
- Cardiovascular infections: Bacteremia/sepsis, endocarditis, pericarditis, thrombophlebitis
- CNS infections: Meningitis, brain abscesses, spinal epidural abscess
- Device-related infections: Central line-associated bloodstream infections, CSF shunt infections

## DIAGNOSTICS

- Culture the organism whenever possible from the infected site (e.g., blood, abscess fluid, bone, synovial fluid, CSF) for identification and antibiotic sensitivities

## MANAGEMENT

- Minor infections such as impetigo or superinfected skin lesions: Mupirocin 2% topical ointment
- For cutaneous abscesses, incision and drainage is the primary treatment. The role of systemic antibiotics is often not necessary after complete drainage of simple, superficial abscesses
- Empiric oral coverage for skin/soft tissue infection includes clindamycin, TMP-SMX, doxycycline (if ≥8 years of age), or linezolid
- Hospitalized patients with suspected MRSA infection should have empiric broad-spectrum antibiotics including vancomycin while awaiting culture data. Stable patients *without* bacteremia or intravascular infection can be treated with clindamycin, as long as local resistance rates are <10%
- Obtain echocardiogram for children with underlying heart disease, persistent bacteremia despite adequate antimicrobial therapy, or clinical signs/symptoms concerning for endocarditis
- Consult with an infectious diseases specialist for invasive infections such as bacteremia, infective endocarditis, device-related infections, or CNS infections

## NEONATAL HERPES SIMPLEX VIRUS INFECTION

**Three main manifestations of neonatal HSV are:**

- **Localized skin, eye, mouth (SEM) involvement (45% of cases)**
- **CNS involvement with or without SEM disease (30% of cases)**
- **Disseminated disease involving multiple organs with or without CNS involvement (25% of cases)**
- **Other TORCH infections are discussed in Neonatology chapter (Chapter 17)**

## EPIDEMIOLOGY

- Incidence of 1 in 3500 live births
- Perinatal transmission rate is higher with maternal primary genital HSV infection (25–60%) than with recurrent infection (0–5%); however, more than 75% of infants with HSV are born to women who have no history or clinical findings of HSV infection
- Disseminated and SEM disease generally present between 7 and 14 days of life, CNS disease generally presents between 14 and 21 days of life
- Additional risk factors for transmission include prolonged rupture of membranes, scalp electrodes, vaginal delivery

## CLINICAL MANIFESTATIONS

- SEM disease: Vesicular rash
- Disseminated disease: Sepsis like syndrome, hypoxia, respiratory or hepatic failure, and DIC; 60–70% have associated encephalitis and 80% have vesicular rash
- CNS disease: Temperature instability, seizures, and irritability; 60–70% have associated vesicular rash
- Though vesicular rash and seizures are most suggestive, symptoms are generally nonspecific and HSV disease should be considered for all cases of suspected neonatal sepsis
- Differential Diagnosis
  ✓ Noninfectious etiologies: Erythema toxicum, miliaria, neonatal lupus, Langerhans cell histiocytosis, epidermolysis bullosa
  ✓ Infectious etiologies: *Staphylococcus aureus*, *Pseudomonas aeruginosa*, group B *Streptococcus*, CMV, *Treponema pallidum*, varicella

## DIAGNOSTICS

- In addition to routine evaluation for neonatal sepsis, obtain:
  ✓ HSV PCR (gold standard) or culture from CSF (PCR is reliable up to 7 days after initiation of acyclovir)
  ✓ HSV culture or PCR of conjunctiva, mouth, nasopharynx, and anus; any positive test after 24 hours of life is diagnostic of disease rather than intrapartum exposure
  ✓ HSV culture or PCR from any skin vesicle
  ✓ HSV PCR from whole blood
  ✓ Serum ALT
- Direct fluorescent antibody (DFA) staining of vesicle scraping is rapid but less sensitive than culture or PCR
- Patients with proven HSV and possible CNS involvement should have an EEG and MRI of head during the acute period

## MANAGEMENT

- High-dose intravenous acyclovir (60 mg/kg/day divided every 8 hours): 21 days for CNS or disseminated disease and 14 days for SEM disease
  ✓ Some experts recommend repeating lumbar puncture before completion of therapy. If HSV PCR remains positive, consider treating for additional 1–2 weeks (limited data available)
  ✓ Suppressive therapy with oral acyclovir for 6 months after IV treatment of neonatal HSV improves neurodevelopmental outcomes and prevents cutaneous recurrences; dose is 300 mg/m²/dose three times daily
- Side effects of acyclovir: Neutropenia, renal failure
- Management of the asymptomatic neonate born to a mother with active HSV lesions: See Kimberlin DW, Baley J, Committee on Infectious Diseases and Committee on Fetus and Newborn. Guidance on management of asymptomatic neonates born to women with active genital herpes lesions. *Pediatrics*. 2013;131:e635–646
- Prognosis:
  ✓ SEM: Mortality and neurologic impairment rare
  ✓ CNS infection: Low risk of death in adequately treated children; >60% of survivors have neurologic impairment
  ✓ Disseminated infection: High risk of death despite treatment; <20% of survivors have neurologic impairment

## PERTUSSIS

**Respiratory disease caused by *Bordetella pertussis*, a fastidious gram-negative rod.**

### EPIDEMIOLOGY

- Occurs year round, peaking late summer through fall
- Increasing in frequency among all age groups likely due to both increasing detection of cases and waning immunity from less immunogenic acellular pertussis vaccine
- Highly transmissible through respiratory droplets and direct or indirect contact with nasal secretions
- Neither natural infection nor vaccination leads to permanent immunity

### PATHOPHYSIOLOGY

- Pertussis toxin is responsible for local epithelial damage, leading to peri-bronchial inflammation and necrotizing bronchopneumonia

### CLINICAL MANIFESTATIONS

- Incubation period is 5–21 days
- Three stages of the disease observed classically, though may be variable in young infants, vaccinated children, and adults:
  ✓ *Catarrhal (1–2 weeks):* Rhinorrhea, low-grade fevers, sneezing; most infectious stage
  ✓ *Paroxysmal (2–6 weeks):* Paroxysmal coughing after which the child may become flushed or cyanotic or have post-tussive emesis. "Whoop" occurs during sudden forceful inspiration. Infants may present with apnea or cyanosis and often lack the characteristic cough or whoop
  ✓ *Convalescent:* Chronic cough can persist for weeks
- Complications: Apnea, superinfection with other bacterial pneumonia, seizures, encephalopathy, pulmonary hypertension, and death (particularly in infants younger than 2 months)

### DIAGNOSTICS

- Clinical case defined as cough illness lasting at least 2 weeks with one of the following: Paroxysms of coughing, inspiratory whoop, or post-tussive vomiting without other apparent cause; confirmed case when *B. pertussis* isolated in culture, detected by PCR, or with an epidemiologic link to laboratory confirmed case
- Leukocytosis with total WBC greater than 15,000/mm$^3$ with absolute lymphocytosis
- Chest x-ray: Perihilar infiltrates, "shaggy right heart border"
- Culture remains gold standard but is insensitive due to the fastidious nature of *B. pertussis* and is often falsely negative in previously immunized individuals, after initiation of antibiotic therapy, or after 3 weeks of illness
- PCR of nasopharyngeal swab specimen is the preferred test at many institutions (high sensitivity and specificity), but no standardized, FDA licensed assay is available
- Direct immunofluorescence is not recommended due to low sensitivity

### MANAGEMENT

**Prevention**

- Immunization with DTaP or TdaP according to vaccine schedule

**Treatment**

- Therapy can curb symptoms if started in the catarrhal stage, but will not improve course of disease or symptoms if started later; however, antibiotic therapy is still recommended to decrease transmission
- Azithromycin, erythromycin, or clarithromycin are first-line agents for both treatment and prophylaxis; azithromycin recommended specifically for infants <1 month due to risk of infantile hypertrophic pyloric stenosis
- Chemoprophylaxis for close contacts with erythromycin, clarithromycin, or azithromycin is recommended, as is pertussis vaccination with age appropriate vaccine
- TMP-SMX is an alternative for macrolide allergic patients >2 months of age
- Respiratory isolation for hospitalized patients until patient is no longer contagious (5 days of treatment; if no therapy is given, until 3 weeks after cough onset). Routine hospitalization to complete treatment is not warranted)
- Consider hospitalization of young infants at risk for apnea

## RICKETTSIAL DISEASES

**Tick-borne illnesses caused by obligate intracellular pathogens that share similar clinical and epidemiologic features and treatment: Includes ehrlichiosis, anaplasmosis, Q fever, rickettsialpox, Rocky Mountain spotted fever (RMSF), and endemic typhus. RMSF, ehrlichiosis, and anaplasmosis are the most common and are discussed subsequently.**

- RMSF is caused by *Rickettsia rickettsii*
- Ehrlichiosis manifests as human monocytic ehrlichiosis (HME; *Ehrlichia chaffeensis*)
- Anaplasmosis manifests as human granulocytic anaplasmosis (HGA; *Anaplasma phagocytophilum*)

### EPIDEMIOLOGY

- RMSF and HME are most prevalent in the southeastern, south central, and northern Rocky Mountain states. HGA occurs predominantly in the northeast and upper Midwest
- Highest prevalence in late spring, summer, and early fall
- Transmission:
  ✓ RMSF: Dog tick (*Dermacentor variabilis*), Wood tick (*Dermacentor andersonii*), and Lone Star tick (*Amblyomma americanum*)
  ✓ HME: Lone Star tick (*Amblyomma americanum*); animal reservoir is the white tail deer
  ✓ HGA: *Ixodes scapularis*; animal reservoir is the white-footed mouse
- Incubation period: 2–14 days for RMSF (median 7 days); 7–14 days for HME and HGA (median 10 days)

### PATHOPHYSIOLOGY

- After inoculation, rickettsia multiply in small vessel endothelium leading to focal areas of small vessel inflammation, thrombus, and capillary leak

### CLINICAL MANIFESTATIONS

- Early phases: Fever, headache, rash, malaise, myalgia, nausea, vomiting, abdominal pain
- RMSF rash: Typically begins on ankles and wrists spreading both centrally to the trunk (within hours) and to the palms and soles; initially blanching, erythematous, and macular but becomes petechial and then hemorrhagic; develops between third and fifth day of illness, but 10% of patients never develop rash

- Rash in 30–50% of HME; rash in less than 10% of HGA; rash can be macular, maculopapular, or petechial with variable distribution
- Other organ systems may be involved:
  - ✓ GI: Diarrhea, hepatomegaly, splenomegaly, jaundice
  - ✓ Renal: Renal failure, acute tubular necrosis
  - ✓ Cardiac: Congestive heart failure, arrhythmias, shock
  - ✓ Neurologic: Meningitis, encephalopathy, seizures, ataxia, aphasia, cranial nerve palsies
  - ✓ Pulmonary and generalized edema, signs of capillary leak
- Duration of illness typically 1–2 weeks; 2–3% mortality

## DIAGNOSTICS

- Thrombocytopenia, anemia, and leukopenia; PT and PTT prolongation; elevated bilirubin, ALT, AST, BUN, and creatinine; low fibrinogen, albumin, and sodium
  - ✓ Leukopenia, anemia, and hepatitis are more frequent in ehrlichiosis than in RMSF
  - ✓ WBC and platelets nadir at 5–7 days of illness and then recover
- CSF pleocytosis and elevated protein in one-third of patients
- Rickettsia-specific serology: Positive titers usually occur 6–10 days into illness. Fourfold increase in titer by indirect fluorescent antibody (IFA) or enzyme immunosorbent assay (EIA) between acute and convalescent sera (2–3 weeks later) confirms diagnosis
- *R. rickettsii (RMSF)* can be identified by direct antibody staining of a rash biopsy specimen
- In HGA and HME, 50% have intraleukocytoplasmic inclusions (morulae) in neutrophils (HGA) and monocytes (HME) on buffy coat or peripheral blood smear
- PCR of blood for HME and HGA are available at commercial laboratories and show promise for early diagnosis of disease

## MANAGEMENT

- Provide supportive management as indicated. Anticipate complications: hypotension, thrombocytopenia, DIC, hypoalbuminemia, and hyponatremia
- Recommended antibiotic is doxycycline. Alternative for RMSF is chloramphenicol, but this has severe side effects and should only be used in rare situations. Alternative for HME and HGA is rifampin (not first line)
- Continue therapy until patient is afebrile for at least 3 days; usual course is 7–10 days (RMSF) and 7–14 days (HME and HGA)
- Because delay of antibiotic treatment greater than 5 days after onset of symptoms (and prior to detection of antibodies) is associated with greater mortality, treat suspected cases empirically
- Expect clinical improvement in 24–36 hours and defervescence in 48–72 hours after initiation of therapy. Mildly ill patients can be treated as outpatients. Hospitalization is recommended for severely ill patients with systemic complications

## TUBERCULOSIS

Caused by *M. tuberculosis*, an acid-fast bacillus

Latent tuberculosis infection (LTBI): Patient has positive tuberculin skin test (TST) or interferon gamma release assay, no physical exam findings, and a chest x-ray that is either negative or reveals only calcifications or granulomas in lung, lymph nodes, or both.

Tuberculosis (TB) disease: Patient with infection in whom symptoms, signs, and/or radiographic findings are apparent.

## EPIDEMIOLOGY

- Increased risk of infection in certain populations: Low income; urban; nonwhite racial groups; foreign born; residence in jails, nursing homes, or homeless shelters; injection drug use; HIV infection; emigration from developing country
- Public health officials should be notified of all active cases of TB early in therapy

## PATHOPHYSIOLOGY

- Transmission is person to person usually via airborne droplets but can occur by direct contact with infected body fluids
- Children rarely infect others because they have sparse bacilli in endobronchial secretions and diminished force of cough
- Adolescents are potentially infectious

## CLINICAL MANIFESTATIONS

### Intrathoracic Disease (Includes Primary Infection and Reactivation)

- Most infected children have positive TST and no symptoms
- Hilar adenopathy, focal infiltrate, and pleural effusion are common
- Extensive pulmonary infiltrates and cavitation are rare
- Symptoms of primary infection and reactivation may include nonproductive cough, hemoptysis, chest pain, dyspnea, fever, night sweats, anorexia, failure to thrive, weight loss

### Miliary Tuberculosis

- Bacteremia leads to disease in two or more organ systems. TST is nonreactive in 30%
- Usually early complication of primary pulmonary tuberculosis in infants
- Initially malaise, anorexia, weight loss, fever
- Progresses to high fever, respiratory distress, hypoxia, and symptoms of other organ system involvement (e.g., hepatomegaly, splenomegaly, diffuse adenopathy)

### Central Nervous System Disease

- Most common in ages 6 months–4 years
- Usually occurs 2–6 months after initial infection
- Clinical manifestations vary widely. Symptoms may be mild (e.g., fever, mild but persistent headache) or severe (e.g., cranial nerve abnormalities, seizures, and decorticate posturing)

### Other Manifestations

- Pericarditis, lymphadenitis, bone or joint infections, abdominal infection (peritonitis, mesenteric adenitis), cutaneous lesions

## DIAGNOSTICS

### Tuberculous Skin Test: Use for Children At Risk of Infection

- Mantoux test containing 5 tuberculin units of purified protein derivative (PPD) administered intradermally
- Delayed hypersensitivity reaction to TST peaks at 48–72 hours
- Nonreactive TST does not exclude infection or disease
- Time from infection to development of positive TST is 2–12 weeks
- Special situations warranting TST include (1) radiographic or clinical findings suggesting TB; (2) vertebral osteomyelitis; (3) pericarditis; (4) prior to initiation of immunosuppressive therapy; (5) contacts of people with confirmed or suspected contagious tuberculosis;

(6) immigration from a country with endemic infection or travel to countries with endemic infection, with contact with indigenous people

## Definition of Positive TST Based on Diameter of Induration

- *Induration 5 mm or greater in diameter:* (1) Contact with infectious cases; (2) abnormal chest x-ray; (3) clinical evidence of tuberculosis disease; (4) HIV infection or other immunosuppressive conditions or therapy (e.g., corticosteroids, chemotherapy)
- *Induration 10 mm or greater in diameter:* (1) Children at risk of disseminated disease (age <4 years or compromising conditions such as diabetes mellitus, chronic renal failure, and malnutrition); (2) birth in or travel to country with high TB prevalence; (3) frequently exposed to adults with TB risk factors
- *Induration 15 mm or greater in diameter:* Children 4 years of age or older without risk factors

   A negative TST does not exclude LTBI or tuberculosis disease

## Immunologic Testing: Interferon Gamma Release Assay (IGRA)

- IGRAs can be used in children ≥5; there is limited experience in younger children
- Sensitivity of IGRAs in children is expected to be comparable to TST; specificity is high and helps distinguish tuberculosis from BCG vaccine and most pathogenic non-tuberculous mycobacteria

## Laboratory Diagnosis

- Acid-fast smear and culture are most important tests for definitive diagnosis but organism may take 2–10 weeks to grow
  - ✓ Early morning gastric aspirates (three specimens on consecutive days) are best for diagnosis of pulmonary TB in young children (positive in <50% of children with pulmonary TB)
  - ✓ Cultures from sputum (in older children), CSF, pleural fluid, urine, or bone marrow biopsy specimen as indicated
  - ✓ Identification of a culture-positive source case (e.g., household member) supports the child's presumptive diagnosis and can be used for drug susceptibility testing
- Chest x-ray to distinguish LTBI from TB disease
- Head CT: In TB meningitis, detects basilar meningitis, increased intracranial pressure, and tuberculomas

## MANAGEMENT

- Exposure to contagious household contact with TB disease, after active TB is ruled out
  - ✓ Treat with INH even if TST is negative for children who are younger than 4 years of age or are immunocompromised, repeat TST in 3 months. If still negative then discontinue INH; if TST becomes positive, continue INH for a total of 9 months
- LTBI
  - ✓ Therapy prevents most cases of progression to TB disease
  - ✓ Isoniazid (INH) for 9 months; consider 12 months of therapy for immunocompromised patients. Alternate regimen for adults: 2 months of rifampin + pyrazinamide
  - ✓ If contact has INH-resistant TB, use rifampin for 6 months
- Pulmonary TB
  - ✓ INH + rifampin + pyrazinamide for 2 months followed by INH + rifampin for 4 months. If drug resistance suspected, add either ethambutol or streptomycin to the three-drug regimen until susceptibility results are available. Supplement pyridoxine with INH for: (1) milk- or meat-deficient diets; (2) HIV-infected children; (3) breast-feeding infants; (4) pregnant females

- ✓ For hilar adenopathy without other pulmonary disease, some experts recommend INH + rifampin for 6 months
- Extrapulmonary TB (including meningitis and miliary TB): Treat in consultation with a tuberculosis or infectious diseases expert
  - ✓ INH + rifampin + pyrazinamide + a fourth agent such as ethionimide or an amino-glycoside for 2 months followed by INH + rifampin for 10 months. Corticosteroids (e.g., dexamethasone or prednisone) for 4–6 weeks in patients with TB meningitis with appropriate tapering; consider for TB pericarditis and pleural effusion to hasten fluid absorption

## VARICELLA ZOSTER INFECTIONS

**Primary infection with varicella zoster virus (VZV) causes varicella (chickenpox). Reactivation of latent VZV causes herpes zoster (shingles).**

### EPIDEMIOLOGY

#### Varicella

- Transmission by airborne route to 90% of unimmunized household contacts
- Transmission to 12–33% during less sustained exposures
- Introduction of varicella vaccine has led to dramatic decrease in disease, though break-through disease can occur

#### Herpes Zoster

- Rare in immunocompetent children younger than 10 years of age
- Primary VZV infection acquired in utero or during first year of life is associated with increased risk of herpes zoster

### PATHOPHYSIOLOGY

#### Varicella

- Mucosal inoculation by respiratory droplets or by direct lesion contact
- Transmission to susceptible contacts exposed 24–48 hours before the appearance of skin lesions

#### Herpes Zoster

- Latent VZV infection in dorsal root ganglion
- Transmission by contact with lesions: VZV is present in skin lesions but is not released into respiratory secretions in immunocompetent host

### CLINICAL MANIFESTATIONS

#### Varicella

- Incubation period of 10–21 days
- Prodrome 24–48 hours before rash appears (fever, malaise, anorexia, headache)
- Generalized pruritic rash begins on scalp, face, or trunk and eventually involves the extremities (less intensely). Initial erythematous macules progress to clear fluid-filled vesicles with a surrounding erythematous irregular margin ("dew drops on a rose petal"). Lesions in multiple stages present on the same are of the body, especially on mucous membranes of the oropharynx, conjunctivae, and vagina

- In 24–48 hours, lesions begin crusting
- New lesions continue to appear for 1–7 days

### Herpes Zoster

- Vesicular lesions in dermatomal distribution of sensory nerve. Usually one to three dermatomal segments involved
- Discrete vesicles appear first and then enlarge and coalesce
- Rash often preceded by pain, pruritis, or hyperesthesia

### Complications

- Complications of varicella: Secondary bacterial infections with *Staphylococcus aureus* or *S. pyogenes* (e.g., cellulitis, necrotizing fasciitis, pneumonia), meningoencephalitis, Reye syndrome, hepatitis, nephritis, postinfectious cerebellitis
- Complications of primary varicella in high-risk populations:
  - ✓ Fetus/newborn: Congenital varicella syndrome if varicella is acquired in first 20 weeks of gestation; neonatal varicella if varicella develops in mother from 5 days before to 2 days after delivery; 30% fatality if untreated
  - ✓ Immunocompromised (lymphoproliferative malignancies, solid tumors, and solid organ transplantation): Visceral dissemination and severe, progressive varicella
- Complications of herpes zoster:
  - ✓ Depends on distribution of involved nerve. Potential complications include conjunctivitis, keratitis, uveitis, iridocyclitis, and facial palsies
  - ✓ Immunocompromised patients with local lesions can continue to transmit virus via aerosolized route and are at risk of visceral dissemination

## DIAGNOSTICS

- Laboratory studies are not routinely indicated but a specific diagnosis of VZV guides treatment in immunocompromised children
- PCR of body fluid/tissue; viral culture if PCR is not available
- Rapid diagnosis: DFA test performed on *epithelial cells* scraped from base of lesions is more rapid and sensitive than culture
- VZV IgG is detectable within 3 days after onset and persists for life after primary infection
- Obtain LFTs and Chest x-ray in immunocompromised patients

## MANAGEMENT

### Varicella

- Varicella vaccination within 72 hours of exposure may prevent or significantly modify disease (administer if no contraindications to varicella vaccination)
- Indications for intravenous acyclovir: (1) Immunocompromised including malignancy, bone marrow or organ transplant, high-dose steroid therapy, HIV infection, and congenital T-lymphocyte deficiency; (2) neonatal varicella; (3) varicella-associated pneumonia or encephalitis
  - ✓ Duration: 7 days or until no new lesions have appeared
- Consider oral acyclovir for infection in the following situations: Chronic cutaneous disorders, cystic fibrosis or other pulmonary disorders, diabetes mellitus, disorders requiring chronic salicylate therapy or intermittent corticosteroid therapy, children older than 12 years
  - ✓ Oral administration within 24 hours after initial lesions appear
- Valacyclovir was licensed in 2008 for varicella infection in children 2 to <18 years of age, which has improved bioavailability compared to oral acyclovir

## Herpes Zoster

- Acyclovir reduces pain and duration of new lesion formation if initiated within 72 hours of infection onset and is recommended for patients at high risk for disseminated disease
- Dose: Same as that for primary infection for total of 7 days or for 2 days after last new lesion

## Passive Antibody Prophylaxis with Varicella Zoster Immune Globulin Following Varicella Exposure

- Recommended for (1) immunocompromised children with no history of VZV; (2) pregnant women with no history of or antibodies to VZV; (3) infants born to mothers whose varicella began within 5 days before or 2 days after delivery; (4) premature infants less than 28 weeks with no maternal history of varicella; or (5) less than 1000 g or hospitalized premature infants regardless of maternal immunity
- Ideally administer within 48 hours of exposure but acceptable if administered within 10 days of exposure
- Dose: 1 vial (125 U)/10 kg body weight (maximum 5 vials) IM

# 16 Metabolism

*Rebecca Ganetzky, MD*
*Can Ficicioglu, MD, PhD*

## FATTY ACID OXIDATION DISORDERS

### GENERAL PRINCIPLES

**Class of metabolic diseases in which enzyme deficiencies in mitochondrial fatty acid import or β-oxidation limit the ability of mitochondria to use fat as an energy source.**

### EPIDEMIOLOGY

- Overall incidence about 1:10,000; autosomal recessive inheritance
- Medium-chain acyl CoA dehydrogenase (MCAD) deficiency is the most common fatty acid oxidation (FAO) defect

### PATHOPHYSIOLOGY

Most significant danger is hypoketotic hypoglycemia, leading to failure of multiple organ systems. General considerations:

- FAO provides energy for heart and liver at baseline, and for skeletal muscle during prolonged exercise. FAO produces ketones used by brain as energy source during prolonged fast
- FAO supports gluconeogenesis by providing ATP, acetyl CoA, and reduced electron carriers
- Risk for hypoketotic hypoglycemia highest when relying on FAO for energy (e.g., prolonged fast, infection)
- Buildup of long-chain fats is toxic to liver, heart, and muscle cells and can result in acute liver injury, cardiomyopathy, or episodic rhabdomyolysis in times of catabolism or excess fat consumption

### CLINICAL MANIFESTATIONS

Varies with syndrome but initial presenting symptoms include hypoketotic hypoglycemia; neonatal neurologic symptoms; coma; Reye-like syndrome; cardiac arrhythmia; cardiomyopathy; sudden death, rhabdomyolysis

### DIAGNOSTICS

**Decompensated Patient**

- Dextrose stick; serum Na, K, Cl, $HCO_3$, hepatic function panel, ammonia, uric acid. CPK, plasma acylcarnitine profile, total and free carnitine
- Blood gas if concern for metabolic acidosis
- Urine for ketones, myoglobin (if blood in U/A), and organic acid profile
- Consider ECG, echocardiography

**Other Studies**

- Acylcarnitine profiles performed in newborn screening programs have identified FAO disorders (FAOD) in many presymptomatic patients
- Mutation (DNA) diagnosis
- Enzyme assays on fibroblasts for some disorders

## MANAGEMENT

### Acute

Goal is to reverse hypoglycemia immediately, to curtail anabolism, and to treat associated morbidities:

- Place widest gauge IV catheter immediately. Some patients require central access to maintain high dextrose infusion rates
- Dextrose bolus (initial bolus of 2 cc/kg with D10; bolus may need to be repeated in older patients), then start dextrose infusion with D10 plus electrolytes at 1.5 × maintenance rate. Insulin surge after dextrose infusion inhibits further lipolysis
- Saline boluses if dehydrated, but should not delay establishing euglycemia
- Do not use intralipids
- Early consultation with biochemical geneticist or other specialist

### Chronic

- Carnitine supplementation for primary carnitine deficiency (e.g., carnitine transporter defect [CTD]). Use in other FAODs is typically done, but benefit is controversial
- For disorders affecting long-chain FAO, low fat, high carbohydrate diet, limit long-chain fatty acid intake. Diet is unrestricted in medium/short-chain disorders
- For disorders affecting long-chain FAO, supplement diet with medium-chain triglycerides (2–3 g/kg/day for infants; 1 g/kg/day in older children)
- Strategies to avoid hypoglycemia include frequent or continuous feeds, evening snacks with glucose polymers (e.g., corn starch), and close clinical monitoring during intercurrent illness
- Immunizations are not contraindicated, but frequent feeds and prophylactic antipyretics are recommended to reduce catabolism associated with febrile reactions. Particularly fragile patients may need IV fluids before and after immunizations
- Any procedure requiring sedation and nothing by mouth period requires admission for IV fluids before procedure

## SPECIFIC DISORDERS

**Important diagnostic laboratory studies for each entity are given in** Table 16-1.

## SHORT/MEDIUM-CHAIN FATTY ACID OXIDATION DISORDERS

### MEDIUM-CHAIN ACYL CoA DEHYDROGENASE (MCAD) DEFICIENCY

A mitochondrial FAOD affecting β-oxidation of medium-chain (e.g., 4–12 carbon length) fatty acids, causing fasting- or stress-induced episodes of hypoketotic hypoglycemia associated with emesis/lethargy.

- Patients who are diagnosed on newborn screen are typically asymptomatic between episodes of hypoglycemia
- Unchecked catabolism may lead to severe hypoglycemia, arrhythmia and death, especially in undiagnosed patients
- Hepatic steatosis generally improves after resolution of decompensation, but acylcarnitine profile is abnormal between episodes in some patients
- Long-term manifestations are unusual, but may include developmental disabilities and seizure disorder, resulting from recurrent hypoglycemia especially in patients with delayed diagnosis
- Newborn screen acylcarnitine analyses detect MCAD deficiency in presymptomatic individuals

| **TABLE 16-1** | Diagnostic Values of Fatty Acid Oxidation Disorders and Disorders of Ketone Metabolism | | |
|---|---|---|---|
| **Disorder** | **Acylcarnitine Profile** | **Urine Organic Acids** | **Plasma-Free Carnitine** |
| Carnitine/acylcarnitine translocase deficiency | ↑ Esters of 16–18 carbons | Normal or ↑ dicarboxylic acids | ↓ |
| Carnitine transporter defect | ↓ Long-chain esters | Dicarboxylic aciduria | ↓ (with paradoxical ↑ urine carnitine) |
| Carnitine palmitoyltransferase I deficiency | ↓ Long-chain esters | Normal | Normal or ↑ |
| Carnitine palmitoyltransferase II deficiency | ↑ Esters of 16–18 carbon length | Usually normal | ↓ |
| Medium-chain acyl CoA dehydrogenase deficiency | ↑ C6:0, C8:0, 4-cis-C8:1, 5-cis-C8:1, 4cis-C10:1 | Medium-chain dicarboxylic acids and hexanoylglycine | Normal to ↓ |
| Mitochondrial trifunctional protein deficiency and long-chain-3-hydroxyacyl CoA dehydrogenase deficiency | ↑ Long-chain esters and long-chain 3-hydroxy esters | Dicarboxylic acids | Usually ↓ |
| Multiple acyl CoA dehydrogenase deficiency* | Globally increased, especially long chains and C5DC | Dicarboxylic, glutaric, 2-hydroxyglutaric, ethylmalonic acids, isovalerylglycine | Normal or ↓ |
| Short-chain acyl CoA dehydrogenase deficiency | ↑ Butyrylcarnitine | Ethylmalonate, methylsuccinate, butyrylglycine | Normal or ↓ |
| Short-chain L-3-hydroxyacyl CoA dehydrogenase deficiency | 3-hydroxy-C4 ester | Dicarboxylic acid (variable) | Variable |
| Beta-ketothiolase deficiency† | ↑ C5:1 acylcarnitine | 2-methylacetoacetate, 2-butanone, 2-methyl-3-hydroxybutyrate | Variable |
| Very long-chain acyl CoA dehydrogenase deficiency | ↑ Very long-chain esters | Dicarboxylic acid | Normal or ↓ |

*Also known as glutaric aciduria type II.
†Also known as methylacetoacetyl-CoA thiolase deficiency and T2 deficiency.

## SHORT-CHAIN ACYL CoA DEHYDROGENASE (SCAD) DEFICIENCY

A mitochondrial FAOD affecting β-oxidation of short-chain (e.g., 4–6 carbon length) fatty acids. The clinical course is incompletely defined. Patients diagnosed on newborn screen are almost exclusively asymptomatic.

- Newborn screen acylcarnitine analyses have detected SCAD deficiency in presymptomatic individuals

## SHORT-CHAIN L-3-HYDROXYACYL CoA DEHYDROGENASE DEFICIENCY

A mitochondrial FAOD affecting β-oxidation of short-chain (e.g., 4–6 carbon length) fatty acids. Hyperinsulinimic hypoglycemia results from a secondary function of the SCAD molecule in the insulin release pathway.

## LONG-CHAIN FATTY ACID OXIDATION DISORDERS

**Included in this category are disorders that affect metabolism of all chain lengths because the majority of dietary fats is long-chain.**

### CARNITINE/ACYLCARNITINE TRANSLOCASE DEFICIENCY

A mitochondrial FAOD affecting transport of acylcarnitines across the inner mitochondrial membrane, limiting ability to use fat as an energy source. Long-chain fatty acylcarnitine and free fatty acid accumulation may contribute to the clinical picture.

- Two clinical subtypes exist:
  - ✓ *Severe:* Neonatal onset hypoketotic hypoglycemia, hypertrophic cardiomyopathy, ventricular arrhythmias, hyperammonemia, myoglobinuria
  - ✓ *Mild:* Fasting- or stress-induced hypoketotic hypoglycemia

### CARNITINE TRANSPORTER DEFECT

The transporter defect impairs transport of carnitine across cytoplasmic membranes into the cell. This results in reduced renal conservation of carnitine (leading to reduced serum carnitine levels) and decreased intracellular carnitine levels (especially muscle cells), both of which contribute to the impairment of FAO.

- Clinical manifestations include hypertrophic cardiomyopathy, progressive cardiac failure, skeletal muscle weakness, and hypoketotic hypoglycemia

### CARNITINE PALMITOYLTRANSFERASE I DEFICIENCY

A mitochondrial FAOD affecting conversion of fatty acyl CoA esters to acylcarnitine. Defective mitochondrial fatty acid import reduces or abolishes ability to use fat as an energy source. The first episode of decompensation usually occurs in infancy or early childhood.

- Manifestations include hypoketotic hypoglycemia, hepatomegaly, and hepatic encephalopathy (Reye syndrome)

### CARNITINE PALMITOYLTRANSFERASE II DEFICIENCY

A mitochondrial FAOD affecting mitochondrial import of long-chain fatty acids, resulting in defective conversion of acylcarnitines to fatty acyl CoA.

- Three clinical subtypes are defined by age at onset of symptoms:
  - ✓ *Classical:* Episodic muscle weakness and rhabdomyolysis after prolonged exercise or other stressors, starting in the second to third decade
  - ✓ *Antenatal:* Fatal multi-organ system disease including hypoglycemia, hepatic and renal insufficiency, congenital malformations, and death often in the neonatal period
  - ✓ *Infantile:* Hypoglycemia, hypotonia, hepatic dysfunction, hepatomegaly, cardiomegaly, and seizures

### MITOCHONDRIAL TRIFUNCTIONAL PROTEIN DEFICIENCY AND LONG-CHAIN-3-HYDROXYACYL CoA DEHYDROGENASE DEFICIENCY

Mitochondrial FAOD affecting β-oxidation of long-chain fatty acids. For long-chain (especially 12–16 carbon length) fatty acids, one enzyme (mitochondrial "trifunctional protein") carries out hydratase, 3-hydroxyacyl CoA dehydrogenase, and thiolase reactions. Some mutations affect all three activities, while others affect only the dehydrogenase. Impaired ability to oxidize long-chain fatty acids severely compromises use of fat as an energy source.

- Isolated long-chain 3-hydroxyacyl CoA dehydrogenase (LCHAD) deficiency is associated with hypoketotic hypoglycemia, fulminant hepatic disease, hypertrophic cardiomyopathy, episodic rhabdomyolysis, peripheral neuropathy, and pigmentary retinopathy
- Mitochondrial trifunctional protein (TFP) deficiency manifests as hypoketotic hypoglycemia, dilated cardiomyopathy, episodic rhabdomyolysis, and hypotonia
- Pregnant mothers carrying fetuses affected with TFP and LCHAD have an increased incidence of fatty liver of pregnancy and HELLP syndrome

## MULTIPLE ACYL CoA DEHYDROGENATION DEFICIENCY (GLUTARIC ACIDURIA TYPE II)

Multiple acyl CoA dehydrogenation deficiency (MADD) affects transfer of electrons from fatty acyl CoA to the electron transport chain, resulting in FAOD. The block also affects oxidation of branched-chain amino acids (leucine, isoleucine, valine) and of glutaryl-CoA (an oxidation product of tryptophan, lysine, hydroxylysine).

- Three clinical subtypes exist:
  - ✓ *Neonatal onset with congenital anomalies* (prematurity, hypoglycemia, metabolic acidosis, hypotonia, hepatomegaly, cardiomegaly, polycystic kidneys, and genitourinary, skeletal, and craniofacial abnormalities)
  - ✓ *Neonatal onset without congenital anomalies* (severe metabolic decompensation in first few days of life)
  - ✓ *Later onset* (variable phenotype including metabolic decompensations and myopathy)

## VERY LONG-CHAIN ACYL CoA DEHYDROGENASE DEFICIENCY

Very long-chain acyl CoA Dehydrogenase (VLCAD) gene mutations result in an impaired ability to oxidize fatty acids longer than 14 carbons in mitochondria and severely compromises use of fat as an energy source.

- Different clinical subtypes exist:
  - ✓ *severe*: neonatal- or infantile-onset hypertrophic cardiomyopathy, hypoketotic hypoglycemia, and/or Reye-like syndrome
  - ✓ *mild*: episodic hypoketotic hypoglycemia during stress or fasting, absence or later-onset cardiomyopathy
  - ✓ *late-onset*: presentation in the second to third decade of life with muscle weakness and rhabdomyolysis after prolonged exercise or other stressors

A "severe" phenotype involves neonatal- or infantile-onset hypertrophic cardiomyopathy and hypoketotic hypoglycemia/Reye-like syndrome. A "mild" phenotype involves episodic hypoketotic hypoglycemia during stress or fasting without cardiomyopathy. A "late" onset form presents in the second to third decade of life with muscle weakness and rhabdomyolysis after prolonged exercise or other stressors.

- Newborn screen acylcarnitine analyses have detected VLCAD in presymptomatic individuals; however, it is important to note that "late-onset" forms may be missed on newborn screen

## KETONE UTILIZATION DEFECTS

## GENERAL PRINCIPLES

**Class of disorders impairing the ability to utilize and clear ketone bodies.**

## EPIDEMIOLOGY

- Overall incidence about 1:1,000,000; autosomal recessive inheritance
- These conditions are likely underdiagnosed

## PATHOPHYSIOLOGY

Ketones that are synthesized are cleared inefficiently and unable to be utilized, resulting in energy failure in the fasted state and episodic ketoacidosis.

## CLINICAL MANIFESTATIONS

- Stresses associated with ketosis (fasting, infection, dehydration) cause severe ketoacidosis
- Ketosis with or without hypoglycemia. Ketosis may persist in the absence of hypoglycemia and even in the face of hyperglycemia. These diseases are important to consider in the differential for diabetic ketoacidosis as well as ketotic hypoglycemia
- Ketoacidosis with Kussmaul respirations and anion gap metabolic acidosis
- *Symptoms of ketoacidosis:* Lethargy, fatigue, malaise, nausea/vomiting/anorexia
- *Hypoglycemia-related complications:* Seizures, mental status changes

## DIAGNOSTICS

- BMP/anion gap, glucose, ketones
- Fasting is not necessary for diagnosis, but supervised safety fasts may be performed to determine the length of time patient can safely fast without developing dangerous ketoacidosis
- Molecular testing confirms suspicion

## MANAGEMENT

- Avoidance of fasting
- Ketogenic diet is absolutely contraindicated
- Sodium bicarbonate may be necessary for normalizing pH
- Any procedure requiring sedation and nothing by mouth period requires admission for IV fluids before procedure

## SPECIFIC DISORDERS

### ß-KETOTHIOLASE DEFICIENCY (METHYLACETOACETYL-CoA THIOLASE DEFICIENCY, T2 DEFICIENCY)

A defect affecting the interconversion of acetyl-CoA and acetoacetyl-CoA. Often there is clearing of ketones and absence of symptoms between episodes. Onset is typically in infancy or early childhood

- Beta-ketothiolase deficiency is characterized by episodic ketoacidosis associated with headaches and malaise
- Basal ganglia involvement including chorea and MRI abnormalities consistent with metabolic stroke have been reported in multiple patients
- Urine organic acids may show subtle elevations in tiglylglycine and 2-methyl-3-hydroxybutyrate in some patients, but absence does not rule out disease

### SUCCINYL-CoA:3-OXOACID CoA TRANSFERASE (SCOT) DEFICIENCY

A defect affecting the addition of a CoA body to acetoacetate to make acetoacetyl-CoA. This is the first step in ketolysis and necessary for any ketolysis to occur. Half of patients present in the neonatal period, with the remainder presenting mostly in early childhood.

- Permanent ketosis/ketonuria is pathognomonic, but not universal
- Even patients with permanent ketosis are asymptomatic between episodes of deterioration

## UREA CYCLE DEFECTS

### GENERAL PRINCIPLES

**Class of metabolic diseases in which an enzyme deficiency compromises activity of the urea cycle, which normally functions to remove waste nitrogen as urea.**

### ETIOLOGY

- Mutations in urea cycle enzymes, including carbamyl phosphate synthetase (CPS), ornithine transcarbamylase (OTC), argininosuccinic acid synthetase (AS), argininosuccinic acid lyase (AL), and arginase
- N-acetyl glutamate synthetase deficiency has also been described
- OTC deficiency is an X-linked disease. Other urea cycle defects (UCDs) are autosomal recessive

### EPIDEMIOLOGY

- *Overall prevalence of UCDs:* About 1:30,000
- *Most common is OTC deficiency:* About 1:40,000

### PATHOPHYSIOLOGY

- The urea cycle is a major mechanism for ammonia ($NH_3$) clearance by converting it to water-soluble urea
- Decompensation states occur during "nitrogen imbalance," when the nitrogen load exceeds the excretion ability, resulting in hyperammonemia
- Conditions of increased nitrogen load include high protein diets, muscle catabolism induced by fasting, stress or exercise, and medicines that increase protein turnover
- Ammonia-stimulated hyperventilation causes respiratory alkalosis
- Hyperammonemia increases tryptophan transport across blood–brain barrier, enhancing serotonin production. Intracerebral glutamine also accumulates, contributing to cerebral edema. The overall effect is an encephalopathy that can include somnolence and coma

### CLINICAL MANIFESTATIONS

- Great variability in clinical spectrum
- *Episodic decompensations with:* Hyperammonemia; cerebral edema; encephalopathy (lethargy, seizures, coma); respiratory alkalosis; other acid/base disturbances
- Neonatal clinical presentation is very similar to sepsis
- *Older patients:* Poor appetite, cyclical vomiting, psychosis
- On exam, focus on ABCs, hydration status, mental status, neurologic exam, and possible sources of infection
- Unexplained tachypnea may be due to hyperammonemia

### DIAGNOSTICS

- Newborn screening programs detect some UCDs in presymptomatic patients; however, OTC and CPS are not diagnosed on newborn screen. Additionally, decompensation in severe cases precedes the results of the newborn screen
- Neonatal presentation is similar to that of sepsis, so it is important to check ammonia levels in septic-appearing newborns

### Decompensated Patient (Initial Hyperammonemic Episode)

- $NH_3$ should be checked urgently; sample should be drawn on free-flowing blood, without a tourniquet and placed on ice
- Initial approach to the differential diagnosis of hyperammonemia includes ruling out sepsis, organic acidopathies, and FAO. Send CBC and differential counts, blood culture, and inflammatory markers, ABG; dextrose stick; basic metabolic panel/anion gap; LFTs; PT/PTT; plasma amino acids; plasma lactate/pyruvate; plasma acylcarnitine profile, total and free carnitine. These studies help determine the cause of hyperammonemia and evaluate for comorbidities of diseases in the differential
- Urine for urinalysis, organic acids, and orotic acid; urine amino acid analysis
- If UCD is confirmed, brain MRI should be performed once stable to ascertain degree of neurologic damage

### Decompensated Patient (Known Urea Cycle Defect)

- $NH_3$, dextrose stick, basic metabolic panel/anion gap, plasma amino acids

### Definitive Diagnostics

- Amino acid profile is unequivocal in some UCDs (AL, AS deficiency); urine orotate; mutation (DNA) analysis; enzyme analysis

### MANAGEMENT (DECOMPENSATED PATIENT)

- *ABCs/fluid management:* Ventilatory and pressor support; wide gauge IV (consider central access); start infusion with 10% dextrose in water at 6–8 mg glucose/kg/min; nasogastric tube. Titrate dextrose infusion upwards as necessary to stop catabolism. As high as 15–20% dextrose at maintenance may be necessary. Do not decrease GIR in the acutely ill patient. If hyperglycemia develops (glucose >150 mg/dL), begin insulin drip at 0.1 unit/kg/h and titrate to target glucose of 100–150 mg/dL
- *Bulk $NH_3$ removal:* Dialysis may be necessary, especially if ammonia exceeds 500 or is rising despite medical management; consider consults with nephrology and critical care; nitrogen scavenging agents (Table 16-2)
- *Reversal of catabolic state:* Stop protein feeds; dextrose infusion as above; consider insulin drip; consider intralipids; amino acids must be provided within 24–48 hours or protein turnover will persist; for total parenteral nutrition, start with 1–1.5 g amino acids/kg/day; if tolerating enteral feeds, use protein-free formula with gradual reintroduction of protein

| TABLE 16-2 | Nitrogen Scavenging Agents | | | | | |
|---|---|---|---|---|---|---|
| | Children (mg/kg) | | | Adolescents/Adults (g/m²) | | |
| **Diagnosis** | **SPA** | **SB** | **Arg-HCl** | **SPA** | **SB** | **Arg-HCl** |
| Presumed UCD | 250 | 250 | 600 | | | |
| CPS/OTC | 250 | 250 | 210 | 5.5 | 5.5 | 4.0 |
| AS/AL | 250 | 250 | 660 | 5.5 | 5.5 | 12 |

Dose size is same for load and maintenance infusion. Deliver loading dose over 90 minutes, then start every 24-hour continuous infusion.

SPA, sodium phenylbutyrate; SB, sodium benzoate; Arg-HCl, arginine-HCl; CPS, carbamyl phosphate synthetase deficiency; OTC, ornithine transcarbamylase deficiency; AS, argininosuccinic acid synthetase deficiency; AL, argininosuccinic acid lyase deficiency.

Data from Summar M. Current strategies for the management of neonatal urea cycle disorders. *J Pediatr.* 2001;138:S30–S39. And Batshaw ML, MacArthur RB, Tuchman M. Alternative pathway therapy for urea cycle disorders: twenty years later. *J Pediatr.* 2001;138:S46–S55.

- *Laboratory monitoring during critical phase:* ABG every 4 hours or as indicated for intu-bated patients; basic metabolic panel every 4 hours; $NH_3$ every 1 hour until less than 300; plasma amino acids every day; other laboratory studies as indicated for dialysis patients
- *Transition/home management:* Enteral nitrogen scavengers include sodium phenylbutyrate or glycerol phenylbutyrate and sodium benzoate; some patients require citrulline (CPS, OTC deficiency) or arginine (AS, AL deficiency) therapy; routine monitoring of nutri-tional markers, plasma amino acids, $NH_3$; consider G-tube placement, especially for neuro-logically impaired patients; normal immunization schedule with prophylactic antipyretics; for procedures requiring sedation and nothing by mouth period, consider admission for IV fluids before procedure; liver transplantation is curative for some patients

## SPECIFIC UREA CYCLE DEFECTS

### ARGINASE DEFICIENCY (ARGININEMIA)

Arginase catalyzes the cytoplasmic production of ornithine and urea from arginine. Arginase deficiency causes arginine elevation and increases risk for hyperammonemia as well as toxic effects of arginine and other guanidino compounds. Unlike other UCDs, arginase deficiency presents primarily as a chronic neurologic disorder with progressive spastic diplegia/quad-riplegia, ataxia, and choreoathetosis.

- Episodic hyperammonemic episodes can occur, but are less prominent than those in other UCDs
- Diagnosis is confirmed by plasma amino acid profile, which shows elevated arginine
- Urinary orotic acid is also increased

### ARGININOSUCCINIC ACID LYASE DEFICIENCY

Argininosuccinic acid lyase (AL) catalyzes the cytoplasmic production of arginine from argininosuccinic acid. In AL deficiency, citrulline accumulates and arginine becomes an essential amino acid.

- Hepatomegaly and hepatic dysfunction/fibrosis may develop
- Diagnosis is confirmed by plasma amino acid profile, which shows elevated citrulline and argininosuccinate with decreased arginine
- The presence of argininosuccinate esters on plasma or urine amino acids is pathognomonic
- Urinary orotic acid is also increased

### ARGININOSUCCINIC ACID SYNTHETASE DEFICIENCY (CITRULLINEMIA)

Argininosuccinic acid synthetase (AS) catalyzes the cytoplasmic production of argininosuc-cinic acid from citrulline and aspartic acid. In AS deficiency, citrulline accumulates and arginine becomes an essential amino acid.

- Plasma amino acids reveal elevated citrulline and decreased arginine
- Urinary orotic acid is also increased

### CARBAMOYL PHOSPHATE SYNTHETASE DEFICIENCY

Carbamoyl phosphate synthetase (CPS) catalyzes production of carbamoyl phosphate from $NH_4^+$, $HCO_3^-$, and ATP. Citrulline and arginine, downstream urea cycle products, become essential amino acids.

- Diagnosis is confirmed by plasma amino acid profile, which shows elevated glutamine with decreased citrulline and arginine
- Urinary orotic acid is normal; this key feature distinguishes CPS deficiency from OTC deficiency

## ORNITHINE TRANSCARBAMYLASE DEFICIENCY (ORNITHINE CARBAMOYLTRANSFERASE DEFICIENCY)

Ornithine transcarbamylase (OTC) is an enzyme encoded on the X chromosome, which catalyzes the entry step into the urea cycle. Citrulline and arginine, downstream urea cycle products, become essential amino acids.

- Classic presentation is a male neonate, well at birth, with progressive emesis, feed refusal, and encephalopathy within a few days. Seizures occur in approximately 50% of patients. Female OTC deficiency carriers have varying degrees of symptomatology depending on X-inactivation pattern in hepatocytes. Older patients may present with cyclic vomiting or behavior disturbances rather than frank metabolic decompensation
- Diagnosis is confirmed by plasma amino acid profile, which shows elevated glutamine and decreased citrulline and arginine
- Urinary orotic acid is also increased

## DEFECTS OF AMINO ACID METABOLISM

### HEREDITARY TYROSINEMIA TYPE 1

**Hereditary tyrosinemia type 1 (HT1) is an inborn error of tyrosine (tyr) metabolism causing progressive liver and renal failure. It is due to mutations in the gene encoding FAH, the terminal enzyme in tyr metabolism.**

#### EPIDEMIOLOGY

- Incidence about 1:100,000; autosomal recessive inheritance
- Incidence much higher in the Lac-St. Jean region of Quebec

#### PATHOPHYSIOLOGY

- Tyr metabolism is both ketogenic (producing acetoacetate) and gluconeogenic (producing fumarate). Tyr metabolism occurs in the hepatocyte and the proximal renal tubule
- Elevated tyr is due to inhibition of upstream biochemical steps, and does not contribute to liver or renal injury
- Blockade at the FAH step causes an accumulation of fumarylacetoacetate (FAA), an alkylating agent that promotes apoptosis and alters gene expression
- Accumulation of succinylacetone, a byproduct of FAA, contributes to renal Fanconi syndrome
- Hypoglycemia may result from hepatic dysfunction, reduced availability of gluconeogenic precursors, and decreased expression of genes required for glucose production
- Porphyria crises occur because succinylacetone inhibits δ-aminolevulinic acid dehydratase in the heme synthetic pathway
- FAA's mutagenic activity may contribute to the development of hepatocellular carcinoma

#### CLINICAL MANIFESTATIONS

- Hepatic failure is progressive, usually beginning in the neonatal period or early infancy. Patients may present with acute hepatic crises, with hypoalbuminemia, ascites, and jaundice
- High risk for cirrhosis and hepatocellular carcinoma if untreated
- Coagulopathy due to compromised liver synthetic function may be the first symptom, sometimes manifested by gastrointestinal bleeding
- Proximal renal tubular dysfunction often presents as a renal Fanconi syndrome

- Neurologic symptoms due to attacks of porphyria include painful peripheral neuropathy, hypertonia, and autonomic instability
- Causes of death include liver failure, hemorrhage, respiratory arrest (porphyria episodes), and hepatocellular carcinoma

## DIAGNOSTICS

- Plasma amino acids may reveal elevated tyr, phenylalanine (phe), and methionine. Definitive diagnosis requires demonstration of succinylacetone on urine organic acid quantitation or on filter-blotted blood specimens. FAH enzyme activity and genetic testing can be used for confirmation
- There are multiple other conditions that can cause elevated tyr; it is important not to make a diagnosis of tyrosinemia 1 on the basis of elevated tyr alone
- Elevation in alpha-fetoprotein (AFP) may predate elevated tyr levels
- Tyr is often not severely elevated, so the sensitivity of newborn screening is poor in the several states that do not measure succinylacetone
- Check coagulation studies and other markers of liver synthetic function. Hepatic transaminases may or may not be elevated

## MANAGEMENT

- 2-(2-nitro-4-trifluoromethyl-benzoyl)-1,3-cyclohexanedione (NTBC, nitisinone) inhibits 4-HPPD, an upstream step in tyr metabolism, reducing production of FAA and succinylacetone. NTBC decreases risk of liver failure and hepatocellular carcinoma. Starting dose is 1 mg/kg/day orally divided twice daily, adjusted for biochemical control
- NTBC treatment increases blood tyr and phe levels, so treated patients require dietary modification
- NTBC can cause corneal erosions and other ocular abnormalities, so baseline and routine ophthalmologic exams are indicated
- Liver transplantation is an option for NTBC nonresponders

## MAPLE SYRUP URINE DISEASE

**Maple syrup urine disease (MSUD) is caused by autosomal recessive mutations in branched-chain ketoacid dehydrogenase, resulting in decreased ability to process branched-chain amino acids (leucine, isoleucine, and valine). Inheritance is autosomal recessive.**

## EPIDEMIOLOGY

- Overall incidence is 1:185,000; however, it is as common as 1:400 in certain Mennonite populations

## PATHOPHYSIOLOGY

- There exist three genes known to cause MSUD
- Accumulation of branched-chain amino acids interferes with entry of other large neutral amino acids into the brain
- Accumulated branched-chain ketoacids result in depletion of brain glutamate and glutamine

## CLINICAL MANIFESTATIONS

Patients may be diagnosed on newborn screening before symptoms develop. Even when detected on screening and placed under good dietary control, episodic deterioration may occur, especially with intercurrent illness

- Episodic encephalopathy/coma associated with cerebral edema

- Characteristic "maple syrup" odor is detectable in urine and cerumen when there is poor dietary control
- Mild intellectual impairment in comparison to family, even when well-controlled

## DIAGNOSIS

- Most patients are detected on newborn screen
- Plasma amino acids show elevations of leucine, isoleucine, and valine, as well as alloisoleucine, whose presence is pathognomonic for MSUD
- Urine organic acids show branched-chain ketoacids

## MANAGEMENT

- Dietary management with restricted branched-chain amino acids. MSUD-specific TPN is available for children who are acutely ill
- *Thiamine:* 25–100 mg/day. Co-factor for branch-chain ketoacid decarboxylase. Few patients respond; trial for approximately 4 weeks
- Liver transplant is used for severe or refractory cases

## PHENYLKETONURIA

**Phenylketonuria (PKU) is an inborn error of phe metabolism associated with mental retardation. Mutations in the gene encoding phe hydroxylase (PAH) account for most cases. Inheritance is autosomal recessive.**

## EPIDEMIOLOGY

- Overall incidence in American children is 1:15,000

## PATHOPHYSIOLOGY

- Increased phe interferes with large neutral amino acid transport in both directions across the blood–brain barrier
- Altered amino acid transport probably affects CNS protein and neurotransmitter (especially dopamine, serotonin) synthesis
- Phe is hydroxylated to form tyr, a precursor of melanin. Relative underpigmentation of PKU patients reflects decreased tyr availability

## CLINICAL MANIFESTATIONS

Due to newborn screening, PKU patients are now diagnosed before symptoms develop. Historically, abnormalities included seizures, infantile spasms, increased tone/spasticity, and microcephaly.

- Patients detected on screening and with good dietary control may have subtle learning-style and behavioral differences, including increased incidence of ADHD
- Tics, parkinsonism, and behavior abnormalities occur in poorly controlled patients
- Light pigmentation of hair, skin, eyes
- Eczema in 20–40%
- Urinary phenylacetic acid causes the classic "mousy odor"

## DIAGNOSIS

- All US neonates are now screened for elevated phe levels
- Confirmatory testing requires plasma amino acid quantitation to verify elevated phe and to determine the phe:tyr ratio. A phe:tyr ratio greater than 3:1 reflects a state of hyperphenylalaninemia

## MANAGEMENT

- Consultation with a biochemical geneticist or other specialist
- Early treatment is associated with better neurodevelopmental outcomes. Dietary therapy should begin immediately after diagnosis, by the end of the first week of life if possible. Dietary management is recommended in patients with phe levels greater than 10 mg% (625 μmole/L). Most physicians also advocate phe-restricted diet in patients with mild hyperphenylalaninemia whose levels are persistently above 6 mg% (360 μmole/L). Phe-reduced formulas and foods form the basis of dietary therapy. Patients also take a small amount of complete protein to provide requisite amounts of phe and tyr
- Goal phe level is controversial, but many experts agree that 2–6 mg% are acceptable levels
- Phe restriction is life-long. Previous liberalization of diet in adults was hypothesized to result in mild cognitive changes
- Kuvan (sapropterin) is a synthetic cofactor for the PAH enzyme, which also acts as a chaperone to stabilize the protein and increase enzyme activity. It is most effective in patients who have residual enzyme activity and can allow liberalization of diet
- Mothers with PKU need strict dietary control before and during pregnancy. Poor first-trimester control increases fetal risk for microcephaly, mental retardation, and congenital heart disease

## DEFECTS OF CARBOHYDRATE METABOLISM

### GALACTOSEMIA

**Galactosemia is an inborn error of galactose metabolism resulting in toxicity after ingestion of lactose or galactose. Mutations may occur in any of three genes involved in galactose metabolism: galactokinase (GK), galactose-1-phosphate uridyltransferase (GALT), and uridine diphosphate-galactose 4' epimerase. GALT deficiency accounts for the majority of cases. "Classical" galactosemia is caused by severe GALT deficiency (<5% activity). "Partial" GALT deficiency (10–25%) is more common and is benign.**

### EPIDEMIOLOGY

- Prevalence of classical galactosemia is 1:50,000
- Inheritance is autosomal recessive

### PATHOPHYSIOLOGY

- Symptoms appear in neonates fed breast milk or cow's milk formulas, both of which contain lactose, a disaccharide of glucose and galactose
- In patients with GALT deficiency, galactose-1-phosphate (gal1P) accumulates. Hypoglycemia occurs because (1) galactose cannot be converted to glucose and (2) gal 1P inhibits phospho-glucomutase, an enzyme required for glycogenolysis

### CLINICAL MANIFESTATIONS

- Newborn screening has allowed for detection of presymptomatic individuals
- Affected children are well at birth with symptoms appearing in a few days
- *In an American series following galactosemic neonates:* 89% had symptoms from hepatocellular damage (jaundice, hepatomegaly, ascites, transaminitis, hyperammonemia, and coagulopathy); 76% had food intolerance (poor feeding, emesis); 29% had failure to thrive; 16% had lethargy; 10% had sepsis (usually *Escherichia coli*); 1% had seizures

- Other neonatal manifestations include hypoglycemia, renal Fanconi, and cataracts. Early death by sepsis, hepatic failure, or renal failure may occur unless patient is diagnosed and treated
- Long-term sequelae include developmental delay, speech dyspraxia, cataracts, and ovarian failure even in children well-controlled on diet

## DIAGNOSTICS

- In some states newborn screening assays detects essentially 100% of affected neonates by GALT enzyme activity directly, which allows diagnosis to be made even in children on lactose-free formulas. However, technique and quality of newborn screening varies by state; also many newborns become symptomatic before the diagnosis is reported by the laboratory, underscoring the need to recognize the clinical picture
- *Evaluation of a sick neonate suspected of having galactosemia:* Dextrose stick, basic metabolic panel, blood culture, liver function tests, PT/PTT, ammonia, urine for reducing substances, galactitol, amino acids, erythrocyte gal1P, GALT activity (whole blood or dried sample on filter paper)
- *Evaluation of an asymptomatic neonate referred because of a presumptive positive newborn screen result:* Urine galactitol, erythrocyte gal1P, GALT activity
- *Interpretation of GALT activity:* Less than 5%: classical galactosemia; 10–25%: Duarte/galactosemia (D/G); 50%: galactosemia carrier (benign); 75–90%: Duarte carrier (benign)

## MANAGEMENT

- ABCs
- In sick neonates, discontinue feeds, reverse hypoglycemia if present, and begin dextrose infusion. If hyperammonemia is present, discontinue protein intake until resolved
- In asymptomatic neonates with a positive galactosemia newborn screen (decreased GALT and increased galactose level), stop lactose/galactose-containing feeds, pending confirmation. Start non-lactose-containing formula (e.g., soy-based)
- Long-term management of classical galactosemia includes avoidance of dietary lactose and galactose (dairy products, some tomato products, many legumes, canned foods, etc.). Calcium supplementation is important. Consultation with a clinical nutritionist is helpful
- In GK deficiency, which causes isolated cataracts, elimination of dairy products alone is sufficient treatment
- Severe epimerase-deficiency galactosemia is difficult to treat, because deficiency impairs not only production of glucose from galactose, but also galactose biosynthesis, which is necessary for processing of some proteins and lipids
- The Duarte allele reduces the enzyme activity of the GALT enzyme, but not as severely as classic disease. Many centers do not do diet modification for children with D/G galactosemia

## HEREDITARY FRUCTOSE INTOLERANCE

**Hereditary fructose intolerance is an inborn error in metabolism resulting in toxicity after fructose ingestion. It is due to a mutation in the gene encoding aldolase B, an enzyme required for conversion of fructose to glucose. Exposure to fructose, sucrose (a glucose–fructose disaccharide), or sorbitol causes symptoms to occur.**

## EPIDEMIOLOGY

- In the United Kingdom, about 1% carry a common disease-causing allele and 1/20,000 are homozygous
- Inheritance is autosomal recessive

## CLINICAL MANIFESTATIONS

- Most affected patients are asymptomatic until weaning, when they are exposed to sucrose or fructose, classically around 6 months
- Symptoms include abdominal pain, vomiting, severe hypoglycemia (diaphoresis, lethargy, seizures, coma), hepatotoxicity (jaundice, coagulopathy, ascites), elevated uric acid, and renal Fanconi
- Untreated patients progress to chronic hepatic and renal failure

## PATHOPHYSIOLOGY

- Aldolase B deficiency primarily affects hepatocytes, mucosa of the small intestine, and the proximal renal tubules, major sites of aldolase B expression. Aldolase B cleaves fructose-1-phosphate (f1P) into 3-carbon products that can be used for glycolysis, glycogen synthesis, or gluconeogenesis
- Aldolase B deficiency leads to accumulation of f1P and depletion of phosphate sources, especially inorganic phosphate ($P_i$) and ATP $P_i$ depletion activates purine degradation, resulting in hyperuricemia. f1P accumulation prevents glycogen breakdown and gluconeogenesis, contributing to hypoglycemia. Inhibition of gluconeogenesis causes precursors (e.g., lactate, pyruvate) to accumulate, resulting in metabolic acidosis, which is compounded by proximal renal tubular dysfunction

## DIAGNOSTICS

- Blood glucose; comprehensive metabolic panel including K, $HCO_3$, BUN, Cr, phosphate, liver function tests; PT/PTT; uric acid
- Urine for reducing substances, glucose, fructose, and amino acids
- Plasma lactate/pyruvate and amino acids may also be helpful
- Definitive diagnosis is based on mutation analysis. IV fructose challenge test under closely supervised conditions may be performed when patient is clinically well

## MANAGEMENT

- *Sick patient after fructose exposure:* ABCs; establish intravenous access; treat hypoglycemia, metabolic acidosis, and electrolyte abnormalities (especially hypophosphatemia)
- *Long-term management:* Avoid fructose and fructose-containing sugars, including sucrose and sorbitol. Consultation with a clinical nutritionist is helpful
- *Sources of sucrose (table sugar) include:* Candies/desserts, canned foods, soft drinks
- *Sources of fructose include* fresh fruits, raw vegetables, new potatoes, whole flour, brown rice
- *Sources of sorbitol include* some medications, diabetic products

## ORGANIC ACIDEMIAS

**Organic acidurias are a group of metabolic disorders due to inborn enzymes deficiencies in metabolism of amino acids to allow entrance to the tricarboxylic acid cyclic, leading to accumulation of non-amino organic acids. Mutations in a variety of enzymes cause these disorders:**

- Propionyl CoA carboxylase (propionic acidemia, PA)
- Methylmalonyl CoA mutase (methylmalonic acidemia, MMA)
- Isovaleryl CoA dehydrogenase (isovaleric acidemia, IVA)
- 3-methylcrotonyl-CoA carboxylase (3-methylcrotonyl-CoA carboxylase deficiency, 3-MCCD)
- Glutaryl-CoA dehydrogenase (glutaric academia type 1, GA1)

## EPIDEMIOLOGY

- *Prevalence:* PA: 1:100,000; MMA: 1:80,000; IVA: 1:100,000; 3-MCCD: 1:40,000; GA1: 1:100,000
- Autosomal recessive inheritance

## DIFFERENTIAL DIAGNOSIS

In patients with acidosis and neurologic dysfunction, consider:

- *Non-metabolic causes:* Sepsis, renal tubular acidosis, congenital cardiovascular or pulmonary malformation, hypocalcemia, other electrolyte abnormalities, toxins, intracranial bleed
- *Metabolic causes:* Biotinidase deficiency and holocarboxylase synthetase deficiency, cobalamin metabolism disorders, primary lactic acidosis syndromes

## PATHOPHYSIOLOGY

- Enzyme deficiency causes organic acid accumulation and consequently a variety of toxic effects on cellular function
- Organic acid accumulation inhibits metabolic pathways including ketogenesis, gluconeogenesis, and ureagenesis
- Organic acids also interfere with hematopoiesis
- Decompensation occurs during states of catabolism (infection, fasting, exercise, other stress) or increased protein turnover (general anesthetics, steroids). Dietary protein overload can also promote decompensation

## CLINICAL MANIFESTATIONS

Perform a comprehensive history and physical exam focusing on: ABCs; hydration status; tachypnea (may be due to acidosis or hyperammonemia); complete neurologic exam including mental status; cardiac exam; epigastric tenderness (vomiting may be due to pancreatitis); superficial skin desquamation; source of infection (if febrile); unusual odor in urine or breath

### Neonatal Presentation

Similar to sepsis; typically a full-term baby, well for the first few days, then with dramatic decompensation:

- Lethargy and progressive neurologic dysfunction (seizures, abnormal tone, unusual movements, coma)
- Poor feeding, hypoglycemia, metabolic acidosis, ketonuria, hyperammonemia
- Stroke-like episodes, which may cause choreoathetoid or dystonic movements (especially GA1)
- Bone marrow suppression, cardiomyopathy (especially PA and MMA), pancreatitis
- Unusual odor of body fluids

### Later Presentation

- Poor appetite, failure to thrive, preference for nonprotein foods
- Episodic vomiting, hypotonia, seizures
- Global developmental delay, especially with regression
- GA1 can present with spontaneous subdural hemorrhage

### Episodic Decompensation

- Catabolic states can cause appearance, recurrence, or exacerbation of any of the previous signs or symptoms

## DIAGNOSTICS

• Newborn screening programs include an acylcarnitine profile

### Decompensated Patient (Initial Presentation)

• *General sepsis workup:* CBC count with differential, blood culture, inflammatory markers
• $NH_3$, ABG with lactate, dextrose stick, basic metabolic panel/anion gap, LFTs, amylase/lipase in vomiting patient, plasma lactate/pyruvate
• *Metabolic tests:* Plasma amino acids; plasma acylcarnitine profile and total/free carnitine; urine for urinalysis and organic acids; CSF for amino acids, lactate/pyruvate, and organic acids if lumbar puncture is performed
• Consider head CT if cerebral edema is suspected
• Perform ECG and echocardiography for signs of cardiac failure

### Decompensated Patient (Known Organic Acidemia)

• ABG; dextrose stick; basic metabolic panel/anion gap; $NH_3$; CBC count and differential; LFTs and lipase/amylase for vomiting/abdominal pain; plasma amino acids; plasma total/free carnitine level; urine for urinalysis

### Definitive Diagnostics

• Enzyme assays, usually on fibroblasts from skin biopsy

## MANAGEMENT

• *ABCs/fluid management:* Ventilatory and pressor support as needed. Place widest gauge IV. Most patients will need multiple access sites and some will require central venous access; start infusion with D10-based solution at 6–8 mg glucose/kg/min; monitor urine output
• *Reverse acidosis:* Maintain $HCO_3$ at 22–25. If severely acidotic (pH <7.22 or $HCO_3$ <14 mEq/L), give $NaHCO_3$ bolus (1 mEq/kg; may be repeated if needed) followed by continuous infusion (2–4 mEq/kg/day). Minimize other sodium sources. If patient becomes hypernatremic, reduce rate of $NaHCO_3$ drip or replace with potassium acetate; THAM is contraindicated
• *Reverse catabolic state:* Stop protein feeds; in patients unable to tolerate enteral feeds, start total parenteral nutrition, with goal intake 20% above maintenance nutrition. Use 10% dextrose (5–10 mg/kg/min) and intralipids (1–3 g/kg/day). Hold amino acids for 24 hours if severely ill, then start gradual reintroduction; if tolerating enteral feeds, use protein-free formula with gradual reintroduction of protein to baseline
• *Reverse hyperammoniemia:* Nitrogen scavenging agents (as in UCDs) may be used; dialysis may be necessary. In severely ill patients, immediate consultations with nephrology and critical care are warranted
• *Laboratory monitoring during critical phase:* ABG every 4 hours or as indicated for intubated patients; basic metabolic panel every 4 hours; NH3 every 1–2 hours until less than 300; daily urine organic and plasma organic acids; daily plasma amino acids; daily CBC count with differential; plasma acylcarnitine profile every other day; other laboratory studies as indicated for dialysis patients
• *Medication therapy:*
  ✓ *Carnitine:* 50–200 mg/kg/day if carnitine deficient (MMA, PA, GA type 1)
  ✓ *Glycine:* 10%: 250–600 mg/kg/day. Favors formation of rapidly excreted isovalerylglycine (IVA)
  ✓ *Hydroxycobalamin:* 1 mg intramuscular injection daily. Co-factor for methylmalonyl CoA mutase (MMA)

- *Transition/chronic care:* Choose appropriate home formula and daily protein allowance with metabolic dietitian; routine monitoring of nutritional markers, plasma and urine organic acids, acylcarnitine profile/carnitine levels, electrolytes, LFTs, CBC count with differential; may require long-term medication and alkalinization therapy; consider gastrostomy tube placement, especially for patients with failure to thrive; early intervention services; yearly developmental assessment; yearly bone density scans after age 4; normal immunization schedule with prophylactic antipyretics and protein-free diet; for procedures requiring sedation and nothing by mouth period, consider admission for IV fluids before procedure

## PRIMARY LACTIC ACIDOSIS

## RESPIRATORY CHAIN DEFECTS

**Inborn errors in assembly, structure, or function of the protein complexes necessary for oxidative phosphorylation. Respiratory chain defects (RCDs) are a large family of rare and incurable disorders, including clinical syndromes such as mitochondrial encephalomyelopathy with lactic acidosis and stroke (MELAS); myoclonic epilepsy with ragged red fibers (MERRF); neuropathy, ataxia, and retinitis pigmentosa (NARP); chronic progressive external ophthalmoplegia (CPEO); myoneurogastrointestinal disorder and encephalomyopathy (MNGIE); Barth syndrome; Pearson syndrome; Kearns–Sayre syndrome; many others.**

### ETIOLOGY

- The respiratory chain of the inner mitochondrial membrane contains five multi-subunit protein complexes
- Complete assembly and maintenance of the electron transport chain requires the mitochondrial genome and hundreds of genes from the nuclear genome
- Inborn errors in nuclear or mitochondrial genes can lead to RCD
- Mutations in mitochondrial DNA are maternally inherited
- RCDs resulting from mutations in nuclear genes are inherited in an autosomal recessive, autosomal dominant or X-linked fashion; mostly autosomal recessive

### EPIDEMIOLOGY

- Estimated prevalence of childhood RCD is 1:10,000

### PATHOPHYSIOLOGY

- Failure of the respiratory chain leads to inability to produce ATP from reduced electron carriers. This affects the efficiency of energy production from essentially all fuel sources
- Decreased ATP production is associated with damage in tissues with high metabolic demand. Failure to reoxidize electron carriers decreases TCA efficiency and leads to lactic acidosis
- Ketosis results from shunting of acetyl CoA away from the TCA cycle and toward ketogenesis
- Increased generation of toxic reactive oxygen species occurs

### CLINICAL MANIFESTATIONS

Phenotypes in RCD are pleiotropic, even within a family. The presence of progressive dysfunction in seemingly unrelated organ systems should raise suspicion for an RCD. Tissues with high requirements for oxidative phosphorylation tend to be the most severely affected. These include:

- *Skeletal muscle:* Weakness, myopathy, rhabdomyolysis, ophthalmoplegia

- *Central nervous system:* Seizure, hearing loss, basal ganglia dysfunction, developmental delay, abnormal tone, retinopathy, stroke-like events
- *Liver:* Steatosis, transaminitis, decreased synthetic function, hepatic failure
- *Bone marrow:* Neutropenia, sideroblastic anemia
- *Pancreas:* Diabetes mellitus, exocrine insufficiency
- *Heart:* Arrhythmias, cardiomyopathy
- *Proximal renal tubule:* Renal tubular acidosis, renal Fanconi
  A wide range of findings are possible on physical exam:

- *Eyes:* Evaluate for ophthalmoplegia and retinal abnormalities
- *Respiratory:* Kussmaul respirations suggest metabolic acidosis, which can be due to lactemia or ketonemia
- *Cardiac:* Irregular rhythms, new murmurs/gallops, signs of congestive heart failure
- *Gastrointestinal:* Hepatomegaly
- *Neurologic:* Evaluate tone, mental status, and focal deficits

## DIAGNOSTICS

### In Patients Suspected of Having a Respiratory Chain Defect

- Basic metabolic panel, liver function tests, and creatine kinase
- Elevated lactate and lactate/pyruvate ratio may be present at baseline, or may be uncovered after glucose loading
- *Plasma ketones:* Ketonemia may be present, even in fed state
- Urine organic acids. May reveal elevated lactate, ketones, and TCA cycle intermediates (e.g., $\alpha$-ketoglutarate)
- *Urine amino acids:* A generalized aminoaciduria reflecting proximal renal tubular dysfunction occurs in some patients. (Generalized aminoaciduria is normal in neonates, limiting the utility of urine amino acids in this age group)
- In patients with CNS disease, CSF lactate/pyruvate
- MRI of brain for structural or degenerative abnormalities
- MR spectroscopy to detect lactate, especially in basal ganglia

### For Definitive Diagnosis

- Mutational analysis with sequencing of both the mitochondrial genome and nuclear genes implicated in mitochondrial disease is the first line of testing
- For patients in whom suspicion is high and molecular testing is unrevealing, functional assays of electron transport chain activity in liver or muscle can be used

## MANAGEMENT

- There is no definitive management for RCDs. Supportive therapies vary according to organ system involvement
- Consultation with a biochemical geneticist is recommended
- A variety of cofactors, antioxidants, and other agents have been attempted. These include CoQ10, vitamin C, vitamin E, thiamine, carnitine, creatine, alpha lipoic acid, riboflavin, and others. No therapy has been conclusively shown to be effective in improving outcome

## MITOCHONDRIAL DEPLETION SYNDROMES

**Inborn errors in mitochondrial DNA replication, or maintenance of mitochondrial nucleotide pools, resulting in inability to replicate mitochondrial DNA. There are 11 described genes, each with a slightly different presentation.**

## ETIOLOGY

- Mitochondria maintain an independent genome, with their own polymerase, helicase, and nucleotide pools
- Each of these genes for maintenance of the mitochondrial genome is nuclearly encoded

## EPIDEMIOLOGY

- Incidence of at least 1:50,000; varies by ethnic group

## PATHOPHYSIOLOGY

- Decreased efficiency of mitochondrial DNA replication results in decreasing numbers of mitochondria and rapid accumulation of mitochondrial mutations over time
- There is secondary loss of ATP production resulting from depletion of mitochondria and accumulation of errors affecting the respiratory chain

## CLINICAL MANIFESTATIONS

Phenotypes in mitochondrial depletion vary by gene involvement, but typical symptoms include:

- Rapid developmental regression in a previously typical patient
- Seizure, especially epilepsia partialis continua
- Rapidly progressive cerebral volume loss
- Steatosis, transaminitis, decreased synthetic function, hepatic failure
- Hypoglycemia may occur in MPV17 mutations

## DIAGNOSTICS

- Basic metabolic panel, liver function tests, and creatine kinase
- Elevated lactate and lactate/pyruvate ratio in blood, CSF or evidenced on MR spectroscopy
- EEG will differentiate EPC from other movement abnormalities
- Urine organic acids. May reveal elevated lactate, ketones, and TCA cycle intermediates (e.g., $\alpha$-ketoglutarate)
- Molecularly testing targeted to the depletion syndromes provides definitive diagnosis

## MANAGEMENT

- Depletion is inevitably progressive and fatal
- Consultation with a biochemical geneticist is recommended
- As in RCDs, a mitochondrial cocktail may be trialed and continued if providing symptomatic relief, but there is no evidence as to its efficacy

## PYRUVATE DEHYDROGENASE DEFICIENCY

**Pyruvate dehydrogenase (PDH) deficiency is an inborn error resulting in decreased activity of PDH, a mitochondrial enzyme complex that converts pyruvate to acetyl CoA. Inefficient oxidation of carbohydrates and a propensity for lactic acidosis occurs. Assembly and activity of PDH require products of at least nine genes, but the vast majority of patients have dysfunction of the E1$\alpha$ subunit.**

## EPIDEMIOLOGY

- Several hundred cases have been described; incidence unknown
- Despite its X-linked inheritance, PDH E1$\alpha$ deficiency has a similar incidence in males and females. The random nature of X-inactivation leads to a different phenotype in females

## PATHOPHYSIOLOGY

- PDH, the biochemical step between glycolysis and the TCA cycle, is exclusively involved in carbohydrate metabolism
- Inability to generate acetyl CoA from glucose severely limits the amount of energy (ATP) produced per mole of glucose
- Involvement of the CNS reflects the exquisite dependence of the brain on aerobic glucose oxidation for cellular functions
- Lactic acidosis results from the conversion of excess pyruvate to lactate by lactate dehydrogenase

## CLINICAL MANIFESTATIONS

- Severity is variable, and is determined both by residual enzyme activity and, for females, the pattern of X-inactivation
- Involvement of the central nervous system is universal and can cause poor feeding, hypotonia, lethargy, and coma in neonates
- *Two general phenotypes exist:* A "metabolic" presentation of overwhelming, refractory neonatal lactic acidosis (especially in boys with profound E1α deficiency), and a chronic "neurologic" presentation causing developmental delay, seizures, and ataxia (typical in affected girls)
- Prenatal complications (low birth weight, decreased fetal movements, facial dysmorphisms) can occur in severely affected patients
- Degenerative changes in the CNS, including subacute neurodegeneration of the brainstem and basal ganglia (Leigh disease) occur in some patients. Apnea and sudden death may occur as a result of brainstem dysfunction
- Hepatomegaly is uncommon and suggests alternative diagnoses

## DIAGNOSTICS

- Plasma lactate and pyruvate. Elevations of both with a normal or near-normal ratio are strongly suggestive
- Plasma amino acids often reveal an elevated alanine in PDH deficiency and other inborn forms of lactic acidosis
- Lactate may also be elevated in other body fluids, including urine and cerebrospinal fluid. CSF lactate and pyruvate are helpful diagnostic aids in children with neurologic symptoms suspected to have a metabolic disease
- Brain MRI to evaluate structural or degenerative CNS abnormalities. Concurrent MR spectroscopy to measure lactate peaks is very helpful
- For definitive diagnosis, enzyme assays can be performed on a variety of tissues including skin fibroblasts, lymphocytes, and muscle. Various PDH components are examined separately in the assays, often allowing for precise biochemical diagnosis

## MANAGEMENT

- Consultation with biochemical geneticist
- Bicarbonate therapy to treat chronic acid load
- Use caution with dextrose-containing fluids, because glucose loads exacerbate lactic acidosis. Generally safe to start with D5-based solutions if necessary
- *Medications:* Alpha-lipoic acid can be used. A small minority of patients respond to thiamine (0.5–2 g/day)
- Ketogenic (i.e., low carbohydrate) diets have in some cases been associated with improved development. They do not appear to reverse the ultimately fatal course of the disease

## PEROXISOMAL DISORDERS

### PEROXISOMAL BIOGENESIS DISORDERS

**Peroxisomes are an essential organelle, which have the key function of controlling metabolism of very long-chain fats and the synthesis of complex lipids, such as plasmalogens from dietary fats.**

#### EPIDEMIOLOGY

- Overall incidence is 1:50,000
- The previously recognized entities Zellweger syndrome, infantile Refsum disease, and neonatal adrenoleukodystrophy are more properly understood to be points along a spectrum

#### PATHOPHYSIOLOGY

- Complex lipid metabolism is important for generating myelin and bile acids
- Peroxisomes are also important in detoxification of reactive-oxygen species
- All peroxisomal proteins must be targeted into the peroxisome using a very complex process. Targeting errors result in disease

#### CLINICAL MANIFESTATIONS

Disease represents a spectrum from mild to severe.

- Dramatic hypotonia may be noted in infancy
- Dysmorphic facies, including large fontanelle, broad forehead, hypertelorism, and epicanthal folds
- Brain anomalies including cerebellar abnormalities (most common), heterotopias, and cerebral dysplasia
- Seizures
- Retinal degeneration or cataracts
- Sensorineural hearing loss
- Transaminitis, jaundice, and hepatic synthetic failures
- Severe patients usually have developmental regression and death within the first few years of life. More mild patients may escape clinical attention for a few years

#### DIAGNOSTICS

- Very long-chain (branched) fatty acid profile is the initial step (normal testing rules out the disease)
- *In a patient with abnormal VLCFA:* Plasmalogens, pipecolic acid, phytanic acid, pristanic acid, and bile acids differentiate the location of the mutation
- Epiphyseal stippling is highly suggestive
- Brain MRI to look for structural defects

#### MANAGEMENT

- Management is largely supportive

### X-LINKED ADRENOLEUKODYSTROPHY

**The exact etiology of X-linked adrenoleukodystrophy is unknown. It is thought to be involved with the importation of fats into peroxisomes for further processing.**

## EPIDEMIOLOGY

- Overall incidence is 1:21,000 (males); 1:17,000 (males and females)
- X-linked adrenoleukodystrophy is the most common peroxisomal disease

## PATHOPHYSIOLOGY

- Not fully understood
- Very long-chain fats accumulate, likely because they cannot be imported into the peroxisome
- Very long-chain fats are directly adrenotoxic
- Errors in complex fat metabolism likely are partially responsible for leukodystrophy
- Inflammatory component to leukodystrophy with lymphocyte infiltration in the CNS

## CLINICAL MANIFESTATIONS

- Phenotypes of patients affected with X-linked adrenoleukodystrophy vary among: Adrenoleukodystrophy, with onset either in childhood, adolescence, or adulthood; adrenomyeloneuropathy; and isolated adrenal insufficiency
- Female carriers can be symptomatic with either adrenomyeloneuropathy or isolated Addison's, but do not have leukodystrophy
- Deterioration of handwriting is the classic harbinger of disease progression

## DIAGNOSTICS

- Very long-chain (branched) fatty acid profile
- ABCD1 sequencing confirms disease
- Brain MRI with gadolinium to assess degree of leukodystrophy

## MANAGEMENT

- Bone marrow transplant before the onset of neurologic symptoms; usually considered at the earliest sign of radiographic changes or handwriting deterioration
- Physiology adrenal replacement
- The "Lorenzo's Oil" diet, replacing normal dietary fats with a mix of oleic acid and erucic acid has been studied, but benefit is controversial and compliance with the diet is extremely difficult

## CONGENITAL DISORDERS OF GLYCOSYLATION

### GENERAL PRINCIPLES

**Glycosylation refers to the addition of sugars to proteins and lipids. This step is important for trafficking of proteins to the right organelles, and correct enzyme functioning. The role and extent of normal glycosylation is currently being studied.**

## EPIDEMIOLOGY

- Overall incidence—at least 1:10,000 with the most common form PMM2-CDG (CDG 1a) occurring in 1:20,000; likely higher
- PMM2-CDG is especially high in the Dutch population, with a carrier frequency of 1:70
- The number of recognized disorders of glycosylation is increasing exponentially

## PATHOPHYSIOLOGY

- Abnormalities in adding sugars to proteins and lipids cause abnormal molecular targeting
- Disease results from the loss of function of the abnormally glycosylated enzymes

## CLINICAL MANIFESTATIONS

Each disease has unique features, related to the particular defect in glycosylation. Because many of these diseases are rare and likely underdiagnosed, the full spectrum is not well-known and a high index of suspicion is required. Testing should be considered in any patient with neurologic or multi-systemic disease without other etiology.

- *Common symptoms include:*
  - ✓ Hypotonia
  - ✓ Structural brain anomalies, especially cerebellar hypoplasia
  - ✓ Abnormal fat pad distribution
  - ✓ Inverted nipples
  - ✓ Hyperinsulinemic hypoglycemia
  - ✓ Protein-losing enteropathy
  - ✓ Coagulopathy
  - ✓ Liver dysfunction
  - ✓ Eye malformations
  - ✓ Congenital myasthenia

## DIAGNOSTICS

- Transferrin isoelectric-focusing is usually diagnostic
- N-linked glycan analysis looks more closely at the glycosylation profile and can be used to differentiate among CDGs

## MANAGEMENT

- Management is largely supportive
- Mannose has been used successfully to treat MPI-CDG (CDG Ib)

# 17

# Neonatology

*Elisabeth Raab, MD, MPH*
*Tawia A. Apenteng, MD*
*Jennifer M. Brady, MD*
*Mary Catherine Harris, MD*

## APGAR SCORES

The Apgar score was designed to provide a quick, reproducible way to evaluate a newborn's condition following delivery. Scores of 0, 1, or 2 are assigned in each of five categories (respiration, color, tone, heart rate, and reflex irritability) at 1 and 5 minutes after birth. The maximum score is 10. If the 5-minute score is less than 7, additional scores are assigned every 5 minutes until the newborn has a score of 7 or more, up to 20 minutes of age.

- The Apgar score itself does not determine the need for resuscitation as such decisions should often begin prior to Apgar score assignment
- The 1-minute score has not been shown to have predictive value, but a 5-minute score of 0–3 is associated with increased mortality in both preterm and full-term infants
- The change between scores at 1 and 5 minutes may reflect the effectiveness of the resuscitation efforts (Table 17-1)

## NEONATAL RECUSCITATION

Approximately 10% of infants will require some form of resuscitation at birth. Therefore, every delivery should have at least one person trained in neonatal resuscitation present. The Neonatal Resuscitation Program updates the algorithm used for clinical decision-making at delivery periodically, the most recent recommends the actions below.

### CLINICAL DECISION-MAKING

- Following delivery, the infant is warmed and dried and the airway cleared
- Is the infant term gestation, breathing/crying, and have good tone?
  - ✓ If yes to the above and if there are no other issues of concern, the infant may remain with the mother
  - ✓ Additional evaluation as necessary
- Heart rate below 100 bpm or presence of gasping or apnea?
  - ✓ Administer positive pressure ventilation (PPV)
  - ✓ Place pulse oximeter

| TABLE 17-1 | Apgar Score | | |
|---|---|---|---|
| | **0** | **1** | **2** |
| Appearance (color) | Blue or pale | Pink body, blue extremities | Completely pink |
| Pulse (heart rate) | Absent | <100 bpm | >100 bpm |
| Grimace (reflex irritability) | No response | Grimace | Sneeze, cough |
| Activity (muscle tone) | Limp, flaccid | Some flexion | Active movements |
| Respiratory effort | Absent | Gasping; slow, irregular | Regular; good, lusty cry |

bpm, beats per minute.

✓ Administer supplemental oxygen as appropriate (see targeted oxygen saturations below under "Important Considerations")
- If heart rate does not increase
  ✓ Assess adequacy of assisted ventilation
- If heart rate remains <60 bpm
  ✓ Continue PPV
  ✓ Continue to assess adequacy of ventilation
  ✓ Begin chest compressions (coordinate with PPV)
  ✓ Consider endotracheal intubation
  ✓ Consider causes of poor response to resuscitation, including hypovolemia and pneumothorax
  ✓ Consider IV epinephrine
- If heart rate above 100 bpm but labored breathing or cyanosis?
  ✓ Clear airway
  ✓ Administer supplemental oxygen as appropriate
  ✓ Consider continuous positive airway pressure (CPAP)

## IMPORTANT CONSIDERATIONS

- *Targeted Oxygen Saturations:* If assisted ventilation is required, a pre-ductal pulse oximeter should be placed on right hand and the fraction of inspired oxygen ($FiO_2$) titrated to goal oxygen saturations by minute of life:
  ✓ 60–65% by 1 minute
  ✓ 65–70% by 2 minutes
  ✓ 70–75% by 3 minutes
  ✓ 75–80% by 4 minutes
  ✓ 80–85% by 5 minutes
  ✓ 85–95% by 10 minutes
  ✓ Full-term infants should initially be resuscitated with 21% $FiO_2$
  ✓ Preterm infants often receive a slightly higher initial $FiO_2$, but rarely 100% when resuscitation is begun
- *Steps to Correct Inadequate Assisted Ventilation:* MRSOPA: M = Mask adjustment, R = Reposition airway, S = Suction nose and mouth, O = Open mouth, P = Pressure increase, A = Airway alternative
- *Meconium Delivery:* An infant needs to meet all three of the following criteria to be considered vigorous: (1) normal respiratory effort, (2) normal muscle tone, and (3) heart rate >100 bpm. If the newborn is vigorous, proceed with routine neonatal resuscitation. If the newborn is not vigorous, do not stimulate. Instead, intubate and suction below the cords for 3 seconds before removing the endotracheal tube. One can repeat tracheal suctioning if meconium is present below the cords and the infant is stable. If no meconium is obtained or the infant becomes unstable, then precede with standard neonatal resuscitation
- *Primary Apnea:* Absence of respiratory effort in the perinatal period that responds to stimulation
- *Secondary Apnea:* Absence of respiratory effort in the perinatal period that does not respond to stimulation, and requires PPV in order to resolve

## APPARENT LIFE-THREATENING EVENT

**Apparent life-threatening event (ALTE) is not a specific diagnosis but rather a general term used to describe an event. ALTE is defined by the National Institutes of Health as "an episode that is frightening to the observer and that is characterized by some combination**

of apnea (central or occasionally obstructive), color change (usually cyanotic or pallid but occasionally erythematous or plethoric), marked change in muscle tone (usually marked limpness), choking, or gagging. In some cases the observer fears that the infant has died."

- *Apnea:* Absence of spontaneous ventilation for 20 seconds or shorter duration if associated with cyanosis or bradycardia
- *Central apnea:* Absence of respiratory effort due to lack of brainstem excitation
- *Obstructive apnea:* Sustained respiratory effort without airflow due to obstruction of the upper airway
- *Mixed apnea:* A combination of central and obstructive apnea
- *Periodic breathing:* A pattern of breathing defined by three or more pauses in respiration, each lasting more than 3 seconds, separated by less than 20 seconds of normal breathing

## EPIDEMIOLOGY

- *Incidence:* 0.5–6%; peaks between 1 and 3 months

## DIFFERENTIAL DIAGNOSIS

- *Normal physiologic variation:* Normal infants may exhibit pauses in breathing of up to 10–20 seconds during sleep
- *Apnea of infancy:* Unexplained pauses in breathing that last longer than 20 seconds or accompanied by cyanosis, pallor, hypotonia, or bradycardia. These events usually cease by 43 weeks postconception
- *Gastrointestinal:* Gastroesophageal reflux, volvulus
- *Infections:* Respiratory viral infections particularly respiratory syncytial virus (RSV), pertussis, pneumonia, sepsis, urinary tract infection, meningitis
- *Metabolic:* Inborn errors of metabolism, hypoglycemia, hypocalcemia
- *Hematologic:* Anemia
- *Cardiovascular:* Conduction disorders (prolonged QT), congenital heart disease, cardiomyopathy
- *Respiratory:* Airway anomalies, foreign-body aspiration, breath-holding spells
- *Neurologic:* Seizures, intracranial hemorrhage, increased intracranial pressure
- *Child abuse:* Non-accidental head trauma, poisoning, suffocation, Munchausen syndrome by proxy, factitious illness, drug effect

## CLINICAL MANIFESTATIONS

- Apnea, cyanosis, and difficulty breathing are most commonly reported
- Pallor, stiffness, floppiness, choking, red face, abnormal limb movements, vomiting
- Physical exam is often normal after the event resolves

## DIAGNOSTICS

- There is no standard ALTE workup. Decisions regarding the appropriate work up are usually driven by the history and physical exam
- *Thorough history:* Determine the exact details of the event, including duration, preceding circumstances, relationship to feeding, location of the infant, and necessary intervention. Ask about the presence of respiratory effort, color change, choking, gasping, emesis, limpness, stiffness, rhythmic movements, eye movements, nasal congestion, hypothermia, and fever. Talk to all caregivers and eyewitnesses. Try to determine the severity of the event
- *Thorough physical exam:* Focus on neurologic, respiratory, and cardiac exams; include pulse oximetry and fundoscopy
- Laboratory and radiology studies are not routinely necessary. The decision to perform testing should be informed by the information obtained through history and physical exam

- *Studies to initially consider based on differential diagnosis:* CBC with differential, serum electrolytes, glucose
- *Other possible initial studies:* Serum ammonia and lactate, chest radiograph, electrocardiogram, urinalysis, urine toxicology screen, nasal swab for pertussis and respiratory viruses
- *Full sepsis evaluation:* If the infant is ill appearing or the event was severe, may need blood, urine, and cerebrospinal fluid cultures
- *Electroencephalogram (EEG):* Obtain if concerned about seizure
- *Head imaging:* Obtain a head ultrasound to evaluate for intraventricular hemorrhage and a head CT if concerned about non-accidental head trauma
- *Metabolic workup:* Newborn screen, plasma ammonia, blood lactate/pyruvate, plasma and urine amino acids, urine organic acids, urine ketones and reducing substances, and consultation with a metabolic disease specialist
- *Gastrointestinal imaging:* Milk scan to evaluate for reflux and upper gastrointestinal series to evaluate the GI anatomy
- *Pneumogram:* Not typically necessary but can help differentiate between central and obstructive apnea. The four-channel pneumogram includes a nasal thermistor to detect airflow, pulse oximeter to detect saturations, and chest leads to monitor heart rate and chest wall movement. A five-channel pneumogram includes a naso-esophageal pH probe to identify acid reflux and its relationship to apneic episodes

## MANAGEMENT

- Consider admission for period of observation and investigation. Place infant on continuous cardiorespiratory monitoring. Record further events and associated factors in detail
- Specific treatment should be directed toward results of the investigation
- Antibiotics are warranted if there is a concern for sepsis
- Risk factors for significant disease include age above 2 months, abnormal findings on physical exam, lactate level greater than 2, and recurrent ALTE
- ALTEs typically cause a high level of parental anxiety. Decisions regarding discharging an infant with a home apnea and bradycardia monitor can be difficult. The American Academy of Pediatrics (AAP) Policy Statement on Apnea, Sudden Infant Death Syndrome (SIDS), and Home Monitoring includes ALTE as an indication for home monitoring. However, parents must be informed that apnea is not predictive of or a precursor to SIDS. There is also no evidence that home cardiorespiratory monitoring prevents SIDS. If a monitor is used, the AAP recommends discontinuing it by approximately 43 weeks postconception or when extreme events cease to occur, whichever comes last

## INFANT OF A DIABETIC MOTHER

**The infant born to a diabetic mother (IDM) is at an increased risk of morbidity and mortality and thus warrants special attention.**

### EPIDEMIOLOGY

- Gestational diabetes (GDM) occurs in 1 and 11.6% of screened pregnancies in countries with advanced economies
- IDMs have a 2–3 times higher risk of congenital malformations compared to the children of nondiabetic mothers. Perinatal mortality is 3–10 times higher than in the general population

### PATHOPHYSIOLOGY

- Glucose crosses the placenta. Maternal hyperglycemia results in fetal hyperglycemia and subsequently increased fetal insulin production during the second half of pregnancy

- Elevated levels of insulin result in fat production (which leads to macrosomia) and increased glycogen content in liver, kidney, skeletal muscle, and the heart (which contributes to visceromegaly). Increased insulin levels also delay fetal lung maturation
- Chronic fetal hyperinsulinism increases the metabolic rate and oxygen consumption, leading to fetal hypoxia. In addition, elevated glycated hemoglobin in women with long-standing diabetes increases the affinity of maternal hemoglobin for oxygen, causing a decrease in oxygen transfer to the fetus. These changes contribute to the greater risk of fetal asphyxia and intrauterine fetal demise in IDMs
- Hypoxia stimulates erythropoietin production, potentially resulting in polycythemia in the neonate
- The exact mechanism(s) underlying the increased risk of malformations is/are unclear. However, the association between malformations and poor maternal glycemic control at the time of conception and early gestation is well established and rigorous maternal glycemic control has been shown to improve perinatal morbidity and mortality

## CLINICAL MANIFESTATIONS

- *Hypoglycemia:* Newborns have transient hypoglycemia after delivery and disruption of the maternal glucose supply. Glucose levels typically stabilize soon after birth. IDMs however, may have earlier, more profound and more persistent hypoglycemia than normal newborns due to elevated insulin levels. Macrosomic infants, though they have plentiful fat stores, may be less able than normal newborns to mobilize glucose from these reserves. The hypoglycemia is often asymptomatic, but symptoms can occur and may include tachypnea, apnea, tremors, diaphoresis, irritability, and seizures
- *Macrosomia and large for gestational age (LGA):* Macrosomia and maternal diabetes are both independent risk factors for shoulder dystocia and coexisting brachial plexus injury. Clavicle and humerus fractures are also associated complications
- *Congenital malformations:* The most common malformations involve the heart, central nervous system, kidneys and urinary tract, skeletal system, and gastrointestinal tract. Presenting signs and symptoms vary depending on the anomaly/anomalies present. Clinicians should maintain a high index of suspicion for underlying anomalies, particularly in the offspring of mothers known to have poor glycemic control
- *Respiratory distress syndrome (RDS):* IDMs born at less than 38 weeks gestation have a six times higher risk of RDS compared to gestational age matched non-IDMs. RDS typically presents as increased work of breathing and/or hypoxia
- *Perinatal asphyxia:* The increased risk of perinatal asphyxia is greatest in the offspring of mothers with preexisting diabetes, most notably those with renal and atherosclerotic disease and/or a long history of unstable glucose control. Clinical findings in asphyxiated newborns include hypotonia and poor respiratory effort at birth and seizures in the neonatal period
- *Hypocalcemia:* Hypocalcemia is a consequence of transient hypoparathyroidism that results from fetal and maternal hypomagnesemia. Hypocalcemia may result in irritability and decreased myocardial function. Hypomagnesemia is typically asymptomatic
- *Hematologic manifestations:* IDMs are at increased risk of polycythemia, hyperbilirubinemia, and venous thrombosis
- *Hypertrophic cardiomyopathy:* The cardiomyopathy typically seen in IDMs is characterized by septal hypertrophy. In severe cases there may be marked hypertrophy of the myocardium as well. Although the hypertrophy typically resolves over the first few months of life, some infants may be critically ill in the newborn period due to outflow tract obstruction and cardiac dysfunction
- *Gastrointestinal issues:* Small left colon and intestinal hypomotility are the most commonly encountered gastrointestinal issues

- Research has raised concerns regarding the possibility of delayed growth and development, impaired psychosocial and intellectual capabilities, and an increased future risk of developing diabetes in IDMs

## DIAGNOSTICS

- The definition of neonatal hypoglycemia is controversial and the level and duration of hypoglycemia that cause injury are unknown. Blood glucose should be monitored for IDMs by at least 2 hours following delivery. The AAP recommends feeding asymptomatic IDMs within 1 hour of birth and checking the first glucose level 30 minutes after the first feed. The report recommends continued monitoring of pre-feed blood sugars in IDMs for the first 24 hours of life or until the glucose levels remain >45 mg/dL. Low values (<40–45 mg/dL) should be confirmed with a serum sample
- Glucose levels should also be checked in symptomatic neonates. Evaluation of calcium and magnesium levels may be appropriate in infants who have demonstrated other metabolic derangements
- Consider a chest x-ray and blood gas if there is concern about respiratory distress, hypoxemia, and/or cardiovascular instability. Echocardiography is useful for patients suspected of having a congenital cardiac anomaly or clinically significant cardiomyopathy
- Consider hematocrit and bilirubin monitoring if there is concern for polycythemia and/or jaundice
- Cranial ultrasound is appropriate when perinatal asphyxia or intracranial thrombosis is suspected

## MANAGEMENT

### Management of Hypoglycemia

- Most transient, moderate hypoglycemia in the newborn can be treated effectively with early enteral feeding. Gavage feeds may be considered in certain patients. The blood sugar should be rechecked 30–60 minutes after an intervention to ensure an adequate response to therapy
- Symptomatic or severe hypoglycemia is typically treated with initiation of continuous intravenous (IV) glucose and a 2 mL/kg bolus of a 10% IV glucose solution. Continuous IV glucose is typically initiated at an infusion rate of 4–6 mg/kg/min and subsequently titrated as needed to maintain euglycemia (often defined as blood glucose greater than 50 mg/dL). Blood sugars are then typically monitored every 30–60 minutes until stable. It may be appropriate in some situations to start a continuous glucose infusion and omit the 2 mL/kg glucose bolus unless hypoglycemia persists
- It is important to remember that hypoglycemia may be a sign of other pathologic processes in the newborn and one should consider other etiologies if symptoms do not abate with therapy (e.g., sepsis, pneumonia, cold stress, polycythemia, inborn errors of metabolism, asphyxia)

### Other Management Issues

- *Metabolic:* Symptomatic or severe hypocalcemia is treated with calcium gluconate. When there is coexisting hypomagnesemia it should be treated with magnesium therapy in order to allow for effective correction of hypocalcemia
- *Cardiorespiratory:* Infants with perinatal asphyxia, RDS, congenital heart disease, and hypertrophic cardiomyopathy may require management in an intensive care setting. Late preterm infants with RDS may benefit from administration of surfactant. Emergent consultation with a cardiologist is appropriate for patients with cyanotic heart disease, in particular to expeditiously determine the need for prostaglandins

- *Hematologic:* Hyperbilirubinemia and polycythemia should be managed as described elsewhere in this chapter. Significant deep vessel thromboses are often treated with low molecular weight heparin with the guidance of a hematologist
- IDMs should be monitored for signs and symptoms of birth injury and congenital malformations

## MECONIUM ASPIRATION SYNDROME

**A common cause of neonatal respiratory pathology characterized by in utero or perinatal aspiration of meconium-stained amniotic fluid (MSAF) that causes respiratory distress.**

### EPIDEMIOLOGY

- Approximately 13% of all deliveries are associated with MSAF
- Approximately 5–12% of neonates delivered through MSAF develop meconium aspiration syndrome (MAS)

### PATHOPHYSIOLOGY

- Passage of meconium seldom occurs before 34 weeks gestational age. It occurs most commonly in full-term and post-dates infants. It is related to fetal distress, which leads to a hypoxia-induced vagal response causing passage of meconium
- The meconium is aspirated during gasping in utero and/or perinatally, causing airway obstruction by ball-valve mechanism. This results in simultaneous atelectasis and overexpansion, potentially leading to air leaks
- Chemical inflammation (pneumonitis) causes alveolar collapse and parenchymal damage. Inhibition of surfactant causes alveolar collapse and decreased lung compliance
- Persistent pulmonary hypertension of the newborn (PPHN) can occur as a result of hypoxia-induced pulmonary artery vasoconstriction and failure to transition to postnatal circulation

### RISK FACTORS

- Post-dates, small for gestational age, placental insufficiency, cord compression, fetal distress

### CLINICAL MANIFESTATIONS

- Meconium staining of nails, skin, umbilical cord, placenta
- *Respiratory exam:* Often presents with initial respiratory depression followed by tachypnea, retractions, grunting, flaring, prolonged expiratory phase, rales, rhonchi, barrel chest with increased antero-posterior diameter, cyanosis
- Neurologic depression may be present

### DIAGNOSTICS

- *Chest x-ray:* Classic appearance is coarse, streaky, nodular pulmonary densities, often distributed asymmetrically. May see hyperinflation with flattening of the diaphragms. Other possible findings include pneumothorax, pneumomediastinum, pleural effusion, and cardiomegaly (secondary to hypoxia)
- *Arterial blood gas:* Hypoxemia, respiratory and/or metabolic acidosis from hypoxia. Can also show respiratory alkalosis from hyperventilation
- *Pre- and post-ductal pulse oximetry:* Used to evaluate right to left shunting through a patent ductus arteriosus (PDA). A difference in saturations of >5% suggests PPHN is present, however if absent, it does not exclude PPHN

## MANAGEMENT

### Prevention (Perinatal Interventions)

- *Amnioinfusion:* Injection of normal saline into the amniotic sac to decrease cord compression and dilute meconium (efficacy unclear)
- Intrapartum suctioning of the oropharynx at the perineum by the obstetrician as soon as the head is visible is no longer routinely recommended as it does not prevent or alter the course of MAS
- Tracheal intubation and suctioning to remove meconium from the airway for "depressed" neonates (absent or depressed respirations, heart rate <100 beats per minute, poor muscle tone) before stimulation and initiation of positive pressure in the delivery room

### Postnatal Management

- Observation and monitoring in the neonatal intensive care unit, as patients can rapidly decompensate
- Correction of acid–base status
- Chest physiotherapy and suctioning
- Noninvasive supplemental oxygen or mechanical ventilation
- Minimal stimulation to prevent hypoxia
- Antibiotic therapy for possible pneumonia
- Maintenance of normal body temperature (unless there is associated asphyxia and encephalopathy that meets criteria for therapeutic hypothermia)
- *Treatment of PPHN:* Liberal use of oxygen, hyperventilation, alkalinization, nitric oxide, vasopressors, fluid resuscitation
- *Additional therapies:* Surfactant, high-frequency mechanical ventilation, sedation, paralysis and in severe cases, extracorporeal membrane oxygenation

## NEONATAL HYPERBILIRUBINEMIA

**A common and often benign problem of newborn infants.**

- *Unconjugated hyperbilirubinemia:* Elevation of indirect serum bilirubin
- *Conjugated hyperbilirubinemia:* Direct bilirubin level greater than 2.0 mg/dL or direct fraction greater than 15–20% of total serum bilirubin
- *Kernicterus:* Pathologic findings of bilirubin toxicity in the brain, associated with staining and necrosis of neurons in the basal ganglia, hippocampus, subthalamic nuclei, and cerebellum. Clinical syndrome is characterized by cerebral palsy, mental retardation, uncoordinated movements, deafness, poor vision, and feeding and speech difficulties. Bilirubin levels greater than 25 mg/dL in otherwise healthy, term, or near-term infants are generally considered to be a risk factor for kernicterus
- *Jaundice:* Yellowing of skin, sclerae, and mucous membranes due to high levels of serum bilirubin
- *Physiologic jaundice:* Elevation of unconjugated bilirubin that occurs in most infants during the first week of life and resolves spontaneously. Mean levels are about 5–6 mg/dL in bottle-fed white and African American infants on the third day of life. Levels in breast-fed infants are higher (mean: 8–9 mg/dL) and peak later (fourth to fifth day)

## EPIDEMIOLOGY

- Jaundice is observed in about 60% of term infants

## ETIOLOGY

### Unconjugated Hyperbilirubinemia

- *Increased Production:* Polycythemia, hemolytic anemia (ABO or Rh incompatibility, glucose-6-phosphate dehydrogenase [G6PD] deficiency, hereditary spherocytosis, sepsis), cephalohematoma
- *Decreased Clearance:* Crigler–Najjar, Gilbert
- *Increased Enterohepatic Circulation:* Breast-feeding jaundice, breast-milk jaundice, intestinal obstruction

### Conjugated Hyperbilirubinemia

- *Anatomic:* Biliary atresia, choledochal cyst, compression of the bile duct, other disorders of the biliary system
- *Infectious:* Sepsis, intrauterine infection, urinary tract infection, other viral and bacterial etiologies
- *Genetic/Inborn errors of metabolism:* Galactosemia, fructosemia, Niemann–Pick disease, cystic fibrosis, Alagille syndrome, many others
- *Miscellaneous:* Total parenteral nutrition-induced cholestasis, medications, hypothyroidism, neonatal hemochromatosis

## PATHOPHYSIOLOGY

- Physiologic jaundice is thought to be due to a combination of increased bilirubin load in neonates (larger RBC volume, shorter RBC life-span), decreased uptake of bilirubin by the liver, defective conjugation of bilirubin, and impaired excretion (bilirubin is excreted in stool and urine)
- Breast-fed infants are at higher risk of indirect hyperbilirubinemia in the first week of life than formula-fed infants due to relative dehydration and increased intestinal reabsorption of bilirubin (breast-feeding jaundice). Additionally, about 2% of breast-fed infants develop indirect hyperbilirubinemia after the first week of life due to factors associated with human breast-milk (breast-milk jaundice)
- Jaundice in the first 24 hours of life is generally pathologic

## CLINICAL MANIFESTATIONS

- *Jaundice:* Clinically visible at bilirubin levels about 5–7 mg/dL; first apparent in the face and then descends as levels increase
- *Early neurologic findings (bilirubin encephalopathy):* Lethargy, poor feeding, emesis, hypotonia
- *Later neurologic findings:* High-pitched cry, hypertonia, opisthotonus, seizures, fever
- *Associated physical findings:* Cephalohematoma, petechiae, purpura, signs of prematurity or intrauterine growth retardation, plethora, hepatomegaly, splenomegaly, light-colored stools, dark urine

## DIAGNOSTICS

- *Serum bilirubin level:* Total, conjugated, unconjugated
- *Initial laboratory tests:* CBC and reticulocyte count, blood smear, blood type (mother and infant), Rh status (mother and infant), direct Coombs test. Laboratory tests to include when bilirubin level found to be extremely elevated: electrolytes (to assess hydration), serum albumin
- *Other laboratory tests to consider:* Urine for reducing substances, G6PD level, hemoglobin electrophoresis, osmotic fragility, thyroid function, liver function, PT/PTT, blood and urine cultures, serum amino acids, urine organic acids

- *Other studies to consider:* Liver ultrasound, hepatobiliary imaging (e.g., DISIDA scan), percutaneous liver biopsy

## MANAGEMENT

### Unconjugated Hyperbilirubinemia

- *Ensure adequate hydration:* Consider supplementation of breast-fed babies with formula and/or IV fluids
- *Phototherapy:* Light energy converts unconjugated bilirubin to a structural isomer, which can be excreted without conjugation. Blue lamps (420–480 nm) are most effective. The AAP recommends initiating phototherapy in *healthy, term, or near-term infants* based on day of life and risk factors (Figure 17-1). Note that nomogram values are based on total serum bilirubin levels. Phototherapy should be initiated at lower levels for premature infants
- *Exchange transfusion:* Double volume exchange transfusions are reserved for infants at high risk of kernicterus. Consider exchange transfusion in healthy, term infants with total bilirubin levels of 25–30 mg/dL. When approaching exchange transfusion levels, a serum albumin level is recommended as bilirubin bound to albumin is less likely to cross the blood–brain barrier. In infants with specific risk factors, consider exchange transfusion at lower bilirubin levels
- *IVIG:* To be considered in cases related to ABO or Rh incompatibility. Studies have shown conflicting evidence as to efficacy. The exact mechanism of action is unknown, but it is thought to block RBC antibody receptors from maternal antibodies
- Treat underlying disorder if jaundice is non-physiologic

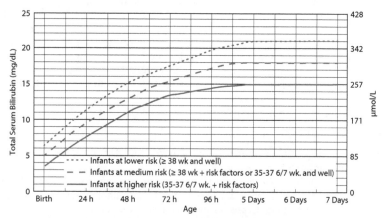

- Use total bilirubin. Do not subtract direct reacting or conjugated bilirubin.
- Risk factors = isoimmune hemolytic disease, G6PD deficiency, asphyxia, significant lethargy, temperature instability, sepsis, acidosis, or albumin < 3.0g/dL (if measured)
- For well infants 35-37 6/7 wk can adjust TSB levels for intervention around the medium risk line. It is an option to intervene at lower TSB levels for infants closer to 35 wks and at higher TSB levels for those closer to 37 6/7 wk.
- It is an option to provide conventional phototherapy in hospital or at home at TSB levels 2-3 mg/dL (35-50mmol/L) below those shown but home phototherapy should not be used in any infant with risk factors.

FIGURE 17-1 **Bilirubin nomogram.** In infants born at ≥35 weeks gestational age, this nomogram designates the total serum bilirubin level at which to initiate phototherapy (based on risk factors and hours of life). (Reproduced with permission from American Academy of Pediatrics Subcommittee on Hyperbilirubinemia: Management of hyperbilirubinemia in the newborn infant 35 or more weeks of gestation, Pediatrics 2004 Jul;114(1):297-316)

### Conjugated Hyperbilirubinemia

- Management is aimed at treatment of the underlying disorder
- Phenobarbital, cholestyramine, and ursodiol may promote bile flow and decrease serum bilirubin levels
- *Dietary management:* Formulas containing medium chain triglycerides are better absorbed; supplement vitamins A, D, E, and K
- Kasai procedure (hepatoportoenterostomy) is used as bridge to transplantation in infants with biliary atresia

## HEMOLYTIC DISEASE: ABO INCOMPATIBILITY

**Hemolysis caused by maternal–fetal ABO blood group incompatibility and resultant transplacental passage of maternal IgG to the fetus is a major cause of neonatal hyperbilirubinemia. Usually the mother is group O, and the newborn is group A or B.**

### EPIDEMIOLOGY

- ABO incompatibility occurs in approximately 20–25% of all pregnancies, but only 0.3–2.2% of infants are symptomatic
- More common if the newborn is blood type B, Asian, or African

### PATHOPHYSIOLOGY

- Mothers with type O blood do not have A or B antigens. Type O mothers produce anti-A and anti-B antibodies throughout life in response to exposure to gram-negative bacteria and other foreign antigens. Sensitization from a previous pregnancy is NOT required to cause disease
- Maternal anti-A and anti-B IgG antibodies cross the placenta
- IgG can attach to fetal red blood cells (RBCs), prompting hemolysis and release of unconjugated bilirubin. Removal of the unconjugated bilirubin in utero occurs via the placenta. After birth, removal occurs via the infant's hepatobiliary system
- Disease is usually mild as compared to disease from Rh incompatibility because A and B antigens are expressed on many tissues other than RBCs. Thus, maternal antibodies attach to the other sites, leaving less to attach to RBCs

### CLINICAL MANIFESTATIONS

- Jaundice in the first 24 hours of life is a hallmark of hemolysis

### DIAGNOSTICS

- Type and screen reveal ABO incompatibility between mother and newborn
- Direct Coombs test result is often, but not always, positive
- CBC (usually normal to mildly decreased hemoglobin)
- Reticulocyte count (can be normal or increased)
- Peripheral smear (spherocytosis is characteristic)
- Conjugated and unconjugated bilirubin levels (usually increased indirect and total bilirubin levels)
- High reticulocyte count, positive Coombs, and previous sibling with neonatal jaundice are predictors for significant or severe disease

### MANAGEMENT

- Maintain adequate hydration
- Initiate phototherapy. Consider IVIG if bilirubin levels are rising rapidly or phototherapy is not sufficient (see Hyperbilirubinemia)

- Exchange transfusion with type O blood of same Rh type as the infant is occasionally required. Type O blood is used (universal donor) because it is compatible with the infant's blood type and also does not react with circulating maternal antibodies
- Follow-up to detect late-onset hemolytic anemia occasionally requiring packed RBC transfusion

## HEMOLYTIC DISEASE: RH INCOMPATIBLITY

**An often severe hemolytic anemia in the fetus and newborn caused by maternal–fetal blood group incompatibility of the Rhesus D antigen (Rh) and resultant transplacental passage of IgG antibodies from a previously sensitized mother to her fetus.**

### EPIDEMIOLOGY

- 11–35% prevalence of RhD(–) phenotype among Caucasians; prevalence is much lower in African American and Asian populations
- Anti-D immunoglobulin for prevention of sensitization has reduced incidence of disease to approximately 10.6 cases per 10,000 live births

### PATHOPHYSIOLOGY

- Mothers who are RhD(–) carry fetuses with paternally derived Rh antigen
- RhD(+) fetal RBCs cross into the maternal circulation during pregnancy or delivery with subsequent maternal antibody production against the foreign Rh antigen. RBCs also cross over with transplacental hemorrhage (e.g., cesarean section, toxemia)
- During subsequent pregnancies, maternal IgG anti-Rh antibodies cross the placenta and attach to fetal RBCs, prompting hemolysis and removal
- Rh disease is usually more severe than disease from ABO incompatibility because Rh antigens are only expressed on RBCs
- ABO incompatibility partially protects against Rh sensitization by causing rapid removal of RhD(+) fetal cells from maternal circulation by anti-A or B antibodies. This is only beneficial if Rh sensitization has not yet occurred

### CLINICAL MANIFESTATIONS

- Fetal hydrops
- Anemia
- Jaundice in the first 24 hours of life
- Hypoglycemia due to islet cell hyperplasia of the pancreas
- Thrombocytopenia from liver dysfunction, disseminated intravascular coagulation, and/or repeated intrauterine transfusions
- *Physical exam:* Jaundice, signs of hydrops (ascites, pleural effusions, edema), pallor, petechia/purpura, hepatosplenomegaly (due to extramedullary hematopoiesis and splenic sequestration)

### DIAGNOSTICS

- Type and Coombs (RhD(+) infant and RhD(–) mother with Positive direct Coombs test)
- CBC (usually decreased hemoglobin with increased nucleated RBCs)
- Reticulocyte count (usually increased)
- Conjugated and unconjugated bilirubin levels (usually increased indirect and total bilirubin levels)

## MANAGEMENT

### Prevention

- Anti-D immunoglobulin prevents Rh sensitization and should be given to RhD(−) mothers at 28–36 weeks estimated gestational age and at delivery. An additional dose of anti-D should be given to mothers when transplacental hemorrhage is suspected

### In Utero Evaluation and Management

- Follow maternal titer monthly throughout pregnancy (titer >16 associated with increased risk of hydrops and death)
- Assessment of fetal anemia:
  ✓ Doppler blood flow in umbilical vein (increased velocity associated with anemia)
  ✓ *Amniocentesis:* To measure hemolytic products (bilirubin) in the amniotic fluid
  ✓ *Cordocentesis:* Ultrasound guided fetal umbilical blood sampling. This also allows access for fetal transfusion if needed

### Postnatal Management

- Initiate phototherapy. Consider IVIG if bilirubin levels are rising rapidly or phototherapy is not sufficient (see Hyperbilirubinemia)
- Exchange transfusion is sometimes required
- *Hydropic infants frequently require intensive care including:* (1) Therapeutic paracentesis or thoracentesis, (2) mechanical ventilation, (3) volume expanders, (4) vasopressors, (5) diuretics, (6) isovolumetric partial exchange transfusion, among other therapies
- Late anemia may develop following Rh isoimmunization

## POLYCYTHEMIA

A venous hematocrit (HCT) greater than 65%. Polycythemic neonates are at risk for hyperviscosity, which can compromise perfusion.

### EPIDEMIOLOGY

- *Incidence of polycythemia:* 1–5%; highest at high altitudes
- More common in small for gestational age neonates (10–15% affected)

### PATHOPHYSIOLOGY

- A normal response to the relative hypoxic intrauterine environment is to increase RBC mass, causing a relative polycythemia
- Polycythemia may occur because of increased red cell mass secondary to chronic intrauterine hypoxia (intrauterine growth retardation, maternal diabetes, maternal smoking). Factors that increase fetal blood volume, such as delayed cord clamping, positioning the infant below the introitus after delivery, maternal–fetal transfusion, and twin–twin transfusion, also increase risk
- Viscosity is directly proportional to HCT but rises logarithmically above an HCT of 60%. When viscosity is increased, blood flow is impaired and tissue perfusion is decreased
- *Other causes of polycythemia include:* Infants of diabetic mothers, congenital hypothyroidism, neonatal thyrotoxicosis, congenital adrenal hyperplasia, Beckwith–Wiedemann syndrome, and trisomies 13, 18, and 21

### CLINICAL MANIFESTATIONS

- Most neonates with polycythemia are asymptomatic
- *Cutaneous symptoms:* Plethora, delayed capillary refill

- *CNS symptoms:* Lethargy, apnea, tremors/jitteriness, poor feeding, hypotonia, an exaggerated startle response. Strokes and seizures are rare
- *Cardiopulmonary symptoms:* Tachypnea, cyanosis, tachycardia, respiratory distress, cardiomegaly. Prominent vascular markings on chest radiograph, elevated pulmonary vascular resistance, and congestive heart failure are also possible
- *Metabolic symptoms:* Hypoglycemia is the most common. Hypocalcemia and hyperbilirubinemia are also possible
- *Renal symptoms:* Renal dysfunction can present as oliguria, proteinuria, or hematuria. Renal vein thrombosis and renal failure are rare
- *Other rare complications:* Thrombus, thrombocytopenia, disseminated intravascular coagulation, necrotizing enterocolitis

## DIAGNOSTICS

- HCT peaks at 2 hours of life and then progressively decreases, stabilizing by 6–24 hours after birth. At 2 hours of life, it is common to use 70% as the upper limit of normal
- Capillary HCTs are significantly higher than venous values, and should only be used as a screening test. If the capillary value is above 65%, repeat with a venous stick. Blood obtained from arterial and umbilical vessels may yield a lower HCT. [HCT level by sample site: Arterial<Venous<Capillary]
- *Other potential studies to obtain in the setting of polycythemia:* Serum glucose, calcium, bilirubin, electrolytes, platelets and blood gas, urine specific gravity

## MANAGEMENT

- *Partial exchange transfusion (PET):* Mainstay of therapy for symptomatic neonates with HCT greater than 65% or any neonate with a venous HCT greater than 70% (although this is controversial). While there is no evidence that PET improves long-term outcomes in neonates with polycythemia, there is a trend toward earlier resolution of symptoms
  ✓ The goal for PET is to decrease HCT to 50%–55%
  ✓ Volume to exchange (mL) is calculated by

$$\frac{\text{Blood volume} \times (\text{Observed HCT} - \text{Desired HCT})}{\text{Observed HCT}}$$

  *Estimated blood volume = 100 mL/kg
  ✓ Normal saline has become the replacement fluid of choice
  ✓ Blood should be removed using a central venous or arterial line. Replacement fluid is infused via a peripheral IV line
  ✓ Repeat HCT at end of procedure and 4–6 hours later
- Asymptomatic neonates with HCT between 60 and 70% can be managed by liberalizing fluid intake and repeating HCT in 4–6 hours

## TORCH INFECTIONS

A group of perinatally acquired nonbacterial infections with overlapping manifestations. Toxoplasmosis, syphilis, rubella, and CMV are discussed here. (See Infectious Diseases chapter [Chapter 15] for detailed discussion on herpes simplex virus infection).

## FINDINGS THAT SUGGEST TORCH INFECTION

- Intrauterine growth retardation, hydrops fetalis, CNS abnormalities (microcephaly, hydrocephalus, intracranial calcifications), hepatosplenomegaly, bone abnormalities (osteochondritis, periostitis), myocarditis, ocular abnormalities (cataracts, chorioretinitis, glaucoma), anemia, and thrombocytopenia

## GENERAL APPROACH TO EVALUATION FOR TORCH

- *Blood:* IgM (rubella, *Toxoplasma*), IgA and IgE (*Toxoplasma*), RPR (syphilis), hepatitis B surface antigen, polymerase chain reaction (PCR) (*Toxoplasma*)
- *Cerebrospinal fluid:* PCR (enterovirus, HSV, *Toxoplasma*), VDRL (syphilis)
- Skin lesion: Direct fluorescent antibody (HSV, varicella), dark-field microscopy (syphilis)
- *Viral culture:* Conjunctiva (HSV); mouth/throat (CMV, enterovirus, HSV, rubella); rectum (enterovirus, HSV); urine (CMV by rapid shell vial, rubella)
- Ophthalmology exam (CMV, HSV, rubella, syphilis, *Toxoplasma*, varicella)
- Hearing screen (CMV, rubella, *Toxoplasma*)
- Head US, Head CT (CMV, *Toxoplasma*)
- *Additional studies:* Liver function tests, complete blood count
- Check the mother's prenatal laboratory results (including rubella, hepatitis B, and syphilis testing)

## TOXOPLASMOSIS

### TRANSMISSION AND DISEASE

- Maternal infection with *Toxoplasma gondii* occurs via ingestion of cysts from infected meat or from contact with cat excrement
- Transmission ensues if primary infection occurs during pregnancy
- The risk of transmission to the fetus increases with advancing gestational age at time of maternal infection, with an overall risk of 20–50%
- The severity of disease in the infant is inversely proportional to the gestational age at time of infection; therefore the disease is most severe if infection occurs in the first trimester

### CLINICAL MANIFESTATIONS

- 70–90% are asymptomatic at birth
- Visual impairment, learning disabilities, or mental retardation become apparent several months to years later
- The most common clinical finding is chorioretinitis
- Other findings include hydrocephalus with generalized calcifications, microcephaly, mental retardation, seizures, opisthotonos, microphthalmia, deafness, lymphadenopathy, hepatosplenomegaly, jaundice

### DIAGNOSIS

- Serologic diagnosis in the infant is based on positive IgM or IgA assay within first 6 months of life or persistently positive IgG titers beyond 12 months
- May detect intracranial calcifications or dilated ventricles on head US
- In utero diagnosis

### MANAGEMENT

- Pyrimethamine combined with sulfadiazine for a prolonged (>1 year) course decreases disease severity. Must supplement with folinic acid

## SYPHILIS

### TRANSMISSION AND DISEASE

- *Treponema pallidum* can cross the placenta at any point in pregnancy
- Infection of the fetus can also occur if there is contact with active genital lesions during labor and delivery
- Infection can be transmitted to the fetus at any stage of maternal disease, however the rate of transmission is highest (60–90%) with primary and secondary syphilis

### CLINICAL MANIFESTATIONS

- Syphilis can cause preterm delivery, nonimmune hydrops, congenital infection or death in the fetus or newborn. Fetal or perinatal death occurs in 40–50% of cases
- Two-thirds of infected liveborn neonates are asymptomatic
- Overt infection can manifest in the fetus, newborn, or later in childhood
- *Early congenital manifestations* (detected before 2 years of age, typically before age 3 months): Nonimmune hydrops, intrauterine growth restriction, hemolytic anemia, jaundice, hepatomegaly, bullous lesions and desquamation on palm and soles, copper-colored maculopapular rash, condyloma lata, chorioretinitis, uveitis, snuffles (persistent, bloody nasal discharge), osteochondritis, periostitis, meningitis, parrot pseudoparalysis (decreased movement of one or both upper extremities due to painful periostitis)
- *Late congenital manifestations* (detected after 2 years of age): Hutchinson teeth (peg-shaped upper central incisors), mulberry molars, rhagades (perioral fissuring), interstitial keratitis, frontal bossing, saddle nose, Clutton joints (chronic painless swelling of the knees), Saber shins (anterior bowing of tibia), mental retardation, hydrocephalus, seizures, and eighth cranial nerve deafness

### DIAGNOSIS

- *Presumptive diagnosis:* Nontreponemal (VDRL or RPR) and treponemal (FTA-ABS or MHA-TP) tests on infant serum
- *Definitive diagnosis:* Identify spirochetes by dark-field microscopy or direct fluorescent antibody tests of lesions, exudate, or tissue
- Long bone radiographs for osteochondritis and periostitis
- CSF evaluation for leptomeningitis

### MANAGEMENT

- Aqueous crystalline penicillin G at 50,000 U/kg per dose IV every 12 hours during first 7 days of life, and every 8 hours thereafter for a total of 10 days OR procaine penicillin G 50,000 U/kg IM once daily for 10 days

## RUBELLA

### TRANSMISSION AND DISEASE

- Transmission to the fetus can occur at any point in the pregnancy but is more likely in the first and third trimesters
- Congenital defects are more likely if infection occurs early in pregnancy (prior to 20 weeks gestation)

### CLINICAL MANIFESTATIONS

- The most common manifestation is sensorineural deafness, followed by mental retardation
- Cardiac malformations (PDA is most common; can also have pulmonary artery stenosis, pulmonary valvar stenosis, aortic valve stenosis, tetralogy of Fallot)

- Ocular abnormalities (cataracts, glaucoma, pigmented retinopathy, microphthalmia)
- Meningoencephalitis
- Blueberry muffin lesions (extramedullary dermal hematopoiesis), thrombocytopenia, and hemolytic anemia can also occur
- Delayed manifestations occur in >20% of individuals with congenital rubella infection. These include insulin-dependent diabetes and thyroid disease

## DIAGNOSIS

- Viral culture of specimens from blood, CSF, urine, and nasopharynx
- Serial serum rubella IgG levels demonstrate an increase over several months
- In utero diagnosis

## MANAGEMENT

- Treatment is solely supportive. Isolate neonate from other newborns as may be contagious

## CYTOMEGALOVIRUS

### TRANSMISSION AND DISEASE

- The most common human intrauterine infection
- 1% of all liveborn infants in the United States have congenital CMV, however only 10% of the infected infants are symptomatic at birth
- Can be transmitted to fetus after maternal primary infection or recurrent infection
- Sequelae are more common in infants after maternal primary infection (25%) than after reactivation of maternal infection (8%)
- Infant is more likely to be symptomatic or to have sequelae if maternal infection occurs during the first half of pregnancy
- Can also be acquired postpartum from infected breast-milk or blood products

### CLINICAL MANIFESTATIONS

- The most common clinical finding is hepatomegaly
- Other findings include microcephaly with periventricular calcifications, chorioretinitis, sensorineural hearing loss, thrombocytopenia, hepatosplenomegaly, hyperbilirubinemia, intrauterine growth retardation, pneumonitis, mental retardation

### DIAGNOSIS

- Proof of congenital infection requires positive viral culture or PCR from specimen (urine, stool, CSF, or respiratory secretions) within 3 weeks of birth
- Presumptive diagnosis can be made by fourfold rise in IgG titer in paired serum samples with positive IgM (infrequently used method)
- In utero diagnosis

### MANAGEMENT

- Ganciclovir may decrease incidence of hearing loss and therefore may also improve developmental outcome. Requires consultation with infectious diseases specialist

*Joann Spinale Carlson, MD*
*Rebecca L. Ruebner, MD, MSCE*

## HEMATURIA

**Microscopic hematuria: Greater than five RBCs per high-powered-field in a urine sample**

### EPIDEMIOLOGY

- *Microscopic hematuria:* 3–4% incidence on single urine sample; falls to 1% or less for two or more positive samples

### DIFFERENTIAL DIAGNOSIS

#### Red Urine with a Negative Dipstick for Blood

- *Medications:* Chloroquine, deferoxamine, metronidazole, nitrofurantoin, pyridium, rifampin, salicylates, doxorubicin
- *Dyes:* Fruits/vegetables (beets, blackberries, food coloring)
- *Metabolites:* Melanin, methemoglobin, porphyrin, urates, tyrosinosis
- *Bacteria: Serratia* urinary tract infection (some strains produce a red/burgundy pigment)

#### Positive Urine Dipstick for Blood, but Absence of Red Blood Cells

- *Hemoglobin:* Suggests a hemolytic process
- *Myoglobin:* Associated with rhabdomyolysis from trauma, infection, prolonged seizures, or severe electrolyte abnormalities

#### Repeatedly Positive Urine Dipstick for Blood and Presence of Red Blood Cells (Hematuria)

- *Urinary tract:* Cystitis/urethritis, hypercalciuria, urolithiasis, trauma, coagulopathy, sports hematuria (may be traumatic or nontraumatic, the latter due either to increased filtration pressure or to increased glomerular permeability as a result of hypoxic damage to the nephron as blood is redistributed to contracting skeletal muscles)
- *Kidney, non-glomerular:* Acute tubular necrosis (ATN), interstitial nephritis, pyelonephritis, sickle cell disease or trait, cysts, tumors (e.g., Wilms), trauma, vascular anomalies (e.g., renal vein thrombosis)
- *Kidney, glomerular:* Glomerulonephritis (GN, see section below)

### PATHOPHYSIOLOGY

- Lesions in the glomerulus, renal interstitium, vasculature, or urinary tract result in bleeding or leakage of red blood cells into urinary tract

### CLINICAL MANIFESTATIONS

- Glomerular hematuria typically presents with brown or cola-colored urine with RBC casts, dysmorphic RBCs, and proteinuria
- Urinary tract or vascular causes present with gross hematuria occasionally with blood clots, eumorphic RBCs (normal appearing), and absent or minimal proteinuria
- Hypertension, edema, and/or acute kidney injury (AKI) suggest acute GN

- Abdominal mass suggests tumor, hydronephrosis, polycystic kidney disease, or obstruction
- Certain rashes are associated with Henoch–Schönlein purpura (HSP) or systemic lupus erythematosus (SLE)
- Fever and dysuria suggest a urinary tract infection (UTI)

## DIAGNOSTICS

The diagnostic pathway depends on whether there is gross or microscopic hematuria as well as other abnormal findings. Begin with a urinalysis with microscopy as well as a thorough history and physical exam.

- *Microscopic hematuria:* In the absence of RBC casts, proteinuria, hypertension, AKI, or other concerning clinical signs, repeat urinalysis weekly ×2 (without exercise)
- *Gross hematuria with proteinuria, dysmorphic RBCs, RBC casts, hypertension, or AKI indicates glomerular origin:* Send serum electrolytes, BUN, creatinine, CBC with differential, and C3/C4. If suspect postinfectious GN, send ASO and/or anti-DNase B titers. Consider further evaluation such as antineutrophil antibody and antineutrophil cytoplasmic antibody based on clinical presentation
- *Gross hematuria without proteinuria or RBC casts:* Suggests an extraglomerular origin. Urine culture if symptoms of infection; renal/bladder ultrasound always indicated to evaluate for stones, tumors, and other structural lesions; consider abdominal CT if strong suspicion for urolithiasis not detected on ultrasound; consider spot urine calcium:creatinine ratio (normal <0.2) if suspicion for stones or hypercalciuria

## MANAGEMENT

- Patients with gross hematuria, persistent microscopic hematuria, or patients with hematuria and with elevated creatinine, proteinuria, hypertension, or hypocomplementemia should be referred to a pediatric nephrologist
- Further management depends on etiology
- Patients with GN often need hospitalization to manage hypertension and AKI

## HYPERTENSION

**Systolic blood pressure (SBP) or diastolic blood pressure (DBP) at 95th percentile or greater for height, age, and gender measured on at least three separate occasions. For children younger than 1 year, systolic BP defines hypertension.**

- *Normotensive:* SBP and DBP less than 90th percentile for age, height, and gender
- *Pre-hypertension:* SBP and DBP between 90th and 95th percentiles (see the Appendix A for normal BP values)

### EPIDEMIOLOGY

- Primary (essential) hypertension is more common in adolescents and adults
- Secondary hypertension (caused by underlying disease process) is more common in children
- *Overall prevalence:* 1% but as high as 11% with body mass index more than 95th percentile

### DIFFERENTIAL DIAGNOSIS

- Inaccurate measurement due to improper technique or cuff size
  - ✓ *Ideal cuff size:* (1) Bladder covers 80% of the upper arm circumference (goal >50%); (2) width of cuff spans at least 40% of the distance between the olecranon and acromion. (Overestimation of BP may occur when cuff is too small)
- Anxiety, white coat hypertension, pain

- *Primary (essential) hypertension:* Genetics, obesity, and diet contribute to risk
- *Secondary hypertension:*
  - ✓ *Renal:* Acute GN, AKI, chronic kidney disease, renal scarring
  - ✓ *Renovascular:* Renal artery thrombosis or stenosis (ask about history of umbilical lines as a neonate), vasculitis, renal artery stenosis (fibromuscular dysplasia)
  - ✓ *Cardiac:* Coarctation of the aorta
  - ✓ *Endocrine:* Pheochromocytoma, Cushings, neuroblastoma, hypo/hyperthyroidisim
  - ✓ *Drugs/Medications:* Cocaine, oral contraceptives, corticosteroids, amphetamines, sympathomimetics, cyclosporine, tacrolimus, heavy metals
  - ✓ *Central/Autonomic Nervous System:* Increased intracranial pressure, dysautonomia

## PATHOPHYSIOLOGY

- Hypertension is caused by dysregulation of one or more of the following mechanisms of blood pressure regulation: Sodium and water balance, renin-aldosterone-angiotensin system, sympathetic nervous system, vascular tone

## CLINICAL MANIFESTATIONS

- In children, hypertension is often asymptomatic
- If there is a prolonged and persistent increase in blood pressure or an acute onset of severe hypertension, patients may develop headache, vision changes, nausea, epistaxis, or seizures
- *Hypertensive emergency:* Severe hypertension (BP >99th% + 5mm Hg) associated with a life-threatening complication or end-organ damage; may present with encephalopathy (stroke, focal deficits), acute heart failure or myocardial infarction, pulmonary edema, aortic aneurysm, or acute kidney injury
- *Hypertensive urgency:* Severe hypertension without end-organ damage. May progress to hypertensive emergency
- Important physical exam findings when evaluating patients with hypertension:
  - ✓ *4 extremity blood pressures: BP lower in legs than arms is suggestive of coarctation*
  - ✓ *General:* Growth failure, obesity
  - ✓ *Skin:* Café-au-lait spots or neurofibromas (suggestive of neurofibromatosis), rashes or flushing (suggestive of endocrine etiologies)
  - ✓ *HEENT:* Moon facies, blurred disk margins on fundoscopic exam, proptosis (hyperthyroidism)
  - ✓ *Chest/CV:* Rales; hyperdynamic chest; rub, gallop, or murmur; decreased lower extremity pulses
  - ✓ *Abdomen:* Hepatosplenomegaly, renal bruit, abdominal mass
  - ✓ *Neurologic:* Focal deficits such as Bell's palsy

## DIAGNOSTICS

Because hypertension is often asymptomatic, blood pressure screening is an important part of the well visit. If the blood pressure is greater than the 90th percentile, follow with two to three readings over at least 6 weeks to document a sustained elevation and to rule out anxiety or issues with technique. If persistently above the 95th percentile:

- Basic metabolic panel with BUN and creatinine, urinalysis to screen for proteinuria or hematuria, renal ultrasound w/Doppler. Consider echocardiogram to look for end-organ damage
- 24-hour ambulatory blood pressure may be helpful to differentiate white coat hypertension from sustained hypertension

*If indicated by initial studies or concern for specific etiology, consider:*

- *Imaging:* CT angiogram for renal artery stenosis, DMSA scan to evaluate for renal scarring
- *Labs:* Plasma renin activity and aldosterone levels, thyroid function, serum metanephrines (if concern for pheochromocytoma)

*If the blood pressure remains between the 90th and 95th percentiles:*

- Monitor every 6 months before initiating an extensive evaluation
- If the child is obese, institute a weight control plan
- If no improvement, additional evaluation may be warranted with referral to Nephrology

## MANAGEMENT

### General Management Issues

Management depends on the severity of the blood pressure and the underlying etiology. The overall goal is to prevent long-term sequelae of hypertension including cardiac disease, retinal damage, and chronic kidney disease.

- *Nonpharmacologic:* For management of mild essential hypertension and for prevention, encourage weight reduction, sodium restriction in diet, exercise, and smoking cessation
- *Pharmacologic:* Initiate when nonpharmacologic efforts fail or if severe elevation of blood pressure or signs of end-organ damage. Type of medication depends on age, comorbid conditions, mechanism of hypertension (e.g., ACE inhibitor for renin-mediated hypertension), and tolerability of side effects
  - ✓ *ACE inhibitors (e.g., captopril, lisinopril):* Renoprotective and anti-proteinuric (beneficial in chronic kidney disease with proteinuria such as focal segmental glomerulosclerosis), side effects include AKI, hyperkalemia, angioedema, cough, and birth defects
  - ✓ *Angiotensin receptor blockers (e.g., losartan):* May have fewer side effects than ACE inhibitors
  - ✓ *Calcium channel blockers (e.g., amlodipine, nifedipine):* Usually well-tolerated
  - ✓ *Diuretics:* Promote salt and water excretion. Main types are loop diuretics, thiazide diuretics, and potassium-sparing diuretics
  - ✓ *Beta-blockers (e.g., atenolol, propranolol):* Limited by adverse side effects including bradycardia. Lack of selectivity results in bronchoconstriction, insulin resistance, and alteration in lipid profiles. Combined alpha/beta blockers (e.g., labetalol) can also be used
  - ✓ *Other types:* Central alpha-2-adrenergic blockers, peripheral alpha-1-adrenergic blockers, direct vasodilators

### Hypertensive Emergency

- Obtain intravenous access and admit to intensive care unit
- Goal is to lower BP promptly (within 1 hour) to prevent a life- or organ-threatening injury, but then gradually to preserve cerebral perfusion
- Reduce mean arterial pressure by one-third of planned reduction over 6 hours, additional third over next 24–36 hours, and final third over next 48 hours
- *Medications:* IV labetalol, esmolol, nitroprusside, nicardipine

### Hypertensive Urgency

- Requires prompt but gradual and controlled reduction in blood pressure over 24 hours
- *Medications:* Hydralazine orally/IV/IM, nifedipine orally, labetalol IV, clonidine orally, enalapril IV

## ACUTE KIDNEY INJURY

Acute kidney injury (**AKI**) **is a decrease in renal function over hours to days that results in the failure to excrete nitrogenous wastes and regulate electrolyte and water homeostasis.**

- *Anuria:* Complete cessation of urine output
- *Oliguria:* Excretion of less than 1 cc/kg/h in infants, less than 0.5 cc/kg/h in children, and less than 500 mL/day in adults

### ETIOLOGY

- *Pre-renal:* Dehydration most common; bleeding; decrease in effective circulating blood volume (shock, hypoalbuminemia, burns, heart failure, liver failure); renal artery or venous occlusion
- Intrarenal:
  - ✓ *Glomerular:* Acute GN (see section), hemolytic uremic syndrome (HUS)
  - ✓ *Tubular:* ATN—dehydration, medications (aminoglycosides), toxins (myoglobin in setting of rhabdomyolysis, uric acid in setting of tumor lysis syndrome, IV contrast)
  - ✓ *Interstitial:* Acute interstitial nephritis—medications (NSAIDs), infections
- *Post-renal:* Bladder outlet obstruction (posterior urethral valves, occluded catheter); upper bilateral ureteral obstruction; intraabdominal tumor obstructing urinary flow

### CLINICAL MANIFESTATIONS

- Depends on etiology of AKI
- *Pre-renal:* May have signs/symptoms of dehydration, hypotension; typically oliguric
- *Renal:* May have hypertension; can be oliguric (e.g., GN) or non-oliguric (e.g., ATN, acute interstitial nephritis)
- *Post-renal:* May have intrabdominal mass (bladder obstruction); will be oliguric/anuric if there is a complete obstruction

### DIAGNOSTICS

#### Urinary Sediment and Indexes

- Obtain urine before fluid resuscitation or diuretic administration
- Calculate the fractional excretion of sodium (FENa):

$$FENa = ([Na_{urine}]/[Na_{plasma}]) \times 100/([Creatinine_{urine}]/[Creatinine_{plasma}])$$

  - ✓ Can only be interpreted in the presence of oliguria
- *Pre-renal etiologies:* High specific gravity; hyaline and fine granular casts; cellular casts unusual; urine [Na] less than 20 mmol/L; FENa less than 1%
- *Renal etiologies:* May see brown granular casts in ATN; RBC casts in GN; FENa more than 1%

#### Laboratory Studies

- Elevated BUN and creatinine, decreased glomerular filtration rate (GFR)
- Schwartz formula for estimation of GFR

$$GFR(mL/min/1.73m^2) = K \times Ht(cm)/SCr(mg/dL)$$

where $K = 0.35$ (preterm infants), 0.45 (term infants), 0.55 (girls and prepubertal boys), 0.70 (postpubertal boys); 0.413 (validated in chronic kidney disease patients); SCr = serum creatinine
- Hypo/hypernatremia; hyperkalemia; hyperphosphatemia; hypocalcemia, acidosis

## Imaging/Other Studies

- Ultrasound for intrinsic and post-renal causes. Further imaging as indicated
- *ECG:* If electrolyte abnormalities

## MANAGEMENT

### Fluid Management

- Daily weights, strict input and output
- *If volume depleted/pre-renal:* Fluid replacement with isotonic fluid (normal saline 20 cc/kg IV, may repeat if clinically warranted)
- *If oliguric and not responding to fluid resuscitation and/or fluid overloaded:* Restrict fluids to insensible losses (300 cc/m²/day) + urine output + GI losses (cc for cc)
- Bladder catheterization may be indicated if there is outlet obstruction

### Electrolyte Management

- Metabolic acidosis should be treated judiciously with sodium bicarbonate; correction of acidosis with bicarbonate can further lower the ionized calcium and precipitate tetany. If hypocalcemic, give calcium before correcting acidosis
- *Hyperkalemia:* No potassium in fluids; (see Management under Hyperkalemia in Fluids and Electrolytes chapter [Chapter 9]). Treatment should include calcium gluconate for cardiac protection

### Other Management Issues

- *Nutrition:* Low potassium, low phosphorous diet
- *Cardiovascular:* Antihypertensive medications may be indicated
- *Renal:* Avoid nephrotoxic medications. *Adjust dosing/schedule of medications for GFR*
- *Indications for dialysis (failure of conservative management of fluid and electrolyte imbalance or cardiopulmonary compromise):* Hyperkalemia ($K^+$ >6.5 or peaked T-waves); acidosis unresponsive to medications ($HCO_3^-$ < 10); symptomatic uremia (symptoms such as seizure, altered mental status, pericarditis); volume overload (congestive heart failure [CHF], pulmonary edema); dialyzable toxins (isopropyl alcohol, methanol, ethylene glycol, salicylates, lithium)
- *Post-renal failure secondary to obstruction:* Place bladder catheter, may require surgical intervention and Urology consultation

## GLOMERULAR DISEASES

## GLOMERULONEPHRITIS

- **Nephritic syndrome: Hematuria with RBC casts, proteinuria, hypertension, and AKI. Due to glomerular injury with glomerular inflammation**
- **Classification according to complement**
  - ✓ *Hypocomplementemic:* **Poststreptococcal** GN, **membranoproliferative glomerulonephritis (MPGN), SLE**
  - ✓ *Normal complement:* **IgA nephropathy, HSP, ANCA-associated vasculitis, anti-glomerular basement membrane syndrome, Alport syndrome**

## POSTINFECTIOUS GLOMERULONEPHRITIS

### EPIDEMIOLOGY

- Most common cause of GN in children. Peak age 2–12 years old; males:females = 2:1
- May occur sporadically or as part of an epidemic

## ETIOLOGY

- Most common after Group A streptococcal pharyngitis or skin infection. Also staphylococci; gram-negative bacteria; viruses

## PATHOPHYSIOLOGY

- Deposition of circulating immune complexes
- Autoimmune response to a self-antigen with molecular mimicry
- Pathology characterized by an acute diffuse proliferative GN with neutrophilic infiltrate in the glomeruli with immune complex deposition in the glomeruli

## CLINICAL MANIFESTATIONS

- Typically presents 7–21 days after strep pharyngitis and 14–21 days after skin infection
- Hematuria (microscopic or gross) with RBC casts, dysmorphic RBCs, proteinuria, hypertension, and AKI
- *Hypertension:* Occurs in greater than 75%; usually secondary to salt and fluid overload; can be treated with diuretics; 50% require antihypertensives
- *Edema:* Typically in face and upper extremities; related to urinary sodium and fluid retention
- *Encephalopathy (headache, mental status change, seizure):* May be related to a concomitant central nervous system (CNS) vasculitis or severe acute hypertension
- Orthopnea, dyspnea, rales, and gallops may be associated with CHF
- Pharyngeal erythema or impetigo has usually resolved
- *Resolution of disease:* Hypertension and edema typically resolve in 1–2 weeks. Microscopic hematuria may persist for up to a year. Persistence of proteinuria longer than 1 year may indicate the persistence of proliferative GN and has a less favorable prognosis

## DIAGNOSTICS

- *Urinalysis:* Urine may have rusty or tea color; presence of heme and protein. Microscopic evaluation reveals RBC casts or dysmorphic RBCs, occasional hyaline or granular casts
- Electrolytes, BUN, creatinine—Patients may have elevated creatinine and hyperkalemia
- *ASO titer, anti-DNase B titer:* Doubling of ASO titer is highly indicative of recent streptococcal infection (70% sensitive). The peak value is found at 3–5 weeks. Anti-DNase B titer increases earlier than ASO therefore sending both increases sensitivity of detecting streptococcal infections
- *Streptozyme:* 95% sensitive; no correlation with disease severity. Positive in skin infection
- *Complement levels (particularly C3):* Reduced in the early acute phase and *usually return to normal in 6–8 weeks*
- *Renal biopsy:* If unclear diagnosis, rapidly progressive renal failure, or if complement levels fail to normalize
- *Renal ultrasound:* If gross hematuria or azotemia
- *Chest x-ray:* To evaluate for pulmonary edema if severe fluid overload or CHF

## MANAGEMENT

- *Fluids:* Restrict fluids if patient has edema or hypertension; consider diuretics (commonly loop diuretics are used in the setting of edema and/or hypertension)
- *Electrolytes:* Salt restriction if edema or hypertension; avoid potassium if acute kidney injury present
- Treat hypertension due to fluid overload with loop diuretics. Calcium channel blockers can also be used. Avoid ACE inhibitors in the setting of AKI and hyperkalemia

- The presence of AKI is not associated with worse prognosis. Children rarely require dialysis for AKI associated with postinfectious GN
- *ID:* If any evidence of a pharyngitis or skin infection persists, treat with a penicillin antibiotic or a macrolide if penicillin allergic
- Long-term prognosis is generally good, with the main sequelae being hypertension. A small proportion has proteinuria, renal insufficiency, and hypertension 10–40 years after presentation

## IgA NEPRHOPATHY

### EPIDEMIOLOGY

- Most common cause of primary GN worldwide. 2–10% of cases of primary GN in the United States
- *Prevalence:* 25–50 per 100,000 individuals; male:female = 2–6:1
- *Onset:* usually 15–35 years of age; uncommon before 10 years

### ETIOLOGY

- Etiology unknown. Genetic factors may lead to an increased susceptibility
- Upper respiratory infection (URI) or mucosal infections often precede onset by a few days

### PATHOPHYSIOLOGY

- Circulating IgA immune complexes and to a lesser extent other immune complexes are deposited in the glomerular mesangium

### CLINICAL MANIFESTATIONS

- Most children present with gross hematuria or with asymptomatic microscopic hematuria on screening urinalysis. Children with macroscopic hematuria often have a history of a URI or gastroenteritis 1–2 days before onset
- At presentation, renal function usually normal and proteinuria can be minimal
- Generally has a benign course in children; however, up to 30% of patients may develop progressive renal failure
- *Indicators of poor prognosis:* Hypertension and renal insufficiency at time of presentation; persistent proteinuria greater than 1 g/day; biopsy with crescents/large areas of fibrosis

### DIAGNOSTICS

- *Urinalysis:* RBCs, proteinuria, RBC casts. Consider 24-hour urine protein collection

## NEPHROTIC SYNDROME

**Composite of clinical findings: Proteinuria, hypoalbuminemia, edema, hypercholesterolemia**

### EPIDEMIOLOGY

- 2–7/100,000 in children with 70–80% cases younger than 6 years old
- About 80–90% of children with nephrotic syndrome (NS) have minimal change disease, about 7% focal segmental glomerulosclerosis. Other causes listed below are less common

### DIFFERENTIAL DIAGNOSIS

- *Minimal change disease:* Most common cause of NS in children. Characterized by normal glomerulus on light microscopy, loss of epithelial foot processes on electron microscopy; possibly related to allergic triggers, atopy. Often triggered by URI, allergies, or immunizations

- *Focal segmental glomerulosclerosis:* More common in adolescents, black race. May be primary (idiopathic), genetic, or secondary (infections, medications). More likely to be unresponsive to steroids and progress to end-stage kidney disease
- *Membranous glomerulopathy:* Primary (idiopathic) or secondary (mainly SLE, infections)
- *Membranoproliferative glomerulonephritis:* May be immune-complex mediated or complement mediated (C3 glomerulopathy). Most commonly idiopathic in children; can also be secondary to infections (e.g., hepatitis), malignancy, and autoimmune disorders. C3 glomerulopathy typically caused by alterations in the regulation of the alternative complement cascade disorders

## PATHOPHYSIOLOGY

- Nephrotic syndrome arises from a permeability defect in the glomerular capillaries that allows protein to be lost from the plasma into the urine

## CLINICAL MANIFESTATIONS

- Facial, periorbital, and pretibial edema; anasarca or ascites
- Vomiting or diarrhea secondary to bowel wall edema. Abdominal pain due to reduced blood flow to the splanchnic bed
- Tachycardia if intravascular volume depleted
- Foamy, frothy urine
- Rales, dyspnea, and orthopnea in severe cases of fluid extravasation and pulmonary edema
- Urinary loss of antithrombin III, increased fibrinogen, and hemoconcentration predispose to hypercoagulability. Lower leg pain or swelling may signify a deep venous thrombosis (DVT). Homan sign (calf pain when ankle is forcibly dorsiflexed while knee is flexed) has poor sensitivity (<50%) and specificity (<50%)
- Urinary loss of IgG may predispose to infection. If abdominal pain present, consider spontaneous bacterial peritonitis

## DIAGNOSTICS

- *Initial studies:* Urinalysis, serum chemistries, lipids, albumin, CBC
- *Urinalysis:* Large protein, possible microscopic hematuria (about 25%)
- *Twenty-four-hour urine collection:* Greater than 40 mg/m$^2$/day of protein
- Urine protein to creatinine ratio greater than 2 mg protein/mg creatinine in first morning void
- Hypoalbuminemia (usually <2 g/dL)
- Serum cholesterol greater than 200 mg/dL—Related to increased liver production of cholesterol and urinary losses of lipoprotein lipase
- Hyponatremia, hypocalcemia (related to hypoalbuminemia)
- Hemoconcentration causes elevated hemoglobin, platelets
- *Consider renal biopsy if:* (1) Older age at presentation; (2) younger than 1 year of age at diagnosis; (3) disease has not responded to 4–6 weeks of steroid treatment (steroid resistant); (4) progressive renal failure; (5) clinical suspicion for diagnosis other than minimal change disease

## MANAGEMENT

- *Fluids:* Due to low oncotic pressure, patients may appear to be fluid overloaded while they are actually intravascularly depleted. If vomiting, diarrhea, hypotensive, or tachycardic, give normal saline bolus IV and maintain on IV fluids to replace losses (monitor strict ins/outs)

- *Albumin:* May be used to increase oncotic pressure in severe cases of edema. Use with extreme caution if patient has respiratory compromise or elevated creatinine. Follow infusion with diuretics
- *Prednisone:* 60 mg/m$^2$ or 2 mg/kg daily for 4–6 weeks followed by taper over 2–3 months. If patients are steroid resistant or frequently relapse, consider alternate immunosuppressive therapy
- *Loop diuretics:* Consider loop diuretics to increase urine output if patient is severely edematous
- *Nutrition:* Low sodium diet to reduce fluid retention
- *Infectious considerations:* Blood culture and empiric antibiotic coverage for fever and/or severe abdominal pain

## OTHER COMMON CONDITIONS

### DIARRHEA-ASSOCIATED HEMOLYTIC UREMIC SYNDROME

**Microangiopathic hemolytic anemia, thrombocytopenia, and acute kidney injury following a prodromal illness of acute gastroenteritis, typically with Shiga toxin-producing *Escherichia coli*.**

### EPIDEMIOLOGY

- *Incidence in the United States:* 1–3/100,000 population/year
- *Peak age:* 6 months–4 years; seasonal peak during summer months

### ETIOLOGY

- Diarrheal HUS caused by infection with Shiga toxin-producing *E. coli* (STEC), especially O157:H7 (90% of cases), which can be found in undercooked hamburger meat, farm animals, alfalfa sprouts; may occur in outbreaks
- *Other Shiga toxin-producing etiologies:* Non-O157 strains of *E. coli*, *Salmonella dysenteriae*
- Differential diagnosis includes *S. pneumoniae* HUS (which accounts for 5% of all HUS), is classically associated with complicated pneumonia; atypical HUS (associated with genetic mutations); secondary HUS (bone marrow transplant, SLE, malignancy, post transplant); thrombotic thrombocytopenic purpura (TTP)

### PATHOPHYSIOLOGY

- Shiga toxin crosses gastrointestinal epithelium, enters bloodstream, and binds neutrophils, which carry the toxin to endothelial cells in other organs
- Shiga toxin preferentially binds to endothelial cell receptors, causing a cascade of intracellular events leading to cell death, tissue ischemia, local activation of coagulation and fibrinolytic reactions and release of inflammatory cytokines, and resulting in multiorgan injury

### CLINICAL MANIFESTATIONS

- *Typical course:* Fever, diarrhea (90% with bloody stools), abdominal pain, vomiting 24–72 hours after exposure to *E. coli*
- 6–9% of children with enterohemorrhagic *E. coli* will develop HUS, about 5–10 days after infection
- Present with pallor, petechiae, jaundice, oliguric AKI; can have volume overload, hypertension
- *Other gastrointestinal disease:* Severe colitis; risk for bowel ischemia; pancreatitis

- *Neurological symptoms:* Irritability, lethargy, restlessness, seizures, ataxia, tremors
- Cardiac failure from myocarditis; cardiomyopathy in rare cases

## DIAGNOSTICS

- *Stool testing:* Stool culture for *E. coli* O157:H7 or direct assay for Shiga toxin
- *CBC every 6–8 hours initially:* Thrombocytopenia often is first manifestation of HUS; hemolytic anemia with schistocytes on peripheral blood smear; leukocytosis in first week
- Serum chemistries and electrolyte panels every 6–8 hours initially
- Elevated amylase/lipase and glucose insensitivity if pancreas involved
- Hypoalbuminemia secondary to enteropathy

## MANAGEMENT

- Early consultation with nephrology and possible admission to intensive care unit
- Once HUS is diagnosed, fluids should be restricted to insensible losses + urine output + stool output
- Meticulous management of electrolytes
- Provide sufficient calories with parenteral nutrition if needed
- Transfuse packed red blood cells only if hemoglobin <6–7 g/dL or cardiovascular compromise
- Transfuse platelets only if active bleeding or before surgery
- Avoid anti-motility medications and, if possible, antibiotics (i.e., when no coexisting bacterial infection)
- May require dialysis

## RENAL TUBULAR ACIDOSIS

**Renal tubular acidosis (RTA) is the failure of the kidney to maintain normal plasma concentration of bicarbonate due to impaired bicarbonate reabsorption or hydrogen ion (urinary acid) excretion which results in a non-anion gap hyperchloremic metabolic acidosis.**

## ETIOLOGY

All forms may be either primary (sporadic or hereditary) or secondary to other conditions:

- *Type I: Distal RTA*
  ✓ Inherited autosomal dominant or sporadic
  ✓ Secondary: Obstructive uropathy, sickle cell nephropathy, autoimmune disorders (Sjögren syndrome, SLE, thyroiditis, chronic hepatitis), toxins/medications
- *Type II: Proximal RTA:* May be an isolated defect in bicarbonate reabsorption or global proximal tubular dysfunction (Fanconi syndrome)
  ✓ *Isolated:* Sporadic, hereditary (autosomal recessive), carbonic anhydrase deficiency
  ✓ *Fanconi syndrome:* Proximal tubular dysfunction with proteinuria, glycosuria, phosphaturia, and aminoaciduria; in children most commonly inherited (i.e., cystinosis, Lowe syndrome, Wilson's disease, galactosemia, tyrosinemia) or secondary to toxins (heavy metals, medications)
- *Type IV: Hyperkalemic RTA*
  ✓ Hypoaldosteronism due to Addison disease, congenital adrenal hyperplasia
  ✓ Pseudohypoaldosteronism; obstructive uropathy; pyelonephritis, interstitial nephritis

## PATHOPHYSIOLOGY

- *Type I: Distal RTA:* Impaired distal hydrogen ion secretion due to poor functioning of or damage to transporters involved in the excretion of $H^+$ in the distal tubule. There is an inability to decrease urinary pH less than 5.5 even in setting of severe acidosis
- *Type II: Proximal RTA:* Impaired proximal tubular reabsorption of bicarbonate due to defective sodium–hydrogen ion exchange. There is retained ability to acidify urine because distal tubule function is maintained. May be primary isolated form but usually associated with more generalized proximal tubule dysfunction (Fanconi syndrome)
- *Type IV: Hyperkalemic RTA:* Hypoaldosteronism or pseudohypoaldosteronism resulting in impaired hydrogen excretion and potassium secretion. Poor response to aldosterone is most common mechanism in children

## CLINICAL MANIFESTATIONS

All forms present with non-anion gap acidosis, may present with growth failure within first few years of life. Distinguishing characteristics are:

- *Type I: Distal RTA:* Acidosis may be more severe (bicarbonate <10), can be associated with nephrocalcinosis
- *Type II: Proximal RTA:* Polyuria and dehydration; anorexia, vomiting, and constipation; hypotonia; in Fanconi syndrome will see signs of phosphate wasting such as rickets. Look for features of inherited disorders associated with Fanconi syndrome
- *Type IV: Hyperkalemic RTA:* Polyuria and dehydration; hyperkalemia; pyelonephritis

## DIAGNOSTICS

- Basic metabolic panel; pH via venipuncture
- Confirm type of metabolic acidosis (anion gap versus non-anion gap)

$$\text{Anion gap} = [Na^+] - [Cl^- + HCO_3^-]$$

  ✓ If anion gap greater than 20, acidosis is most likely NOT due to RTA
- *Urinalysis:* In distal RTA, unable to acidify urine in setting of acidosis, so urine pH will be greater than 5.5. In proximal RTA, urine pH may be appropriately <5.5 in setting of acidosis as distal acidification is still intact
- *Urine anion gap (UAG):* UAG = [UrineNa$^+$] + [UrineK$^+$] − [UrineCl$^-$]
  ✓ *Negative UAG:* Normal, GI bicarbonate losses, possible proximal RTA
  ✓ *Positive UAG:* Suggests type I. Can have a falsely positive UAG if there is low urine volume and/or low urine Na in the setting of dehydration

## MANAGEMENT

- Bicarbonate replacement is the most important therapeutic step:
  ✓ Usually as sodium bicarbonate, sodium citrate (Bicitra), or sodium/potassium citrate (Polycitra). Divide replacement into 3–4 doses per day. Titrate dose to maintain normal bicarbonate levels. Proximal RTA usually requires higher daily doses of alkali. Consider phosphate replacement for Fanconi syndrome. Give mineralocorticoids for hypoaldosteronism

## UROLITHIASIS

**Stones can be found in the lower (bladder, urethra) or upper (kidney, ureter) urinary tract.**

## EPIDEMIOLOGY

- *In United States:* Less than 1% in children under 10 years old and less than 3% in children under 19 years old
- In children, most due to metabolic and genitourinary abnormalities or infection

## ETIOLOGY

- *Calcium stones (calcium oxalate and calcium phosphate):* Most common stones in children
  - ✓ *Normocalcemic hypercalciuria:* Distal RTA, loop diuretics, formulas high in calcium or parenteral calcium
  - ✓ *Hypercalcemic hypercalciuria:* Increased absorption from bone (hyperparathyroidism, immobilization) or increased absorption of calcium from the gut
  - ✓ *Promoters of calcium stone formation:* Hypocitraturia, hyperuricuria, hyperoxaluria, hyperphosphaturia
- *Uric acid stones:*
  - ✓ Urinary pH less than 5.8 promotes uric acid crystal precipitation
  - ✓ *Idiopathic:* Normal serum uric acid concentration
  - ✓ Inborn errors of metabolism that cause hyperuricemia (i.e., Lesch–Nyhan)
  - ✓ High cell turnover from myeloproliferative, lymphoproliferative, or chronic hemolytic disorders can cause hyperuricemia
  - ✓ Ketogenic diet, inflammatory bowel disease, chronic diarrheal conditions
- *Cystinuria:*
  - ✓ Autosomal recessive disorder characterized by the failure of the renal tubules to reabsorb cystine, ornithine, lysine, and arginine
  - ✓ pH less than 7 precipitates cystine
- *Struvite stones:*
  - ✓ Related to UTI with organisms that can split urea and increase $NH_4$, resulting in increased urinary pH
  - ✓ *Proteus* (70%), *Pseudomonas, Klebsiella, Streptococcus, Serratia species*
  - ✓ Tend to grow rapidly and form staghorn calculi
  - ✓ More common in children with anatomic abnormalities of the urinary tract

## CLINICAL MANIFESTATIONS

- Sudden onset of severe, crampy abdominal or flank pain that radiates to scrotum or labia
- May have nausea, vomiting, dysuria, frequency, urinary retention
- Hematuria (microscopic or gross) in 90%
- May have fever if associated with UTI

## DIAGNOSTICS

- *Urinalysis:* Hematuria, signs of concomitant UTI
- *Urine microscopy:* May reveal crystals; normal RBC morphology
- If febrile, send blood and urine cultures
- Urine calcium/creatinine ratio
- Serum electrolytes and creatinine
- Abdominal film may pick up radio-opaque stones
- Renal/bladder ultrasound can reveal shadowing of stones, nephrocalcinosis, and obstruction
- Gold standard for diagnosis is CT without IV contrast
- Attempt to obtain stone by straining urine stream

- If first episode, every child should have renal and bladder ultrasound and complete metabolic panel. Children <3 years old should have spot urine for calcium, oxalate, citrate, and creatinine. Children >3 years old should have 24-hour urine collection. Further testing and follow up based on initial evaluation

## MANAGEMENT

- Intravenous fluids
- Narcotic pain medication if needed
- *Uric acid stones:* Increase fluid intake, alkalinization, allopurinol
- *Hypercalciuria:* Increase fluid intake, dietary sodium restriction. Dietary calcium restriction is NOT recommended. Thiazide diuretics will decrease urinary calcium excretion. Consider citrate. Dietary oxalate restriction if calcium oxalate stones
- *Cystinuria:* Urinary alkalinization with potassium citrate; low methionine and sodium diet. If this fails, consider penicillamine and Thiola
- Stone removal by Urology may be needed if stone is obstructing the urethra and causing hydronephrosis, is causing a chronic UTI, or is a struvite stone
  - ✓ *Stones below the pelvic brim:* Ureteroscopy with direct stone removal or lithotripsy
  - ✓ *Upper tract stones:* Extra corporeal shock wave lithotripsy
  - ✓ Open surgical stone removal is rarely needed

## RHABDOMYOLYSIS

### ETIOLOGY

- *Physical:* Compression and trauma, occlusion or hypoperfusion of vasculature, muscle overuse, electrical current, hyperthermia
- *Nonphysical:* Infection (i.e., influenza, coxsackievirus), drug-induced (i.e., antipsychotics, statins), electrolyte abnormalities, metabolic myopathies, endocrinopathies, rarely inflammatory myopathies

### PATHOPHYSIOLOGY

- Regardless of etiology, muscle cell membrane integrity is compromised. There is a decrease in available intracellular ATP necessary for Na–K exchanger and calcium-exchanger, and calcium moves from the extracellular to intracellular space. This results in sustained contraction, energy depletion, and cell death as well as the release of enzymes and oxygen-free radicals
- Myoglobin, released in large amounts, is unbound in serum and is filtered by the kidney. When urine flow is decreased (hypotension) myoglobin can precipitate, leading to ATN, tubular obstruction, and AKI
- Release of intracellular potassium and phosphorous
- Damage and cell death of muscle also results in large fluid shifts into the affected areas with ensuing hypernatremia, shock, and AKI

### CLINICAL MANIFESTATIONS

- Clinically have myalgias, weakness, pain, muscle tenderness. Urine can be dark/brown/red
- Fluid shifts may result in hypotension, shock, tachycardia, hypernatremia
- Oliguric or non-oliguric AKI
- May progress to compartment syndrome
- *Electrolyte abnormalities:* Hypocalcemia initially; hypercalcemia during recovery phase; hyperkalemia; hyperphosphatemia
- Seizure, cardiac arrhythmia from electrolyte abnormalities

## Chronic Rhabdomyolysis

- *In metabolic myopathies:* Low-grade chronic muscle pain, episodic dark urine with exercise
- Muscle cramps precipitated by exercise, followed by weakness

### DIAGNOSTICS

- *Labs show elevated creatinine phosphokinase (MM fraction):* From striated muscle breakdown; peak concentrations greater than 50,000–100,000 U/L; elevated lactate dehydrogenase (LDH); elevated uric acid; basic metabolic panel can have multiple electrolyte abnormalities; anion gap acidosis; hematological parameters may reflect DIC
- Urine shows myoglobinuria. Urinalysis, positive dipstick for blood, no or few RBCs, reddish-golden pigmented granular casts
- *ECG:* Changes consistent with electrolyte abnormalities

### MANAGEMENT

- Strict monitoring of intake and output, daily weights, chemistries, urine pH with each void
- Mainstay of therapy is aggressive fluid resuscitation with isotonic fluid. Use of bicarbonate-based fluid to alkalinize the urine is controversial, but may be indicated in patients with low urine pH and/or severe rhabdomyolysis
- Frequent neurovascular exams of affected muscle groups to detect compartment syndrome
- Consider dialysis if severe renal failure or refractory electrolyte abnormalities

# 19 Neurology

*Annapurna Poduri, MD, MPH*
*Renée A. Shellhaas, MD*
*Dennis J. Dlugos, MD*
*Peter H. Berman, MD*
*Gihan I. Tennekoon, MD*

## GENERAL PRINCIPLES

### ACUTE WEAKNESS

**Acute weakness is the acute loss of strength.**
- *Bulk:* Assess symmetry of muscle bulk
- *Tone:* Assess by passive movement of limbs with patient relaxed; may be normal, increased (spastic or rigid), decreased
- See Table 19-1

### ETIOLOGY (BY LOCALIZATION)

- *Central Nervous System (CNS)-Brain:* Acute stroke, unilateral or bilateral
- *CNS-Spinal cord (anterior horn cell body):* Cord infarction, cord compression, trauma, contusion, infection (e.g., enterovirus), transverse myelitis, spinal epidural abscess, syringomyelia
- *Spinal root of peripheral nerve:* Acute inflammatory demyelinating polyneuropathy (Guillain–Barré)
- *Peripheral nerve (axon):* Intensive care unit (ICU) neuropathy, HIV or zidovudine therapy, hereditary tyrosinemia, acute intermittent porphyria, medication-related (e.g., phenytoin, vincristine, nitrofurantoin, INH), toxins (heavy metals, glue), metabolic (uremia-mixed sensory and motor, or pure motor after dialysis), autoimmune (lupus), other vasculitis, chronic juvenile rheumatoid arthritis
- *Neuromuscular junction:* Myasthenia gravis, botulism, tic paralysis, pharmacologic blockade, aminoglycoside toxicity
- *Muscle:* Myositis (infectious, dermatomyositis, polymyositis), metabolic (hypocalcemia, hypokalemia, hypothyroid state), medication-related (especially steroids), ICU myopathy, familial periodic paralysis (hypo/hyperkalemic)

| TABLE 19-1 | Scales for Strength and Deep Tendon Reflexes | | |
|---|---|---|---|
| **Scale** | **Strength** | **Scale** | **Deep Tendon Reflexes** |
| 5 | Full, normal strength | 4+ | Increased with clonus |
| 5− | Nearly full strength | 3+ | Increased without clonus |
| 4 | Able to meet some resistance | 2+ | Normal |
| 3 | Able to overcome gravity but not resistance | 1+ | Diminished |
| 2 | Able to move in space but not overcome gravity | 0 | Absent |
| 1 | Flicker of movement but no movement in space | | |
| 0 | No movement | | |

| TABLE 19-2 | Summary of Examination for Weakness by Localization | | | | |
|---|---|---|---|---|---|
| **Examination Summary** | **Strength** | **Tone** | **DTRs** | **Sensory Loss** | **Fasciculations** |
| Spinal cord | ↓ | ↓ then ↑ | ↓ then ↑ | + | +/− |
| Anterior horn cell | ↓ | ↓ | — | — | + |
| Spinal root | ↓ | ↓ | — | — | — |
| Peripheral nerve | ↓ | ↓ | ↓/− | + | — |
| Neuromuscular junction | ↓ | ↓ | + (nl) | — | — |
| Muscle | ↓ | ↓ | + (nl) | — | — |

DTRs, deep tendon reflexes.
+ (nl) indicates that the finding is present and its presence is what is normally expected in healthy children.

## CLINICAL MANIFESTATIONS

- *Central nervous system:* Stroke; typically unilateral weakness in a cerebrovascular distribution; expected concomitant language, cranial nerve, or sensory changes; initial low tone then spastic; extensor plantar response ("upgoing toe") on affected side (Table 19-2)
- *Spinal cord:* Acute flaccid paraparesis ("spinal shock") then spastic, bowel or bladder symptoms, incontinence, evolving spasticity, sensory level, back pain or trauma, fasciculation, fever (epidural abscess), hypotension (infarction), decreased rectal tone, extensor plantar responses ("upgoing toes")
- *Spinal root of peripheral nerve:* Symmetric length-dependent weakness, often concomitant sensory disturbance, distal more than proximal weakness, areflexia, +/− back pain, normal to decreased tone
- *Peripheral nerve:* Weakness and sensory loss in distribution of specific nerve, in several discrete nerve distributions (mononeuritis multiplex), or diffusely in polyneuropathy (may be painful); may have decreased deep tendon reflexes (DTRs)
- *Neuromuscular junction:* Hypotonia; DTRs present; no sensory loss (see Myasthenia Gravis and Botulism sections)
- *Muscle:* Proximal more than distal weakness; normal tone; myalgias; normal to decreased DTRs

## DIAGNOSTICS

### Imaging

- Immediate brain imaging if stroke or hemorrhage is suspected
  - ✓ CT or MRI, depending on availability for emergent imaging; MRI is preferred
  - ✓ MRI of brain if stroke is suspected
- MRI of spine if spinal cord compression, infarction, or transverse myelitis is suspected; can confirm diagnosis of Guillain–Barré syndrome by demonstration of enhancement of nerve roots after administration of gadolinium

### Electrophysiology (Electromyography and Nerve Conduction Velocities)

- May show evidence of anterior horn, peripheral nerve axon, neuromuscular junction, or muscle process; may show evidence of demyelination
- Abnormalities appear >1 week after symptom onset

### Laboratory Studies

- Creatine phosphokinase (CPK) if myopathy is suspected
- Lumbar puncture (LP) if Guillain–Barré is suspected

- Lyme titers for mononeuritis multiplex, a painful, asymmetrical, and asynchronous sensory and motor peripheral neuropathy that involves at least two separate nerves
- Amino-levulinic acid for porphyria
- *Muscle biopsy:* Performed as needed to evaluate for evidence of myopathy

## Management

Management depends on clinical setting.

- *Stroke:* Prompt recognition and management are important
- *Spinal cord emergencies:* Early steroids may stem evolution to compression; neurosurgical intervention may be needed; antibiotics if suspect abscess
- *Uremic neuropathy:* May respond to dialysis early in course
- *Neuromuscular weakness:* Close monitoring of respiratory status; specific treatments for Guillain–Barré, botulism, myasthenia
- *With elevated CPK:* Monitor for rhabdomyolysis, monitor renal function, and maintain hydration

## ALTERED MENTAL STATUS

**Decreased alertness or consciousness resulting from a pathologic process affecting the brain, whether an intrinsic central nervous process or diffuse metabolic derangement.**
**Normal: Awake, easy to arouse, and maintain alertness**
**Lethargic: Difficult to maintain alertness**
**Obtunded: Decreased alertness, responsive to pain, other stimuli**
**Stuporous: Decreased alertness, responsive only to pain**
**Comatose: Unresponsive even to pain**
**Orientation to person, place, time, and medical situation**
**Language: Fluency, comprehension, naming, and repetition**

### ETIOLOGY

- *Metabolic derangement:* Low or high glucose, $Na^+$ or $Ca^{2+}$, low $Mg^{2+}$, thyroid dysfunction, hypoparathyroidism, hepatic or renal encephalopathy, hypotension, hypertensive encephalopathy, hyperammonemia, sepsis, hypoxemia, hypercarbia, adrenal insufficiency, inborn error of metabolism
- Toxin or overdose (e.g., CO, cyanide, acetaminophen, narcotics, benzodiazepines, barbiturates)
- *Seizure:* Nonconvulsive seizures or post-ictal state
- *Infection:* Meningitis, encephalitis, CNS abscess
- *Increased ICP:* Space-occupying lesion, obstructed VP shunt, cerebral edema
- *Vascular:* Subarachnoid, subdural, intracerebral hemorrhage; stroke; migraine
- *Trauma:* Concussion, contusion, hemorrhage

### PATHOPHYSIOLOGY

- Dysfunction in both cerebral hemispheres, and/or the ascending reticular activating system

### CLINICAL MANIFESTATIONS

- Abnormal mental status exam, change in breathing pattern
- Possible loss of brainstem reflexes, including pupillary, corneal, vestibuloocular
- Vesicular lesions suggest herpes simplex virus
- Evaluate on coma scale (see Table 19-3)

## DIAGNOSTICS

- Glucose, electrolytes, liver function tests, ammonia, arterial blood gas, complete blood count, thyroid function tests, toxin screen, blood culture, urine culture
- LP unless obvious cause identified; avoid LP if concern for herniation (clinically or radiologically)
  - ✓ CSF HSV PCR, in addition to glucose, protein, cell count, and bacterial culture
- Head CT to evaluate for mass lesions and evidence of increased intracranial pressure (ICP)
- ECG to evaluate for arrhythmia
- EEG to evaluate for subclinical seizures, post-ictal state (or if normal, to suggest brainstem pathology, e.g., a "locked-in" state that may be present with a pontine lesion and create the appearance of altered mental status)

## MANAGEMENT

- *Treatment of reversible causes:*
  - ✓ Correct electrolyte, acid–base, ABCs, glucose disturbances
  - ✓ Antibiotics (see Meningitis in Infectious Diseases chapter [Chapter 15]); consider empiric acyclovir
  - ✓ Anticonvulsants when seizures are ongoing clinically or subclinically
  - ✓ Maintain normal body temperature
  - ✓ Consider naloxone
  - ✓ Consider specific antidotes

## ATAXIA

**Impaired control of coordination, movement, and balance**

### ETIOLOGY

- Intrinsic cerebellar disturbance
- Disturbance of input to cerebellum (from frontal lobes, posterior columns, and/or spino-cerebellar tracts)
- Vestibular dysfunction

### DIFFERENTIAL DIAGNOSIS

- Acute ataxia
  - ✓ Post-infectious cerebellitis
  - ✓ *Infectious cerebellitis:* Usually viral
  - ✓ *Drug ingestion:* Alcohol, phenytoin, carbamazepine, sedatives, hypnotics, phencyclidine, thallium
  - ✓ *Other:* Head trauma, cerebellar hemorrhage, neuroblastoma (opsoclonus-myoclonus-ataxia), acute disseminated encephalomyelitis [ADEM], hydrocephalus, Miller–Fisher variant of Guillain–Barré syndrome, meningitis, labyrinthitis, seizure or post-ictal state, basilar migraine, posterior circulation stroke, conversion
- *Intermittent ataxia:* Metabolic disorder (e.g., pyruvate dehydrogenase deficiency), acute paroxysmal vertigo
- Subacute, chronic, or progressive ataxia: Brain tumor, congenital anomaly, degenerative spinocerebellar diseases (e.g., Friedreich ataxia, ataxia-telangiectasia)

### CLINICAL MANIFESTATIONS

- *Manifestations depend on location of the lesion:*
  - ✓ *Cerebellar vermis:* Truncal ataxia

✓ *Cerebellar hemispheres:* Gait veers toward involved side, dysmetria of ipsilateral extremity
✓ *Sensory ataxia (peripheral nerve or posterior columns):* Abnormal sensation of light touch, proprioception, vibration, high-stepping gait, + Romberg, difficulties with fine motor movements, no dysmetria when eyes open, + dysmetria when eyes closed

## PHYSICAL EXAM

- *Cerebellar exam:* Coordination, truncal ataxia, limb ataxia
- *Cranial nerves:* Lower brainstem abnormalities raise concern for tumor or vascular insufficiency; vermis lesions cause direction-changing nystagmus; opsoclonus (concern for neuroblastoma)
- *Motor:* Unilateral weakness is concerning for posterior-fossa lesions; loss of DTRs suggests sensory ataxia
- *Sensory:* Afferent sensory input abnormalities are exacerbated by eye closure (not true of cerebellar ataxia)
- *Mental status:* Consider encephalitis if abnormal

## DIAGNOSTICS

### Radiology

- *Brain imaging:* CT acutely to rule out hemorrhage or space-occupying lesion; MRI best for posterior fossa and for leptomeningeal enhancement
- Body CT if concern for neuroblastoma

### Laboratory Studies

- CBC, electrolytes, toxin screen
- LP
- Urine VMA/HVA (if opsoclonus-myoclonus)
- Consider metabolic/genetic evaluation (especially if intermittent or progressive ataxia)

## MANAGEMENT

- Treat underlying etiology
- Post-infectious cerebellitis is self-limited (begins to resolve in 1–4 weeks). Steroids are not indicated
- Physical and occupational therapy

## BRAIN DEATH

**Irreversible loss of cortical and brainstem function, including respiratory drive**

- Death by Neurological Criteria protocols differs, and physicians must act in accordance with their own institution's policies
- Does NOT apply to children younger than 7 days (41 weeks conceptional age)
- A comatose patient with intact circulatory function must be declared dead by neurologic criteria before organ donation can be pursued

*Guidelines for the Determination of Brain Death in Children*

- Eliminate reversible causes of coma (e.g., opiates)
- *Physical exam criteria (see below):* Coma, absent brainstem reflexes, apnea
- In some institutions, at least one exam must be performed by a neurology or neurosurgery attending physician
- A second exam consistent with death by neurologic criteria at a specified time, depending on age

- Apnea test (to be performed as part of the last exam)
- Ancillary testing may be required (see below)
- *Age-specific requirements:*
  - ✓ *7 days–2 months:* Two exams and EEGs 48 hours apart
  - ✓ *2 months–1 year:* Two exams and EEGs 24 hours apart OR one exam and initial EEG demonstrating electrocerebral silence plus no cerebral blood flow on a radionuclide angiogram
  - ✓ *More than 1 year:* Two exams 12–24 hours apart with other studies optional

## PHYSICAL EXAM

- Normal temperature and blood pressure
- Mental status = coma (unresponsive to any stimulus)
- *Absent brainstem function:* Midposition or fully dilated pupils; no oculocephalic (doll's eye) response; no vestibulo-ocular response to (cold) caloric testing; no corneal, gag, or cough reflexes; no suck or root reflex
- Flaccid tone, no spontaneous or induced movements (except spinally mediated reflex movements)
- Persistence of this exam consistent with death by neurological criteria for appropriate length of time, as above
- *Apnea test (performed as part of the second or last exam):* Give 100% $O_2$ for 10 minutes before test. Allow hypercapnia (maximal respiratory stimulus) to develop by holding assisted ventilation. Monitor for spontaneous respirations. Monitor $CO_2$ level every 5 minutes, and continue to observe until $pCO_2$ is 60 torr or greater. Stop test if $pO_2$ less than 50 torr

## DIAGNOSTICS

- Workup for reversible causes of coma should be negative
- Drug levels should not be in toxic range
- If required, EEG must be done using special protocol and must determine electrocerebral silence to be consistent with death according to neurologic criteria
- Radionuclide angiogram must demonstrate lack of cerebral blood flow to be consistent with death according to neurologic criteria

## MANAGEMENT

- If patient satisfies definition for death by neurologic causes, physician should explain to family that patient is dead
- Consider organ donation, depending on wishes of family

## COMA

**A state of profound unconsciousness from which one cannot be aroused; Glasgow Coma Score less than 8** (Table 19-3).

## ETIOLOGY

- Trauma, infection, vascular, metabolic, increased ICP, seizure, toxin, or overdose

## DIFFERENTIAL DIAGNOSIS

- Profound neuromuscular disease, severe akinetic mutism, locked-in state, catatonia

| | | | |
|---|---|---|---|
| **TABLE 19-3** | | The Glasgow Coma Scale | |
| **Response** | **Score** | **Infants** | **Children** |
| **Ocular** | 4 | Open spontaneously | Open spontaneously |
| | 3 | To sound | To sound |
| | 2 | To pain | To pain |
| | 1 | Not at all | Not at all |
| **Verbal** | 5 | Coos, babbles | Oriented |
| | 4 | Cries but consolable | Confused |
| | 3 | Cries to pain, irritable | Inappropriate words |
| | 2 | Moans to pain, inconsolable | Nonspecific sounds |
| | 1 | None | None |
| **Motor** | 6 | Normal spontaneous movement | Follows commands |
| | 5 | Withdraws to touch | Localizes pain |
| | 4 | Withdraws to pain | Withdraws to pain |
| | 3 | Decorticates (abnl flexion) to pain | Decorticates (abnl flexion) to pain |
| | 2 | Decerebrates (abnl extension) to pain | Decerebrates (abnl extension) to pain |
| | 1 | Flaccid | Flaccid |

abnl, abnormal.

## PHYSICAL EXAM

- ABCs, vital signs, primary survey
- *Normal aggregate Glasgow Coma Score, based on age:* Birth–6 months: 9; older than 6–12 months: 11; older than 1–2 years: 12; older than 2–5 years: 13; older than 5 years: 14
- Focused neurologic exam

## MANAGEMENT

### Resuscitation

- ABCs, correct glucose, electrolytes
- Control seizures, consider naloxone and mannitol
- IV fluids: Normal saline at maintenance unless fluid–electrolyte disturbances
- There is no evidence to support hyperventilation measures

### Medical Management

- Empiric antimicrobials (e.g., third-generation cephalosporin + vancomycin + acyclovir) if concern for bacterial or treatable viral cause of meningitis. Do not wait for neuroimaging and LP if suspicion for infection is high

### Surgical Management

- Neurosurgical consultation
- Decompression of space-occupying lesion (hemorrhage or tumor) or shunt for acute hydrocephalus
- Ventriculostomy to monitor ICP, if indicated

## CRANIAL NERVES

Problems with cranial nerve (CN) function suggest brainstem abnormalities. For localization, consider the Rule of Fours: CN I–IV arise at midbrain level; CN V–VIII arise at pons level; CN IX–XII arise at medulla level.

- *CN I:* Olfactory: smell of non-noxious scents (e.g., coffee)
- *CN II:* Optic: pupillary response, visual acuity, visual fields, fundus exam
- *CN III:* Oculomotor: eye movements: vertical and horizontal adduction
- *CN IV:* Trochlear: eye movements: intorsion with adduction (down and in)
- *CN V:* Trigeminal: facial sensation (three distributions)
- *CN VI:* Abducens: eye movements: abduction
- *CN VII:* Facial: closure of muscles of facial expression
- *CN VIII:* Auditory: cochlear-hearing; vestibular-balance
- *CN IX:* Glossopharyngeal: palate elevation, phonation
- *CN X:* Vagus: palate elevation, phonation
- *CN XI:* Spinal accessory: trapezius and sternocleidomastoid strength
- *CN XII:* Hypoglossal: tongue symmetry, strength

## DERMATOMES

The surface of the skin is divided into dermatomes, areas of skin innervated by sensory fibers derived from a single spinal nerve root (Figure 19-1).

## ACQUIRED NEUROLOGIC DISEASE

## ACUTE DISSEMINATED ENCEPHALOMYELITIS

Monophasic inflammatory demyelinating condition of the CNS resulting in scattered focal white matter greater than deep gray matter lesions; typically occurs after viral illness and very rarely after vaccination (rabies, hepatitis, measles vaccines)

### EPIDEMIOLOGY

- *70% have prodromal illness:* Usually upper respiratory infection or nonspecific febrile illness
- About 90% of children recover completely

### DIFFERENTIAL DIAGNOSIS

- Meningitis, cerebellitis, sarcoidosis, CNS vasculitis, embolic events, acute hemorrhagic leukoencephalitis, multiple sclerosis (Table 19-4)

### PATHOPHYSIOLOGY

- *Vasculitis:* Probably complement-mediated, with antigen–antibody complexes causing endothelial damage
- *Demyelination:* Immune-mediated destruction of myelin

### CLINICAL MANIFESTATIONS

- Multifocal neurologic deficits (ataxia, hemiparesis, optic neuritis, CN palsies)
- Impaired consciousness (about 65%), ataxia (about 60%), meningismus (about 25%), fever (about 50%), headache (about 45%), seizures

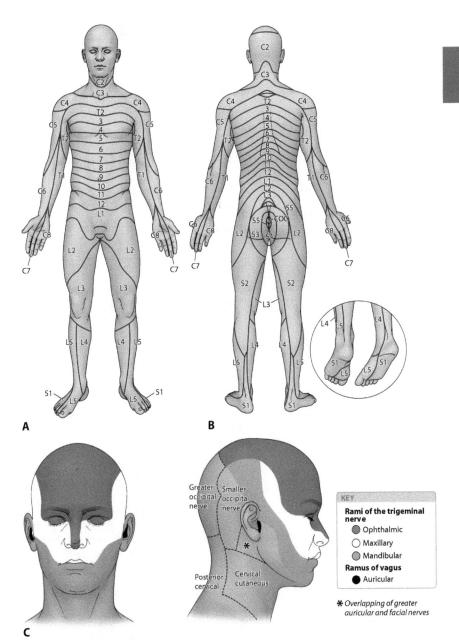

**FIGURE 19-1 Dermatomes.** The cutaneous fields of peripheral sensory nerves. (Reproduced with permission from Wolff K, Johnson RA, & Saavedra AP (Eds): *Fitzpatrick's Color Atlas and Synopsis of Clinical Dermatology,* 7th edition. New York, NY: McGraw-Hill; 2013.)

| TABLE 19-4 | Distinguishing Acute Disseminated Encephalomyelitis from Multiple Sclerosis |
|---|---|
| **ADEM** | **Multiple Sclerosis** |
| Monophasic | Multiple episodes |
| Lesions throughout (white and gray) | Peri-ventricular white matter lesions |
| Viral prodrome | Viral prodrome unusual |
| Ataxia common | Ataxia uncommon |
| Thalamic involvement common | Thalamic involvement very rare |
| Lesions may resolve on subsequent MRI | May find new lesions on subsequent MRI |
| More often in children | More often in adults |

ADEM, acute disseminated encephalomyelitis; MRI, magnetic resonance imaging.

- Perform general exam to evaluate for infection
- Detailed neurologic exam reveals multifocal deficits

## DIAGNOSTICS

### Laboratory Studies

- *LP:* Increased protein, increased WBCs (usually <50/mm³, lymphocyte predominance), culture negative, glucose normal. CSF findings normal in about 25%
- If history or distribution of lesions is suspicious for multiple sclerosis, send CSF for myelin basic protein and oligoclonal bands
- Other laboratory studies as indicated by clinical situation

### Radiology

- Early imaging may be normal
- MRI should be done in the acute setting if available. If MRI is not available, CT may be helpful to rule out other pathological processes
- *T2-weighted MRI:* Scattered increase signal white greater than gray matter lesions. Lesions are typically bilateral, asymmetric, and variable in size

## MANAGEMENT

- May resolve over 2–4 weeks without treatment, but most neurologists will opt to treat in an acute presentation
- *Pulse methylprednisolone:* Dose varies but some use 15–30 mg/kg/dose given once daily for 3 days
- IVIG may also be useful if response to steroids is incomplete (consider Neurology consultation)
- Physical and occupational therapy

## ACUTE MYOPATHY

**Motor dysfunction at the level of muscle**
**Acute weakness, typically proximal, may be painful or painless.**

## ETIOLOGY

- *Myositis:* Infectious (e.g., influenza), benign acute childhood myositis, idiopathic inflammatory progressive myopathies (dermatomyositis, polymyositis)

- *Metabolic myopathy:* Hypocalcemia, hypokalemia, inherited disorder of carbohydrate metabolism, critical illness myopathy

## DIFFERENTIAL DIAGNOSIS

- Joint disease, peripheral neuropathy (Guillain–Barré, axonal neuropathy), neuromuscular junction disorder (neuromuscular blockade, botulism, myasthenia gravis)

## DIAGNOSTICS

- *Laboratory studies:* CPK, BUN, and creatinine (if CPK is elevated), erythrocyte sedimentation rate (ESR) (may be elevated), Mi-2 antibodies (+ in 25% of dermatomyositis patients)
- *Nerve conduction studies and electromyography (EMG):* Normal conduction velocities, myopathic features can be seen from 1 week after onset, EMG reveals small and polyphasic motor unit potentials
- *Muscle biopsy:* Inflammatory changes, fiber necrosis replaces muscle by fat, dermatomyositis leads to perifascicular atrophy, polymyositis leads to endomysial inflammation, lipid myopathy
- *Muscle MRI:* Can help define extent of edema or fatty infiltration

## MANAGEMENT

- Management is variable; consider consultation with neurology service or experts in neuromuscular disease management
- Generally, analgesia and systemic corticosteroids are used
- *Immunosuppression:* Methotrexate, azathioprine, or cyclophosphamide (consider consultation with neurology service/neuromuscular experts for indications and dosing)
- IVIG for refractory inflammatory myopathies (2 g/kg acutely then monthly)
- Monitor for rhabdomyolysis and hydrate if CPK is elevated (see Rhabdomyolysis, in Nephrology chapter [Chapter 18])
- Physical therapy to avoid contractures from inactivity
- *Dermatomyositis:* Consider evaluation for malignancy, especially testicular cancer in males

## BOTULISM

**Neuroparalytic illness caused by neurotoxins produced by *Clostridium botulinum* (anaerobic, spore-forming, bacillus)**

### EPIDEMIOLOGY

- *Clostridium botulinum* is found in soil, honey, and home-canned foods
- *Four types:* Foodborne, wound, infant, adult
- Seventy to 100 cases of infant botulism are reported annually to Centers for Disease Control
- 70–90% of cases occur in breast-fed infants
- *Typical age:* 6 weeks–9 months (90% younger than 6 months)

### DIFFERENTIAL DIAGNOSIS

- Sepsis, toxin ingestion (e.g., organophosphates), Guillain–Barré, myasthenia gravis, stroke

### PATHOPHYSIOLOGY

- *Infant botulism:* Ingested spores germinate and colonize GI tract (infection) then release toxin
- *Children and adults:* Ingested toxin from contaminated food

- Neurotoxin binds irreversibly to presynaptic nerve endings, inhibiting acetylcholine release. Toxin does not cross the blood–brain barrier

## CLINICAL MANIFESTATIONS

- Symmetric, descending flaccid paralysis
- Infants classically present with constipation; they may also present with poor feeding, and weak cry, followed by respiratory compromise
- Cranial nerves (ophthalmoparesis, ptosis, disconjugate gaze, diminished gag, difficulty swallowing, weak suck) involved initially and then descends to upper extremities and respiratory muscles
- Neurologic sequelae are rare
- Progressive weakness and hypotonia (typically over 1–2 weeks) with bulbar and spinal nerve abnormalities; hyporeflexia develops later in course
- Deep tendon reflexes are initially normal despite profound hypotonia; hyporeflexia develops later in the course
- Autonomic dysfunction is common including decreased tearing and salivation
- Normal pupillary light reflex fatigues with repeated stimulation over 1–2 minutes

## DIAGNOSTICS

### Laboratory Studies

- Stool for *C. botulinum* toxin assay; use water enema to facilitate obtaining stool for testing
- Rule-out sepsis workup in infants
- Serum toxic screen
- *EMG:* Not routinely necessary but when performed reveals incremental response in muscle action potential with high-frequency stimulation; normal nerve conduction velocity
  - ✓ No response to injection of edrophonium chloride or neostigmine, which distinguishes it from myasthenia gravis
- Brain and/or spine imaging if diagnosis unclear

## MANAGEMENT

- Human-derived botulinum immune globulin for infants
- Trivalent equine antitoxin for adults (risk of anaphylaxis)
- To obtain antitoxin or immune globulin (in any state), call California Department of Health Services: 510-540-2646 (www.infantbotulism.org)
  - ✓ Administration within 3 days of hospitalization is ideal though administration within 4–7 days yields better outcomes than no treatment
- Avoid aminoglycosides because they can potentiate neuromuscular blockade, precipitating rapid clinical deterioration
- Contact state/local public health authorities for suspected or documented cases of botulism (except infant botulism)
- *Supportive care:*
  - ✓ Up to 70% may require mechanical ventilation, nasogastric feeds
  - ✓ Suppositories often required for constipation
  - ✓ Nasogastric tube feedings are usually required during course of illness to prevent aspiration of formula
    - Small volumes of continuous enteral feeding stimulates gut motility and may obviate the need for central venous catheterization
    - Resume oral feedings when gag, swallow, and suck reflexes return
    - Strict monitoring of intake/output and weight given risk of SIADH, which complicates up to 15% of cases

- Typical hospitalization is 2–3 weeks though full recovery may take up to 2 months
- Case fatality rates are less than 1%

## GUILLAIN–BARRÉ SYNDROME

**Acute inflammatory demyelinating polyradiculoneuropathy**
**Affects spinal nerve roots and peripheral nerves**
**May affect axons in acute motor axonal neuropathy**
**Classic Guillain–Barré syndrome: Progressive often ascending weakness in more than one limb, areflexia**
**Miller–Fisher variant: Ataxia, ophthalmoparesis, areflexia**
**Classic CSF finding: Albumino-cytologic dissociation (markedly elevated protein level with normal or trivially elevated CSF WBCs)**

### EPIDEMIOLOGY

- *Incidence:* 0.6–1.9 cases per 100,000 children/year
- Slight male predominance
- Most common paralytic illness in children in developed countries

### ETIOLOGY

- Follows viral infection in over 50% of cases
- May follow bacterial infection (e.g., *Campylobacter jejuni*), surgery
- Seen in a higher-than-expected rate in patients with sarcoidosis, SLE, lymphoma, HIV infection, Lyme disease, and solid tumors
- Often no clear trigger

### DIFFERENTIAL DIAGNOSIS

- Transverse myelitis, spinal cord compression, myositis, myopathy, posterior fossa lesion, acute cerebellar ataxia, bilateral strokes
- *Infections:* Poliomyelitis (LP with elevated WBCs), HIV seroconversion (LP with elevated WBCs), diphtheria
- Tick paralysis, porphyria
- *Drugs:* INH, vincristine, amitriptyline, hydralazine, nitric oxide
- *Toxins:* Lead, mercury, arsenic, thallium, organophosphates, glue, acrylamide
- *Neuromuscular blockade:* Botulism, myasthenia gravis

### PATHOPHYSIOLOGY

- Immune-mediated inflammation and demyelination of spinal nerve roots and peripheral nerves
- Likely molecular mimicry
- Anti-GM1 Ab and *C. jejuni*
- Anti-GQ1B Ab in Miller–Fisher variant

### CLINICAL MANIFESTATIONS

- *Progressive, often ascending weakness in the limbs:* 50% plateau by 2 weeks, 80% by 3 weeks
- Numbness or paresthesias in the extremities in a classic stocking-glove distribution. Children *often* complain of pain
- Facial weakness in 50%, weakness of respiratory muscles
- Ataxia, ophthalmoparesis, may have autonomic instability

- Back pain from spinal nerve root inflammation
- Constipation or bowel/bladder incontinence
- *Clinical recovery is the rule with good supportive care:* May take weeks to months; complete recovery in 80%
- Acute relapses occur in 1–5% of patients in large series
- Chronic inflammatory demyelinating polyradiculoneuropathy (CIDP) can begin with a rapid onset of weakness indistinguishable from Guillain–Barré syndrome
- *Vital signs:* May have instability
- Preserved mental status
- *Cranial nerves:* Facial weakness, may have ophthalmoparesis
- *Motor:* Weakness, usually distal greater than proximal, loss of DTRs
- *Sensory:* Length-dependent loss of sensation
- Check gait for degree of weakness and for ataxia

## DIAGNOSTICS

- *LP required:* Albumino-cytologic dissociation = elevated CSF protein (typically 80–200 mg/dL); normal or mildly elevated CSF WBC (<10 mononuclear cells/mm$^3$); may be normal in first week of disease
- *EMG:* For confirmation of diagnosis; abnormal in 50% of patients in the first 2 weeks and in 85% of patients afterwards; evidence of segmental demyelination
- *MRI:* If suspicion for spinal cord compression; Guillain–Barré syndrome pattern: enhancing nerve roots

## MANAGEMENT

- Admit patient for observation
- *Supportive therapy:* Monitor respiratory status with serial negative inspiratory force (NIF); intubation if necessary
- *Hastening of recovery:* IVIG 2 g/kg divided into five daily doses OR *plasmapheresis:* plasma exchange volume 200–250 mL/kg divided in three to five treatments over 7–14 days
- Pain control (mostly back, limb; pain control often achieved with gabapentin and sometimes with opioids or NSAIDs), bowel regimen, Foley catheter if voiding limited, deep venous thrombosis prophylaxis if immobile

## INCREASED INTRACRANIAL PRESSURE

**Abnormal elevation of pressure inside the skull, caused by an increase in brain volume, intracranial blood, CSF, and/or mass. Normal ICP varies with age: neonate: less than 2 cm H$_2$O; younger than 12 months: 1.5–6 cm H$_2$O; child: 3–7 cm H$_2$O; adolescent: less than 15 cm H$_2$O; adult: less than 20 cm H$_2$O**

### DIFFERENTIAL DIAGNOSIS

- Brain tumor, meningitis, pseudotumor cerebri, hydrocephalus due to ventriculo-peritoneal (VP) shunt malfunction, intracranial hemorrhage, metabolic derangement, seizure

### PATHOPHYSIOLOGY (OF EDEMA)

- *Vasogenic edema:* Impaired blood–brain barrier; increased capillary permeability; increased capillary transmural pressure; retention of extravasated fluid in interstitial space; occurs near tumors, hemorrhages, inflammatory foci
- *Cytotoxic edema:* Impaired Na$^+$-K$^+$-ATPase pump due to decreased cerebral blood flow; causes increased extracellular K$^+$ and increased intracellular Ca$^{2+}$, leading to cell death secondary to membrane dysfunction; occurs near areas of ischemia and hypoxemia

- *Interstitial edema:* High pressure obstructive hydrocephalus leading to ischemia
- *Hydrostatic edema:* Increased transmural vascular pressure resulting in increased extracellular fluid; may result from abrupt loss of cerebral autoregulation
- *Osmotic edema:* Decreased serum osmolality and hyponatremia ($Na^+$ <125 mEq/L)

## CLINICAL MANIFESTATIONS

- *Mental status changes:* May progress to coma
- *Headache:* Especially early morning and positional
- Irritability, nausea, vomiting, diplopia
- Focal neurologic findings depending on etiology
- Glasgow Coma Scale score (see Table 19-3)
- *Cushing's triad:* Bradycardia, hypertension, irregular respirations
- Acutely increasing head circumference; full or bulging fontanel or increased separation of sutures
- Detailed cranial nerve, motor, sensory, and cerebellar exam
- Infants rarely have papilledema

## DIAGNOSTICS

### Radiology

- VP shunt series in patients with ventricular shunt
- *Emergent head CT or brain MRI with and without contrast:* Can have normal head CT with increased ICP; ultrasound usually sufficient for diagnosis in infants with open fontanel

### Laboratory Studies

- If clinically indicated, LP only if neuroimaging excludes mass lesion or effaced ventricles
- Serum electrolytes and osmolarity
- Ammonia level if diffuse cerebral edema

### Intracranial Pressure Monitoring (Intensive Care Unit Setting)

- *Indicated if:* Glasgow Coma Scale score less than 8; rapidly deteriorating neurologic status; pharmacologic paralysis; mechanical ventilation with increased mean airway pressures or increased pulmonary end-expiratory pressure

## MANAGEMENT

### Resuscitation

- ABCs, control seizures
- *Maintain adequate mean arterial pressure (MAP) because:*
  ✓ Cerebral perfusion pressure: CPP = MAP−ICP
- Low CPP results in ischemia (aim for CPP greater than 50 mm Hg)
- *Goal CPP:* Greater than 60 mm Hg in adolescents; greater than 50 mm Hg in infants and children

### Reduce Cerebral Blood Volume

- Elevate head of bed
- Hyperventilation to $PaCO_2$ 25–30 mm Hg recommended in acute setting, but avoid chronic hyperventilation
- Cerebral vasoconstricting sedation (thiopental, pentobarbital)
- Avoid hyperthermia

## Reduce Brain and Cerebrospinal Fluid Volume

- *Mannitol:* 0.25–1.0 mg/kg IV (effect seen in 10–15 minutes and lasts up to 8 hours); must monitor blood pressure, electrolytes, serum osmolarity
- *Furosemide:* 0.5–1.0 mg/kg IV (or 0.15–0.3 mg/kg IV when used along with mannitol)
- *Acetazolamide:* 30 mg/kg/day IV/orally in four to six divided doses, maximum 1 g/day (may cause transient increased ICP due to $CO_2$ release, but then decreases CSF production significantly)
- *Dexamethasone:* 1–2 mg/kg IV/orally loading dose (maximum 10 mg) followed by 1 mg/kg/day in four divided doses (maximum 16 mg/day) to decrease vasogenic edema
- Ventriculostomy drain or VP shunt (Neurosurgery consultation)
- Consider decreasing fluid infusion to two-thirds of maintenance requirements using 0.9% normal saline rather than 0.45% normal saline

## Reduce Intracranial Volume

- Surgical decompression, VP shunt

## For Suspected Shunt Malfunction

- Head CT, shunt series, sterile shunt tap to assess proximal and distal flow; emergent shunt revision

## MULTIPLE SCLEROSIS

**Multiple demyelinating episodes in time and space. Multiple sclerosis (MS) is a lifelong disease with variable course.**

- *Clinically Definite MS:* Two clinical attacks at least 24 hours long and separated by 1 month AND clinical evidence (on neurological exam) of two lesions OR clinical evidence of one lesion AND paraclinical evidence of a second lesion (see subsequent section)
- *Laboratory Supported Definite MS:* Two attacks AND clinical or paraclinical evidence of one lesion AND lumbar puncture evidence of MS

### EPIDEMIOLOGY

- Geographic variation in prevalence. Northern United States, greater than 30/100,000; Southern United States, 5–30/100,000; children who move before age 15 acquire risk of new environment
- Pediatric cases are 1.8–5% of all cases
- Female:male ratio: 1:1 before puberty; 2.2–3:1 after puberty
- *Youngest reported case:* 10 months

### ETIOLOGY

- Likely multifactorial; genetic component
- Possible viral or environmental trigger
- 25% risk of developing MS if monozygotic twin has MS
- In patients with MS, family history is positive in 10–26%

### DIFFERENTIAL DIAGNOSIS

- Systemic lupus erythematosus, Sjögren, neurosarcoidosis, HIV, syphilis, CNS infection, Lyme, vitamin $B_{12}$ deficiency, CNS vasculitis, autoimmune disease, Behcet, recurrent ADEM, antiphospholipid antibody syndrome

## PATHOPHYSIOLOGY

- Immune-mediated inflammation and demyelination of central white matter
- *Lesions are plaques:* 1 mm–4 cm in diameter; loss of myelin, sparing of axons; T cells, macrophages; evolution to gliosis
- Likely molecular mimicry and attack of myelin basic protein

## CLINICAL MANIFESTATIONS

- Attacks tend to last days to weeks and may be precipitated by acute infection or metabolic derangement
- Loss of sensation, coordination, or gait; nystagmus
- *Motor:* Weakness (acute or chronic), spasticity
- Frequent brainstem involvement; sensory greater than motor dysfunction
- *Optic neuritis:* Painful; usually unilateral loss of vision; on exam may see swollen disc, decreased color saturation, and decreased acuity with acute optic neuritis; a pale disc is seen with previous optic neuritis
- Transverse myelitis or spinal cord syndrome
- Ataxia, other cerebellar dysfunction, bladder dysfunction
- *Seizures:* 10–22% of children with MS, more with younger age of onset
- *Mental status:* Usually normal at disease onset, possible cognitive difficulties
- *L'Hermitte's phenomenon:* Neck flexion yields electrical sensation down arms
- *Uhthoff's phenomenon:* Symptoms worsen or brought on by heat
- *Progression of disease:* Two-thirds of children with MS have relapsing-remitting form;
- *Other forms:* primary or secondary progressive, progressive relapsing

## DIAGNOSTICS

- *Magnetic resonance imaging of brain and spinal cord with gadolinium:* Classic periventricular white matter lesions; in isolated optic neuritis, helps predict progression to MS; active lesions enhance; old lesions do not enhance
- LP: Oligoclonal bands, elevated IgG index
- Paraclinical evidence (extensions of the neurological exam): MRI, brainstem auditory evoked responses, visual-evoked response, documented urologic dysfunction
- Laboratory studies to rule out other processes. *Antibodies:* anti-nuclear antibody (ANA), anti-neutrophil cytoplasmic antibodies, anti-ssA, anti-ssB, ACE, anti-scl70, anticardiolipin antibody.
  ✓ *Inflammatory markers:* ESR, CRP
  ✓ *Infectious:* RPR, HIV, Lyme; vitamin $B_{12}$ level
- *If history of oral and genital ulcers:* Skin pathergy test for Behcet

## MANAGEMENT

### Acute Management of an Attack

- Evaluate and treat precipitating infection (temp, urinalysis, chest x-ray, etc.)
- If symptoms are severe and progressive (e.g., non-ambulatory), consider pulse steroids (methylprednisolone 15–30 mg/kg/dose given once daily for 3 days; maximum 1 g/day) and taper to hasten recovery from attack
- *Optic neuritis:* IV steroids hasten recovery (no effect on final vision) and may slow progression of MS (IV only)

### Prevention of Disease Progression

- *IFN1α weekly injections:* First line as it has been evaluated as safe and tolerable in children
- *Other agents studied in adults:* Glatiramer acetate, IFN1β

## MYASTHENIA GRAVIS

**An antibody-mediated autoimmune disease resulting in depletion of nicotinic ace-tylcholine (ACh) receptors at the neuromuscular junction and subsequent fatigable weakness**

- *Myasthenic crisis:* Life-threatening respiratory weakness

### EPIDEMIOLOGY

- 50–125 cases per million population (approximately 10% are children)
- Develops at any age
- Girls affected more often than boys postpuberty
- 15% of adults with MG will have thymomas but rare in children; 85% of adults have thymic lymphofollicular hyperplasia
- 10% of children will have associated autoimmune disease

### DIFFERENTIAL DIAGNOSIS

- Congenital myasthenic syndrome, transient neonatal myasthenia, drug-induced myasthenia, hyperthyroidism, Lambert–Eaton syndrome, botulism

### PATHOPHYSIOLOGY

- Auto-antibodies cause deficit of ACh receptors at neuromuscular junctions leading to accelerated degradation, functional blockade of the binding sites, and complement-mediated damage to the receptors
- Abnormal ACh receptors (simplified membrane folds) and wide synaptic space also contribute
- Resulting decreased amplitude of end-plate potentials causes failure to trigger action potentials, reducing muscle power

### CLINICAL MANIFESTATIONS

- Weakness and fatigability of skeletal muscles, ptosis, dysphagia, shortness of breath, blurred vision
- Muscles usually strongest early in the morning. Symptoms improve with rest
- *Diplopia, ptosis most often:* 50% at presentation, 80–90% later
- *Generalized weakness in 2/3 of children:* Bulbar, truncal, limb
- Intact DTRs, sensation, and coordination
- *Closed eye rest test:* Rest with eyes closed for 15 minutes. Observe degree of ptosis before and after test

### DIAGNOSTICS

#### Anticholinesterase Test (Edrophonium, Tensilon)

- Tensilon, 0.1–0.2 mg/kg (maximum 10 mg) IV: Start with 20% as test dose and wait 2 minutes, then 30% and wait 2 minutes, then 50%
- Positive if unequivocal improvement in objectively weak muscle
- Monitor for bradycardia, hypotension, respiratory compromise
- Have atropine ready STAT if patient becomes bradycardic

#### Radioimmunoassay for ACh-receptor Antibodies

- Positive in 50–90% of pediatric patients

#### Other

- *Thyroid function studies:* 3–8% will have hyperthyroidism

- Consider screening for other autoimmune disorders, especially diabetes mellitus
- Purified protein derivative test before immune therapy
- Serum vitamin $B_{12}$ level
- *EMG:* Repetitive nerve stimulation, single fiber EMG if unclear
- Consider chest CT to evaluate thymus
- If isolated CN weakness, consider brain imaging to rule out mass

## MANAGEMENT

### Chronic Medical Management

- *Anticholinesterase agents:* Pyridostigmine (Mestinon) is first-line therapy:
  - ✓ Initial dosing in children is every 4–6 hours. In adults, usually given three times a day but sustained release formulations permit every day to twice-daily dosing
  - ✓ Titrate dose to effect
- *Immunosuppression:* Prednisone, azathioprine, others
- *Other immunotherapy:* Plasmapheresis, IVIG; used for myasthenic crisis, preparation for thymectomy, or failure to respond to medications

### Crisis

- Criteria to consider mechanical ventilation include forced vital capacity less than 15 mL/kg, less than 30% predicted for age, severe aspiration, or labored breathing; consider plasmapheresis or IVIG

### Surgical Management

- Thymectomy has a therapeutic effect in childhood generalized myasthenia gravis; prevention of spread of thymoma in adults (rare in childhood)

## PSEUDOTUMOR CEREBRI

**Syndrome characterized by increased ICP, normal CSF, normal/small ventricles, no intracranial mass. Often used synonymously with the term idiopathic intracranial hypertension.**

- ICP greater than 200 mm $H_2O$ if non-obese, greater than 250 mm $H_2O$ if obese patient

### EPIDEMIOLOGY

- Classically, obese women of child-bearing age
- *Prepuberty:* No gender difference, less commonly associated with obesity, less often chronic

### ETIOLOGY

Associated conditions and possible risk factors include:

- *Neurologic:* Venous sinus thrombosis, meningitis (including Lyme)
- *Systemic:* Malnutrition, refeeding, SLE, hypertension, vitamin $B_{12}$ or iron deficiency, hypervitaminosis A, renal failure, significant weight change
- *Medications:* Steroid withdrawal, tetracycline, doxycycline, minocycline, vitamin A, isotretinoin, ciprofloxacin, lithium, thyroxine, nalidixic acid, oral contraceptive pills
- *Endocrine:* Obesity, hyper/hypothyroid, hypoparathyroidism, Addison, pregnancy

### PATHOPHYSIOLOGY

Theories include decreased CSF absorption by arachnoid granulation tissue versus CSF overproduction.

## CLINICAL MANIFESTATIONS

- Headache worse in morning or lying flat, +/− nausea, vomiting, and photophobia
- Diplopia, blurry vision (common in children), loss of central vision (central scotoma), may progress to blindness
- Transient visual obscurations likely due to optic nerve ischemia
- May have normal level of consciousness and intellectual functioning
- Strabismus, pulsatile tinnitus, neck/back pain, irritability, somnolence
- Papilledema (not universal); visual field loss (central scotoma)
- Visual acuity and color vision spared initially
- CN VI palsy (resolves when ICP normalized)
- Symptoms may improve immediately post-LP

## DIAGNOSTICS

*Pseudotumor cerebri is a diagnosis of exclusion:*

- *Neuroimaging:* Emergent imaging to evaluate for mass or hydrocephalus; MRI/MRV best for venous sinus thrombosis
- *Laboratory Studies:*
  - ✓ LP with opening pressure, cell count, glucose, protein, cultures (should be normal except pressure; protein can be low)
  - ✓ Specific laboratory tests to evaluate for specific etiologies (e.g., vitamin A)
  - ✓ Consider electrolytes, BUN, creatinine, ANA, urinalysis, hypercoagulability tests
- *Vision Testing:* Visual acuity and quantitative perimetry testing at diagnosis and at regular intervals thereafter

## MANAGEMENT

### Medical

- If substantial visual field loss: Admit, administer steroids such as dexamethasone (see Increased Intracranial Pressure) or prednisone (1–2 mg/kg/day up to 60–100 mg/day with a gradual taper over 2 weeks), follow serial visual field exams
- Stop any precipitating agents
- No specific treatment if headache resolves in 24–48 hours
- Acetazolamide (Diamox) for symptomatic children (see Increased Intracranial Pressure topic for dosing guidelines). Watch for dose-dependent paresthesias

### Surgical

- For patients who fail medications and are symptomatic
- Optic nerve sheath fenestration
- Lumbar peritoneal shunt

### Other

- Weight loss in obese patients
- Serial LPs are NOT effective long-term

## SPINAL CORD EMERGENCY

## ETIOLOGY

- *Trauma:* Breech or traumatic delivery; in older children, mostly cervical spine in order of decreasing frequency: motor vehicle accidents, diving, falls; may occur in setting of head injury or other trauma

- *Infection:* Epidural abscess, tuberculosis, HIV, often after trauma or vertebral osteomyelitis
- *Infarction:* Hypotension (e.g., after arrest), aortic dissection, anterior spinal artery occlusion
- *Hemorrhage:* Arteriovenous malformation, intramedullary tumor
- *Inflammation:* Demyelinating spinal cord process (e.g., transverse myelitis), vasculitis

## CLINICAL MANIFESTATIONS

- Sudden flaccid paraparesis (spinal shock)
- Evolution to spastic paresis or plegia
- Neck or back pain, fever if abscess
- Bowel and bladder compromise
- History of trauma
- A fall may occur as a result of the spinal cord process and resultant weakness and may not be the inciting factor
- *Vital signs:* May have diaphragm paralysis if C3–C5 are involved
- Femoral pulses
- Preserved mental status unless there is concurrent head injury
- Cranial nerve function should be preserved
- *Motor:* Weakness with a spinal level; initial low tone, then increased; initial loss of DTRs, then increased
- *Sensory:* Spinal level

## DIAGNOSTICS

- MRI of the spine
- *Depending on clinical suspicion:* Electrolytes, CBC, ESR, CRP, ANA, bone radiographs, LP

## MANAGEMENT

- Immobilization of the spine
- ABCs (minimal neck extension if cervical trauma)
- Emergent neurosurgical consultation
- *Steroids within 8 hours of injury:* Methylprednisone 30 mg/kg IV bolus, then 5.4 mg/kg/h for 23 hours
- Monitor respiratory status with serial measurements of NIF
- *Other:* Supportive therapy, pain control, bowel regimen, Foley catheter, DVT prophylaxis, intubation if necessary

## STROKE

**Stroke: Prolonged or permanent dysfunction of brain due to interruption of blood flow Transient Ischemic Attack (TIA): Symptoms last less than 24 hours**

## EPIDEMIOLOGY

- 2–3 cases/100,000 children/year
- *Neonatal stroke (infants <30 days old):* 1/4000 live births
- Approximately 50% have persistent neurologic abnormality or seizure disorder after stroke; 5–10% of affected children die, about 30% have a recurrence, about 30% have no sequelae
- Incidence of ischemic stroke is similar to hemorrhagic stroke, but mortality rate is 41% in hemorrhagic and 5% in ischemic

## ETIOLOGY

- Thrombosis, embolism, hemorrhage, hypoperfusion
- No cause detected in 20%

- *Risk factors for arterial ischemic stroke:* Congenital heart disease, sickle cell disease, coagulation disorders, infection (e.g., endocarditis, varicella), moyamoya, arterial dissection
- *Risk factors for hemorrhagic stroke:* Arteriovenous malformation, cerebral aneurysm, cavernous malformations, head trauma, bleeding diathesis
- *Risk factors for venous sinus thrombosis:* Severe dehydration, sepsis, hypercoagulability

## PATHOPHYSIOLOGY

- *Arterial ischemic stroke:* Decreased cerebral blood flow causes ischemia. Cell death causes edema and surrounding damage. Patients may have hemorrhage into stroke territory
- *Hemorrhagic stroke:* Mass effect causes local damage and may result in midline shift or herniation
- *Venous sinus thrombosis:* Venous hypertension, venous infarction with hemorrhages
- Maximal edema occurs 2–3 days after stroke

## CLINICAL MANIFESTATIONS

- *Ischemic stroke:* Focal neurologic deficit
- *Hemorrhagic stroke:* Headache, mental status change, focal neurologic deficit
- Children often present hours or days after symptoms begin
- *Vital signs:* Watch for signs of herniation including Cushing's triad of hypertension, bradycardia, and abnormal respirations
- Perform detailed neurologic exam to identify focality and evaluate level of consciousness
- May have papilledema
- Evidence of trauma or predisposing disease
- Serial exams are required

## DIAGNOSTICS

### Radiology

- Non-contrast head CT
- Brain MRI better for early infarcts (diffusion-weighted MRI)
- *MR Angiography/Venography to evaluate vascular abnormalities:* Include MRA of neck if suspect arterial dissection and MRV if suspect venous sinus thrombosis
- Cerebral angiography if further information required after MRA
- Transcranial Doppler ultrasound can predict increased risk in patients with sickle cell disease

### Laboratory Studies

- CBC, PT/PTT/INR, lipid profile, HIV, RPR
- *Hypercoagulability workup* (see Box 12-1): Protein C and protein S levels, AT-III, factor V Leiden, homocystine level and MTHFR gene, antiphospholipid, prothrombin 20210 gene mutation, lipoprotein a, $\beta$-2 glycoprotein 1
- *Screen for vasculitis:* ESR, C3, C4, ANA
- *Toxicology screen:* Cocaine
- *Hemoglobin electrophoresis:* Sickle cell disease
- Blood culture if suspect endocarditis
- *If infarct not in typical vascular distribution:* Plasma ammonia, lactate, pyruvate, amino acids, urine organic acids, CSF lactate
- Also consider ECG and echocardiography

## MANAGEMENT

- *For initial resuscitation:* ABCs, treat hypoglycemia, treat seizures, maintain temperature 36.5–37°C

## Acute Medical Management

1. *Arterial ischemic stroke:* Lay flat (maximize cerebral perfusion); liberal IV normal saline (avoid dextrose to minimize edema); correct electrolyte abnormalities (avoid hyperosmolality); maintain normotension; monitor ICP; if arterial dissection or cardiac clot, consider heparin
2. *Hemorrhagic stroke:* Monitor vital signs, ICP; elevate head 45 degrees; maintain normotension; correct electrolyte imbalances; *avoid* anticoagulation
3. *Venous sinus thrombosis:* Monitor ICP; liberal IV normal saline; if not contraindicated, start heparin (no *bolus*)

## Anticoagulation

- *Aspirin (ASA)* (acute and chronic therapy): 2–3 mg/kg/day causes antiplatelet effect ("low-dose" = 1 mg/kg/day)
- *Heparin* (risk of recurrence or extension versus risk of bleed): Do NOT bolus; younger than 12 months: 28 U/kg/h; older than 12 months: 20 U/kg/h; target aPTT: 60–85 seconds
- *Low-molecular-weight heparin (Enoxaparin):* Children and adults use 1 mg/kg/dose every 12 hours; neonates use 1.5 mg/kg/dose every 12 hours
- *Warfarin* is most effective long-term anticoagulant in children: Avoid contact sports; target International Normalized Ratio (INR) is 2.0–3.0
- *Thrombolytics* have not been well studied in children with stroke and are not recommended at this time

## Surgical

- Emergent evacuation of large hemorrhage and/or increased ICP
- May require ventriculostomy to monitor ICP
- Consider surgery for vascular malformations, large middle cerebral artery infarcts, and hydrocephalus

## TRANSVERSE MYELITIS

**Acute or subacute inflammatory process involving both gray and white matter of the spinal cord, resulting in bilateral motor, sensory, and autonomic dysfunction**

### EPIDEMIOLOGY

- One to four new cases/million/year; seasonal clustering (winter)
- Peak incidence at ages 10–19 and 30–39 years
- No gender or familial predisposition
- One-third recover completely, one-third moderate permanent disability, one-third severe persistent disability

### DIFFERENTIAL DIAGNOSIS

- Guillain–Barré syndrome, ADEM, MS, compressive lesions of spinal cord, fibrocartilaginous emboli
- *Ischemia; if symptom nadir occurs in less than 4 hours:* Arteriovenous malformation, vasculitis

### PATHOPHYSIOLOGY

- *Anatomic changes:* Edema, demyelination, necrosis of spinal cord
- *Post-infectious:* Associated with numerous infections, including viral URI, herpes zoster, HIV, EBV, influenza, *Mycoplasma*, and mumps
- *Post-vaccination:* Polio, cholera, typhoid, rabies
- *Autoimmune:* Abnormal cell-mediated response to myelin sheath component

## CLINICAL MANIFESTATIONS

- Back pain, then weakness and sensory changes develop over days
- Usually legs more than arms
- Voiding dysfunction common
- Often fever, nuchal rigidity
- Deficits progress quickly, usually reaching maximum in 2 days
- *May see signs of recovery after 6 days:* Full in 50%, partial in 40%, and none in 10%
- *On physical exam:* Flaccid (early) or spastic (late) paraplegia or quadriplegia; sensory level (often mid-thoracic); sphincter abnormalities; abnormal DTRs (decreased early, increased late); perform ophthalmologic exam for optic nerve involvement

## DIAGNOSTICS

### Laboratory Studies

- *LP:* Increased WBC (lymphocytic predominance), normal or increased protein, normal glucose. Send bacterial and viral cultures, oligoclonal bands, IgG index. Consider cytology, specific viral studies (e.g., VZV, EBV, Lyme titer, *Mycoplasma*)
- Serum/CSF viral titers if clinically indicated
- Screening for autoimmune disease
- HIV, HTLV-1, RPR tests
- U/A and culture if urinary retention

### Other Studies

- *Gadolinium-enhanced MRI of spine:* Fusiform swelling of spinal cord
- *Gadolinium-enhanced MRI of brain:* To evaluate for multifocal disease
- *EMG:* Denervation associated with poor prognosis

## MANAGEMENT

- High-dose IV methylprednisolone (15–30 mg/kg/dose, maximum 1 g/day) for 5 days is standard of care
- *Sphincter dysfunction:* Intermittent catheterization; treat constipation
- *Supportive:* Physical and occupational therapy

## SEIZURES AND EPILEPSY

### GENERAL PRINCIPLES

**Seizure:** Paroxysmal event caused by abnormal electrical discharges in the brain
**Epilepsy:** Recurrent unprovoked seizures, usually stereotyped
**Simple partial:** Motor signs, sensory or psychic experience with preserved awareness
**Complex partial:** Partial seizure with impairment of awareness (often staring)
**Generalized seizures:** Tonic–clonic, tonic, clonic, atonic, myoclonic, or absence
**Simple seizures may evolve to complex partial seizures, and either may evolve to a generalized seizure.**

### EPIDEMIOLOGY

- 1% of children will have an afebrile seizure by age 14 years
- 2–4% of American children will have a febrile seizure
- *Active epilepsy:* 0.4–0.9% of children, 1% overall population

## ETIOLOGY

- Fever, hypoxia, ischemia, head trauma, hemorrhage, CNS infection, hyperammonemia, toxin, medication, medication withdrawal, inborn error of metabolism
- Structural abnormality (tumor or malformation)
- *Electrolyte disturbance:* Low or high glucose, Na or Ca, low Mg
- *Idiopathic:* Presumed genetic
- *Symptomatic:* Following hypoxic-ischemic injury, trauma, hemorrhage, stroke, CNS infection; associated with brain tumor, neurological syndrome
- Cryptogenic

## DIFFERENTIAL DIAGNOSIS

- *Syncope:* Anoxia may precipitate a provoked seizure
- Breath-holding spell, tic, cardiac dysrhythmia with collapse, myoclonus, behavioral event (e.g., staring), parasomnia, conversion disorder (nonepileptic), gastroesophageal reflux (GERD)

## PHYSICAL EXAM

- *During a seizure, the following are possible:* Impaired awareness, change in vital signs, focal seizure activity
- *After a seizure, the following are possible:* Decreased awareness and responsiveness, Todd's paresis (transient post-ictal paresis that resolves within 24–48 hours), eye deviation toward the side of seizure focus

## MANAGEMENT

- Acute management focuses on maintaining control of ABCs and, when appropriate, cessation of seizures with benzodiazepines, for example, lorazepam (0.05–0.1 mg/kg IV); maximum dose is 4 mg for children and 8 mg for adults. Chronic management consists of raising the seizure threshold and should be initiated after a second seizure
- *Medications that can be loaded by IV route:*
  - ✓ *Phenytoin* 20 mg/kg IV SLOWLY (no faster than 1 mg/kg/min, usually over 1 hour) in non-dextrose-containing solution; monitor for cardiac arrhythmia. Fosphenytoin: same dose given as "phenytoin equivalents," but can be administered either IM or as a faster IV infusion compared to phenytoin
  - ✓ *Phenobarbital* 20 mg/kg IV; monitor for hypotension and respiratory suppression
  - ✓ *Valproic acid* 15 mg/kg IV above 2 years old and if no suspicion for metabolic disease
- Outpatient anticonvulsant can be chosen based on seizure type, EEG, and side effect profile. If one of the above medications has been loaded, continue orally and check a level in 1 week
  - ✓ *Phenytoin* 5 mg/kg/day divided three times a day
  - ✓ *Phenobarbital* 5 mg/kg/day divided twice daily (8 mg/kg/day for neonates)
  - ✓ *Valproic acid* 20 mg/kg/day divided three times daily
  - ✓ *Carbamazepine* or oxcarbazepine for partial epilepsy

## FEBRILE SEIZURES

**Simple febrile seizure: A brief (<15 minute), generalized seizure in a 6-month to 5-year-old child who has a fever (>38.4°C). To classify as simple, there can only be one seizure in 24 hours, and there can be no intracranial infection or significant metabolic abnormality. Complex febrile seizure: Prolonged (>20 minutes), focal, or recurrent (greater than one in 24 hours) seizure in 6-month to 5-year-old child with fever**

## EPIDEMIOLOGY

- 2–5% of all children have a febrile seizure
- Peak age of onset is 18–22 months
- *Recurrence risk:* Age younger than 12 months: 50%; age older than 12 months: 30%; second febrile seizure: 50% have at least one additional recurrence
- Overall risk of epilepsy in children with simple febrile seizures is similar to 1% risk in general population. Children with multiple febrile seizures and the first seizure at younger than 12 months of age have about 2% risk

## DIAGNOSTICS

- *LP:* Should always be performed if age less than 12 months; often, if age 12–18 months; only if clinical suspicion of intracranial infection if age greater than 18 months; if risk factors: complex febrile seizure, suspicious findings on exam, lethargy, concurrent antibiotic treatment
- *Laboratory studies:* Electrolytes, $Mg^{2+}$, $Ca^{2+}$, CBC count, glucose: only if age less than 6 months, suspicious history, or abnormal findings on physical exam
- *CT/MRI:* Not indicated for simple febrile seizure if recovery is complete and exam is normal
- *EEG:* Not indicated for simple febrile seizure in a normal child

## MANAGEMENT

- Antipyretic medications do *not* prevent recurrent febrile seizures
- Daily *phenobarbital* and *valproate* can reduce the risk of recurrence, but they have significant side effects (especially sedation) and are *rarely* used as prophylaxis against febrile seizures
- *Continuous or intermittent anticonvulsant medications are not recommended for prevention of simple febrile seizures*
- In cases of prolonged febrile seizures, it may be appropriate to prescribe rectal diazepam (for age less than 5 years, 0.5 mg/kg; for 5 years or older, 0.25 mg/kg, maximum 10 mg) for use as abortive therapy

## INFANTILE SPASMS

**Generalized epilepsy characterized by seizures with brief bilateral contractions of neck, trunk, and extremities, often occurring in clusters (flexor, extensor, or mixed). Seizures often occur on awakening or falling asleep:**

- *Idiopathic/Cryptogenic* (10–45%): Normal prenatal and postnatal history before onset of seizures, normal brain imaging
- *Symptomatic* (50–90%): Directly related to risk factors (e.g., periventricular leukomalacia, congenital infections, brain malformations, head trauma, hypoxic-ischemic encephalopathy); associated with 80–90% risk of mental retardation
- *West syndrome:* Infantile spasms, developmental plateau/regression, and hypsarrhythmia on EEG

## EPIDEMIOLOGY

- One in 4000–6000 live births
- 85% begin before age 1 year (peak age of onset 3–5 months)
- Normal development occurs in about 25% of patients with idiopathic infantile spasms (fewer if symptomatic)

## CLINICAL MANIFESTATIONS

- Brief symmetric contractions of head, neck, and extremities
- Often occur in clusters on falling asleep or awakening
- Often associated with loss of developmental milestones

## DIAGNOSTICS

- *EEG:* Hypsarrhythmia (disorganized, high-amplitude multifocal epileptiform pattern); electrodecremental seizures
- *Brain MRI:* Evaluates for malformations, bleeds, etc

## MANAGEMENT

- *Goals include disappearance of hypsarrhythmia, reduction in seizures, and stabilization of development:*
  - ✓ *ACTH:* Suppresses CRH synthesis; must be given IM; 70–80% will respond; adverse effects include hypertension, irritability, weight gain, hyperkalemia, hyperglycemia, risk of sepsis, risk of infection at injection sites
  - ✓ *Vigabatrin:* First line in many countries because of good response and fewer side effects, but not available in United States due to retinal toxicity and peripheral vision loss
  - ✓ *Topiramate, pyridoxine, valproate,* and *benzodiazepines* have all been used to treat infantile spasms
  - ✓ Excision of focal lesion can occasionally be curative

## NEONATAL SEIZURES

**Seizure that occurs in the first month of life**

### EPIDEMIOLOGY

- Occurs in 4.4/1000 live births; incidence increases with earlier gestational age
- Approximately 50% of infants with seizures due to hypoxic-ischemic encephalopathy have moderate to severe neurologic abnormalities at follow-up

### ETIOLOGY

- Most common cause in first 24 hours of life is hypoxic-ischemic encephalopathy
- *Other causes:* Metabolic abnormality, infection (TORCH, meningitis), trauma, structural abnormality, hemorrhage, pyridoxine dependency, inadvertent local anesthetic injection during delivery, familial neonatal convulsions

### PATHOPHYSIOLOGY

- Electric discharges in the neonatal brain are regional and rarely spread to contralateral hemisphere; therefore, generalized tonic–clonic seizures are rare in neonates

### DIAGNOSIS

#### History

- Family history of neonatal seizures, metabolic disorders
- Maternal drug use
- Apgar less than 5 at 5 minutes, base deficit greater than 10 at birth

#### EEG

- Normal EEG in term infant or mildly abnormal EEG = good prognosis
- Flat or burst-suppression pattern on EEG = poor prognosis
- EEG abnormal for greater than 2 weeks in newborn with asphyxia = always poor prognosis
- If EEG positive for subclinical seizures, consider continuous EEG during medication loading until subclinical seizures cease

## Laboratory Studies

- Glucose, electrolytes, BUN, creatinine, $Ca^{2+}$, $Mg^{2+}$, $PO_4$, bilirubin, ammonia
- Blood gas (rule out acidosis)
- If metabolic acidosis and increased ammonia, send urine organic acids
- Check state newborn metabolic screening results
- Consider serum amino acids, lactate, pyruvate, long-chain fatty acids
- Consider karyotype
- TORCH titers
- *LP:* Cell count, protein, glucose, culture, HSV, metabolic laboratory studies
- Serum/urine toxicology screen from mother and/or neonate

## Radiology

- Head ultrasound to evaluate for intraventricular hemorrhage; brain MRI with and without contrast to evaluate structural lesions

## Evaluate for Pyridoxine Dependency

- Give 100 mg IV pyridoxine during EEG monitoring, then continue 100 mg orally every day for 1 week. Positive if all clinical seizures stop (minutes) and EEG normalizes (hours)

## MANAGEMENT

- If identifiable, treat underlying disorder
- Seizures due to hypoxic-ischemic encephalopathy subside after 72 hours, regardless of therapy
- *Antiepileptic drugs:*
  - ✓ *Phenobarbital* is first-line therapy. Load 15–20 mg/kg IV, then maintenance 5–8 mg/kg/day
  - ✓ *Phenytoin* is second-line therapy. Load 20 mg/kg IV to achieve level 15–20 μg/mL, then maintenance 4–6 mg/kg/day. *Fosphenytoin:* same dose given as phenytoin equivalents, but can be administered either IM or as a faster IV infusion compared to phenytoin
  - ✓ *Benzodiazepines* are useful to acutely stop seizures while loading other medications, and for breakthrough seizures
  - ✓ Check levels after loading and follow levels regularly if seizures continue or if subclinical seizures are noted on EEG

## STATUS EPILEPTICUS

**A seizure lasting more than 20 minutes or multiple seizures without return to baseline**

## EPIDEMIOLOGY

- Greater than 50% in patients not previously known to have seizures
- 10% of epilepsy presents with status epilepticus
- Occurs in approximately 25% of children with epilepsy, most within the first 5 years of diagnosis
- Most common pediatric neurology emergency

## DIAGNOSTICS

- After stabilizing the patient (ABCs), check STAT glucose
- Electrolytes, BUN, Cr, LFTs, ABG, anticonvulsant levels, urine toxin screen
- *In a patient without known epilepsy:* $NH_3$, metabolic screens

- CT head once patient is stable
- LP when patient is stable; blood and urine cultures (especially if fever); also consider CSF HSV, enteroviral, or arboviral PCR testing

## MANAGEMENT

Acute management focuses on maintaining control of ABCs and cessation of seizures. Successive doses of anticonvulsants may suppress respiration and necessitate intubation

### Convulsive Status Epilepticus

- ABCs
- Check glucose and give 50% glucose solution 1 mg/kg
- *Anticonvulsants to be loaded parenterally:*
  1. *Ativan (lorazepam)* 0.05–0.1 mg/kg IV or IM (maximum dose 8 mg) or *Versed* 0.2 mg/kg IV or 0.2–0.5 mg/kg PR. Doses may be repeated every 5–10 minutes, but if seizures persist after approximately three doses, proceed to:
  2. *Phenytoin* 20 mg/kg IV SLOWLY (no faster than 1 mg/kg/min, usually over 1 hour) in non-dextrose-containing solution; monitor for cardiac arrhythmia or *fosphenytoin* (same dose but can be given either IM or as a faster IV infusion compared to phenytoin)
  3. *Phenobarbital* 20 mg/kg IV; monitor for hypotension and respiratory suppression
  4. *Valproic acid* 15 mg/kg IV if patient is above 2 years old and no suspicion for metabolic disease
- If these are ineffective, *pentobarbital* can be loaded with concurrent EEG monitoring. Dose with 10 mg/kg boluses and titrate to EEG burst suppression
- If there is concern for ongoing subclinical seizures after convulsive seizures have stopped, an EEG should be obtained
- Consider empiric antibiotics and acyclovir if concern for CNS infection

### Nonconvulsive Status Epilepticus

- ABCs, check glucose
- Anticonvulsants should be given judiciously. The longer the seizures continue, the harder it may be to stop them. However, these seizures do not pose the same immediate danger as convulsive status epilepticus
- Consider *Ativan* or *Versed, valproic acid, phenobarbital,* or *phenytoin* as described above

## UNPROVOKED SEIZURE, FIRST

**A seizure for which no specific trigger is identified**

### EPIDEMIOLOGY

- In the United States, 25,000–40,000 children have a first unprovoked afebrile seizure each year
- Overall recurrence risk −1/2; remote symptomatic seizure recurrence greater than 2/3; cryptogenic seizure recurrence about 1/3
- If unexplained seizure, normal physical exam, and normal EEG, recurrence risk is 15–20%

### DIAGNOSTICS

#### Laboratory Studies

- Selection of laboratory studies based on clinical circumstances (e.g., vomiting, dehydration, mental status)
- Electrolytes, BUN, creatinine, ionized calcium, magnesium

- Urine toxicology screen if prolonged post-ictal state or high suspicion
- CBC if infection suspected
- *LP*: Required in infants younger than 6 months, for failure to return to mental status baseline, or for meningeal signs
- If increased ICP suspected, obtain head CT before LP

### Neuroimaging

- *Indications for emergent head CT*: Focal deficit on exam; patient does not return to baseline within several hours of the seizure
- *Indications for outpatient brain MRI*: Age younger than 1 year; unexplained cognitive or motor deficits; abnormal neurologic exam; partial onset seizure; focality on EEG

### EEG

- *Urgent/Inpatient*: If patient does not return to baseline
- *Outpatient (within 1–2 weeks)*: Indicated for all children with first unprovoked seizure

## MANAGEMENT

- Outpatient neurologic consultation within 1–2 weeks
- No evidence that antiepileptic drugs (AEDs) change natural history of seizure disorders. Usually, AEDs are not indicated after a first unprovoked seizure

## UNPROVOKED SEIZURE, SECOND

**Epilepsy: Recurrent unprovoked seizures, usually stereotyped**

### EPIDEMIOLOGY

- Affects 0.4–0.9% of children, 1% of overall population
- Occurs in 40% of those who had a first unprovoked seizure

### DIAGNOSTICS

- *Neuroimaging*: CT only if patient looks ill or has new focal neurologic exam. Obtain MRI with gadolinium to evaluate for seizure focus
- *EEG*: To identify features of generalized epilepsy or focality; if there is doubt as to the nature of the paroxysmal events, consider prolonged monitoring with ambulatory EEG or inpatient video EEG
- *Laboratory studies*: If patient is unstable and/or is in the emergency department, check glucose, electrolytes, and calcium. Consider a metabolic screening workup if suspicion is raised by developmental regression or other worrisome features in the history

# 20 Nutrition

*Jamie Merves, MD*
*Diane Barsky, MD*
*Maria R. Mascarenhas, MBBS*

## ASSESSMENT OF NUTRITIONAL STATUS

**Information gathering, growth assessment, estimation of needs, determination of risk factors, identification of goals and provide recommendations and education**

### ASSESSMENT

- Nutrition-focused medical history
  - ✓ Usual intake including types and portion sizes of foods consumed
  - ✓ *Fluid intake:* Juice, milk, water over 24-hour period
  - ✓ For Breast-fed children, assess minutes on each breast and frequency of feeding
  - ✓ *Formula:* Type, changes, and response
  - ✓ Oral supplements or tube feedings (delivery method, tolerance, formula, length of time)
  - ✓ Herbal, vitamin, or mineral supplements
  - ✓ Food aversions, allergies, appetite, and religious/ethnic restrictions
  - ✓ *Access to food:* Food insecurity, Women, Infants and Children (WIC), food stamps
  - ✓ Note specific conditions that may affect absorption, metabolism, and digestion or increase the caloric needs of the patient (fever, increased respiratory rate and effort, cardiac disease, etc.)
  - ✓ Deficiencies from inadequate intake or comorbidities: Vitamin D, iron deficiency anemia, zinc
- Gastrointestinal history including defecation patterns, nausea, vomiting, gastroesophageal reflux treatment, abdominal surgeries
- Medications and potential food/drug interactions:
  - ✓ Note side effects of drugs that may cause electrolyte wasting, change in stool patterns or malabsorption
  - ✓ Note whether the drug's efficacy is reduced by food or food interferes with absorption or mechanism of action
- *Family history:* Food allergies/atopic disease, celiac disease, diabetes, obesity, heart disease, stroke
- *Birth history:* Prematurity, intrauterine growth retardation, small for gestational age, necrotizing enterocolitis
- *Laboratory values:*
  - ✓ Consider evaluating electrolytes, albumin, prealbumin, CBC, and hepatic function and lipid panels if indicated (e.g., in the setting of emesis, diarrhea, poor growth, obesity, supplemental nutrition or when otherwise warranted based on clinical evaluation)
  - ✓ *Deficiencies (if diet history indicates):* 25-OH vitamin D, zinc, iron profile
- *Growth parameters:*
  - ✓ *Unintentional weight loss:* 5–10% loss is moderate, >10% is severe
  - ✓ Length/height, weight, head circumference (if younger than 3 years) percentiles
    - Up to 2 years of age—Use 2006 World Health Organization (WHO) growth chart for weight, supine length, and head circumference
    - 2–20 years of age—Plot weight and standing height on the Center for Disease Control (CDC) 2000 growth charts and calculate BMI and plot

- ■ Plot on CDC growth chart or specialty chart (prematurity, disease specific, etc.) until 20 years of age
- ■ Correct for prematurity until 3 years of age
- ✓ *Optional:* Obtain triceps skinfold and mid-arm circumference to calculate muscle and fat stores. Measure lower leg length, knee height, or arm span (when unable to obtain accurate height)
- ✓ Typical growth velocity presented in Table 20-1
- ✓ Use z score to express individual anthropometrics in relation to population standard (i.e., 25th percentile weight-for-age= z score of 1 indicates that weight-for-age is 1 standard deviation from the mean)

## Stunting and Wasting

- • Wasting is an indicator of acute malnutrition
- • Stunting is an indicator of chronic malnutrition

## Grading Malnutrition

- • Acute (<3 months) and chronic (>3 months) malnutrition includes both undernutrition and obesity. Undernutrition can be classified based on a variety of measures including anthroprometrics: weight for length z score, BMI for age z score, length/height z score, mid-upper arm circumference, weight gain velocity, weight loss, deceleration of weight for length or BMI for age as well as nutrient intake
- • *Classification based on weight for length and BMI for age z scores:* mild malnutrition – 1.0 to 2.0 z score, moderate malnutrition – 2.0 to 3.0 z score and severe malnutrition – <3.0 z score (also including length/height z score)

## Body Mass Index

- • Body mass index (BMI) = Weight (kg)/(Height (cm))$^2$ × 10,000
- • Used for children older than 2 years of age for assessment of obesity
- • BMI percentile 85–95% = overweight and BMI percentile >95% = obese

## Estimating Nutrition Needs

There are a variety of methods to estimate energy (calorie) needs.

- • The recommended daily allowance (RDA) guideline is recommended for infants and may be used to estimate calorie (Table 20-2) and protein (Table 20-3) needs for healthy children
- • *Dietary Reference Intakes (DRI):* A set of reference values for recommended intake of vitamins, minerals, and nutrients in healthy populations of Americans and Canadians
  - ✓ *Estimated Average Requirements (EAR):* Average daily intake of nutrient that will meet nutritional needs of half the individuals in the group

| TABLE 20-1 | Growth Velocity* | |
|---|---|---|
| **Age** | **Weight (g/day)** | **Length (cm/month)** |
| <3 months | 25–35 | 2.6–3.5 |
| 3–6 months | 15–21 | 1.6–2.5 |
| 6–12 months | 10–13 | 1.2–1.7 |
| 13 years | 4–10 | 0.7–1.1 |
| 4–6 years | 5–8 | 0.5–0.8 |
| 7–10 years | 5–12 | 0.4–0.6 |

*For children <2 years of age, please review the WHO website for more detailed weight and length velocity charts.

| TABLE 20-2 | RDA Guidelines for Daily Calories |
|---|---|
| **Age** | **Kcal/kg** |
| 0–6 months | 108 |
| 6–12 months | 98 |
| 1–3 years | 102 |
| 4–6 years | 90 |
| 7–10 years | 70 |
| *Males* | |
| 11–14 years | 55 |
| 15–18 years | 45 |
| *Females* | |
| 11–14 years | 47 |
| 15–18 years | 40 |

| TABLE 20-3 | Daily Recommended Intake for Protein | | |
|---|---|---|---|
| **Age** | **AI (g/kg/day)** | **EAR (g/kg/day)** | **RDA (g/kg/day)** |
| 0–6 months | 1.52 | — | 2.2 |
| 7–12 months | — | 1.1 | 1.2 |
| 1–3 years | — | 0.88 | 1.05 |
| 4–10 years | — | 0.76 | 0.95 |
| 11–13 years | — | 0.76 | 0.85 |
| Boys: 14–18 years | — | 0.73 | 0.85 |
| Girls: 14–18 years | — | 0.71 | 0.85 |

AI, adequate intake (protein intake sufficient if above this level); EAR, estimated average requirement (half of the healthy individuals in this group would meet their protein requirements at this level); RDA, recommended daily allowance (risk of inadequate intake is very small at this level).

✓ *Recommended Dietary Allowance*: Amount of nutrition that meets needs of 97–98% of healthy individuals
✓ *Adequate Intake (AI)*: Expected to meet nutritional need of everyone in the group to give guidance but is not a defined calculation
- The WHO equation (Table 20-4) provides a more detailed calculation of energy requirements for children and adolescents to provide the resting energy expenditure (REE). The REE is then modified by activity levels and stress factors, which are important considerations in hospitalized children
- Once the REE is calculated, an activity or stress factor must be incorporated to account for additional calorie needs under special circumstances. (REE × [Activity or Stress Factor] = estimated caloric needs)
  ✓ REE × 1.3: Well-nourished child at bed rest with mild-to-moderate stress
  ✓ REE × 1.5: Normally active child with mild-to-moderate stress; inactive child with severe stress (trauma, sepsis, cancer) or child with minimal activity and malnutrition requiring catch-up growth
  ✓ REE × 1.7: Active child requiring catch-up growth or active child with severe stress

| TABLE 20-4 | WHO Equation for Resting Energy Expenditure |
|---|---|
| **Age** | **kcal/Day** |
| *Males* | |
| 0–3 years | $(60.9 \times Wt) - 54$ |
| >3–10 years | $(22.7 \times Wt) + 495$ |
| >10–18 years | $(17.5 \times Wt) + 651$ |
| >18–30 years | $(15.3 \times Wt) + 679$ |
| *Females* | |
| 0–3 years | $(61.0 \times Wt) - 51$ |
| >3–10 years | $(22.5 \times Wt) + 499$ |
| >10–18 years | $(12.2 \times Wt) + 746$ |
| >18–30 years | $(14.7 \times Wt) + 495$ |

Wt, weight in kilograms.

## OBESE POPULATION

- Caloric needs vary significantly in the obese population and equations do not always accurately predict needs; consider evaluating REE if available
- Schofield height and weight equation is most accurate for calculating calorie needs
- When calculating calorie needs for an obese patient, consider using an adjusted body weight (BW) instead of the actual BW in the WHO equation
- Adjusted BW = Ideal BW + 0.25 × (Actual BW − Ideal BW)

## CATCH-UP GROWTH

- Calorie requirements for catch-up growth can be calculated using the RDA Guideline table (see Table 20-2) and the following equation:

$$\text{Daily Calorie Requirement for Catch-up Growth} = \frac{\text{RDA for Weight Age} \times \text{Ideal Weight for Height}}{\text{Actual Weight}}$$

- Protein requirements for catch-up growth can be calculated using the DRI for Protein table (see Table 20-3) and the following equation:

$$\text{Protein Requirement for Catch-up Growth} = \frac{(\text{Protein for Weight Age} \times \text{Ideal Weight for Height})}{\text{Actual Weight}}$$

✓ Use weight in kilograms
✓ Weight-age = kcal/kg/day = age at which present weight would be at the 50th percentile on the growth chart
✓ To determine ideal weight for actual height, use the patient's height to find the 50th-percentile point on the height curve, and then drop down vertically to the weight curve

to the corresponding 50th-percentile point on the weight curve. Follow that point horizontally to determine the corresponding weight

## ENTERAL NUTRITION

### TUBE FEEDING

Tube feeding should be considered if the patient has a functional gastrointestinal (GI) tract but is unable/unwilling to consume sufficient calories/protein intake for weight maintenance/growth. Feedings may be intermittent or continuous. Many children benefit from a combination of daytime bolus and overnight continuous feeding thus the regimen should be based on the individual child's needs.

- Due to risk of bacterial contamination, hang time of formula should not exceed 4 hours for hospitalized patients, especially neonates

### CONTINUOUS FEEDS

- *Advantages of continuous feeds:*
  - ✓ Enhanced tolerance and absorption (especially in short bowel patients)
  - ✓ Used for nocturnal supplemental feedings (with daytime oral intake)
  - ✓ Less likely to cause abdominal distention
  - ✓ Physiologic for small bowel feeds
- *Disadvantages of continuous feeds:*
  - ✓ Requires a pump and therefore decreases mobility
  - ✓ Risk of bacterial contamination if feeds are left at room temperature for a long period
  - ✓ May suppress appetite thus consider limiting to overnight feeds if possible
- *Suggested initial regimen and advancement for continuous feeding:*
  - ✓ *For age 1 month–7 years:* Initial regimen, 0.5–2 mL/kg/h; *advance by* 0.5–1 mg/kg/h every 4–24 hours as tolerated
  - ✓ *For age greater than 7 years:* Initial regimen, 10–20 mL/h; *advance by* 10–20 mL/h every 4–8 hours as tolerated
  - ✓ Individual tolerance must be closely monitored

### INTERMITTENT (BOLUS) FEEDS

- *Advantages of bolus feeds:*
  - ✓ *Easier to administer:* Faster and do not always require a pump
  - ✓ *Physiologic for gastric feeds:* Pattern is similar to mealtimes
  - ✓ *Enhances mobility:* Not continuously connected to a pump
- *Disadvantages of bolus feeds:*
  - ✓ May worsen gastroesophageal reflux
  - ✓ Aspiration risk due to volume of feeding in stomach
  - ✓ May impinge on respiratory effort with large bolus feeds
- Suggested initial regimen and for advancement, refer to Table 20-5; individual tolerance must be closely monitored

### MONITORING

- *Elevated BUN/creatinine:* Check for increased protein content of formula, decreased renal function, or inadequate fluid intake
- *GI tolerance:*
  - ✓ *Constipation:* Evaluate for inadequate fluid and fiber intake, inactivity, and consider evaluating for a fecal impaction

| TABLE 20-5 | Guidelines for Intermittent Enteral Feeding Regimens | |
|---|---|---|
| **Age** | **Initial** | **Advance By** |
| 1 month–7 years | 2–5 mL/kg/feed every 3–4 hours<br>*Usually full strength* | Advance volume by 5–10 mL/feed every 3–12 hours as tolerated OR if hypertonic formula is used increase caloric density q 8–24 hours as tolerated. Do not advance both volume and caloric density at the same time.* |
| >7 years | 90–120 mL/feed every 3–4 hours<br>*Usually full strength* | Advance volume by 30–60 mL q 4–8 hours as tolerated OR if hypertonic formula is used increase caloric density every 8–24 hours as tolerated. Do not advance both volume and caloric density at the same time.* |

*Feeding advance should be tailored according to the patient's clinical circumstances and feeding tolerance.

✓ *Diarrhea:* Etiologies to consider: hyperosmolar medication or formula, rapid infusion, intolerance to particular component of formula (i.e., carbohydrate and fat content) or modular supplements, tube migration (i.e., from stomach to duodenum with bolus feeds), inadequate fiber intake, low albumin, impaction leading to overflow diarrhea, possible bacterial contamination of formula

✓ *Vomiting:* Etiologies to consider: delayed gastric emptying; GER; displacement of tube (i.e., in the distal esophagus); gastritis; intolerance of a particular component of formula (i.e., fat content or allergy); rapid infusion rate; also consider a behavioral component

• *Hydration status:* Monitor urine specific gravity, input, and output and check whether regimen meets the child's free water requirements

• *Glucose homeostasis:* If high blood glucose or glucosuria, consider possible infection or medication side effect (i.e., steroids), check carbohydrate intake

• *Anthropometrics:* Weight, height, and head circumference (as appropriate for age); adjust calorie/protein intake accordingly

✓ Consider following weights closely or daily while inpatient to guide adjustments

## MECHANICAL PROBLEMS

### Clogged Tube

• Usually avoided by scheduled water flushes, especially after interruption of feeds or following instillation of medications

✓ Attempt to flush with warm water using progressively smaller syringes (e.g., 5, 3, 1 mL)

✓ If the tube does not clear with warm water, consider using an enzymatic solution according to your institutional protocol (e.g., Clog Zapper™) to unclog the tube

✓ If attempts to clear the clog fail, consider replacement of tube

### Leakage of Gastric Contents Around the Gastrostomy Site

• Prevent leakage by minimizing tube movement (e.g., using a foam [Mepilex®] dressing) and using protective skin care (such as gauze, petroleum jelly, Stomahesive® protective powder)

• Check the amount of water in balloon (refer to manufacturer's instructions)

- Ensure the tube size is appropriate. Do not increase the tube size to avoid progressive enlargement of the stoma site
- Consider calling the service that placed device to decide if further action needed

### The Tube has Fallen Out

- If the tube has never been changed or the tract is immature (review your hospital policy, consider <12 weeks old for tubes placed in Interventional Radiology [IR] and 4 weeks old for surgically placed tubes), the patient should contact the team that placed the tube as soon as possible. If the team that placed the tube cannot be reached, the patient should go to the ER for evaluation and to preserve the stoma site. In the ER, a 10 Fr Foley can be carefully placed (without inflating the balloon) to maintain patency but should not be used for feeding. Once the appropriate team replaces the tube, consider obtaining a dye study to confirm placement to avoid complications such as peritonitis and death
- If the tube has been changed before and is >12 weeks old (or 4 weeks if surgically placed), the family should replace the tube or place a foley in the stoma to keep it patent until an appropriate tube is available

### Granulomas at Gastrostomy Tube Site

- Consider a trial of silver nitrate or triamcinolone cream 1–2 times per day for up to 1–2 weeks. If not improved, contact the G-tube Nurse or the service that placed the tube
- Gastric mucosa prolapse through the stoma is not a granuloma and is a problematic complication that may require temporary removal of tube or surgical revision of site. Surgical consultation is recommended

**Formula Choice: A variety of infant and pediatric formulas are available based on the individual child's needs. Refer to** Table 20-6 **for a summary.**

**Modular Supplements: Can be used to add macronutrients and calories. Refer to** Table 20-7 **for a summary.**

## PARENTERAL NUTRITION

**Indication: To maintain nutritional status and achieve growth in patients who cannot receive adequate nutrition enterally. Remember that enteral nutrition is the route of choice.**

**Peripheral parenteral nutrition (PPN): Used in peripheral veins and therefore is limited to maximum dextrose concentration of 10% (in some circumstances, 12.5%) and osmolality less than 1000 mOsm/L. It is intended for nutritional support of less than 10 days' duration.**

**Central parenteral nutrition: Used in central veins, which allows for higher dextrose concentrations and osmolality greater than 1000 mOsm/L. It is used when the anticipated need is greater than 7–10 days.**

*Parenteral Energy Intake*

- 10–20% lower than estimated enteral needs due to reduced energy cost for digestion/absorption (see estimating nutritional needs earlier in the chapter)

## PARENTERAL NUTRITION (PN) COMPONENTS

- *Carbohydrates:* Given as dextrose (glucose)
  - ✓ *Calorie density:* 3.4 kcal/g
  - ✓ Goal of 40–55% of caloric intake

| TABLE 20-6 | Enteral Formula Selection | | |
|---|---|---|---|
| | **Infant–1 Year** | **1–10 Years** | **Greater than 10 Years** |
| Healthy | Standard intact age appropriate formula | Standard intact age appropriate formula | Standard intact age appropriate formula |
| Fluid restricted | Concentrate to 22, 24 or 27 kcal/ounce | Choose formula with 1.5 or 2.0 kcal/mL | Choose formula with 1.5 or 2.0 kcal/mL |
| Food allergy | Milk protein allergy: trial of protein hydrosylate and switch to amino acid (AA) based if not improved. If IgE mediated, start with AA based | If IgE mediated, use an AA based | If IgE mediated, use an AA based |
| Constipation | Not applicable | Fiber enriched | Fiber enriched |
| Malabsorption* | Protein hydrosylate or AA based | Protein hydrosylate or AA based | Protein hydrosylate or AA based |
| Renal failure | Low protein, concentrate volume, adjust electrolytes | Low protein, concentrate volume, adjust electrolytes | Low protein, concentrate volume, adjust electrolytes |
| Critically ill | Consider a partially hydrolyzed formula | Consider a partially hydrolyzed formula | Consider a partially hydrolyzed formula |
| Pancreatitis | Low-fat formula | Low-fat formula | Low-fat formula |
| Chylothorax | Low fat, high MCT formula | Low fat, high MCT formula | Low fat, high MCT formula |

*Use a formula high in MCT in children with cholestasis

✓ *Calculation of Glucose infusion rate (GIR) (mg/kg/min):*

$$\text{GIR (mg/kg/min)}: \frac{\text{\% Dextrose (g/dL)} \times \text{(Infusion Rate mL/h)} \times 0.167}{\text{Weight (kg)}}$$

✓ Begin at 10–12.5% and advance daily by 2.5–5.0% to a goal of about 20–25% (maximum GIR: 12.5 mg/kg/min in infants, 6 mg/kg/min in children and adolescents)
✓ Monitor urine for glucose when PN is started and after changing GIR—If positive, check serum glucose and reduce GIR as appropriate
• *Protein:* Given as amino acids
✓ *Calorie density:* 4 kcal/g
✓ Goal of 10–16% of total calories
✓ Protein goals as per Table 20-8. Neonates can start at 2 g/kg/day and advance daily by 1.0 g/kg/day to goal, whereas non-neonates can be started at or near goal
*Exceptions:* Less protein is indicated in the setting of renal or hepatic failure. More protein may be indicated in the setting of trauma, sepsis, or increased protein needs (i.e., ongoing losses, healing from injury or surgery)

| TABLE 20-7 | Modular Supplements | | |
|---|---|---|---|
| **Modular Type** | **Name** | **Components** | **Amount per Serving** |
| Calorie boosters | Duocal, Super soluble | Carbohydrate and fat | 25 calories per scoop (5 g)<br>42 calories per tablespoon (8.5 g) |
| | BeneCalorie | Fat (91%) and protein (9%)<br>NOT recommended for tube feeding. | 330 calories/1.5 oz serving cup |
| | Pro-Cal | Carbohydrate, protein, and fat<br>For ages 1 year and up. | 100 calories and 2 g of protein per scoop or packet (15 g) |
| Carbohydrate-based additive | Solcarb | Soluble form of powdered carbohydrate (maltodextrin). Can be added to formula, liquids, and moist foods. | 23 calories per tablespoon (6 g) |
| Fat-based additive | Microlipid | Fat emulsion of both long-chain and medium-chain fatty acids. Used to add calories with minimal increase in total volume and osmolality | 4.5 calories/mL |
| | MCT oil | Medium-chain triglycerides, used in patients with decreased bile flow, defective lymphatic transport. | 7.7 calories/mL |
| | Liquigen | Medium chain triglycerides emulsion (50% MCT, 50% water), indications as above for MCT | 4.5 calories/mL |
| Protein-based additive | ProMod Liquid Protein | Liquid protein and carbohydrate | 10 g of protein and 100 calories per 30 mL |
| | BeneProtein | Whey protein powder, for ages 3 years and up. | 6 g protein and 25 calories per scoop or packet (7 g) |
| | Complete Amino Acid Mix | Essential and nonessential amino acid source, used to add additional protein to formulas. | 7.8 g or protein and 31 calories per tablespoon (9.5 g) |
| | Essential Amino Acid Mix | Essential amino acids, used to add additional protein to formulas. | 7.2 g of protein and 28.4 calories per tablespoon (9 g) |

(continued)

| TABLE 20-7 (continued) | | | |
|---|---|---|---|
| **Modular Type** | **Name** | **Components** | **Amount per Serving** |
| | Liquid Protein Fortifier (Infant) | Extensively hydrolyzed protein source for infants, can be added to human milk or formula. | 1 g of protein and 4 calories per 6 mL |
| Fiber additive | BeneFiber Non-flavored Powder | Soluble fiber source: wheat dextrin | 1.5 g of fiber and 7.5 calories per teaspoon |
| | BeneFiber Non-flavored Stick Packs | Soluble fiber source: wheat dextrin, in prepackaged packets. | 3 g of fiber and 15 calories per packet or 2 teaspoons (3.5 g) |
| | NutriSource Fiber (previously Resource BeneFiber) | Soluble fiber source: partially hydrolyzed guar gum. For ages 3 and up. | 3 g of fiber and 15 calories per tablespoon or packet (4 g) |

Adapted with permission from the Clinical Nutrition Department, Children's Hospital of Philadelphia, 2015.

| TABLE 20-8 | Protein and Lipid Requirements for Parenteral Nutrition | | | |
|---|---|---|---|---|
| | **Protein (g/kg/day)** | | **Lipid (g/kg/day)** | |
| **Age/Weight** | **Initial** | **Goal** | **Initial** | **Goal** |
| Preterm | 2 | 2.5–4.0 | 2.0 | 3.5 |
| Term infant | 2 | 2.2–3.5 | 2.0 | 3.5 |
| Child 5–20 kg | 1.0–2.5 | 1.0–2.5 | 1.0 | 2.0 |
| Child 20–40 kg | 1.0–2.0 | 1.0–2.0 | 1.0 | 2.0 |
| Adolescent >40 kg | 0.8–2.0* | 0.8–2.0* | 0.5 | 1.0 |

*A maximum of 150 g of protein/day is recommended.

- *Fat:* Given as intravenous lipid
  - ✓ *Calorie density:* 2 kcal/mL of 20% solution (20 g/100 mL)
  - ✓ Goal lipid content should account for 25–40% of calories. A minimum of 1–2% total calories is needed to prevent essential fatty acid deficiency. Lipid content should generally not exceed 3.0 g/kg/day or 50% of total daily calories
  - ✓ *Initial rate of lipid administration:* Refer to Table 20-8
  - ✓ Neonates can advance daily by 1.0 g/kg/day to goal, whereas non-neonates can be started at or near goal. Do not advance beyond 1 g/kg/day in patients with cholestasis
  - ✓ *Volume of lipid solution needed is calculated as follows:*

  Weight(kg) × Goal Grams IV Fat/kg/day × 100mL/20g IV Fat = mL of 20% IV Fat

  - ✓ Triglyceride level should be monitored with a goal <200 mg/dL in neonates, <400 mg/dL in children and adolescents. Consider reducing lipid dose if the triglyceride level is elevated. Carnitine may be added to improve lipid tolerance (however data is limited).
- *Minerals and electrolytes:* Refer to Tables 20-9 and 20-10

| TABLE 20-9 | Parenteral Nutrition Mineral Requirements for Children Based on Weight (kg) | | | |
|---|---|---|---|---|
| Element | <5 kg | 5–40 kg | >40 kg | Maximum |
| Chromium | 0.2 µg/kg | 0.2 µg/kg | 8 µg | 15 µg |
| Copper | 20 µg/kg | 20 µg/kg | 800 µg | 1500 µg |
| Manganese | 1 µg/kg | 1 µg/kg | 40 µg | 150 µg |
| Selenium | 2 µg/kg | 2 µg/kg | 80 µg | 120 µg |
| Zinc | 400 µg/kg | 125 µg | 5000 µg | 16,000 µg |

| TABLE 20-10 | Parenteral Nutrition Electrolyte Requirements | | | |
|---|---|---|---|---|
| Electrolyte (mEq/kg/day) | Infants (0–5 kg) | Children (5–20 kg) | Children (20–40 kg) | Adolescents (>40 kg) |
| Acetate | PRN* | PRN* | PRN* | PRN* |
| $Ca^{2+}$ | 1.0–4.0 | 0.5–1.0 | 10–25† | 10–20 |
| $Cl^-$ | 2.0–5.0 | 2.0–5.0 | 2.0–3.0 | 80–150 |
| Mg | 0.3–0.5 | 0.3–0.5 | 0.3–0.5 | 10–30 |
| Phos | 2.0–4.0 | 1.0–2.0 | 1.0–1.5 | 30–60 |
| $K^+$ | 2.0–4.0 | 2.0–3.0 | 1.5–2.5 | 40–60 |
| $Na^+$ | 2.0–5.0 | 2.0–6.0 | 2.0–3.0 | 60–150 |

*As needed for acidosis.

†mEq/day for $Ca^{2+}$ in this age group.

Other considerations:

1. If the patient's serum calcium is low, correct the value based on serum albumin (Corrected Calcium = (0.8 × (Normal Albumin – Patient's Albumin)) + Serum Ca) and obtain an ionized calcium prior to adjusting calcium in TPN.
2. If a patient requires an increasing potassium dose due to hypokalemia, they should be closely monitored for arrhythmia during infusion (in an ICU setting if appropriate).
3. When adjusting sodium content, please note the patient's total body sodium status. For example, a patient may have hypervolemic hyponatremia and additional sodium may exacerbate edema. Also, correct sodium for hyperglycemia (e.g., in the setting of diabetic ketoacidosis).
4. In patients with renal failure, magnesium, potassium, and phosphorus should be monitored closely to avoid toxicity due to decreased excretion.
5. Check solubility of your electrolytes (e.g., calcium and phosphorus) with your TPN pharmacy to avoid precipitation.
6. There are currently shortages of several intravenous electrolytes. Consider monitoring electrolytes more frequently if your electrolyte supply is limited and a patient is TPN dependent. Also consider enteral supplementation if possible.
7. When choosing phosphorus salts for supplementation in premature infants, choose those with minimal aluminum content to avoid toxicity.

- *Vitamins:* A pediatric multivitamin should be added for children <11 years of age and <40 kg (dose is 5 mL/day for children and 2 mL/kg/day to a maximum of 5 mL/day for neonates). For children >40 kg or >11 years of age, use adult multivitamin (10 mL/day)

## MONITORING LABORATORY STUDIES

- *Initial laboratory studies (within 48 hours of PN initiation):* CBC, electrolytes, calcium, phosphorus, magnesium, triglycerides, alanine transaminase (ALT), gamma-glutamyl transferase (GGT), total and conjugated bilirubin, albumin, prealbumin. Severe abnormalities in electrolytes should be corrected before initiating PN

- *Daily or every-other-day laboratory studies:* Electrolytes, phosphorus, magnesium, and calcium until stable and at full kcal and protein goal. Check a triglyceride level with every increase in IV fat
- *Weekly laboratory studies (once stable):* Electrolytes, calcium, phosphorus, magnesium, triglycerides, ALT, GGT, albumin, prealbumin, total and conjugated bilirubin
- *Long-term PN and minimal enteral nutrition:* Check vitamin status, trace elements, cholesterol, iron panel, CBC, reticulocyte count, and triene to tetraene ratio in patients receiving a low-fat regimen

## SPECIAL CIRCUMSTANCES: PARENTERAL NUTRITION CYCLE REGIMEN

- Cycling is used in long-term PN to promote normal daily activity and oral intake and to possibly lower the risk of PN-associated steatosis
- The infusion rate of PN solutions with greater than 10% dextrose should be decreased by 50% during the last hour of the infusion to prevent rebound hypoglycemia
- Complications of Total Parenteral Nutrition and Central Venous Catheters
- *Metabolic and electrolyte imbalances:* Follow laboratory monitoring as above
- *Catheter occlusion:* May be related to clot, fibrin deposition, or precipitate. Review your hospital policy regarding management
- *Air embolus:* Presents with sudden onset of respiratory distress. Clamp the catheter and place the patient left side down in the Trendelenburg position and seek emergent care
- *Catheter breakage, crack, or aneurysm:* Stop infusion, clamp catheter, and contact the team that placed the catheter
- *Catheter related blood-stream infection (CR-BSI):* After routine treatment cultures and treatment, consider central line lock therapies (i.e., ethanol) according to your hospital policy to prevent recurrent infections
- *Malpositioning of a central catheter with extravasation of fluid:* Stop infusion, clamp the catheter, and evaluate catheter position
- *Parenteral Nutrition-Associated Liver Disease (PNALD):*
  - ✓ Prevent overfeeding
  - ✓ *Cycle PN:* Decrease the duration of PN (e.g., decrease from 24 hours per day to a goal of 10–12 hours per day) to rest the liver from constant exposure to glucose and other nutrients
    - ▪ Blood sugar should be monitored while cycling TPN
  - ✓ Decrease IV fat (to a goal of 1 g/kg/day)
    - ▪ Monitor for essential fatty acid deficiency in this circumstance
  - ✓ Copper and magnesium are both excreted in bile and can accumulate in liver disease. Consider decreasing the copper dosage (generally by 50%) and consider removing magnesium
  - ✓ Start enteral trophic feeds as soon as possible

# CHAPTER 21

# Oncology

Jason L. Freedman, MD
Benjamin R. Oshrine, MD
Naomi Balamuth, MD

## PRINCIPLES OF TREATING CANCER

### CHEMOTHERAPY

#### GENERAL PRINCIPLES

- Cancer cells are rapidly dividing, and therefore more susceptible to cytotoxic agents
- Combination therapy is useful for preventing the development of resistance and overcoming existing resistance by using agents with different mechanisms of action
  - ✓ Also permits more intensive overall therapy by using agents with nonoverlapping toxicities
- Dose-intensification effective as most malignancies have a steep dose-response curve
  - ✓ *Two main approaches:* Increase dose (per cycle or by increasing the total number of chemotherapy cycles) or decrease interval between treatment cycles
  - ✓ Increases supportive care requirements
- *Adjuvant therapy:* Administration of systemic chemotherapy in the absence of overt disease
  - ✓ Targeted at micrometastases (see Solid Tumor section)
- *Toxicities:* Myelosuppression, alopecia, nausea/vomiting are most common acute toxicities (see Principles of Supportive Care for management of specific toxicities)
  - ✓ Long-term many agents affect fertility and can cause secondary leukemia
  - ✓ See Table 21-1 for specific toxicities relevant to commonly used agents in pediatric oncology

### RADIATION THERAPY (RT)

#### GENERAL PRINCIPLES

- Delivery of ionizing radiation typically by external beam
- Biologic effect achieved by inducing direct and indirect DNA damage
- Different tumor types have different required doses for efficacy
  - ✓ Wide range (e.g., 21 Gy for neuroblastoma/lymphoma, up to 60+Gy for sarcomas)
- Normal tissues have different dose tolerance thresholds before toxicity is seen
- Effect (and toxicity) can be potentiated by concomitant chemotherapy (e.g., doxorubicin, dactinomycin)
- *Radiation recall:* Inflammation in previous radiation field after administration of certain chemotherapy (days to years after original treatment)
- Photons versus protons
  - ✓ Photons are standard, but deliver radiation to all structures in path (i.e., entry and exit doses)
    - ▪ Intensity-modulated RT (IMRT) is used to carve out treatment volume to minimize exposure to normal tissues
  - ✓ Protons are heavier and deposit radiation more precisely at target
    - ▪ Decreased exposure to normal tissues as they enter/exit target areas

**TABLE 21-1** Commonly Used Chemotherapy Agents and Important Agent-Specific Toxicities

| Agent(s) | Class | Mechanism of Action | Specific Toxicities | Prevention/Treatment |
|---|---|---|---|---|
| Cyclophosphamide | Alkylators | DNA cross-linking | Hemorrhagic cystitis | Hydration |
| Ifosfamide | | | Fanconi syndrome (Ifosfamide) | Mesna |
| Cisplatin | Platinum | Platination/Cross-linking | Ototoxicity | Hydration and electrolyte replacement |
| Carboplatin | | | Nephrotoxicity (↓Cr and electrolyte wasting) | |
| Doxorubicin, daunorubicin, mitoxantrone, idarubicin | Anthracycline | DNA intercalation | Cardiac (cardiomyopathy and arrhythmia) | Dexrazoxane (cardioprotectant) |
| | | | Mucositis | |
| Vincristine, Vinblastine | Vinca alkaloids | Inhibition of microtubule spindle formation | Constipation | Bowel regimens |
| | | | Peripheral neuropathy | Decreased dose if necessary |
| Methotrexate | Antimetabolites | DNA precursor analogues | Nephrotoxicity, hepatotoxicity | Hydration, urine alkalization, and leucovorin for high dose |
| 6-Mercaptopurine | | | Hepatotoxicity | TPMT genotyping for slow metabolizers to dose correctly |
| Thioguanine | | | | |
| Etoposide | Epipodophyllotoxin | Topoisomerase inhibitor | Hypotension | Slow the infusion rate if hypotension |
| | | | Anaphylaxis | |
| Asparaginase | Enzyme | Asparagine depletion | Pancreatitis | Can switch to another type/hypoallergenic form |
| | | | Thrombosis | |
| | | | Anaphylaxis | |
| Imatinib | Tyrosine kinase inhibitors | Inhibit certain tyrosine kinases | Hypertension | Switching to another agent in same class |
| Sorafenib | | | Rash | |

## INDICATIONS

- *Local control:* Can be used as sole or complementary way to control disease around primary site of tumor (e.g., in Ewing sarcoma, when margins are positive after resection)
- *Metastatic disease:* Targeting metastatic sites and bone lesions, or total lung radiation for persistent lung metastases (e.g., Ewing sarcoma and Wilms tumor)
- Cranial/craniospinal
  - ✓ Brain tumors with metastatic disease or potential
  - ✓ ALL with CNS involvement (particularly T-cell)
- *Total body irradiation:* Conditioning option for HSCT (particularly in ALL)
- *Symptom management:* In relapsed disease, can control cancer-related pain, particularly at bony sites
- *Emergencies:* Occasionally used to manage impending organ-function threats of tumors (e.g., spinal cord compression, ocular tumors, mediastinal masses)

## TOXICITY

- Proportional to dose-intensity and radiation field (area exposed). Younger children are generally more susceptible to late effects (neurocognitive, growth, etc.)
  - ✓ Acute
  - ✓ Dermatitis
  - ✓ Mucosal damage
  - ✓ Cytopenias from marrow damage
  - ✓ Fatigue
- Chronic
  - ✓ *CNS:* Neurocognitive impairment, second tumors, endocrinopathies
  - ✓ *Musculoskeletal:* Growth impairment (especially if growth plate involved), arthritis, avascular necrosis
  - ✓ *Cardiopulmonary:* Cardiac dysfunction, pulmonary fibrosis
  - ✓ *Second malignant neoplasms:* Often sarcomas, particularly osteosarcoma; breast

## SURGERY

- Typically employed for biopsy of suspected mass to obtain histological diagnosis and aid with staging a patient via exploration of peritoneal washings and lymph nodes sampling in certain settings (e.g., pelvic masses)
- Depending on the type of tumor, surgery occurs at different points in therapy (typically up front in brain tumors or germ cell tumors) or after several weeks of therapy as local control in other tumors (some sarcomas and neuroblastoma)
- The goal of surgery may be complete resection, removal of discrete metastatic lesions (e.g., lung metastases in osteosarcoma) or in a palliative setting, debulking the tumor to decrease pressure or symptoms from compression of local structures

## BONE MARROW TRANSPLANTATION

### TYPES AND INDICATIONS

- *Allogeneic:* Replacing recipient's marrow with hematopoietic stem cells from another person (allograft)
  - ✓ Indications
    - ▪ *Malignancies:* ALL (mostly ≥CR2), AML, CML, JMML, MDS
    - ▪ *Bone marrow failure:* Aplastic anemia, Fanconi, severe congenital neutropenia, etc.
    - ▪ *Hemoglobinopathies:* β-thalassemia major, severe sickle cell disease

- *Primary immunodeficiencies:* SCID, HLH, WAS, CGD, NEMO, etc.
- *Metabolic disorders:* Mucopolysaccharidoses, leukodystrophies, osteopetrosis
- *Autologous:* Infusing patient's previously stored stem cells after delivery of high-dose chemotherapy—better thought of as a rescue after high-dose chemotherapy
  - ✓ *Indications:* Treatment of certain tumors that are chemosensitive but at high risk for relapse
    - High-risk neuroblastoma and medulloblastoma
    - Relapsed lymphomas

## PRINCIPLES OF ALLOGENEIC TRANSPLANTATION

- Approach depends on goal of transplant
  - ✓ Hematologic malignancy
    - Treat cancer with high-dose chemotherapy +/− radiation
    - Immunosuppress recipient to accept allogeneic graft
    - Make space in marrow
  - ✓ Defective hematopoietic cell(s)
    - Only need to immunosuppress and make space
- *Conditioning regimen:* Prepares the patient to receive the allograft
  - ✓ *Myeloablative:* High-dose chemotherapy +/− radiation to completely ablate marrow
  - ✓ *Reduced-intensity:* Less toxic regimen that is sometimes used for nonmalignant indications or heavily pretreated patients; still highly immunosuppressive
- *Donors:* Chosen based on best available HLA match, and other factors (gender, CMV status, etc.)
  - ✓ Matched siblings preferred
  - ✓ *Alternative donors:* Unrelated voluntary donors; umbilical cord blood; parent (mismatched related, haploidentical)
- *Stem cell sources:* Bone marrow, mobilized peripheral blood stem cells, umbilical cord blood
  - ✓ Chosen based on availability and type/purpose of transplant
  - ✓ Sources differ by engraftment kinetics, immune reconstitution, risk of GVHD, etc.
- *Graft-versus-host disease (GVHD):* Process by which donor T-cells recognize recipient antigens as foreign and induce tissue damage
  - ✓ Increased risk with decreased HLA matching
  - ✓ Allograft recipients receive prophylaxis with calcineurin inhibitor +/− steroids or methotrexate or mycophenolate
  - ✓ *Acute:* Skin (erythema→desquamation), liver (cholestasis), and/or GI tract (diarrhea)
  - ✓ Chronic form resembles autoimmune diseases like scleroderma
  - ✓ Treatment with immunosuppression (1st line=steroids)
- Immune function and opportunistic infections
  - ✓ Patients at very high risk for infection, even after engraftment
  - ✓ *Viruses:* CMV, adenovirus, HSV, VZV, EBV, HHV6
  - ✓ *Fungus:* Candida, Aspergillus, mucormycosis
  - ✓ *Bacteria:* GNR, *Strep mitis*, Staph species; bacteremia most common early post-transplant
  - ✓ *Pneumocystis jirovecii* pneumonia: Universal prophylaxis
- BMT-specific organ toxicities
  - ✓ *Veno-occlusive disease (VOD):* Disorder of vascular damage/thrombosis in small vessels of liver that occurs in first several weeks after transplant
    - Painful hepatomegaly, ascites, weight gain, direct hyperbilirubinemia, portal vein flow reversal, splenomegaly, refractory thrombocytopenia, kidney injury
  - ✓ *Idiopathic pulmonary syndrome:* Noninfectious noncardiac respiratory insufficiency occurring in first weeks after transplant

## ONCOLOGIC EMERGENCIES

## FEVER AND NEUTROPENIA

### GENERAL PRINCIPLES

- Bone marrow suppression from cancer and its treatment decrease granulocytes and thus cancer patients lack a first line of defense against bacterial infection
- Patients with fever and neutropenia (ANC <500/mm³) deserve critical attention
- *Definitions of fever and neutropenia vary by treating center but commonly:*
  - ✓ *Fever:* A single temperature taken orally that is greater than 38.3–38.5°C or three temperatures greater than 38.0°C in a 24-hour period
  - ✓ *Neutropenia:* An absolute neutrophil count (ANC) less than 500 cells/mm³ or less than 1000 cells/mm³ and falling

### CANCER AND THE IMMUNOCOMPROMISED HOST

- Cancer can increase infectious risk by inherent immunosuppression (leukemia) or by a mass creating obstruction of an organ (bladder, biliary tree, etc.) and subsequent development of infection
- Therapy disrupts normal barriers to infection including myelosuppression, disruption of the mucosal epithelium, local tissue breakdown, skin disruption, and the presence of foreign bodies such as a central venous catheter
- Many febrile, neutropenic patients have an occult infection but symptoms may be subtle or inapparent due to lack of inflammatory reaction
- When pathogens are documented, bacteria are the most common (85–90%)
- Infections with mold or fungi are most common in patients exposed to chronic broad-spectrum antibiotics or with prolonged neutropenia
- *High-risk features:* Inpatient at the time of diagnosis, uncontrolled cancer, comorbidities (hypotension, tachypnea, hypoxemia, mucositis), prolonged neutropenia (>5 days), higher fever, lower absolute neutrophil count (i.e., ANC <100/μL)

### APPROACH TO THE HISTORY AND PHYSICAL EXAM

- *Key pieces of the history and physical exam:*
  - ✓ Determine the date of the most recent chemotherapy to predict the expected direction of the WBC trend as most agents cause suppression 7–10 days after infusion
  - ✓ Note any recent blood transfusions (transfusion reaction can cause fever), and history of other infections (may guide antibiotic choices)
  - ✓ Critical to assess what type of indwelling catheter the child has (none, PIV, PICC, Broviac®, Port-A-Cath®), as these carry various risks of infection and antibiotic coverage may differ
- *Perform a thorough physical examination focusing on:*
  - ✓ The oropharynx (looking for mucositis, gingival involvement)
  - ✓ The central venous line sites (looking for signs of infection, such as erythema, tenderness, or discharge at the site of insertion)
  - ✓ Skin (looking for lesions that could indicate opportunistic fungus or molds)
  - ✓ *Abdominal exam:* A neutropenic patient is also at risk for neutropenic colitis (typhlitis), a fatal complication, so perform a thorough abdominal examination and consult with a surgeon if there is any concern. Hepatosplenomegaly should also be assessed

✓ The perineum (looking for perianal abscesses)
✓ Physical exam findings may be subtle or absent in profoundly neutropenic patients

## DIAGNOSTICS

- At least one set of blood cultures from each lumen of the central venous catheter and, in some institutions, a culture from a peripheral site before initiation of antibiotics
- If the catheter site is inflamed or draining, send Gram stain and culture for bacteria and fungi
- If lesion is persistent or chronic, send acid-fast stain and culture
- CT scan (head/sinuses, chest, abdomen) for evaluation of fungal disease with WBC count recovery in patients who have prolonged febrile neutropenia or in patients on longstanding broad-spectrum IV antibiotics who develop a new fever

## MANAGEMENT

- *Empiric Antibiotic Therapy:*
  ✓ Since gram-positive or gram-negative organisms can cause infection, empiric therapy must be broad spectrum (including anti-pseudomonal coverage) and bactericidal. Antibiotic choice depends on the individual institutional resistance patterns and the combinations used are quite varied and are institution specific. Typical empiric combinations include:
    - Monotherapy with cefepime, ceftazidime, or imipenem/meropenem
    - Two drug therapy with a third- or fourth-generation cephalosporin or an anti-pseudomonal penicillin in addition to an aminoglycoside
    - *Consider addition of vancomycin for gram-positive coverage if:*
      ▷ High institutional rate of gram-positive organisms leading to severe infection; suspected central line infection; receipt of intensive chemotherapy known to result in severe mucositis (SCT, AML); recent infection sensitive to vancomycin; colonization with vancomycin-sensitive organisms; patients presenting with hypotension
  ✓ If there are signs of a specific infection on exam, add appropriate coverage (i.e., gram-positive coverage for skin infection or anaerobic coverage for perirectal or oral infection)
  ✓ If no organism can be identified, broad coverage (usually with a third- or fourth-generation cephalosporin) should continue until the patient is afebrile with evidence of bone marrow recovery (e.g., ANC above 200–500 cells/mm$^3$ on 2 consecutive days and rising)
- *Empiric Antifungal Therapy:* Should be started in patients who have persistent febrile neutropenia (>3–5 days) or a new fever while on broad-spectrum empiric antibacterial coverage. Risk is greatest in HSCT and hematologic malignancy patients; solid organ patients with expected duration of neutropenia <5 days are a low risk
- *Remove central venous catheters:* If there is evidence of a subcutaneous tunnel infection, periportal infection, fungemia, atypical mycobacteremia, or persistently positive bacterial blood cultures, despite IV antibiotics, or in a critically ill patient
- Fever with a true infection may not develop in patients receiving steroids as part of their therapy or for chronic symptom management. Empiric antibiotic coverage should be considered in afebrile patients taking steroids that are neutropenic and have signs or symptoms suggestive of infection
- Avoid rectal interventions (taking temperature or giving medicines) in a patient with neutropenia, except in an emergency

## HYPERLEUKOCYTOSIS

### DEFINED AS WBC ON PRESENTATION >100,000/mm³

- Often seen in AML, ALL, and CML in decreasing order
- Sometimes asymptomatic, but symptoms arise from WBC sludging, stasis, and increased blood viscosity and can include:
  - ✓ *CNS:* Confusion, headache, focal neurologic symptoms, somnolence
  - ✓ *Respiratory:* Dyspnea, respiratory insufficiency, hypoxemia
  - ✓ *Renal:* From severe tumor burden and associated lysis
- Despite profound anemia, transfusions of packed red cells in patients with hyperleukocytosis have been associated with poor outcomes. (Transfusions must be discussed with oncology and intensive care teams)
- Interventions are made in any symptomatic patient, or if WBC>200,000/mm³ in AML or 300,000–400,000/mm³ in ALL
  - ✓ *Early options include:* Leukopheresis, low-dose cytoreductive chemotherapy (hydroxyurea or cytarabine). Careful attention to risk of tumor lysis syndrome (see below) is mandatory
  - ✓ Definitive therapy is initiation of cancer-directed treatment

## SPINAL CORD COMPRESSION

**A mass that compromises the integrity of the spinal cord, conus medullaris, or cauda equina.**

### EPIDEMIOLOGY

- Acute compression of the spinal cord develops in 3–5% of children with cancer. (This must be differentiated from back pain of other etiologies that develops in 5–10% of patients with cancer)
- Sarcomas (especially Ewing) account for about 50% of cases. Other commonly involved tumors include neuroblastoma, leukemia, and lymphoma

### ETIOLOGY

- Tumor in the epidural or subarachnoid space
- Metastatic spread to the cord parenchyma or the vertebrae with secondary cord compression
- Extension of paravertebral tumor through the intervertebral foramina leading to epidural compression
- Subarachnoid spread down the spinal cord from a primary CNS tumor

### PATHOPHYSIOLOGY

- Physical compression of the spinal cord, conus, or cauda equina leads to impaired blood flow, which results in venous hypertension and vasogenic cord edema, hemorrhage, ischemia, and eventually, infarction

### CLINICAL MANIFESTATIONS

- Back pain with localized tenderness is presenting sign in 80% of patients
- Radicular pain
- Abnormalities of bowel or bladder dysfunction (i.e., incontinence, retention)
- Most have objective motor loss
- *Patent/parent report of:* Night-waking, weakness, pain, tingling, bowel or bladder dysfunction

## DIAGNOSTICS

- *Spine radiographs:* May be helpful, but are abnormal in less than 50% of cases
- *Radionuclide bone scanning:* More sensitive than plain films, but are not appropriate with evolving neurological dysfunction
- *MRI with and without gadolinium:* Detects presence and extent of epidural involvement, intraparenchymal spread of tumor, and small lesions compressing nerve roots in the cauda equina
- *Cerebrospinal fluid analysis:* Important in the evaluation of subarachnoid disease and meningeal leukemia or carcinomatosis, but is not appropriate before the initial imaging

## MANAGEMENT

- Perform detailed neurologic exam
- If patient has focal spinal tenderness or neurologic deficit, determine the nature of symptoms and if they are progressive
- If neurologic symptoms are evolving, discuss initiation of steroids (see below) with an oncologist and perform MRI with and without gadolinium
- If evidence of spinal cord compression by imaging, consider urgent chemotherapy, surgery, or local radiation only after careful discussion with all disciplines as initial management decisions can have a profound effect on future therapy and patient function. Escalation to an intensive care unit is recommended
- *Empiric management with dexamethasone:*
  - ✓ For progressive dysfunction with significant physical deficits, administer 1–2 mg/kg/day as loading dose followed by 1.5 mg/kg/day divided every 6 hours
  - ✓ For mild stable deficits, administer 0.25–1 mg/kg/dose every 6 hours
- Definitive therapy is initiation of appropriate cancer-directed treatment, so diagnostic biopsy should be pursued emergently, and often *empiric chemotherapy* is initiated to treat most likely histologies while awaiting a definitive pathologic diagnosis

## SUPERIOR VENA CAVA SYNDROME AND SUPERIOR MEDIASTINAL SYNDROME

**Signs and symptoms that result from compression, obstruction, or thrombosis of the superior vena cava (SVC). Superior mediastinal syndrome (SMS) includes SVC syndrome (SVCS) with associated tracheal compression.**

### ETIOLOGY

- *Malignant (90%):* Most commonly seen with non-Hodgkin lymphoma, Hodgkin disease, T-cell ALL, and germ cell tumors
- *Nonmalignant:* Vascular thrombosis secondary to central venous line, thrombotic complications of cardiovascular surgery for congenital heart disease, infectious masses (i.e., tuberculosis, histoplasmosis, aspergillosis), bronchogenic cyst; hamartoma; ganglioneuroma

### PATHOPHYSIOLOGY

- Tumor or infection in the nodes or thymus can compress the SVC, causing venous stasis
- The trachea and right main stem bronchus in infants and children are smaller than that in adults and minimal compression/swelling can result in obstructive symptoms. Compression, clotting, and edema decrease airflow and reduce venous return from the head, neck, and upper thorax, leading to the signs and symptoms of SVCS and SMS

## CLINICAL MANIFESTATIONS

- 75% of children with mediastinal masses have respiratory symptoms that are aggravated when the patient is supine
- *Signs:* Edema and/or cyanosis of the face, neck, and upper extremities; plethoric appearance; conjunctival suffusion; cervical and thoracic venous distention; wheezing; stridor; pleural/pericardial effusion
- *Symptoms:* Cough, dyspnea, dysphagia, orthopnea, hoarseness, wheezing, stridor, chest pain, anxiety, headache, confusion secondary to carbon dioxide retention

## DIAGNOSTICS

- Chest x-ray demonstrates mass
  - ✓ *Laboratory evaluation:*
  - ✓ *CBC:* Pancytopenia, leukocytosis, blasts on smear (leukemia, lymphoma), left shift (infection)
  - ✓ *Chemistry panel:* Potassium, calcium, phosphorus, creatinine, uric acid, LDH (can be elevated with leukemia, lymphoma)
  - ✓ *α-fetoprotein, β-hCG:* Elevated in germ cell tumors
  - ✓ *Urine catecholamines:* Elevated in neuroblastoma
  - ✓ *ESR:* Can be elevated with lymphoma
- *Assess risk for general anesthesia/surgery:*
  - ✓ *If respiratory distress or orthopnea at presentation:* High risk for anesthesia
  - ✓ *If even minimal symptoms, full evaluation is necessary before sedation:* CT scan, echocardiography, pulmonary function testing including a volume flow loop to assess reserve
- **Sedation or general anesthesia in patients with a mediastinal mass may be contraindicated because they can decrease respiratory drive and result in respiratory failure, decreased venous return, and circulatory collapse**

## MANAGEMENT

- Clinical Decision-Making
  - ✓ General principle is to establish diagnosis/staging with the least invasive test possible, particularly if high risk for anesthesia
  - ✓ If CBC and other studies confirm diagnosis, begin tumor-specific treatment in consultation with oncology team
  - ✓ If no diagnosis is made after initial noninvasive studies, continue evaluation and assess risk of patient for anesthesia to safely obtain tumor tissue
    - ■ If patient is at low risk for anesthesia, perform diagnostic procedures and then begin tumor-specific treatment
    - ■ If patient is at high risk for anesthesia, perform necessary procedures unsedated or treat empirically with chemotherapy or radiation based on the most likely disease, although this is can complicate the eventual diagnostic procedure. Empiric therapy should only be done after consultation with an oncologist if possible
- General Management Issues
  - ✓ Control the airway, give oxygen, and avoid intubation if possible
  - ✓ *Extreme care in handling the patient:* Minimize stress, sedation, and avoid the supine position
  - ✓ If tissue diagnosis is not possible, empiric therapy may be necessary
  - ✓ Empiric use of steroids, RT, and chemotherapy can all affect masses and lymph nodes making subsequent tissue diagnosis and treatment more difficult, but these interventions are sometimes medically indicated

## TUMOR LYSIS SYNDROME

**Metabolic abnormalities that result from dying tumor cells and the rapid release of intracellular metabolites into circulation that exceeds the excretory capacity of the kidneys. Tumor lysis syndrome (TLS) often occurs at presentation or within 12–72 hours after the start of chemotherapy. The classic triad involves hyperuricemia, hyperkalemia, and hyperphosphatemia**

- *Hyperuricemia:* Results from the release of nucleic acids from malignant cell breakdown. Uric acid is soluble at physiologic pH, but precipitates in the acidic environment of the kidney and can lead to acute renal failure
- *Hyperkalemia:* Potassium is the principal intracellular cation and serum levels can also increase with acute renal failure. High serum potassium can cause fatal dysrhythmias
- *Hyperphosphatemia:* Lymphoblasts have four times the content of phosphate as normal lymphocytes; leads to hypocalcemia by decreasing production of calcitriol, decreasing absorption of calcium from the GI tract and from precipitation; if $Ca^{+2} \times PO_4^{-3}$ product reaches 60, calcium phosphate crystals form and precipitate in the microvasculature, leading to acute renal failure

### ETIOLOGY

- *Most common:* Burkitt lymphoma (BL), lymphoblastic lymphoma, ALL (T-cell)
- *Predisposing factors:* Tumors with high growth fraction and sensitivity to chemotherapy, bulky tumors, high pre-therapy uric acid or LDH, poor urine output, high WBC count

### CLINICAL MANIFESTATIONS

- Usually have no signs or symptoms; most commonly occurs in the 24 hours after starting treatment
- May present with vomiting or diarrhea
- *May present with evidence of hypocalcemia:* Muscle weakness, spasms, tetany, seizures, renal failure
- **Strategies for the prevention and management of TLS are outlined in** Table 21-2

| TABLE 21-2 | Prevention and Management of Tumor Lysis Syndrome |
|---|---|
| **Diagnosis and monitoring** | • CBC, electrolytes, creatinine, uric acid every 4–6 hours |
| | • Cardiac monitoring if hyperkalemia or hypocalcemia |
| | • Urine pH, specific gravity, and output |
| | • Chest x-ray to evaluate for mediastinal mass |
| | • Abdominal ultrasound if concern of abdominal mass or renal failure |
| **Hydration** | • D$_5$1/4 NS with 40 mEq/L sodium bicarbonate or sodium acetate (without K$^+$, Ca$^+$, PO$_4$) at 2–4 times maintenance fluid rate to maintain urine output at >100 mL/m$^2$/h, urine specific gravity <1.010 |
| | • Close monitoring of weight/fluid status |
| | • If patient has renal failure and cannot be hydrated appropriately, consider dialysis. |

| TABLE 21-2 | (continued) | |
|---|---|---|
| **Alkalinization** | • Maintain urine pH at 7.0–7.5 | |
| | • Increase sodium bicarbonate or sodium acetate as needed. Not required if urate oxidase is used | |
| | • Stop $NaHCO_3$ when cytotoxic therapy is initiated (to prevent precipitation of calcium-phosphorous calculi) or when the urine pH >7.5 | |
| **Uric acid reduction** | • Allopurinol: xanthine oxidase inhibitor that prevents uric acid synthesis (10 mg/kg/day divided three times daily) | |
| | • Urate oxidase (rasburicase): converts uric acid to allantoin, which is much more soluble. Consider use if the uric acid level remains highly elevated, evidence of renal insufficiency, and/or uric acid is rising rapidly despite allopurinol administration. As this agent causes significant hemolysis in patients with G6PD deficiency, use with caution if G6PD status unknown. | |
| **Treatment of metabolic abnormalities** | | |
| *Hyperkalemia* | • Calcium gluconate (100–200 mg/kg) | |
| | • Kayexalate (1 g/kg with 50% sorbitol) | |
| | • Insulin (0.1 U/kg) and 25% glucose (2 mL/kg) to increase cellular uptake of potassium | |
| | • Consider furosemide or other loop diuretics | |
| *Hyperphosphatemia* | • Aluminum hydroxide (15 mL q4–8h) or | |
| | • Sevelamer (adult dosing of 800–1600 mg three times daily) | |
| | • Insulin and glucose as above | |
| *Hypocalcemia* | • Calcium gluconate slow IV infusion *only* if symptomatic | |
| *Dialysis indications* | • Volume overload: pleural, pericardial effusions | |
| | • Renal failure | |
| | • Hyperkalemia | |
| | • Hyperphosphatemia | |
| | • Hyperuricemia | |
| | • Symptomatic hypocalcemia | |
| | • Uncontrolled hypertension | |
| | • Oliguria or anuria | |

# PANCYTOPENIA AND ACUTE LEUKEMIA

## GENERAL PRINCIPLES

### PRESENTATION

- Manifestations of a single or multiple cytopenias
  - ✓ *Anemia:* Headache, light-headedness, dyspnea on exertion, palpitations, fatigue, pallor, irritability
  - ✓ *Thrombocytopenia:* Mucosal bleeding, petechiae, purpura, easy bruising
  - ✓ *Leukopenia/neutropenia:* Fevers, mucosal ulceration, invasive bacterial infections

## DIFFERENTIAL DIAGNOSIS

- Broad division between decreased bone marrow production and peripheral destruction (or combination)
  - ✓ *Decreased production:* Bone marrow failure (inherited or acquired), leukemia, lymphoma, metastatic solid tumor, infection (CMV, EBV, HHV6, parvovirus, etc.), hemophagocytosis (HLH)
  - ✓ *Destruction/consumption:* Evan's syndrome, hypersplenism, combinations of causes of individual cytopenias

## EVALUATION

- *History:* Fever pattern, bone pain, weight loss, night sweats
- *Physical examination:* Lymphadenopathy, hepatosplenomegaly
- CBC/differential/reticulocyte count with review of peripheral blood smear
  - ✓ Smear review critical for blasts and evidence of stressed marrow (nucleated RBCs or teardrop) that may suggest infiltrative process
- Electrolytes (with Mg, Ph), BUN/Cr, hepatic panel
- LDH and uric acid to evaluate for TLS
- PT/INR and PTT; fibrinogen if abnormal
- CXR for mediastinal mass or adenopathy
- Bone marrow examination (aspirate and biopsy) for definitive diagnosis
- Features suggestive of a malignancy include prominent constitutional symptoms, bone pain, adenopathy, hepatomegaly, mediastinal mass, or laboratory evidence of TLS

## ACUTE LEUKEMIA

**Accounts for approximately 30% of childhood cancer. Characterized by excessive proliferation of early hematopoietic cells (blasts) whose maturation has been arrested. Lymphoid leukemia (ALL) represents 80% of cases; myeloid leukemia (AML) 20%.**

### CLINICAL MANIFESTATIONS

- *Bone marrow replacement:* Cytopenias and their associated symptoms
- *Uncontrolled proliferation:* Bone pain, adenopathy, organomegaly, fever
- *Unique presentations:* Coagulopathy (APML), anterior mediastinal mass (T-cell ALL), chloromas (collections of myeloid blasts), leukemia cutis (cutaneous infiltrates—often bluish), testicular mass (ALL)

### INITIAL MANAGEMENT

- Two priorities are to obtain a prompt diagnosis and address existing or potential oncologic emergencies
  - ✓ *Diagnosis:* Bone marrow aspirate/biopsy and LP with intrathecal chemotherapy (if confident in malignancy based on presentation/smear)
  - ✓ *Emergencies:* TLS, infection, hyperleukocytosis, cytopenias, anterior mediastinal mass, coagulopathy
- Once diagnosis is established, disease-specific therapy (see below) is implemented

### ALL: ACUTE LYMPHOBLASTIC LEUKEMIA

- *Divided into two groups based on immunophenotype of blasts:* B-cell (80%) and T-cell (20%). T-cell ALL tends to affect older patients, have more extramedullary disease (CNS involvement, lymphadenopathy, mediastinal mass, hepatosplenomegaly), and be more difficult to treat

- Prognostic factors
  - ✓ Immunophenotype (T-cell worse than B-cell)
  - ✓ CNS status (involved is worse)
  - ✓ Initial total WBC (≥50,000/mm³ is worse)
  - ✓ Age (≥10 years is worse than age 1–9.99 years; infants ≤1 years have very poor prognosis)
  - ✓ Cytogenetics
    - *Favorable:* Hyperdiploid, t(12;21)
    - *Unfavorable:* Hypodiploid, Ph+—t(9;22), MLL rearranged, other molecular markers
  - ✓ Response to therapy
    - Failure to achieve remission by end of induction is very poor prognostic factor
    - Minimal residual disease (MRD) is very sensitive measure of remission status now used to identify patients who need augmented therapy
- Treatment
  - ✓ Conventional chemotherapy is capable of curing the majority (>80%) of childhood ALL, is typically delivered over a 2–3 year period, and is divided into phases each having a specific purpose. Exact treatment regimens are based on risk stratification, which is dictated by above prognostic factors
  - ✓ *Induction:* Establish a complete remission
    - *Drugs:* Steroid, asparaginase, vincristine +/− daunorubicin
    - *Duration:* 1 month
  - ✓ *Consolidation:* Increased CNS-targeted therapy and consolidation of systemic remission
    - *Drugs:* Incorporates different agents than induction; protocol-specific
    - *Duration:* 1–2 months
  - ✓ *Interim maintenance:* Continued CNS treatment; systemic treatment with less myelosuppression
  - ✓ *Delayed intensification:* Period of intensive treatment, essentially repeating induction and part of consolidation
    - *Duration:* 2 months
  - ✓ *Maintenance:* Prevent relapse and eradicate residual disease with continuous low-intensity chemotherapy
    - *Drugs:* Mostly oral chemotherapy (6-MP and methotrexate) with monthly VCR and steroid pulses
    - *Duration:* 1–2 years
  - ✓ *CNS treatment:* All patients receive CNS-targeted therapy with intrathecal chemotherapy
    - If CNS+ at diagnosis, CNS therapy more intensive +/− cranial radiation
    - T-cell patients more likely to be CNS+ and receive cranial radiation
  - ✓ Relapse
    - Relapsed ALL is the fourth most common childhood cancer, occurring in approximately 20% of all ALL patients. Treatment approach is dictated by risk, which is based on timing and site of relapsed disease:
    - *Low risk:* Late (>18 months) isolated extramedullary (CNS/testes)→conventional chemotherapy
    - *Intermediate risk:* Early (<18 months) extramedullary; late (>36 months) bone marrow or combined relapse →decision re: chemo versus HSCT at discretion of family/oncologist and based on donor availability
    - *High risk:* Early (<36 months) bone marrow/combined→HSCT with any available donor
    - *T-cell:* HSCT generally recommended regardless of timing or site

✓ Special groups
- *Infants:* ALL occurring in children <1 year is a biologically unique disease with frequent MLL rearrangements, and is very difficult to cure, with the majority of children dying of relapsed disease. The role of HSCT is controversial given that optimal conditioning involves total body irradiation to a very young child, and survival benefit has not been definitively established
- *Trisomy 21:* Confers a much higher risk of ALL; generally similar treatment is utilized, although effort made to de-intensify and reduce methotrexate toxicity

## AML: ACUTE MYELOID LEUKEMIA

- Generally divided into de novo AML (occurring in previously well child), secondary AML (occurring in child with history of exposure to certain chemotherapy agents, or in child with bone marrow failure syndrome or MDS), and acute promyelocytic leukemia (APML)
- Prognostic factors
  - ✓ Cytogenetics and molecular features
    - *Low risk:* t(8;21), inv16, *CEPB*, *NPM*
    - *High risk:* Monosomy 7, 5q-, *FLT3* ITD
      ▷ All therapy- or MDS-related AML is considered high risk
    - *Intermediate risk:* All others
  - ✓ Response to therapy
    - Failure to achieve remission after first induction cycle is poor prognostic factor
    - MRD is increasingly used to evaluate quality of remission and assign subsequent treatment courses
- Treatment
  - ✓ *General approach:* Cure rates vary from 20 to 80% based on risk
  - ✓ 3–4 intensive chemotherapy cycles +/− HSCT for consolidation
  - ✓ Decision regarding stem cell transplant in first remission (CR1)
    - *Low risk:* No
    - *Intermediate risk:* If end-induction remission status poor or MSD
    - *High risk:* Any available donor
  - ✓ Structure
    - *Induction I and II:* Cytarabine, daunorubicin, and etoposide
    - *Intensification I and II:* Cytarabine with either etoposide, mitoxantrone, or asparaginase
    - If HSCT used, typically after three cycles of chemotherapy
- Relapse
  - ✓ All children with relapsed AML are treated with intensive chemotherapy followed by HSCT if remission can be achieved; prognosis is very poor
- Special groups
  - ✓ *APML:* Unique form of AML that has a characteristic cytogenetic abnormality—t(15;17)—making it amenable to targeted therapy with the differentiating agent all-trans retinoic acid (ATRA)
    - Therapy with ATRA on top of induction and maintenance chemotherapy
  - ✓ *Trisomy 21:* Generally seen in ≤4 years old and associated with very good prognosis even with decreased intensity of therapy. Generally AMKL (acute megakaryocytic leukemia)
    - *TMD:* Transient myeloproliferative disorder seen in first weeks to months of life associated with increased peripheral blasts +/− organomegaly
    - Only requires therapy if respiratory compromise, but increases risk of acquiring AML later in life

## LYMPHADENOPATHY AND LYMPHOMA

### GENERAL PRINCIPLES

#### PRESENTATION

- Features suggestive of a malignant etiology
  - ✓ Generalized or ≥2 nodal regions or any supraclavicular
  - ✓ Firm (rubbery), painless, enlarging, no overlying erythema/cellulitis
  - ✓ Constitutional symptoms, organomegaly, mediastinal mass

#### DIFFERENTIAL DIAGNOSIS

- Based on pattern (focal/diffuse), characteristics (size, pain, firmness, etc.), associated symptoms, and other physical exam findings
- Other masquerading etiologies
  - ✓ EBV, CMV, toxoplasmosis
  - ✓ Cat-scratch disease
  - ✓ Atypical mycobacterium
  - ✓ Kawasaki disease

#### EVALUATION

- History and physical
- CBC/differential, review of peripheral blood smear, electrolytes, LDH, uric acid, infection testing
- CXR
- CT of affected areas (if concern for lymphoma, include neck, chest, abdomen, pelvis)
- Biopsy if concern for malignancy or diagnostic uncertainty in ill child
  - ✓ Should be in consultation with oncologist
  - ✓ Excisional biopsy preferred as nodal architecture important in lymphoma diagnosis
- Staging of lymphomas
  - ✓ CT (as above)
  - ✓ PET/CT
  - ✓ Bone marrow aspirates and biopsies (bilateral)
  - ✓ LP (if NHL)

### LYMPHOMA

**Generally divided into Hodgkin (40%) and non-Hodgkin (60%) lymphoma based on immunophenotype of malignant cells. Comprises about 10–15% of childhood cancers, and up to 25% in adolescent age group.**

#### HODGKIN LYMPHOMA (HL)

- Malignant cell represents the minority of cellular composition of lymph node; remainder is mixed infiltrate of mature lymphocytes, eosinophils, and monocytes/macrophages. In classical HL, the malignant cell is termed the Reed–Sternberg cell and is giant, multi-nucleated with prominent nucleoli
- Presentation
  - ✓ Lymph node enlargement is often more indolent than in NHL
  - ✓ Cervical and supraclavicular nodes are most frequently involved and anterior mediastinal masses are common (60%) (See Oncologic Emergencies section)

✓ Constitutional symptoms of fever, night sweats, and unintentional weight loss (B symptoms) occur in 20–30%

✓ Oncologic emergencies in HL are uncommon. Anterior mediastinal masses usually do not enlarge quickly enough to case cardiopulmonary compromise and the malignant cell does not turnover rapidly enough to cause TLS

- Staging and risk stratification

✓ Staging based on site(s) of nodal involvement (Ann Arbor system)
  - *Stage I:* 1 region
  - *Stage II:* ≥2 regions on same side of diaphragm
  - *Stage III:* ≥2 regions on both sides of diaphragm
  - *Stage IV:* Diffuse disease or bone marrow involvement

✓ *Risk stratification:* Based on stage, presence of B symptoms, and bulk (specific measurements done by radiology in conjunction with oncologist)
  - *Low risk:* Stage I or II without B symptoms or bulk
  - *High risk:* Stage III or IV with B symptoms
  - *Intermediate risk:* All other stages

- Treatment

✓ Multi-agent chemotherapy +/− radiation of involved lymph node areas

✓ Since cure of HL is successful in >90% of children, current regimens focus on de-intensifying therapy (typically by removal of radiation) in children at lower risk of relapse to avoid late effects

✓ For low and intermediate risk, if there is a good response to chemo, omission of XRT should be strongly considered

- Relapse

✓ Most children with relapsed HL can be salvaged. Treatment involves initial chemotherapy followed by autologous HSCT +/− radiation

- Late effects

✓ Long-term adverse effects of therapy occur with all childhood cancers, but survivors of HL are among those at highest risk

✓ *Second cancers:* Breast, thyroid, skin, soft tissue sarcomas (XRT); AML (chemotherapy/radiation)

✓ *Cardiac:* Anthracycline-exposure/radiation

✓ *Pulmonary:* Bleomycin/radiation

✓ *Fertility:* Alkylating agents (boys>girls; young>older)

## NON-HODGKIN LYMPHOMA (NHL)

- Subtypes

✓ Based on phenotype (B versus T) and differentiation (mature versus precursor) of lymphoma cells
  - *Mature B-cell:* Burkitt lymphoma and diffuse large B-cell lymphoma (DLBCL)
  - *Mature T-cell:* Anaplastic large cell lymphoma (ALCL)
  - *Precursor:* Lymphoblastic lymphoma (LL) (T>>B)

- Presentation

✓ Can present with symptoms similar to HL with a generally more aggressive pattern, or in relatively unique ways based on subtype

✓ *Burkitt:* Abdominal lymphadenopathy that can serve as lead-point for intussusception

✓ *Lymphoblastic lymphoma:* Mediastinal mass, effusions, and bulky adenopathy

✓ *ALCL:* Nonspecific presentations, with skin findings, waxing and waning fevers/adenopathy

- Staging
  - ✓ Staging is based on number of nodal areas and sites involved (St. Jude system)
    - *Stage I:* 1 region (not abdomen or mediastinum)
    - *Stage II:* ≥2 regions on same side of diaphragm; resectable abdominal tumor
    - *Stage III:* ≥2 regions on both sides of diaphragm; any chest, paraspinal, or unresectable abdominal tumor
    - *Stage IV:* CNS or bone marrow involvement
- Treatment
  - ✓ *BL/DLBCL:* Short, but intensive, therapy with multi-agent systemic and intrathecal chemotherapy
  - ✓ *LL:* Treated like ALL, with up-front intensive therapy followed by maintenance, over 2–3 years
  - ✓ *ALCL:* Intermediate intensity and length
- Relapse
  - ✓ Difficult to cure in general; treatment with intensive chemotherapy followed by autologous HCT +/− radiation
- Special groups
  - ✓ *Immunocompromised hosts:* Children with acquired or inherited immunodeficiencies are at increased risk of developing NHL (particular B-cell)
  - ✓ *Recipients of solid organ transplants:* Post-transplant lymphoproliferative disease (PTLD)
    - EBV driven
    - *Management:* Reduction in immunosuppression, EBV-targeted therapies (e.g., rituximab), and antineoplastic therapy if indicated based on histologic type
  - ✓ *Primary mediastinal B-cell lymphoma (PMBCL):* Biologically unique form of DLBCL that originates from thymic tissue, is locally invasive, and relatively resistant to conventional chemotherapy

## SOLID TUMORS

## ABDOMINAL MASSES

### HISTORY

- Duration, pain, vomiting/diarrhea, obstruction, B symptoms (fever, night sweats, weight loss), age, underlying genetic syndrome

### PHYSICAL EXAM

- Location, size, mobility, consistency

### EVALUATION

- Labs include CBC, LFTs, uric acid, LDH, urinalysis, tumor markers (AFP, bHCG, urine HVA/VMA)
- Diagnostic imaging (CT/MRI, PET, MIBG)

## WILMS TUMOR

### EPIDEMIOLOGY

- Represents about 6% of childhood cancer
- Most commonly diagnosed in children less than 5 years old

- Can be associated with other congenital anomalies
  - ✓ Cryptorchidism, hypospadias
  - ✓ WAGR (Wilms tumor, aniridia, genitourinary malformation, mental Retardation)—germline deletion at 11p
  - ✓ Denys–Drash—Pseudohermaphroditism, renal disease, Wilms tumor—WT1 mutation
  - ✓ Beckwith–Wiedemann—macroglossia, omphalocele, visceromegaly
  - ✓ Perlman syndrome
  - ✓ Simpson–Golabi–Behmel syndrome

## ETIOLOGY/GENETICS

- *WT1*—Wilms tumor suppressor gene
  - ✓ Patients with bilateral disease may have constitutional *WT1* mutations
- *WT2*—Genomic imprinting within the *WT2* locus may account for BWS
  - ✓ Loss of heterozygosity at 16q and 1p are hypothesized to portend a worse outcome
- Deregulation of the Wnt pathway also plays a role in WT

## CLINICAL MANIFESTATIONS

- Pain, hematuria, fever, and hypertension
- Varicoceles can be seen in males with spermatic vein compression
- Note any signs of syndromes associated with Wilms tumor including aniridia, facial abnormalities of Beckwith–Wiedemann syndrome, hemihypertrophy, or GU anomalies

## DIAGNOSIS AND STAGING

- *Laboratory evaluation:* Complete blood count, urinalysis, electrolytes, BUN/creatinine, liver function
- *Primary tumor imaging:* CT/MRI, ultrasound to assess involvement of IVC
- *Metastatic evaluation:* CT chest. Bone scan and brain MRI can be considered if histology shows clear cell sarcoma or rhabdoid tumor of kidney
- *Staging:*
  - ✓ *Stage I:* Tumor confined to the kidney, completely resected
  - ✓ *Stage II:* Tumor extends beyond the kidney, but is completely resected
  - ✓ *Stage III:* Gross or microscopic residual tumor remains postoperatively
  - ✓ *Stage IV:* Hematogenous metastases or lymph node metastases outside the abdomen
  - ✓ *Stage V:* Bilateral tumors

## PROGNOSIS

- Tumor size, young age, histology, absence of metastases and favorable features of the primary tumor (lack of capsular or vascular invasion) are predictive of more favorable outcome

## TREATMENT

- Surgery
  - ✓ When feasible, an up-front nephrectomy is preferred for unilateral tumors. This allows for examination of histology as well as complete staging of lymph nodes
  - ✓ Unresectable, unilateral tumors may be biopsied, although special consideration should be made for the possibility of "up-staging," should there be intra-operative spillage. In certain circumstances, treatment without biopsy is preferred
  - ✓ Nephron-sparing surgery is being investigated for patients with bilateral disease
- Chemotherapy
  - ✓ *Stage I/II favorable histology:* Vincristine/actinomycin for 6 months
  - ✓ *Stage III:* Vincristine/actinomycin/doxorubicin + radiation (see below)

✓ *Stage IV*: As stage III + lung irradiation for lung metastases
✓ *Stage V*: Special considerations based on extent of local stage
• Radiation therapy
  ✓ *Stage III*: Flank radiation, extending across vertebral column to avoid scoliosis
  ✓ *Stage III + peritoneal spill/rupture*: Whole abdomen irradiation
  ✓ *Stage IV*: Stage III radiation + whole lung radiation

## NEUROBLASTOMA

**A malignant tumor derived from neural crest cells that can be found anywhere along the sympathetic chain, including the adrenal medulla. Variations in location and histologic differentiation result in a wide range of biologic and clinical characteristics.**

### EPIDEMIOLOGY

• Neuroblastoma (NBL) is the most common extracranial solid tumor in children
• Most commonly diagnosed in children less than 5 years old; median age is 17 months

### ETIOLOGY/GENETICS

• MYCN amplification is associated with advanced disease and a worse outcome
• *1p* and *11q* loss of heterozygosity is independently associated with a worse outcome
• ALK (anaplastic lymphoma kinase)—Activating mutations in ALK have been shown to be a cause of hereditary neuroblastoma. Mutations and amplifications are also found in about 10% of sporadic cases
  ✓ Associated syndromes
  ✓ Hirschsprung disease
  ✓ Central hypoventilation
  ✓ Neurofibromatosis

### CLINICAL MANIFESTATIONS

• Classic signs and symptoms include fever, weight loss, limp, periorbital ecchymosis/proptosis, bone pain, and pancytopenia
• Tumors can occur anywhere along the sympathetic chain
  ✓ Abdomen/adrenal—Can be detected as an asymptomatic mass or with abdominal pain; more common in younger children
  ✓ Thoracic/paraspinal—Can present as an asymptomatic mass or with spinal cord compression
  ✓ Cervical—Can present with Horner's syndrome (ptosis, myosis, anhidrosis); more common in infants
• Elevated catecholamines (HVA, VMA) can lead to hypertension or flushing
• Most common sites of metastases are regional nodes, bone, bone marrow, liver, and skin. Rarely, metastases can occur in lung and brain
• Infants can present with skin involvement (stage 4S) with bluish, non-tender subcutaneous nodules
• Paraneoplastic manifestations
• Opsoclonus myoclonus ataxia syndrome—Presumed secondary to anti-neural antibodies
• Secretory diarrhea—Associated with vasoactive intestinal peptide (VIP) secretion

### DIAGNOSIS/STAGING/RISK STRATIFICATION

• Biopsy is preferred, whenever possible, for histologic confirmation, as well as to have tissue for molecular diagnostic studies

- Laboratory evaluation
- CBC with differential, electrolytes, BUN/creatinine, liver function tests, urinary HVA/VMA, LDH
- Bilateral bone marrow aspirates and biopsies
- Imaging
- CT/MRI of primary tumor including chest/abdomen/pelvis
- MIBG scan
- Staging (International Risk Group Neuroblastoma Staging System)
  - ✓ *L1:* Localized tumor not involving vital structures as defined by a list of image-defined risk factors and confined to one body compartment
  - ✓ *L2:* Locoregional tumor with presence of one or more image-defined risk factors
  - ✓ *M:* Metastatic disease (except stage MS)
  - ✓ *MS:* Metastatic disease in children younger than 18 months with metastases confined to skin, liver, and/or bone marrow
- *Risk stratification (low, intermediate, or high):* Complex algorithm based on age, stage, MYCN status, histology, and ploidy

## PROGNOSIS

- *Age/Stage:* Age greater than 2 years and increased stage are the most important factors predictive of unfavorable disease outcome
- *Pathology:* Undifferentiated tumors with high mitotic rate have a poor prognosis
- *Molecular genetics:* MYCN amplification (unfavorable), hyperdiploid (favorable), chromosomal deletion of allelic loss (unfavorable)

## TREATMENT (RISK-RELATED)

- *Low risk:* Surgery alone
- Intermediate risk
  - ✓ Surgery
  - ✓ Chemotherapy—Carboplatin, cyclophosphamide, etoposide, doxorubicin
  - ✓ Radiation—Can be considered in cases where tumor bulk precludes surgery and tumor does not respond to chemotherapy
- High risk
  - ✓ *Chemotherapy:* Topotecan, cyclophosphamide, vincristine, doxorubicin, cisplatin, etoposide
  - ✓ *Surgery:* Best possible resection of primary tumor
  - ✓ Autologous stem cell transplant
  - ✓ Radiation therapy—To primary tumor site and other sites not responding to induction chemotherapy
  - ✓ *Immunotherapy:* Ch14.18 monoclonal antibody combined with IL-2 or GM-CSF
  - ✓ *Isotretinoin:* 6-month course to promote maturation of any remaining malignant neuroblastoma cells
- Relapsed disease
  - ✓ No known cure
  - ✓ I$^{131}$ MIBG can be used as a form of RT to palliate painful sites of disease
- Neonates with MS disease often require urgent treatment secondary to respiratory distress and abdominal competition
  - ✓ Chemotherapy
  - ✓ Radiation therapy—Reserved for cases where tumor does not respond rapidly enough to chemotherapy

## BONE TUMORS

Osteosarcoma (OS) is a malignant bone tumor arising from mesenchymal cells. It is unique in its production of immature bone (osteoid) by cell stroma.

Ewing sarcoma (ES) is part of a family of tumors comprising a histologic spectrum ranging from undifferentiated small round blue cells to differentiated cells resembling peripheral neuroectodermal tissue (PNETs).

## OSTEOSARCOMA

### EPIDEMIOLOGY

- Most common bone tumor in adolescence
  ✓ Likely relationship between rapid bone growth and development of OS
- More common in boys than girls
- More common in blacks than whites
- Usually occurs in metaphyseal portions of long bones (distal femur, proximal tibia, proximal humerus)

### ETIOLOGY/GENETICS

- Only known factor that increases risk for OS is ionizing radiation

### ASSOCIATED CLINICAL SYNDROMES

- *Rothmund–Thomson (autosomal recessive):* Poikioderma, small stature, and skeletal dysplasia
  ✓ Mutation in RECQL4 gene
- Hereditary retinoblastoma
  ✓ Germline mutation in Rb gene
- *Li–Fraumeni syndrome:* Cancer predisposition
  ✓ P53 mutation

### CLINICAL MANIFESTATIONS

- Pain over involved site with or without associated soft tissue mass
- Can have erythema, warmth, or swelling that mimics infection
- Can result in pathologic fracture

### DIAGNOSIS/STAGING

- *Biopsy:* Open biopsy should be performed by an experienced orthopedic surgeon (ideally should be the surgeon who will perform later definitive surgery). Incision and technique are extremely important and can affect the subsequent surgery as well as the patient's prognosis if not performed properly
- *Staging:*
  ✓ *Imaging of primary tumor:* MRI should include both the joint above and the joint below to examine for skip lesions
  ✓ *Metastatic evaluation:* Chest CT, bone scan

### PROGNOSIS

- Extent of disease at diagnosis (metastatic disease unfavorable)
- Location of primary tumor
  ✓ Axial skeleton is unfavorable, due to difficulty in obtaining a full resection

- Tumor size (>15 cm is unfavorable)
- Young age (<10 years is unfavorable)
- Histologic response at the time of local control (<90% tumor necrosis is unfavorable)

## TREATMENT

- *Pre-surgical (neoadjuvant) chemotherapy:* Cisplatin/doxorubicin/methotrexate
  - ✓ Allows evaluation of tumor responsiveness to chemotherapy in a uniform manner, eradication of micrometastases early instead of waiting until postoperative recovery and demonstrated improvement in outcome

## SURGERY

- Removal of all gross and microscopic tumor is essential to prevent local recurrence. Surgical procedures include either amputation or limb-salvage procedures (allografts, vascularized grafts, endoprostheses, rotationplasty)
- The type of surgical procedure depends on tumor location, size, presence of metastatic disease, age, skeletal development, lifestyle preference, and desired activities
- *Post-surgical (adjuvant) chemotherapy:* Cisplatin/doxorubicin/Methotrexate

## EWING SARCOMA

### EPIDEMIOLOGY

- Second most common bone tumor in adolescence
- More common in boys than girls
- More common in whites than blacks
- Usually diaphyseal

### ETIOLOGY/GENETICS

- T(11;22) is present in about 85% of tumors
  - ✓ Results in a chimeric EWS-FLI1 transcription product
  - ✓ Detection by RT-PCR and FISH

### CLINICAL MANIFESTATIONS

- Constitutional symptoms—Fever, weight loss
- Pain over involved site with or without associated soft tissue mass
- Paraspinal tumors can present with spinal cord compression
- Can have erythema, warmth, or swelling that mimics infection
- Can result in pathologic fracture

### DIAGNOSIS/STAGING

- *Biopsy:* Open biopsy should be performed by an experienced orthopedic surgeon (ideally should be the surgeon who will perform later definitive surgery). Incision and technique are extremely important and can affect the subsequent surgery as well as the patient's prognosis if not performed properly
- *Staging:*
  - ✓ Imaging of primary tumor—For bony primaries, MRI should include both the joint above and the joint below to examine for skip lesions
  - ✓ Metastatic evaluation—Chest CT, bone scan +/− PET scan, bilateral bone marrow aspirates, and biopsies

## PROGNOSIS

- Presence of metastatic disease is the most important adverse prognostic factor
- Primary site (pelvis is unfavorable)
- Larger tumor size is unfavorable
- Poor response to initial therapy is unfavorable
- Older age is unfavorable

## TREATMENT

- *Pre-surgical (neoadjuvant) chemotherapy:* Vincristine, doxorubicin, cyclophosphamide alternating with etoposide/ifosfamide on a compressed, every 2 week, schedule
- Every patient is assumed to have micrometastatic disease at diagnosis and the primary treatment involves combination chemotherapy. Goal is to decrease primary tumor volume for both eventual local control and immediate control of micrometastatic disease
- *Local control:* Approach depends on the site and whether radiation would cause significant growth or functional difficulty. Each potential site of disease is associated with varied options for surgery and radiotherapy. Final decision balances the need for complete tumor eradication with the goal of maintaining function
- Post-surgical (adjuvant) chemotherapy

## RHABDOMYOSARCOMA

**Tumor derived from primitive mesenchyme that may develop into muscle, fat, fibrous tissue, bone, or cartilage.**

### EPIDEMIOLOGY

- Two-thirds of cases diagnosed in children less than 6 years (largely embryonal histology)
- Small second peak in adolescence (largely alveolar histology)
- Relationship between age at diagnosis and site of primary tumor/histology
  - ✓ Head and neck tumors most common in children less than 8 years
  - ✓ Orbital tumors almost always embryonal
  - ✓ Extremity tumors more common in adolescents and usually alveolar

### ETIOLOGY/GENETICS

- Vast majority of cases are sporadic
- *Associated syndromes:*
  - ✓ Neurofibromatosis Type I
  - ✓ Li-Fraumeni—p53 mutation, cancer predisposition
  - ✓ Costello syndrome (growth retardation, coarse facies, developmental delay)
  - ✓ *Alveolar disease has characteristic translocation:* t(2;13)
    - ▪ Fusion of PAX3 or PAX7 with FKHR (transcription factor)
  - ✓ Embryonal disease has loss of heterozygosity at 11p15

### CLINICAL MANIFESTATIONS

- Disturbance in normal function due to mass effect
- *Head/neck:* Proptosis, ophthalmoplegia, visual disturbance, chronic sinus obstruction
- *Genitourinary tract:* Dysuria, hematuria, pain, urinary obstruction, constipation. Testicular disease often presents with painless unilateral enlargement
  - ✓ *Extremity:* Pain, tenderness, and erythema of the affected limb
  - ✓ *Other less common sites:* Biliary tract, perineal, intrathoracic, retroperitoneal

- Metastatic disease (present in <25% at diagnosis)
  - ✓ Lymph nodes, lung, bone/bone marrow are most common sites

## DIAGNOSIS/STAGING

- Biopsy/surgical resection if feasible without excessive morbidity
- CBC with differential, comprehensive metabolic panel including renal function and liver function testing
- *Group:* Depends on extent of initial resection
- *I:* Complete resection, negative margins
- *II:* Microscopic residual disease
- *III:* Gross residual disease
- *IV:* Metastatic disease
- *Stage:* Depends on primary site, size of primary tumor, and involvement of nodes
  - ✓ *I:* Favorable site (orbit, superficial head and neck, biliary tree, paratestis, vagina)
  - ✓ *II:* Unfavorable site, <5 cm, no nodal involvement
  - ✓ *III:* Unfavorable site and >5 cm OR <5 cm with nodal involvement
  - ✓ *IV:* Metastatic disease
- *Staging evaluation:*
  - ✓ Primary site imaging (CT/MRI)
  - ✓ Chest CT
  - ✓ Bone scan/PET scan
  - ✓ Bilateral bone marrow aspirates and biopsies

## FAVORABLE PROGNOSTIC FACTORS

- Absence of metastatic disease
- Favorable site (orbit, superficial head and neck, biliary tree, paratestis, vagina)
- Low group/stage
- Embryonal histology
  - ✓ Age <10 years

## TREATMENT

- *Surgery:* Always use unless impaired function or cosmetic result. Up-front aggressive surgery or wide excision should not be used in the female genital tract, orbit, bladder, or biliary tract
- *Chemotherapy:* Combination depends on risk group stratification (combination of group and stage)
  - ✓ *Most common agents:* Vincristine, actinomycin, cyclophosphamide
- *Radiation therapy:* Dose, fractionation, and therapy for certain tumor locations (orbit/cranial tumors) are variable and controversial. In general, RT is given for patients with large tumors, alveolar histology, and for those without surgical options for local control

## CENTRAL NERVOUS SYSTEM TUMORS

Approach to the patient with a suspected brain tumor

- Patients with brain tumors may be asymptomatic, but commonly diagnosis is made after clinical symptoms such as new onset seizure, intractable headache, persistent nausea or vomiting (especially in the morning), or new onset focal neurologic symptoms (visual loss, ataxia, confusion, etc.) lead to imaging studies

- Tumor location will dictate presenting signs and symptoms. Initial care is directed at emergent management of increased intracranial pressure, spinal cord compression, respiratory or cardiovascular compromise, if present
- Involvement of neurosurgical, oncology, and critical care services is mandatory

## EPIDEMIOLOGY

- Second most common group of all pediatric malignancies (about 20% of total)
- *Age:* Incidence peaks in first decade
  ✓ *Supratentorial tumors:* Most common in patients younger than 1 year and older than 11 years
  ✓ *Infratentorial tumors:* More common in patients 1–11 years of age
- *Sex:* Slightly higher in male predominance overall
- *Risk factors and predisposing conditions:*
  ✓ *Genetic disorders (<10% of cases):* NF-1, NF-2, tuberous sclerosis, von Hippel–Lindau, Turcot syndrome, Gorlin syndrome, Li-Fraumeni syndrome, Cowden syndrome, retinoblastoma
  ✓ *Ionizing radiation immunosuppression:* Higher risk of CNS lymphoma in patients with inherited or acquired T-cell dysfunction (CVID, Wiskott–Aldrich syndrome, ataxia/telangiectasia, AIDS, and solid organ transplant patients)
  Clinical presentation of tumors based on location (Table 21-3)
- *Supratentorial (cerebrum, basal ganglia, thalamus/hypothalamus, pituitary pineal, optic):* Increased intracranial pressure (ICP), seizures, visual loss, hemiparesis, headache, emesis; new need for glasses; difficulty in school; behavioral difficulty, personality changes; failure to thrive; change in dominant hand; diencephalic syndrome (failure to thrive with increasing appetite and good mood); endocrinopathies such as diabetes insipidus, short stature; Parinaud's syndrome (poor upward gaze, poor pupillary light reflex but normal to accommodation and convergence nystagmus)
- *Infratentorial (cerebellum, brainstem):* Ataxia, clumsiness, worsening handwriting, dysarthria; nystagmus; head tilt; cranial nerve palsy; increased ICP from ventricular compression (morning headache and vomiting); extreme vomiting if near area postrema
- *Nonspecific signs and symptoms:* Change in activity level, change in appetite with associated weight gain or loss, delayed or precocious puberty, macrocephaly in infants, vomiting, complaints consistent with spinal cord involvement such as back pain or bowel/bladder dysfunction (see Oncologic Emergencies section)

## DIAGNOSTICS

- CT scan of brain with and without contrast (useful as a quick screen, especially in unstable patients) evaluates ventricular size, midline shift, and hemorrhage; inadequate for anatomic detail and often misses smaller tumors or those in the posterior fossa
- Brain MRI with gadolinium
- Spinal MRI to evaluate for drop metastases/leptomeningeal spread (sometimes seen in PNET, medulloblastoma, germ cell tumors, ependymoma, GBM
- Magnetic resonance spectroscopy (MRS) and positron emission tomography (PET) being used more, but not uniformly
- Lumbar puncture (only after scan and evaluation for increased intracranial pressure) for glucose, protein, culture, cytology, and markers such as α-fetoprotein and B-HCG
- Bone marrow aspirate/biopsy for some PNETs

- Surgical biopsy for histological diagnosis is critical prior to treatment except in cases of diffusely infiltrating pontine gliomas, visual pathway gliomas (in kids with NF1), and tectal gliomas, which are diagnosed from neuroimaging findings and in cases of elevated B-HCG and AFP

## MANAGEMENT

- Initial management of increased intracranial pressure, respiratory or cardiovascular stabilization if present, with involvement of neurosurgical and critical care services
- Tumor-directed therapy
  - ✓ Approach is based on biologic potential of tumor and method of spread (see table 12-3). In general, tumors with higher biologic potential require therapy directed at the entire neuroaxis (e.g., CSI/chemotherapy) and those with lower biologic potential or only local invasion may be treated with surgery or local XRT alone
  - ✓ An ideal approach includes an experienced, multidisciplinary team including a pediatric neurosurgeon, oncologist, radiation oncologist, neurocognitive specialist, endocrinologist, and neuro-ophthalmologist
- *Observation:* Some benign tumors like optic pathway/hypothalamic gliomas can remain stable for years and can be monitored with surveillance imaging, opting for treatment for visual decline or significant tumor progression
- *Surgery:* Balance preservation of function and maximization of tumor removal. For some tumors (JPA), surgery alone is adequate therapy. Diffuse tumors are not amenable to complete resection, but biopsy and identification of the tumor are often critical and may be achieved using CT- or MRI-guided stereotactic surgical techniques
- *Chemotherapy:* Used in combination and specific to tumor type
  - ✓ Presence of the blood–brain barrier is an obstacle to effective therapy, although this may be disrupted in the setting of active neoplasm
  - ✓ Active agents include alkylating agents (cyclophosphamide, ifosfamide, thiotepa, cisplatin, carboplatin, and temozolomide), antimetabolites (methotrexate), and plant alkaloids (vincristine, etoposide)
  - ✓ For aggressive or recurrent tumors, high-dose (marrow ablative) chemotherapy with stem cell rescue has been used
  - ✓ Use of chemotherapy has enabled a decrease in the doses of radiation, sparing late effects to the developing brain
- Radiation therapy
  - ✓ Aimed at tumor bed and/or craniospinal area for spread or prophylaxis
  - ✓ Proton beam therapy (versus traditional photon) is being used increasingly in children for its precise targeting and potential for fewer late effects
  - ✓ Age, comorbidities, and balance of early and late toxicity must be considered
  - ✓ Radiation is used most commonly in medulloblastoma, PNET, ependymoma, high-grade gliomas, diffuse brainstem glioma, and germ cell tumors
  - ✓ In some tumor types, radiation is reserved for residual tumor, if chemotherapy fails or progression occurs
- *Newer modalities:*
  - ✓ Antiangiogenic agents are part of many therapies now
  - ✓ *Other promising agents under investigation include:* Differentiating agents (cis-retinoic acid, histone-deacetylase inhibitors), tyrosine kinase inhibitors, molecular targets, and immunotherapy

**TABLE 21-3** Classification of CNS/Spinal Tumors

| Cell Type | Tumors | Most Common Locations | Estimated Incidence* | Spread | Approach to Treatment[1] |
|---|---|---|---|---|---|
| Embryonal | Medulloblastoma | Cerebellum | 15–20% | Seeding | Surgery<br>Radiation (focal/CSI[2])<br>Chemotherapy |
| | PNET | Supratentorial | | | |
| | Pineoblastoma | Pineal gland | 0.5–2% | | |
| Glia[3] (*Gliomas*) | Low-grade astrocytoma (pilocytic, fibrillary) | Any site | 15–20% | Focal | Surgery<br>±Radiation (focal)<br>±Chemotherapy |
| | High-grade astrocytoma (anaplastic/glioblastoma) | | 10–12% | | Surgery<br>Radiation (focal)<br>Chemotherapy |
| | Ependymoma | | 5–10% | | Surgery<br>Radiation (focal) |
| | Oligodendroglioma | | 1% | | Surgery<br>±Radiation (focal)<br>±Chemotherapy |
| | Brainstem glioma | Brainstem | 10–20% | | Radiation (focal) |

*(continued)*

**TABLE 21-3** *(continued)*

| Cell Type | Tumors | Most Common Locations | Estimated Incidence* | Spread | Approach to Treatment[1] |
|---|---|---|---|---|---|
| Choroid plexus | Papilloma | Ventricles | 3% | | Surgery ±Radiation |
| | Carcinoma | | | Seeding | ±Chemotherapy (for carcinoma) |
| Rathke's pouch | Craniopharyngioma | Suprasellar | 3–5% | Focal | Surgery ±Radiation (focal) |
| Germ cell | Germinoma | Suprasellar, pineal | 4–5% | Seeding | Surgery (for mature teratoma) Radiation (focal ±WV[4] ±CSI) ±Chemotherapy |
| | Non-germinomatous germ cell tumors | | | | |

*In ages 0–14 years old.

[1]Treatments differ based on location/spread of disease and age of patient (radiation is often avoided in very young children). In some tumors, treatments vary based on presence or absence of high-risk features (e.g., in medulloblastoma: high-risk features include residual tumor >1.5 cm$^2$, age <3 years old, supratentorial location, and metastatic disease).

[2]CSI, craniospinal irradiation.

[3]WHO classification of gliomas: Low grade (I=pilocytic astrocytoma, II=fibrillary) and high grade (III=anaplastic, IV=glioblastoma multiforme). Treatment varies by grade.

[4]WV, whole ventricle irradiation.

## PRINCIPLES OF SUPPORTIVE CARE

### INFECTIOUS PROPHYLAXIS

- *Streptococcus mitis:* Patients with a history of *Strep mitis* require prophylaxis when they become neutropenic, typically with clindamycin, vancomycin, or the narrowest antibiotic their strain of *S. mitis* was sensitive to
- *Pneumocystis pneumonia:* Patients receiving chemotherapy or other forms of immunosuppressive therapy are at risk for *Pneumocystis jirovecii* pneumonia
  - ✓ Most effective prophylactic agent is cotrimoxazole (sulfamethoxazole/trimethoprim), usually given twice a day × 2 days a week
  - ✓ Other agents available include dapsone, aerosolized pentamidine (IV for patients <5 years old), and atovaquone, but are inferior as there is increased potential for *Pneumocystis* breakthrough with these second-line agents
  - ✓ PCP prophylaxis is typically continued for 3–6 months after therapy or longer (12 months) in stem cell transplant patients
- *Fungal prophylaxis:*
  - ✓ Increased risk correlates to prolonged/profound neutropenia (AML, relapsed ALL, stem cell transplant) or to profound lymphopenia (transplant patients with GVHD, alemtuzumab exposure, etc.) in patients receiving the most intense chemotherapy
  - ✓ When neutropenic, patients are typically started on an antifungal agent like fluconazole or another at the discretion of the treating team
  - ✓ Studies are ongoing to determine the best fungal prophylaxis for this population

## MUCOSITIS

**Any rapidly dividing cell, like gastrointestinal or oral mucosa, can suffer effects of chemotherapy and break down, become ulcerated or inflamed causing mucositis. Doxorubicin, daunorubicin, methotrexate, and cytarabine are most commonly associated with mucositis.**

### SIGNS AND SYMPTOMS

- Pain, drooling, dysphagia, abdominal pain, diarrhea, melena, or hematochezia
- Mucositis can interfere with adequate oral hydration and also create an entry point for infectious agents
  - ✓ Patients receiving high-dose cytarabine or HSCT are at particularly high risk for a mucositis-related infection, including *Streptococcus mitis*, which can cause life-threatening sepsis

### TREATMENT

- Debridement with sponges dabbed in sterile saline
- Analgesia with "magic mouthwash" (2% viscous lidocaine, liquid Maalox®, and liquid diphenhydramine) every 4 to 6 hours
- Oral mucositis can also be complicated or worsened by oral thrush so an antifungal agent (nystatin or fluconazole) may be indicated
- *Treatment modalities for anal mucositis:* Stool softeners, creams applied to the anal verge (nystatin cream, zinc oxide)
- Mucositis can cause significant discomfort and patients may require intravenous fluids, parenteral nutrition, or IV opioid therapy

## NAUSEA AND VOMITING

### GENERAL PRINCIPLES

- Nausea and vomiting can be caused by chemotherapy and radiation, or can occur postoperatively
- Consequences include dehydration, electrolyte imbalance, anorexia, weight loss, and increased susceptibility to infections
- *Chemotherapy-induced nausea vomiting (CINV) is defined by when it occurs:*
  - ✓ *Acute:* Occurs within the first 24 hours after receiving chemotherapy
  - ✓ *Delayed:* Occurs >24 hours after administration and can persist up to 1 week after therapy (common with platinum-based chemotherapy)
  - ✓ *Breakthrough CINV:* Defined as more than three episodes of emesis or retching within 24 hours and occurs despite proper prophylaxis
  - ✓ *Anticipatory CINV:* A preconditioned emetic response often related to anxiety surrounding treatments due to prior poor control of nausea/emesis. Can also be triggered by tastes, odor, or sights

### EMETOGENICITY AND TREATMENT GUIDELINES

- Emetogenicity varies among commonly used chemotherapeutic agents (Table 21-4)
  - ✓ If multiple chemotherapy agents or radiation are given on a single day, the emetogenicity is generally classified based on the most highly emetogenic agent
  - ✓ If multiple days of chemotherapy are being given consecutively, the emetogenicity is generally classified by the most highly emetogenic agent given each day of therapy
- Prophylactic antiemetic regimens
  - ✓ Consider oral before IV antiemetics
  - ✓ Requires administration of 5HT3-antagonist (e.g., ondansetron, granisetron) antiemetics "around the clock" (i.e., scheduled) rather than symptomatically (or as needed) for patients actively receiving chemotherapy. This may include dexamethasone
  - ✓ *Common regimens:*
    - *Low:* No routine antiemetics recommended
    - *Moderate:* Promethazine, prochlorperazine + diphenhydramine
    - *Moderate/High:* 5HT3 antagonist* (e.g., ondansetron) +/− dexamethasone orally/ IV q24h (maximum 8 mg q24h)
    - *High:* 5HT3 antagonist* + dexamethasone orally/IV q12h (maximum 8 mg q12h). May also include an NK-1 receptor antagonist (aprepitant)
    
    *Based on new recommendations due to QTc prolongation, no more than 16 mg/dose IV of ondansetron should be administered in a single dose. Patient may still have daily total of 24 mg.*

- *Breakthrough emesis:*
  - ✓ Requires as needed rescues or adjunct medications, which can include dexamethasone, benzodiazepines (lorazepam), cannaboids, antihistamines, anticholinergics, phenothiazines, promotility agents (metoclopramide), or additional 5HT3 antagonist if daily maximum dose not reached
- Bone marrow transplant patients usually receive antiemetics until 24 hours after the last dose of chemotherapy or irradiation
- Antiemetic regimens are usually institution specific, so please consult the formulary at treating center for dosing guidelines

### NUTRITIONAL SUPPORT

- Malnutrition is very prevalent in oncology patients
- *Is often multifactorial:* Decreased intake, poor absorption, increased caloric losses, and/or increased metabolic demand

| TABLE 21-4 | Emetogenic Potential of Each Drug in the Chemotherapy Regimen or by the Site of Radiation | | |
|---|---|---|---|
| **Minimal** | **Low** | **Moderate** | **High** |
| <10% frequency of emesis in absence of prophylaxis | 10–30% frequency of emesis in absence of prophylaxis | 30–90% frequency of emesis in absence of prophylaxis | >90% frequency of emesis in absence of prophylaxis |
| Alemtuzumab | Cytarabine | Busulfan | Carboplatin |
| Asparaginase | ($<200\,mg/m^2$) | Carmustine (low dose) | Carmustine |
| Bevacizumab | Etoposide | Clofarabine | Cisplatin |
| Bleomycin | Fludarabine (oral) | Cyclophosphamide | Cyclophosphamide |
| Cladribine | 5-Fluorouracil | (low dose) | ($>1\,g/m^2$) |
| Dasatinib | Gemcitabime | Daunorubicin | Cytarabine ($>3\,g/m^2$) |
| Dexrazoxane | Mitoxantrone | Doxorubicin | Dactinomycin |
| Erlotinib | Nilotinib | Etoposide (oral) | Methotrexate |
| Gemtuzumab | Paclitaxel | Idarubicin | ($>12\,g/m^2$) |
| Hydroxyurea | Thiotepa ($<300\,mg/m^2$) | Ifosfamide | Procarbazine |
| Lenalidomide | Topotecan | Imatinib | Thiotepa |
| Nelarabine | | Intrathecal therapy | Total body irradiation |
| Rituximab | | Irinotecan | Brain/Craniospinal |
| Sorafenib | | Methotrexate | radiation |
| Temsirolimus | | ($<12\,g/m^2$) | Abdomino-pelvic |
| Thioguanine | | Temozolamide | radiation |
| Vinblastine | | Vinorelbine | |
| Vincristine | | | |
| 6-Mercaptopurine | | | |

Data from Hesketh PJ: Defining the emetogenicity of cancer chemotherapy regimens: relevance to clinical practice, *Oncologist*. 1999;4(3):191–196 and Basch E, Prestrud AA, Hesketh PJ, et al: Antiemetics: American Society of Clinical Oncology clinical practice guideline update, *J Clin Oncol*. 2011 Nov 1;29(31):4189–4198

- Malnutrition is associated with increased risk of infection, prolonged hospitalization, and poorer outcomes as compared to healthy weight patients
- When supplemental nutrition is required, the enteral route, by mouth, is preferred
- Patients with mucositis or severe nausea may require tube feedings via nasogastric or other routes
- Placing a gastrostomy tube for nutritional and medication delivery purposes may be beneficial in certain patients (where radiation or severe mucositis may impair eating/taking medications)
- Appetite stimulants can be considered in appropriate patients
- Total parenteral nutrition (TPN) is less favored, but often times necessary for weight maintenance
- Being overweight has also been associated with poor outcomes, so maintaining a healthy weight is critical

## PAIN

### Somatic or Visceral Pain

- Typically managed with opioid therapy, as anti-inflammatory medications like ibuprofen, which can affect platelet function, are contraindicated in patients with actual or expected thrombocytopenia

- Begin with oral regimens and proceed to IV as needed, following the WHO two-step opioid ladder, with some patients requiring a PCA (patient controlled analgesia device)
- Proper bowel regimens (stool softeners plus cathartic agents) are required for patients being started on opioid therapy to prevent significant constipation associated with opioid use (which is, of note, the only side effect of opioids to which patients do not become tolerant)

## Neuropathic Pain

- Neuropathic pain is a common side effect of several chemotherapy and immunotherapy regimens
- GABA analogs like gabapentin and pregabalin are helpful for these symptoms, but require a slow titration to be effective
- Depending on the length of pain therapy, a slow taper off of the medication may be required

## PSYCHOSOCIAL AND PSYCHIATRIC SUPPORT

- Patients with cancer are at increased risk of psychological distress, including anxiety, adjustment disorder, and depression. They are also more likely to experience sleep disturbances as a result of treatment factors, hospitalizations, medication side effects, and psychosocial stressors
- Appropriate attention should be made to addressing these symptoms and their management. Consultation with psychosocial support teams and child life staff is prudent and can be beneficial

## TRANSFUSION

- There is wide variation in practice, so please consult the oncologic team at a given institution. Patients with clinical indications for blood products (bleeding, anemia, gallops, etc.) should be transfused at the discretion of the treating provider

## Packed Red Cell Transfusions

- Typically indicated if the patient is symptomatic from anemia or the hemoglobin is <7–8 g/dL
- Prior to procedures and radiation, some centers aim for hemoglobin closer to 9–10 g/dL (mainly for anesthesia purposes)
- Ensure that all blood products are irradiated and leukoreduced; in addition, for a CMV-negative or pre/post bone marrow transplant patient, blood should also be CMV antibody negative

## Platelets

- Transfusion of platelets is typically indicated when platelet counts are <10,000/mm$^3$ or there is active bleeding
- In bone marrow transplant or neuro-oncology patients with residual tumor, or children who are very active, higher thresholds of 20,000/mm$^3$ are typically followed
- Platelets should be >20,000–30,000/mm$^3$ for lumbar puncture
- Prior to neurosurgical procedures or other procedures with significant risk bleeding, platelet goal should be over 50,000/mm$^3$
- There is no accepted platelet requirement for bone marrow aspirate or biopsy

## Special Situations

- Patients at risk for hyperviscosity syndrome (new diagnosis of leukemia with elevated WBC >100,000/mm$^3$) should only be transfused in discussion with oncology given high risk of vascular sludging and sequelae (stroke, pulmonary failure, cardiac dysfunction)

- Patients on concurrent anticoagulation for history of thrombosis are typically maintained at platelet count >50,000/mm³
- Provision of fresh frozen plasma, cryoprecipitate, or vitamin K is sometimes required for correction of severe coagulopathy in specific cases (e.g., preoperative or in DIC associated with APML) but is not a standard practice in all patients

## VACCINATION

- Aside from the yearly inactivated influenza vaccine, routine immunizations should be deferred in all patients undergoing cancer chemotherapy
- Revaccination should not begin until at least 6 months after therapy is complete, and longer (12 months) post-allogeneic bone marrow transplantation

## VASCULAR ACCESS

- Patients undergoing treatment for chemotherapy typically require indwelling central lines
- Temporary lines such as IVs are not typically used for certain chemotherapy, given concerns for subcutaneous extravasation into skin or joints
- Peripherally inserted central catheters (PICC) can provide up to 2 weeks of continued access but are less favored than more permanent options such as subcutaneous ports (Port-a-cath®) or tunneled central venous line (Broviac®, Hickman®)
- The choice of line depends on diagnosis and treatment protocol (based on type and rate of administration of chemotherapy and supportive care requirements), as well as planned future care (stem cell transplant, etc.)

# CHAPTER 22

# Ophthalmology

*Gil Binenbaum, MD, MSCE*
*Stefanie L. Davidson, MD*

## OCULAR EXPOSURE

**The surface of the eye needs to stay well lubricated or it can lead to vision-threatening complications in the ICU**

### PATHOPHYSIOLOGY

- Normal ocular surface protective mechanisms include tear production, intact corneal sensation, blinking, and complete eyelid closure
- Impaired protective mechanisms result in corneal exposure and drying
- Corneal "dryness" (subclinical epithelial breakdown) may progress to corneal abrasion, ulceration, infection, scarring, thinning, and/or perforation if untreated

### CLINICAL MANIFESTATIONS

- Risk factors for corneal exposure include loss of protective mechanisms due to deep sedation, neurologic impairment, or eyelid abnormality; overhead warmers; treatments causing air to blow over the eyes
- *Risk increases with poor eyelid closure:* Low risk with eyelids that close completely, increasing with white sclera showing, highest with cornea or underlying iris showing
- Eye exam may reveal conjunctival redness or swelling, corneal haze or opacity, blunted red reflex

### DIAGNOSTICS

- Slit lamp biomicroscope exam and fluorescein staining may reveal punctate erosions, corneal abrasion, opacity (ulcer), thinning, or perforation

### MANAGEMENT

- *Prophylaxis for at-risk patients (e.g., intubated and sedated) is critical:*
  - ✓ Lubricating eye ointment (Lacri-lube ointment which consists of mineral oil and white petrolatum) with frequency according to eyelid position
  - ✓ Closed lids every 6–8 hours, sclera showing every 4–6 hours, cornea showing every 2–4 hours; the frequency of ointment administration may be reduced if the eye and ointment are then covered with a piece of non-sticky plastic wrap (e.g., saran wrap) to form a "moisture chamber"
  - ✓ Artificial tear drops evaporate quickly and are not useful
- Prompt ophthalmology consultation for red conjunctiva, corneal haze or opacity, or if the cornea is visible due to incomplete eyelid exposure in an at-risk patient
- Antibiotic ophthalmic ointment (erythromycin, polysporin) if there is corneal epithelial staining with fluorescein
- Complicated cases may require tarsorrhaphy (suturing of eyelids), bandage contact lens, corneal gluing, or emergent corneal transplantation

## CORNEAL CLOUDING AND GLAUCOMA

**The cornea should always be clear with visible iris details and a bright red reflex, and any opacity, whether diffuse or focal, is a sign of serious eye disease.**

**Glaucoma is irreversible optic nerve damage due to increased intraocular pressure.**

### DIFFERENTIAL DIAGNOSIS OF CORNEAL CLOUDING IN AN INFANT

- *Trauma:* Forceps injury, corneal perforation with amniocentesis
- *Infection:* Syphilis, rubella, HSV, bacterial ulcer
- *Infantile glaucoma:* Associated with enlarged eye (buphthalmos)
- Corneal or limbal dermoid, associated with Goldenhar syndrome
- *Anterior segment dysgenesis:* Peters anomaly (central corneal opacity), sclerocornea
- *Corneal dystrophy:* Congenital hereditary endothelial dystrophy (CHED), congenital hereditary stromal dystrophy (CHSD)
- *Metabolic:* Mucopolysaccharidoses (Hurlers, MPS IH; Type IV, mucolipidoses), cystinosis, tyrosinemia

### EPIDEMIOLOGY AND ETIOLOGY

#### Primary Glaucoma

- *Primary infantile glaucoma (congenital glaucoma):* 1:10,000–1:15,000; 90% sporadic
- Caused by developmental defect in the structure of the anterior chamber
- Associated systemic syndromes include Sturge–Weber, neurofibromatosis type 1, Marfan, Stickler, Lowe, Rubinstein–Taybi, Wolf–Hirschhorn
- Also associated with ocular syndromes such as aniridia, Peters anomaly

#### Secondary Glaucomas

- Secondary glaucomas of childhood are more common than primary glaucomas
- *Traumatic:* Acute glaucoma related to a hyphema (see Hyphema) or glaucoma years after trauma secondary to damage of drainage angle in the eye (angle recession)
- *Inflammatory:* Caused by trabecular meshwork inflammation or clogging with inflammatory debris; for example, uveitis associated with juvenile idiopathic arthritis
- *Steroid-induced:* Can be caused by topical, systemic, or inhaled forms of glucocorticoids, by decreasing aqueous outflow
- *Aphakic:* Absence of the natural lens usually due to cataract extraction; 8% to 41% chance of developing glaucoma
- *Intraocular neoplasms* such as retinoblastoma, juvenile xanthogranuloma

### PATHOPHYSIOLOGY

- Intraocular pressure (IOP) is maintained by the balance of aqueous humor production by the ciliary body and drainage by the trabecular meshwork
- When this drainage system is impaired, IOP increases
- Elevated IOP causes loss of the nerve fiber layer of the retina, optic nerve damage, and, if left untreated, irreversible blindness

### CLINICAL MANIFESTATIONS

- Children younger than 3 years present with enlarged eye (buphthalmos), photophobia, epiphora (tearing), blepharospasm (repetitive involuntary closure of the lids), and cloudy cornea (corneal edema)

- Children older than 3 years may have completely asymptomatic glaucoma until advanced, irreversible visual loss occurs
- Check ocular size (typically by measuring corneal diameter, see Diagnostics below), corneal clarity, and visual acuity
- *Haab's striae:* Breaks in Descemet's membrane (basement membrane of the cornea) that occur as the cornea enlarges. Typically seen as horizontal lines in the cornea and develop in children younger than 3 years
- *Cupping of the optic nerve:* Cup to disc ratio greater than 0.4 is suggestive of glaucoma
- Look for evidence of associated syndromes

## DIAGNOSTICS

- *Tonometry:* Pressure greater than 21 mm Hg in a calm infant is abnormal
- *Gonioscopy: Visually* assess the angle anatomy
- Measure corneal diameter and axial length to follow response to treatment: Normal corneal diameter is 9.5–10.5 mm in newborns and 11–12 mm in adults

## MANAGEMENT

- Ophthalmology should be consulted on all patients with a clinical suspicion of glaucoma or with any corneal opacity regardless of concern for glaucoma

### Medical

- *Topical Therapy:*
  ✓ Beta-blocker (e.g., timolol maleate 2 times per day) is a common first-line agent
  ✓ Initial IOP >30 mm Hg or insufficient lowering of IOP to <21 mm Hg requires addition of a carbonic anhydrase inhibitor (e.g., dorzolamide or brinzolamide 2 or 3 times daily) and/or prostaglandin (latanoprost once daily)
- *Oral therapy:* Acetazolamide for highly or persistently elevated IOP
- Duration of therapy is lifelong unless surgical treatment is performed

### Surgical

- Primary congenital glaucoma is a surgical disease
- 80% of children can be cured with:
  ✓ *Goniotomy:* An incision is made in the trabecular meshwork with a blade inserted into the anterior chamber. Improves trabecular outflow and reduces IOP. Can only be performed if the cornea is clear
  ✓ *Trabeculotomy ab externo:* External dissection of Schlemm's canal to increase exit of aqueous fluid. Can be done even if corneal is cloudy (corneal edema)

  *When primary infantile glaucoma fails above surgeries and other types of glaucomas fail medical management then:*

  ✓ *Trabeculectomy:* Filtration procedure creating a communication between the anterior chamber and subconjunctival space to allow drainage of aqueous
  ✓ *Glaucoma drainage device:* Similar purpose to trabeculectomy but uses an implant
  ✓ *Photocyclocoagulation and cyclocryotherapy:* Destroys the ciliary body, thereby reducing production of aqueous fluid; usually a last resort

## ABNORMAL RED REFLEX AND LEUKOCORIA

**Red reflex testing should be done on all newborns, infants, and young children**
**"Leukocoria" is from Greek meaning "white pupil"**

## EPIDEMIOLOGY

- *Congenital cataracts are most common cause of leukocoria:* 1/2500 live births
- Retinoblastoma in 1/15,000 people; extremely rare after 6 years of age

## DIFFERENTIAL DIAGNOSIS

- Cataract (lens opacity) may result in permanent vision loss if not treated early
- Retinoblastoma is life threatening and the most concerning diagnosis
- Advanced retinopathy of prematurity and retinal detachment
- Strabismus will cause asymmetric red reflexes
- High refractive errors cause blunted red reflex
- Other ocular disorders, including retinal dysplasia (developmental anomaly, present at birth), coloboma (missing piece of tissue in the eye, such as a chorioretinal or optic nerve head coloboma), and Coats disease (retinal vascular abnormalities and lipid exudates)

## PATHOPHYSIOLOGY

- The vascular choroid behind the retina reflects light, forming the normal "red reflex"
- Light passes through the cornea, aqueous humor, pupil, lens, and vitreous to get to the retina. Interference by any of these structures may lead to a diminished, irregular, absent, white, or asymmetric red reflex

## CLINICAL MANIFESTATIONS

- *Red reflex exam:* Use a direct ophthalmoscope an arm's length from the infant's eyes in a dark room
  - ✓ A normal exam has clear, bilaterally symmetric reflexes with equal color, intensity, and clarity
  - ✓ Any white spots, opacities, or asymmetry are abnormal and require evaluation
  - ✓ Darker pigmented children will have reflexes that appear darker

## DIAGNOSTICS

- A patient with abnormal or asymmetric red reflexes or leukocoria urgently requires a full eye exam, including a dilated fundus examination by an ophthalmologist
- Ocular ultrasound by an ophthalmologist and MRI of the eye may help to rule out retinoblastoma

## MANAGEMENT

- Depends on etiology
- Congenital cataracts are typically surgically removed by 4–6 weeks of age and require ongoing amblyopia treatment
- Retinoblastoma treatment is begun immediately because mortality is tied to spread of disease; untreated children will die from extension to the brain
- Children with bilateral congenital cataracts may require evaluation for congenital infections (TORCH), metabolic diseases, and chromosomal abnormalities

## UVEITIS

**Uveitis is intraocular inflammation of the uveal tract (iris, ciliary body, choroid)**

## CAUSES OF UVEITIS

- Idiopathic

- *Systemic inflammatory disorders:* JIA (especially pauciarticular, ANA positive, rheumatoid factor negative), sarcoidosis, Behcet's, inflammatory bowel disease, HLA-B27 associated disease
- *Infection:* Lyme, HSV, CMV, HIV, TB, toxoplasmosis, toxocara, syphilis
- *Tubular interstitial nephritis and uveitis (TINU)*
- *Trauma*
- *Neoplasm (masquerade syndrome)*—Retinoblastoma, leukemia, lymphoma

## DIFFERENTIAL DIAGNOSIS

- *Conjunctivitis or extra-ocular inflammation* does not affect corneal or red reflex clarity
- *Key warning signs that a red eye is not a simple conjunctivitis:* Vision loss, photophobia, eye pain, eye surgery, contact lens use, chronic (>2 weeks), hyper-purulent discharge, corneal opacity, irregular pupil, poor red reflex, vesicles on lids

## CLINICAL MANIFESTATIONS

- *Symptoms:* Photophobia, pain, redness, decrease in vision, floaters
- Children may be completely asymptomatic (no conjunctival redness, no pain), especially with JIA
- *Signs:* Conjunctival injection, corneal endothelial deposits, anterior chamber cells, hypopyon (grossly visible collection of white cells behind the cornea), irregular pupil from synechiae (scarring between iris and lens behind it), blunted red reflex, inflammatory lesions on fundus exam

## DIAGNOSTICS

- Diagnosis is made visually by slit lamp biomicroscopic and fundus examinations
- Laboratory and radiographic workup for recurrent, bilateral, or posterior uveitis or suspicion of systemic disease

## MANAGEMENT

- Uveitis is a site-threatening condition requiring diagnosis and management by an ophthalmologist, often jointly with a pediatric rheumatologist
- Aggressive control of intraocular inflammation with topical steroids (e.g., prednisolone acetate 1% every hour until inflammation is controlled)
  ✓ Systemic steroids if topical steroids do not adequately control the inflammation or if the posterior structures of the eye are involved
  ✓ Steroid-sparing immunosuppressive agents (e.g., methotrexate, infliximab) if oral steroids cannot be tapered off without recurrence of uveitis
- Cycloplegic eyedrops (e.g., atropine) while active inflammation is present
- Antibiotics as indicated for infectious causes

## HYPHEMA

**Blood in the anterior chamber of the eye**

### EPIDEMIOLOGY

- Annual incidence of 17–20 per 100,000; mostly younger than 20 years old

### PATHOPHYSIOLOGY

- Blunt or penetrating trauma damages iris blood vessels, causing blood to leak into the anterior chamber with potential to increase IOP

- Bleeding stops when a clot forms
- Re-bleeding risk is highest during first 5 days post-trauma when the clot weakens, and can result in pressure spike
- Spontaneous (non-traumatic) hyphema may be caused by intraocular tumors

## CLINICAL MANIFESTATIONS

- Patients present with a history of eye trauma, eye pain, and vision loss
- Children may be somnolent
- Some patients have history of bleeding disorders, sickle cell disease, or anticoagulation therapy
- Blood in the anterior chamber appears as a red or dark meniscus in the aqueous humor behind the cornea and in front of the iris

## DIAGNOSTICS

- Small hyphemas may only be seen with magnification, best provided by a slit lamp biomicroscope
- Assess visual acuity and IOP
- Rule-out an open-globe injury (see below)
- Sickle cell testing for African Americans, because patients with sickle cell trait or disease are at much greater risk for acute glaucoma with hyphema

## MANAGEMENT

- Ophthalmology should be consulted on all patients with hyphema
- *Prevent re-bleeding with the following measures:*
  - ✓ Bed rest
  - ✓ Avoid NSAIDs
  - ✓ Protect the eye with a plastic or metal shield, which covers but does not touch the eye. Do not apply gauze patches, as these touch the eye
- Admission and/or sedation may be required for young, active children
- Topical mydriatics (e.g., atropine 1% twice per day) and topical steroids (prednisolone acetate 1% four times per day)
- Glaucoma medications for elevated IOP (see Glaucoma management above, but note that topical and systemic carbonic anhydrase inhibitors are relatively contraindicated in sickle cell or sickle trait positive patients with hyphema)
- *Consider surgical intervention if:* Elevated IOP unresponsive to medications, patients with sickle cell disease, corneal blood staining
- *Surgical procedures:* Anterior chamber washout and clot removal

## ORBITAL FRACTURE

**Fracture of one or more of the orbital bones due to trauma, including from assault, falls, motor vehicle accidents, and sports**

## DIFFERENTIAL DIAGNOSIS

- Bruised extraocular muscles, cranial nerve palsy, and orbital edema all present with double vision
- Eye trauma may result in open globe injury, hyphema, retinal detachment, vitreous hemorrhage, lens dislocation or cataract, and/or choroidal rupture

## PATHOPHYSIOLOGY

- *The orbit is composed of seven bones:* Maxilla, zygoma, lacrimal, ethmoid, palatine, sphenoid, and frontal. The walls are thin; the rims are thick
- Most fractures occur in the medial wall or posteromedial floor, near the infraorbital groove, which contains the infraorbital nerve (V2), providing sensation to the cheek and upper alveolus/teeth (**Figure 22-1**)
- Extraocular muscle may become entrapped in a fracture, causing oculocardiac reflex (vagal nerve) induced bradycardia
- Open globe injuries (full thickness hole in the wall of the eye) may result from penetrating trauma (laceration) or blunt trauma (ruptured globe), in which increased IOP causes a sclera break and may not be accompanied by an orbital fracture
- Extensive retrobulbar (orbital) hemorrhage with orbital fracture may cause an orbital compartment syndrome and ischemic injury to the optic nerve and retina

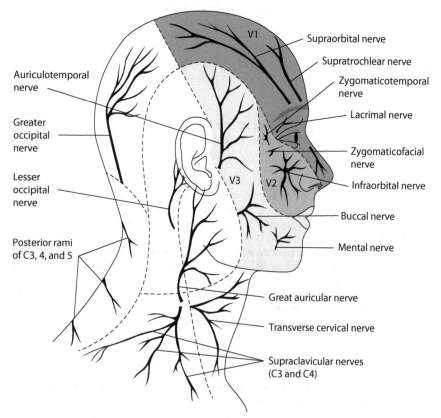

**FIGURE 22-1 Sensory innervation of the head.** The figure shows distribution of the three components of the trigeminal nerve. V1, ophthalmic, sensory; V2, maxillary, sensory; V3, mandibular, sensory, and motor. (Adapted with permission from Lalwani AK (Ed). *Current Diagnosis & Treatment in Otolaryngology-Head & Neck Surgery*, 3rd ed. New York, NY: McGraw-Hill; 2012.)

## CLINICAL MANIFESTATIONS

- Patients may be asymptomatic ("white-eyed" blow out fracture) or present with periorbital ecchymosis and swelling, pain on vertical gaze, double vision, and/or decreased sensation in the V2 cranial nerve distribution
- Check ocular motility, which may be decreased if there is muscle entrapment, and palpate orbital rims for a step off
- Extraocular muscle entrapment may cause a symptomatic oculo-cardiac reflex with bradycardia, and pre-syncopal symptoms, particularly with eye movement
- *Signs of an open globe injury* include
  - ✓ Obvious laceration site
  - ✓ Protruding uvea (appears as brown tissue)
  - ✓ Large amount of subconjunctival hemorrhage
  - ✓ Collapsed anterior chamber (cornea and iris come close to one another)
  - ✓ Peaking of the pupil toward wound site
  - ✓ Decreased vision
- *Signs of an orbital compartment syndrome* include
  - ✓ Decreased vision
  - ✓ Proptosis
  - ✓ Increased eye pressure with an eye that feels hard to palpation

## DIAGNOSTICS

- Thin cut CT in both axial and coronal planes is the study of choice
- Plain film x-rays are insufficient for ruling out an orbital fracture; MRI depicts bones poorly

## MANAGEMENT

### Nonsurgical

- Ice compresses for 48 hours; elevation of head in bed
- Avoid aspirin and NSAID use, minimize coughing and nose blowing
- The following medications have not clearly been shown to improve outcomes, and some ophthalmologists do not use any of these approaches
  - ✓ Some ophthalmologists consider the use of nasal decongestants to prevent or minimize nose blowing
  - ✓ Oral steroids to reduce edema, particularly if ocular motility is decreased
  - ✓ Antibiotics covering sinus flora (e.g., ampicillin-sulbactam), particularly if there is a concomitant sinus infection

### Surgical

- Immediate canthotomy and cantholysis for orbital compartment syndrome with decreased vision
- Urgent surgery for entrapped muscles, particularly if a symptomic oculocardiac reflex is present
- Otherwise, fracture repair is recommended within 1–3 weeks if patient has diplopia, enophthalmos, soft tissue herniation into maxillary sinuses, or if greater than 30% of orbital floor is fractured
- Open globe injuries should be shielded (not patched) and the patient made NPO for surgical repair

## WHEN TO CONSIDER AN OPHTHALMOLOGY CONSULTATION

- Discuss exam location and timing with the ophthalmology team. For some conditions, a slit lamp biomicroscope exam is important and best performed in the ophthalmology clinic. It may be advantageous to wait until the patient is well enough to travel to the office or to arrange an outpatient visit
- Pupillary dilation with mydriatic eye drops will prevent a reliable pupil exam for 4 or more hours but is necessary for a complete exam

### Symptoms or signs as an inpatient
- Red eye
- Vision loss or blurry vision
- Eye pain
- Diplopia (double vision)
- Risk for corneal exposure
- Corneal opacity
- Irregular pupil
- Abnormal red reflex
- New onset strabismus
- Nystagmus

### Based on suspected or confirmed systemic disease (Finding)
- CARDIOLOGY
  - ✓ Congenital heart disease
  - ✓ CHARGE syndrome
  - ✓ PHACES syndrome
- CHILD ABUSE
  - ✓ *Intracranial hemorrhage in an infant:* Retinal hemorrhages with abusive head trauma
- CRANIOFACIAL
  - ✓ *Pierre Robin sequence:* Stickler syndrome
  - ✓ *Hydrocephalus:* Papilledema
- DERMATOLOGY
  - ✓ Stevens–Johnson syndrome, toxic epidermal necrolysis
  - ✓ Peri-ocular capillary hemangioma
  - ✓ PHACES syndrome
  - ✓ Incontinentia pigmenti
  - ✓ Juvenile xanthogranuloma
  - ✓ Oculocutaneous albinism
- GASTROENTEROLOGY
  - ✓ *Wilson's disease:* Kayser–Fleischer ring, cataracts
  - ✓ *Alagille syndrome:* Posterior embryotoxon
- GENETICS
  - ✓ *Marfan syndrome:* Lens subluxation
  - ✓ *Neurofibromatosis:* Iris Lisch nodules
  - ✓ Tuberous sclerosis
  - ✓ *Trisomy 21:* Nystagmus, strabismus, cataracts, glaucoma, blocked tear ducts, high refractive error
  - ✓ 22q11.2 deletion syndrome
- HEMATOLOGY
  - ✓ *Hermansky–Pudlak syndrome:* oculocutaneous albinism

- IMMUNOLOGY
  - ✓ *Chediak–Higashi syndrome:* oculocutaneous albinism
- INFECTIOUS DISEASE
  - ✓ HIV
  - ✓ Preseptal or orbital cellulitis
  - ✓ Neonatal conjunctivitis
  - ✓ Neonatal herpes simplex virus infection
  - ✓ Periocular herpes simplex virus or varicella virus infection
  - ✓ *Cat-scratch disease:* Parinaud's oculoglandular syndrome, neuroretinitis, focal chorioretinitis
  - ✓ *Lyme:* Optic neuritis, cranial nerve palsies, uveitis
  - ✓ *Fungemia*
  - ✓ *Endocarditis:* Retinal hemorrhages and septic emboli
  - ✓ *TORCH infections:* Toxoplasmosis, Rubella, CMV, Herpes, Syphilis
- METABOLISM
  - ✓ *Galactosemia:* Cataract
  - ✓ *Tyrosinemia:* Type 2 with corneal deposits causing redness, tearing, photophobia
  - ✓ *Cystinosis*
- MITOCHONDRIAL DISEASE
  - ✓ MERFF (myoclonic epilepsy with ragged red fibers)
  - ✓ MELAS (mitochondrial encephalomyopathy with lactic acidosis and stroke-like episodes)
  - ✓ Kearns–Sayre
  - ✓ *NARP:* Neuropathy, ataxia, retinitis pigmentosa
- NEONATOLOGY
  - ✓ Neonatal conjunctivitis
  - ✓ Extreme prematurity (birth weight ≤1501 g, gestational age ≤30 weeks; guidelines vary for middle income countries)—Retinopathy of prematurity exams
- NEPHROLOGY
  - ✓ *Tubular interstitial nephritis:* Uveitis
- NEUROLOGY
  - ✓ Seizures, especially infantile spasms
    - *Tuberous sclerosis:* Retinal hamartomas
    - *Aicardi syndrome (X-linked dominant, primarily affecting girls):* Retinal lacunae
    - Use of vigabatrin for seizure control
  - ✓ *Myasthenia gravis:* Ptosis, strabismus, ocular motility deficits
  - ✓ *Cranial nerve palsies:* 3rd, 4th, 6th, and 7th nerve palsies
  - ✓ *Multiple sclerosis:* Optic neuritis, internuclear ophthalmoplegia
- RHEUMATOLOGY
  - ✓ *JIA:* Uveitis, slit lamp exam essential, patients generally asymptomatic
  - ✓ *Kawasaki disease:* Conjunctivitis and uveitis

# Orthopedics 23

*Christian Turner, MD*
*Matthew Grady, MD*
*Theodore Ganley, MD*

## BASICS OF PEDIATRIC ORTHOPEDICS

Musculoskeletal complaints and injuries are some of the most commonly encountered problems in pediatrics. In addition, children have immature musculoskeletal systems that pose particular challenges that are quite different than those of adults.

- Children have open growth plates, or physes, located between the epiphysis and the metaphysis
- Fractures most commonly occur near the metaphysis or physis
- An open growth plate is cartilaginous, and has not yet calcified, which makes it the weakest part of the immature bone
- Pediatric bones are less brittle than adults leading to some distinct fracture patterns
- In a buckle fracture, compression force leads to partial failure, but the fracture does not traverse the entire bone
- A greenstick fracture occurs due to tension or torsion force that leaves the cortex and periosteal sleeve intact of one side of the bone
- Angulated fractures in children have a much greater potential to remodel back to original shape than fractures in adults. Remodeling potential is greatest in: younger patients, injuries near a growing physis, and those in the plane of motion congruent to an associated joint
- Open fractures require consultation with Orthopedic Surgery
- Consider child abuse as a factor in pediatric fractures. Injuries concerning for abuse include: Bucket-handle (metaphyseal corner) fractures, multiple fractures of different ages, posterior rib or scapular fractures, and long bone fractures in children that do not walk

## FRACTURES

**Management of fractures depends on the type, location, and amount of displacement present. Displacement, or loss of normal alignment of the distal fragment, is usually described in terms of translation (repositioning away from but remaining parallel to the long axis), angulation (degrees of bending from a straight line), shortening (overlap) or distraction (increased distance), and rotation (twisting).**

### FRACTURES OF THE PHYSIS

Physeal fractures are more common than isolated ligament or tendon injuries in skeletally immature patients because the surrounding connective tissues are stronger than the open physis. Injuries involving the physis are described with the Salter–Harris (SH) classification as shown in Figure 23-1, and described in Table 23-1.

- Physical exam findings in physeal fractures: Tenderness over long bone physis following an injury, swelling, difficulty bearing weight
- Diagnosis: Commonly made by plain radiographs

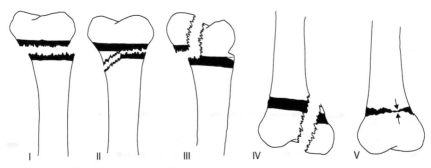

FIGURE 23-1 **Salter–Harris types I–V.**

| TABLE 23-1 | Salter–Harris Classification for Fractures Involving the Physis | |
|---|---|---|
| **Fracture Type** | **Characteristics** | **Comments** |
| SH-I | Shearing injury to the physis without apparent bony fracture | Most common in toddlers; may not be recognized on radiographs |
| SH-II | Fracture at physis that extends into the metaphysis | Overall the most common pattern |
| SH-III | Fracture at physis that extends into the epiphysis | Intraarticular extension can lead to joint instability; should be managed by Orthopedic Surgery |
| SH-IV | Fracture involving the metaphysis, physis, and epiphysis | About 10% of physis fractures. One example is the triplane fracture. |
| SH-V | Crush injury of the physis | Rare, <1% of fractures |

- SH-I fractures may not be visible on initial films. Look for soft tissue swelling adjacent to the physis in question
- In equivocal cases, consider imaging the contralateral joint to compare physeal widths
- Injuries to the physis should be monitored for several months after injury to monitor for growth arrest
- Injuries that result in some measure of disability, along with tenderness at a physis on exam, should be treated as SH-I fractures even if there is no abnormality demonstrated on the radiographs

## UPPER EXTREMITY

### Clavicle Fractures

- The most frequently fractured bone in children; most are in the midshaft
- Mechanism of injury: Trauma at birth due to difficult delivery; fall onto shoulder or outstretched arm in older children
- Physical exam: Tenderness at clavicle; patient may have visible deformity
- Shoulder range of motion (ROM) likely limited, especially forward flexion and abduction
- Assess for associated injuries, especially at the sternoclavicular (SC) joint

*Diagnostic Workup:*

• Plain radiographs: True anterior-posterior (AP) view of both clavicles, and AP view with beam at 30-degree cephalad angle ("serendipity view")

*Management:*

• Infants: Pinning the sleeve to the body of their shirt for comfort; avoid direct pressure on the clavicle
• Older children: Sling, or figure of eight splint, typically for 3–4 weeks
• A palpable bony callus often remains after healing, but should not affect function
• Orthopedic referral required for open fractures, injuries adjacent to the SC or acromio-clavicular (AC) joint, or when significant skin tenting is present

## Proximal Humerus Fractures

This is a rare injury in children, accounting for <5% of pediatric fractures. Patients with proximal humerus fractures need to be seen by Orthopedic Surgery service within 24–48 hours.

• Mechanism of injury: Backwards fall onto outstretched arm in older children and adolescents
• Children >11 years old usually have SH II pattern
• Assess neurovascular status, especially the axillary nerve (lateral shoulder sensation)

*Diagnostic Workup:*

• Plain radiographs: AP, lateral, and oblique views

*Management:*

• Consult with Orthopedic Surgery
• Infants: Nearly all do well with nonsurgical care
• Older children and adolescents: Most can be managed with sling and swathe
• Surgical indications: >50% translation, and angulation of >30–40 degrees in adolescents or >60–70 degrees in younger children

## Fractures About the Elbow

**All elbow fractures require consultation with Orthopedic Surgery**. Elbow fractures do not remodel so alignment for healing fractures needs to be near perfect.

• The lateral epicondyle is the last ossification center to appear, around age 8–11 in girls and 9–13 in boys
• The medial epicondyle is the last to fuse, at age 14 in girls and 17 in boys

**Supracondylar humerus fracture:** Account for 60–80% of elbow fractures in children. Most occur in children <8 years old. Up to 15% may be associated with nerve injury, especially the anterior interosseous (Flynn). Evaluate by having patient flex thumb interphalangeal (IP) joint, and index finger distal IP joint (making the "OK" sign).

*Diagnostic Workup:*

• Plain radiographs: AP, lateral, oblique
• In the presence of a posterior fat pad (Figure 23-2), there is about a 75% chance of fracture

*Management:*

• If there is little to no posterior translation of the distal humerus, cast alone may be appropriate
• Most other fracture patterns require closed reduction and pinning

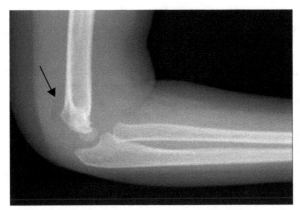

**FIGURE 23-2 Presence of the posterior fat pad indicates high likelihood of supracondylar humerus fracture.** (Reproduced with permission from Rudolph CD, Lister GE, First LR, & Gershon AA (Eds): *Rudolph's Pediatrics*, 22nd ed. New York, NY: McGraw-Hill; 2011.)

**Lateral condyle fracture:** The second most common elbow fracture, accounting for about 15% of elbow fractures in children. Injury is often due to varus force to the elbow during a fall.

*Diagnostic Workup:*

• Plain radiographs: AP, lateral, oblique
• Oblique view is paramount to properly assess for displacement

*Management:*

• Most are treated surgically, and the amount of displacement is a key factor
• If <2 mm displaced, consider long-arm cast for 4–6 weeks with repeat radiographs in cast at 1 and 2 weeks
• Fractures displaced >2 mm require surgical treatment
• Unlike most pediatric fractures, these can show nonunion that may lead to cubitus valgus

**Medical condyle fracture:** More likely in boys (nearly 80%) with peak incidence in early adolescence. The mechanism is valgus force with associated firing of forearm flexor and pronator muscles. There is an association with elbow dislocation in 50% of cases. The ulnar nerve may be compromised in rare cases.

*Diagnostic Workup:*

• Plain radiographs: AP, lateral, oblique

*Management:*

• Most surgeons accept treatment with cast for displacement 2–5 mm. Internal fixation is advised if displaced >5mm
• May be associated with loss of terminal extension, which is more common with dislocation injuries and prolonged immobilization

### Forearm Fractures

Forearm fractures account for nearly 50% of fractures in skeletally immature children, and nearly 80% involve the distal 1/3 of the forearm. Typical mechanism of injury is a fall onto an outstretched hand ("FOOSH").

- Most fractures are buckle, greenstick, or SH-II pattern, and displacement is often dorsal
- Fractures involving both bones (radius and ulna) are more complex, as are diaphyseal and proximal injuries
- Be sure to evaluate distal vascular status
- Monteggia fractures are a proximal ulna fracture with an associated dislocation of the radial head. These require management by Orthopedic Surgery

*Diagnostic Workup:*

- Plain radiographs: AP and lateral views of the forearm to include both the elbow and wrist
- Assess distal and proximal articulations of the radius, ulna, and humerus

*Management:*

- Non-displaced injuries: Can be initially managed with volar splint (proximal forearm to metacarpal heads) (Figure 23-3B)
- Reduction attempt with sedation is warranted for displaced distal fractures, followed by long-arm splint or cast for 4 weeks
- Up to 50% translation is likely acceptable if >2 years of growth remains
- Most metaphyseal fractures are managed successfully in short-arm cast for 4 weeks

## Hand Fractures

A fall onto an outstretched hand and direct blows are common mechanisms. Overall the thumb and little finger are most likely to be injured. Tendon and ligament injuries are uncommon until skeletal maturity.

- Distal phalangeal fractures are common
- Metacarpal fractures most often occur at the neck. Evaluate for rotational displacement by having patient make a fist, which should show all fingers pointing to scaphoid
- Carpal bone fractures are rare. The scaphoid is the most commonly fractured carpal bone. Patients have snuffbox tenderness, and radiographs may be negative

*Diagnostic Workup:*

- Plain radiographs: AP, lateral, oblique
- Consider "scaphoid view" with wrist in ulnar deviation

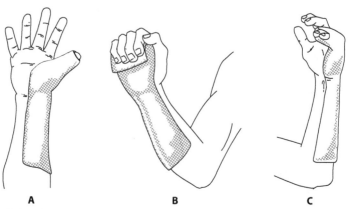

**A**          **B**          **C**

FIGURE 23-3 **Splints.** A. Thumb spica. B. Volar splint (proximal forearm to metacarpal heads). C. Safe position splint for metacarpal fractures (10 degrees wrist extension, 60–70 degrees flexion at MCP joints, extension at IP joints).

*Management:*

- Most metacarpal fractures are treated with closed reduction and splint in the "safe position" (10 degrees wrist extension, 60–70 degrees flexion at MCP joints, extension at IP joints) (Figure 23-3C)
- Displaced fractures usually require open reduction and pinning
- Snuffbox tenderness, even with negative radiographs requires thumb spica (Figure 23-3A) immobilization for 2–3 weeks then repeat evaluation with radiographs out of cast. If fracture is present then total immobilization is usually 6–12 weeks

## LOWER EXTREMITY

Fractures of the lower extremity are more often seen in older children and adolescents.

### Femur Fractures

- Most femur fractures are due to low energy events in middle childhood (6–10 years) with falls during play being the most common cause (Wells)
- In children less than 1 year, 80% may be due to abuse
- In adolescents most are due to motor vehicle accidents
- With a femoral shaft fracture, the patient is likely unable to bear weight, and may have visible deformity
- Distal femur physis fractures are most likely SH-I or II. Knee may be held in flexion due to hamstring spasm. Exam may reveal tenderness at the distal physis, which is just proximal to the joint line near the superior pole of the patella

*Diagnostic Workup:*

- Plain radiographs: AP, lateral; obtain oblique view for distal injuries. Include the ipsilateral hip and knee
- For fractures into the joint, consider CT scan to assess displacement in multiple planes
- Infants often warrant a skeletal survey to evaluate for child abuse

*Management:*

- Birth–5 years: Treat with spica cast or Pavlik harness for infants. Most show significant healing in 4 weeks, but may need up to 8 weeks immobilization
- 5–10 years: Consider conservative management with inpatient traction then spica casting. Surgical options include intramedullary nails, plates with screws, and external fixation devices
- >11 years: Surgery is the primary treatment; intramedullary nails are often used and facilitate early weight bearing (Wells)
- There is high risk for growth arrest with distal femur physeal fractures, and treatment of distal physeal injuries depends on fracture pattern
- SH-I injuries may be treated with long-leg or spica cast with knee at 15–20 degrees flexion
- SH-II fractures may require percutaneous pinning if unstable
- SH-III and IV require open reduction and internal fixation (ORIF) with long-leg cast postoperatively

### Tibia Fractures

The tibia is the most commonly fractured bone of the lower extremity in children, and these injuries are frequently accompanied by ipsilateral fibula fracture. Most proximal tibia physeal fractures are SH-I or II, and if displaced can compromise the surrounding vascular structures.

- Tibial tubercle avulsion fractures are rare, and occur with a jumping or landing mechanism that typically produces a pop sensation and presents with significant swelling over the tubercle and an inability to do straight leg raise

- The Toddler's fracture is a non-displaced spiral fracture of the tibial metaphysis in children 1–4 years old. It occurs with an apparently innocuous twist and fall that is often unwitnessed. Child may limp or stop weight bearing
- The Cozen fracture involves the proximal tibia metaphysis, and is seen in children 2–10 years old. It can lead to progressive valgus deformity
- Both Tillaux and triplane fractures are fractures of the distal tibia in adolescents near skeletal maturity. They most often occur due to external rotation of a planted foot and may be mistaken for an ankle sprain
- The Tillaux fracture is an SH-III injury to the anterolateral distal tibial epiphysis
- A triplane fracture involves coronal, sagittal, and transverse components at the distal tibia. It appears as an SH-II fracture on lateral radiographs and as an SH-III on anterior posterior radiographs

*Diagnostic Workup:*

- Plain radiographs: AP, lateral, oblique views to include the ipsilateral knee and ankle
- CT scan may be indicated for Tillaux and triplane fractures to assess the degree of displacement at the joint surface

*Management:*

- Most tibial shaft fractures are treated with cast; consider closed reduction as needed
- Non-displaced tibial tubercle avulsions are managed with cast above the knee; if displaced, they warrant ORIF
- Cozen fractures are treated with closed reduction and casting
- Proximal physeal fractures are treated with cast above the knee if non-displaced. If displaced they require closed reduction, often under general anesthesia
- Treat Toddler's fracture with above the knee cast, weight bearing as tolerated, for 3 weeks (Wells)
- Closed reduction may be attempted for Tillaux and triplane fractures, but ORIF is indicated for residual joint step-off greater than 2 mm

## Foot Fractures

Most metatarsal fractures are due to a direct blow. Fractures at the base of the 5th metatarsal require special attention.

- The apophysis at the 5th metatarsal base appears on radiographs as a line parallel to the shaft of the bone. A lucency perpendicular to this is consistent with a fracture
- Avulsion of the apophysis at the base of the 5th metatarsal occurs with inversion of the foot and ankle with tension from the lateral cord of the plantar aponeurosis pulling on the apophysis
- Jones' fracture is injury at the junction of the metaphysis and diaphysis, distal to the apophysis. It occurs in adolescents, and is often seen as an acute on chronic injury

*Diagnostic Workup:*

- Plain radiographs: AP, lateral, oblique
- Obtain weight-bearing views if tolerated

*Management:*

- Most non-displaced metatarsal fractures are treated with short-leg walking cast
- Immobilization is preferred for avulsion at the base of the 5th metatarsal
- Nonoperative care can be considered with acute Jones' fracture and consists of non-weight bearing cast for 6–8 weeks. There is a relatively high nonunion rate, and some patients will require internal fixation with a screw

## SIGNIFICANT ORTHOPEDIC ISSUES

### COMPARTMENT SYNDROME

Compartment syndrome occurs when increased pressure within an osseofascial compartment leads to impaired blood flow with ischemia of muscle and nerve tissue.

- Most often seen in the lower leg or the forearm
- May result from trauma and hemorrhage, or postsurgically. Especially likely in the setting of a crush injury
- 75% of cases are associated with a fracture
- Pain apparently out of proportion to injury, or pains with passive stretching are hallmarks that warrant further evaluation
- Late findings include diminished pulse and pallor

*Diagnostic Workup:*

- For proper assessment (visualization, palpation, ROM) removal of cast or splint is necessary
- Clinical concern can be corroborated with compartment pressure measurement

*Management:*

- If suspected, immediate surgical consultation is advised
- Remove any restrictive dressings including cast material
- Keep affected limb at the level of the heart. Do not elevate the limb as this can decrease arterial blood flow
- Fasciotomy is the definitive intervention

### SLIPPED CAPITAL FEMORAL EPIPHYSIS (SCFE)

SCFE is a disorder in which the femoral neck slides up and outward along the femoral physis, consistent with an SH-I injury. The femoral head remains in place within the acetabulum.

- Typically seen from late childhood (9–10 years) through middle adolescence (15–16 years)
- More likely in obese youth
- May be acute (symptoms <3 weeks), chronic, or a combination thereof
- Symptoms: Unilateral hip, groin, thigh or knee pain. Patients with chronic picture have more vague pain and often limp
- Up to 60% can be bilateral
- It is stable if the patient can ambulate, either with or without crutches
- Exam reveals limited internal rotation, abduction, and flexion, with pain upon hip ROM. The affected limb may be held in external rotation, and may appear slightly shortened

*Diagnostic Workup:*

- Plain radiographs: AP and frog-leg lateral (hips flexed and abducted) views of the pelvis with assessment of both hips
- A line (Klein's line) drawn along superior aspect of the femoral neck should intersect the lateral capital epiphysis. As the femoral neck slips up and outward, the line will intersect progressively less of the epiphysis, until it no longer contacts it at all. This is the radiographic finding in SCFE (Figure 23-4)

*Management:*

- Upon diagnosis, contact Orthopedic Surgery

- Make patient non-weight bearing with either crutches, or a wheelchair for bilateral involvement. Transfer to Emergency Department, and/or hospital admission is warranted
- Definitive treatment for non-displaced lesions is in situ fixation using a pin or screw. Surgical intervention for the unaffected hip, whether symptomatic or not, may be considered, but remains controversial

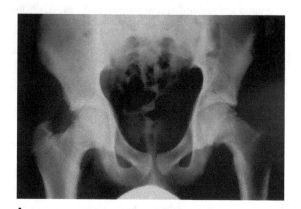

A

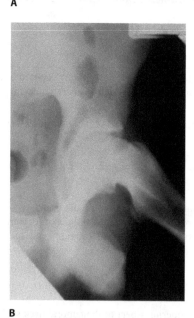

B

FIGURE 23-4 **Left slipped capital femoral epiphysis on plain radiographs (AP and frog-leg lateral).** Klein's line in image A fails to intersect the femoral head on the affected side. (Reproduced with permission from Skinner HB & McMahon PJ (Eds). *Current Diagnosis & Treatment In Orthopedics*, 5th ed. New York, NY: McGraw-Hill; 2014.)

## TRANSIENT SYNOVITIS VERSUS SEPTIC ARTHRITIS

This remains a potential diagnostic dilemma. Both are primarily seen in the hip with unilateral pain at hip, groin, thigh, or knee, often with a limp. The affected limb may be held with hip flexed and abducted.

- Transient synovitis is the most common cause of hip pain and usually affects children 3–8 years old. It is often associated with recent or current illness. Children are nontoxic appearing, and are able to bear weight on the effected limb
- The child with septic arthritis may appear more ill, and have higher fever. (**See Infectious Diseases chapter for management of septic arthritis**)

*Diagnostic Workup:*

- History and physical, along with complete blood count (CBC) for white blood count (WBC), and erythrocyte sedimentation rate (ESR)
- The four primary criteria to consider are: Fever, inability to ambulate, WBC count >12,000/mm$^3$, and ESR of 40 mm/h or higher
- If all four criteria are met, there is up to a 99% chance that the patient has septic arthritis. The likelihood decreases to 93% if three of four criteria are positive, 40% if two of four are positive, and down to <5% if only one of four present (Kocher criteria)
- Joint aspiration is indicated if two or more criteria are met
- An aspirate is considered indicative of bacterial infection if the fluid has >50,000 WBCs/mm$^3$ or if bacteria are present on Gram stain

*Management:*

- Most transient synovitis will resolve spontaneously within 2 weeks. Weight bearing is limited for comfort, and nonsteroidal anti-inflammatory drugs (NSAIDs) are used as needed
- Despite its efficacy for pain relief, joint aspiration is reserved for diagnostic purposes as fluid often rapidly reaccumulates
- The septic joint must be explored surgically, and is a relative emergency

# Otolaryngology 24

*Pamela Mudd, MD*
*John Germiller, MD, PhD*

## ADENOTONSILLAR HYPERTROPHY

**Enlargement of palatine tonsils and adenoid lymphoid tissue that contributes to obstruction of the upper airway**

• Results in sleep disordered breathing defined as an abnormal respiratory pattern during sleep including snoring, mouth breathing, and pauses in breathing which may be symptoms of obstructive sleep apnea (OSA)

### EPIDEMIOLOGY

• Volume of lymphoid tissue increases from 6 months of age to puberty; peak of OSA in preschool years, when tissue makes up greatest proportion of upper airway
• Associated craniofacial and neuromuscular disorders and obesity increase likelihood of symptomatic adenotonsillar hypertrophy

### PATHOPHYSIOLOGY

• The underlying etiology of adenotonsillar hypertrophy is unknown
• Upper airway obstruction is multifactorial; includes hypertrophied lymphoid tissue, compliance and elasticity of pharyngeal soft tissue, facial morphology, and changes to the pharyngeal musculature during sleep
• Cyclic airway obstruction during sleep causes hypoxia and hypercapnia, leading to arousals to restore respiration
• Repeated arousals interrupt rapid eye movement sleep, which can lead to daytime somnolence

### CLINICAL MANIFESTATIONS

• *Nighttime:* Snoring, apnea, restless sleep, enuresis, nightmares
• *Daytime:* Somnolence, behavioral changes, learning difficulties, nasal obstruction, mouth breathing, hyponasal speech; in severe cases, dysphagia, failure to thrive
• *Degree of tonsillar enlargement:* Tonsil within fossa = 0; less than 25% obstruction = 1+; less than 50% obstruction = 2+; less than 75% obstruction = 3+; greater than 75% obstruction = 4+ (Brodsky grading scale) (Figure 24-1)

### DIAGNOSTICS

• Overnight polysomnography is definitive test for OSA
• Lateral neck radiograph versus flexible nasopharyngolaryngoscopy (NPL) to assess adenoid size and airway caliber; however, volume of tonsils and adenoids do not always correlate well with severity of OSA
• ECG and/or echocardiogram in severe, longstanding OSA to rule out cor pulmonale—Right heart strain, right ventricular hypertrophy

454

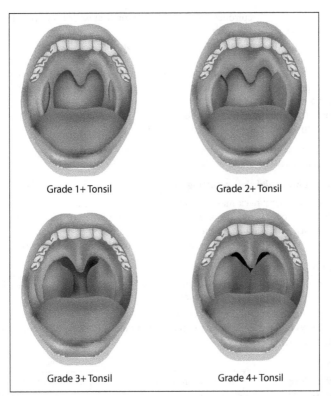

Grade 1+ Tonsil

Grade 2+ Tonsil

Grade 3+ Tonsil

Grade 4+ Tonsil

FIGURE 24-1 **Assessing the degree of tonsillar enlargement using the Brodsky grading scale.** (Reproduced with permission from Brodsky L: Modern assessment of tonsils and adenoids, *Pediatr Clin North Am.* 1989 Dec;36(6):1551–1569.)

## MANAGEMENT

### Medical

- Nasal corticosteroids decrease nasal turbinate and adenoid hypertrophy, and may decrease severity of OSA, improve snoring, and improve nighttime symptoms such an enuresis, though long-term effectiveness unclear. Dosage—1 spray each nostril daily (if under 2 years give every other day)
- Noninvasive positive pressure ventilation (e.g., continuous positive airway pressure)
- Weight loss for obese patients

### Surgical

- Indications for adenotonsillectomy
  ✓ Sleep disordered breathing leading to daytime and nighttime symptoms, and all children with documented OSA
  ✓ Nasal obstruction causing discomfort in breathing and distortion of speech, or recurrent otitis media (adenoidectomy only)
  ✓ Dysphagia or speech disturbance (dysarthria or hypernasality) due to large tonsils (tonsillectomy only)

✓ *Chronic tonsillitis:* 7 episodes in the past year or 5 episodes per year for 2 years or 3 episodes per year for 3 years

✓ Prior complications of tonsillitis (peritonsillar abscess, post-streptococcal glomerulonephritis)

- Risks of surgery include postoperative hemorrhage (0.1–3%), airway obstruction due to edema, prolonged pain and dehydration, anesthesia risks, speech change, and post-obstructive pulmonary edema
- Tracheostomy (temporary or permanent) may be needed in severe, refractory OSA or for children with complex medical/anatomic conditions

## BRANCHIAL CLEFT ANOMALIES

**Persistence of branchial cleft resulting in cysts, sinuses, or fistulae of the lateral neck**

- *Cyst:* Persistent lateral neck mass; usually painless unless it is infected
- *Sinus:* External opening to neck along the anterior border of the sternocleidomastoid muscle (SCM), extending along the tract. May intermittently drain fluid
- *Fistula:* Opening both externally in neck and internally in tonsillar fossa or hypopharynx

### EPIDEMIOLOGY

- Branchial cleft anomalies are present from birth, but are often not recognized until acute infection, usually in the first decade of life
- 90% arise from the second branchial cleft
- Almost always unilateral. Bilateral branchial anomalies may suggest an underlying genetic syndrome (branchio-oto-renal)

### ETIOLOGY

- Anomalies develop from ectodermal remnants in the tract of the second branchial cleft, which arises from the anterior-superior border of the SCM, passes between the internal and external carotids and over the 10th and 12th cranial nerves to end at the tonsillar fossa
  ✓ Third branchial cleft remnants are less common and have a slightly different course, terminating in the hypopharynx. Fourth cleft anomalies are very rare and are almost exclusively on the left side; they also terminate in the hypopharynx

### DIFFERENTIAL DIAGNOSIS

- Differential diagnosis of neck masses is affected by location (Figure 24-2)
- *Congenital:* Hemangioma, cystic hygroma, thyroglossal duct cyst, SCM pseudotumor of infancy (fibromatosis colli), remnant of branchial arch cartilage, enlarged or ectopic thyroid, epidermoid cyst (usually lateral), neurofibroma (usually lateral), lipoma
- *Following trauma:* Hematoma, subcutaneous emphysema
- *Infectious:* Reactive adenopathy, adenitis (see Infectious Diseases chapter [Chapter 15]), Kawasaki, infectious mononucleosis syndrome, toxoplasmosis, sarcoid
- *Malignant:* Leukemia, lymphoma, neuroblastoma, Langerhans cell histiocytosis, others

### CLINICAL MANIFESTATIONS

- Cystic neck mass or opening anterior to mid-portion of SCM
- May have tenderness, redness, swelling, purulent drainage if infected
- Internal opening of fistula may be visible near tonsillar fossa
- Third and fourth branchial anomalies may present with unilateral acute thyroiditis
- *Pertinent negative:* Branchial cysts are never midline. A midline mass that moves upward with tongue protrusion or swallowing suggests a thyroglossal duct cyst

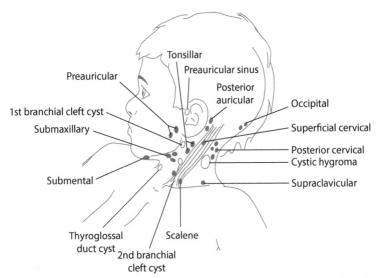

**FIGURE 24-2 Typical locations of cystic and solid neck masses.** Key: o = Cysts/sinuses; ● = lymph nodes.

## DIAGNOSTICS

- CT or MRI (preferred) usually delineates the mass and any associated tract
- Ultrasound can establish cystic versus solid masses
- Rarely, instillation of radiopaque material is needed to demonstrate the extent of the fistula or sinus

## MANAGEMENT

- Acute infection/abscess is treated with systemic antibiotics (e.g., ampicillin-sulbactam, amoxicillin-clavulanate, or clindamycin) and, if needed, incision and drainage
- Complete surgical excision is the definitive treatment, but is usually deferred until after resolution of acute inflammation

## CLEFT LIP/PALATE

### CLEFT LIP

- Complete = Extends into floor of the nose
- Incomplete = Extends part way through the lip

### CLEFT PALATE

- Always involves uvula
- Unilateral or bilateral
- Severity depends on degree of soft and hard palate involvement

### EPIDEMIOLOGY

- One in 1000 white births; 1:400 Japanese births; 1:3000 African births
- *Cleft lip*: 80% unilateral, 20% bilateral; 75% have associated cleft palate

- Facial clefting associated with approximately 300 syndromes including van der Woude, Stickler, and associated Pierre Robin sequence
- Both genetic and environmental factors have been implicated

## PATHOPHYSIOLOGY

- *Embryology:* Palatogenesis occurs between 5th and 12th week of gestation
- Clefting results from incomplete closure of upper lip, with or without incomplete closure of the two halves of the hard palate, and the overlying soft palate
- Feeding difficulties are due to inability to create adequate negative oral pressure with sucking
- Poor Eustachian tube function results from the incomplete sling of palatal musculature. Results in middle ear effusion and conductive hearing loss. Most children with cleft palate require pressure equalization tubes
- Speech problems found in most cleft palate patients mostly due to velopharyngeal insufficiency (VPI) with air escape from nose (hypernasal speech) with associated articulation errors
- Other congenital abnormalities common

## MANAGEMENT

- *Multidisciplinary approach:* Surgeon, dentist, speech pathologist, audiologist, geneticist, social worker, nurse, nutritionist, psychologist

### Feeding

- Breast-feeding is possible with cleft lip and palate
- Bottle feeding with special nipples such as Habermann feeder or Mead-Johnson cleft bottle
- Frequent burping required due to increased air swallowing
- Nasogastric feeding or gastrostomy tube may be required, more likely with associated syndromes

### Surgical

- Cleft lip repair around 10 weeks of age (*rule of 10s*—10 weeks, 10 lbs, 10 g/dL hemoglobin)
- Lip adhesion may be performed as initial procedure to facilitate later definitive closure
- Presurgical nasoalveolar molding (NAM) is an orodental appliance which can aid in closure of cleft lip and palate and improve nasal symmetry
- *Cleft palate repair:* Goals include separation of nasal from oral cavity, a competent velopharyngeal valve, elongation of the palate, and restoration of palate musculature. All are aimed at yielding improved speech quality. Eustachian tube function also eventually improves
- Cleft palate repair typically completed by 9–18 months of age

## EPISTAXIS

## PATHOPHYSIOLOGY

- Anterior septum (Little's area) is most common site due to vascularity (Kiesselbach's plexus) and exposure (dry air, trauma)
- Epistaxis from trauma (digital or impact), inflammation, dryness, or less often tumor, vascular abnormality, or coagulopathy

## CLINICAL MANIFESTATIONS

- Active bleeding or dry blood +/− identifiable source
- *Mucosa:* Dry, cracked, pale, boggy, prominent vessels

- *Localize active bleeding:* Anterior, posterior, unilateral, or bilateral. Unilateral epistaxis without obvious source on anterior septum raises suspicion for discrete masses or vascular lesions further posteriorly in nose
- Check for masses, polyps, foreign bodies
- *Signs of underlying bleeding disorder:* Petechiae, ecchymosis
- *Hypertension:* Very rarely a factor in children
- *History:* Bruising, bleeding, or family history of same; use of anticoagulants or platelet inhibitors. Long-term use of nasal steroids can increase risk of epistaxis

## DIAGNOSTICS

- *None routinely required but clinical situation may warrant the following:*
  ✓ Hematologic/coagulation studies, and/or hematology consultation. Use if no typical, focal bleeding source is identified, or if additional bleeding sites besides epistaxis, or family history of coagulopathy. Initial studies should include prothrombin and partial thromboplastin times and platelet count
  ✓ Sinus CT or MRI if neoplasm suspected
  ✓ Arteriography or MR angiography if vascular anomaly suspected or embolization is considered

## MANAGEMENT

### Medical

- Hold external direct pressure on soft tissue of nostrils for 5–15 minutes
- Oxymetazoline (0.05%; Afrin) spray to affected nostril for local vasoconstriction (up to twice daily for maximum 3 days)
- Anterior nasal packing with absorbable hemostatic agents including Surgicel, Merogel, or Gelfoam, or with ointment-coated sponges which require removal after 72 hours
- Posterior packing (gauze, nasal tampons/balloons) rarely needed except for severe trauma or tumor bleeding
- Antibiotics (e.g., cephalexin, clindamycin, amoxicillin-clavulanate) while packing in place due to risk of toxic shock syndrome and sinusitis
- Treat underlying process (e.g., allergic rhinitis, bleeding diathesis)
- ENT consult for severe epistaxis, suspicion of occult nasal lesion, or underlying hemorrhagic diathesis
- *For chronic recurrent epistaxis from identified source:* Petrolatum ointment nightly and humidifier use during dry air seasons; moisten/lubricate with saline spray and gel, keep petrolatum quantity small and avoid long-term use of antibiotic ointments

### Surgical

- Chemical cautery (e.g., silver nitrate) of bleeding site. Moderately high rate of recurrence
- Electrocautery of bleeding site (avoiding excessive cautery of both sides of nasal septum due to risk of septal ischemia and perforation). Lower recurrence rate than chemical cautery but requires general anesthesia
- Limited septoplasty. The mucoperichondrium is simply elevated off the septal cartilage and allowed to heal back into place; the surgical trauma induces enough scarring to reduce the rate of epistaxis
- Embolization, laser excision, or arterial ligation in severe cases (e.g., tumor, vascular malformation)

## FOREIGN BODY ASPIRATION/INGESTION

### EPIDEMIOLOGY

- Highest incidence 1–3 years of age
- Twice as common in boys
- *Most common foreign body (FB):* Food matter/nuts (aspiration), coins (ingestion)

### ETIOLOGY

- Toddlers have less control of swallowing and immature chewing ability, laryngeal elevation, and glottic closure. Cannot grind foods until molars develop, and dentition ability continues to mature throughout childhood
- Mental retardation, autism, and neurologic or seizure disorders increase risk

### CLINICAL MANIFESTATIONS

- History of FB in mouth or close to child or unobserved period before appearance of symptoms
- May be asymptomatic for weeks or months before presentation
- *Airway foreign body:* Wheezing, unexplained coughing spells, significant respiratory distress, pneumonia, decreased breath sounds in obstructed lobe/lung
  - ✓ *Upper airway symptoms:* Hoarseness, aphonia, stridor, inspiratory wheeze
  - ✓ *Lower airway symptoms:* Expiratory wheeze, asymmetric aeration of lung fields
  - ✓ Unilateral wheezing or migrating wheeze on physical examination is highly suspicious for FB as opposed to reactive airway disease
- *Ingested foreign body:* Drooling, throat pain, dysphagia, odynophagia, localizable anterior neck pain, less commonly respiratory distress due to compression of the airway from esophageal FB
- *Food impaction:* Raises suspicion for chronic esophagitis, notably eosinophilic esophagitis, especially if repeat episodes
- *Disc battery ingestion:* Full-thickness esophageal wall injury, due to electrical discharge and caustic chemical leakage, begins within minutes and rapidly progresses; can result in permanent stricture, perforation

### DIAGNOSTICS

- Posteroanterior and lateral chest and neck films together are used to localize radiopaque objects in airway or esophagus
- Chest CT if erosion or extraluminal extension suspected
- *Aspiration:* Acutely, failure of affected lobe to deflate may be seen on inspiratory/expiratory (hyperinflation on expiratory film) or lateral decubitus (air trapping in dependent lung) chest x-ray. Subacutely or chronically, the chest x-ray may show resorptive post-obstructive atelectasis, compensatory emphysema of nonobstructed lobes, pneumonia, pneumothorax, shift of mediastinum during expiration, or abscess
- *Ingestion:* Most common objects such as coins are often radiopaque, esophageal air may delineate tissue-density FB on plain film. Barium swallow may identify radiolucent esophageal FB. Must rule out presence of disc battery (halo sign on AP view and step off on lateral view) as true emergency and delay in removal can be fatal
- *Repeated episodes:* Consider evaluation of swallowing function (presence of gag reflex, observed feedings, modified barium swallow with speech therapy), or esophageal anatomy (upper endoscopy, biopsy to rule out eosinophilic esophagitis, barium swallow)

## MANAGEMENT

- *Complete airway obstruction is an absolute emergency. Perform the Heimlich maneuver on children older than 1 year of age, and back blows/chest thrusts on children younger than 1 year of age*
- *Disc battery/Button battery ingestion is an emergency requiring emergent operative endoscopy. Do not delay diagnosis or treatment*
- Endoscopy can be both diagnostic and therapeutic. General anesthesia is required
- *Rigid bronchoscope:* Allows visualization of the trachea and bronchi, with removal of the FB through the scope. Ventilation occurs through the scope
- *Rigid esophagoscopy:* Allows visualization of the entire esophagus with removal of the FB through the scope
- FBs that cannot be removed endoscopically may require thoracotomy for direct removal

## HEARING LOSS

**Decreased hearing may be present at birth (congenital), or may begin later in childhood. Hearing loss can be stable or progressive.**

**May be sensorineural (inner ear, nerve, or central source) or conductive (mechanical sound conduction, from outer or middle ear disease).**

- *Most commonly picked up at newborn hearing screen, school, or well visit screening tests, or by caregiver concern for hearing or speech delay*

### EPIDEMIOLOGY

- Prevalence of congenital or childhood hearing loss is 1–2 per 1000

### ETIOLOGY

- *Genetic:* 50% congenital loss is genetic. 1/3 of these associated with syndrome
  - ✓ *Recessive:* Usher (vestibular dysfunction, retinitis pigmentosa), Pendred (thyroid goiter, cochlear dysplasia), Jervell and Lange-Nielsen (prolonged QT, sudden death)
  - ✓ *Dominant:* Waardenburg (heterochromia, white forelock), branchio-oto-renal (auricular deformity, preauricular pits or tags, branchial cleft anomalies [commonly bilateral], and renal anomalies), Stickler (retinal detachment, cleft palate, arthritis), Treacher Collins (midface hypoplasia, down sloping eyes, conductive hearing loss), neurofibromatosis
  - ✓ *Other syndromes:* Fetal alcohol, Down's syndrome, Goldenhar
  - ✓ 2/3 of congenital hearing loss is non-syndromic [that is, no other anomalies]
  - ✓ Connexin 26 (GJB2) gap-junction protein mutation—Most common cause of non-syndromic genetic hearing loss in North America
- Nongenetic
  - ✓ In utero exposure to cytomegalovirus (CMV) most common cause, often otherwise asymptomatic and mother may experience minimal or no symptoms—May account for 1/3 of congenital hearing loss
  - ✓ Bacterial meningitis, fetal alcohol, congenital rubella, trauma (e.g., temporal bone fracture)
- Other
  - ✓ Cerumen impaction, acute infection, and persistent middle ear fluid (otitis media with effusion) can lead to conductive hearing loss, which is treatable or self-resolving. Other disease such as ear drum retraction, formation of middle ear mass or cholesteatoma can also lead to hearing loss

## DIFFERENTIAL DIAGNOSIS

- Congenital (present since birth)—May be stable or progressive thereafter
- External ear causes—Cerumen impaction, foreign body, outer ear infection
- Middle ear causes—Acute otitis media (AOM), middle ear effusion (OME), cholesteatoma (skin cyst, which can be either congenital or more commonly acquired from repeated infections or retraction) or other middle ear mass, scarring from infection, sclerosis or abnormal formation of the ossicles, trauma
- Inner ear causes—Congenital or progressive sensorineural hearing loss, malformed cochlea or cochlear nerve (cochlear hypoplasia), enlarged vestibular aqueduct, rare mass lesions

## CLINICAL MANIFESTATIONS

- Failed screening testing, speech delay, poor school performance, social isolation

## DIAGNOSTICS

- Otoscopy—May reveal external or middle ear causes
- Audiogram—"Gold standard"—can distinguish sensorineural and conductive hearing loss. May be followed over time and with intervention. Different testing available depending on age, cooperation
- Otoacoustic emissions (OAE)—Show inner ear hair cell function. May be used as a screening test, does not require patient participation. Simple, noninvasive. However, not definitive; will miss auditory nerve dysfunction or central hearing loss (auditory neuropathy spectrum)
- Tympanogram—Assess movement of ear drum and pressure of middle ear—can determine if there is fluid in middle ear or a perforation
- Auditory brainstem response (ABR)—Objective testing on the inner ear and brainstem to assess hearing ability. For children unable to perform standard audiogram; often requires sedation after 6 months of age. Used in many centers for newborn screening
- CT or MRI to assess for middle or inner ear abnormalities in some cases
- Medical workup for suspected genetic causes may include genetic testing (connexin 26/30 most common), CMV testing in neonates, ECG for bilateral deaf patients (detects long QT abnormalities such as Jervell and Lange-Nielsen syndrome), eye exam

## MANAGEMENT

### Medical

- Cerumen or foreign body removal, treatment of external or middle ear disease
- Hearing aids standard for permanent hearing loss
- FM systems, preferential classroom seating, early intervention services for all children with hearing loss

### Surgical

- Ventilating ear tubes for repeated infections or persistent ear fluid (>3 months duration, associated with hearing loss or in high-risk populations), Eustachian tube dysfunction with retraction
- Surgery may be required for cholesteatoma, retraction, ear drum perforation, middle ear mass, or other causes
- Cochlear implantation for those with bilateral profound hearing loss who do not benefit from hearing aids

## INFECTED PREAURICULAR CYST OR SINUS

**Preauricular sinuses or pits, located near the front of the ear, mark the entrance to a sinus tract that travels under the skin near the ear cartilage. These tracts may sequester to produce epithelial-lined subcutaneous cysts or may become infected.**

### EPIDEMIOLOGY

- Congenital anomalies that may be sporadic or inherited (autosomal dominant with variable penetrance)
  ✓ Inherited cases are more likely bilateral
- 3–5% occur in association with other syndromes, including deafness and branchio-oto-renal syndrome

### PATHOPHYSIOLOGY

- Infection occurs when the opening of the sinus is occluded with bacteria and desquamated skin
- *S. aureus* is most commonly isolated; other pathogens include viridans group streptococci, *Peptostreptococcus* spp, and *Proteus* spp

### CLINICAL MANIFESTATIONS

- Sinus appears as a pinpoint hole anterior to ear, usually just above tragus
- Cyst appears as a preauricular mass, often adjacent to an associated sinus
- Signs of infection include
  ✓ Preauricular erythema, swelling, and tenderness
  ✓ Purulent drainage or preauricular granulation tissue may be present
- Superinfected cyst may manifest as a tender, enlarging preauricular mass

### DIAGNOSTICS

- Clinical diagnosis from symptoms and physical exam
- Imaging rarely needed
- Consider hearing screen and renal ultrasound if dysmorphic features or other congenital abnormalities are also present

### MANAGEMENT

- Oral antibiotics (e.g., amoxicillin-clavulanate, clindamycin) for uncomplicated cases, IV antibiotics if recalcitrant cases or associated with facial cellulitis or high fever
- May require needle aspiration (21-gauge needle); incision and drainage should be avoided if possible as inflammation may impair wound healing and increases recurrence risk
- Definitive management is excision of the preauricular sinus and tract once acute infection resolved
  ✓ Recurrence after surgical excision varies by center; typically 5–15%
  ✓ Factors associated with recurrence include
    ▪ Excision performed during active infection or inflammation
    ▪ Excision under local anesthesia
    ▪ Poor delineation of sinus tract during surgery

## LARYNGOMALACIA

**Congenital flaccid larynx**

## EPIDEMIOLOGY

- Most common laryngeal anomaly in infants
- Accounts for 65–75% of infant stridor

## ETIOLOGY

- Exact etiology unknown. Theories include hypotonia or dyscoordination of laryngeal or supralaryngeal structures
- Gastroesophageal reflux may be contributing factor

## PATHOPHYSIOLOGY

- Prolapse of loose laryngeal tissues into airway on inspiration. Causes inspiratory airway noise/obstruction
- Prolapse is caused by excess compliance of the laryngeal cartilages with an omega-shaped epiglottis, short aryepiglottic folds, and possible excess mucosa over the arytenoids
- Laryngomalacia can be secondary to other airway lesions, from increased work of breathing and negative airway pressures. Examples include cysts of the tongue base or vallecula, glottic or subglottic stenosis, tracheomalacia (collapse of trachea on inspiration)
- With normal growth, symptoms typically worsen initially, then gradually resolve between 6 and 18 months of age

## CLINICAL MANIFESTATIONS

- Onset of "noisy breathing" or inspiratory stridor within the first few weeks of life, which worsens with agitation and/or supine positioning
- Inspiratory stridor that is typically positional, louder when supine or during sleep; also with agitation or exertion (e.g., feeding, crying, laughing)
- Cry/phonation is typically normal (expiratory process)
- *Evidence of increased work of breathing:* Nasal flaring, retractions, pectus excavatum
- Strong association with gastroesophageal reflux

## DIAGNOSTICS

- *Flexible NPL:* Confirms diagnosis and assesses extent of prolapse/obstruction. Allows detection of secondary airway lesions above the vocal cords. Noninvasive, is done in office or at bedside, without sedation
- Airway fluoroscopy may reveal laryngomalacia, but much less useful than flexible endoscopy
- For severe cases, rigid laryngoscopy and bronchoscopy under general anesthesia may be warranted
- Evaluation for additional congenital tracheobronchial anomalies is important in severe or unusual cases. Airway fluoroscopy is useful here, to detect coincident tracheomalacia. Diagnosis of other secondary lesions requires rigid bronchoscopy under anesthesia

## MANAGEMENT

### Medical

- Depends on severity of symptoms
  - ✓ *Mild:* No feeding problems; symptoms not progressive
  - ✓ *Moderate:* Feeding difficulties but thriving; progressive stridor
  - ✓ *Severe:* Apnea, cyanosis, failure to thrive
- *Mild/Moderate:* Conservative management with reassurance to family that condition is self-limited, complete resolution may take up to 18 months. Consider proton pump

inhibitor and change in formula. CPR education for caretakers. Home pulse-oximetry monitoring may be indicated
- *Severe:* Surgery may be necessary
- Treatment of gastroesophageal reflux often helps, regardless of severity

## Surgical

- *Supraglottoplasty:* Excision of the obstructive aryepiglottic folds and/or redundant supraglottic tissues
- Rigid laryngoscopy and bronchoscopy is done at time or surgical intervention to detect any secondary lesions
- *Tracheotomy:* Rarely indicated, in most severe cases

## TRACHEOSTOMY

**Tracheostomy: The actual hole in the trachea following tracheotomy**
**Tracheotomy: The surgical incision in the trachea used to gain access to the airway**
**Indications for Tracheostomy**

- Ventilator dependency (40%)
- Extrathoracic obstruction (30%)
- Neurologic dysfunction (20%)
- Intrathoracic obstruction (10%)

### TRACHEOSTOMY VERSUS PROLONGED ENDOTRACHEAL INTUBATION

- Risks of prolonged intubation include injury to glottis, subglottis, and trachea due to pressure of tube
- Endotracheal tube irritation can be minimized by avoiding cuffed tubes and use of nasotracheal placement to minimize tube movements
- Endotracheal tubes can easily become blocked due to small lumen of pediatric tubes
- Typical recommendation is for tracheostomy after 2–4 weeks of intubation in child, longer in neonates
- *Advantages of tracheostomy:* Hospital discharge on ventilator support, avoid damage to larynx and subglottis, easier replacement if decannulated, ease of suctioning and pulmonary toilet, improved ability to wean ventilator and associated sedation
- *Disadvantages of tracheostomy:* Need for frequent cleaning, suctioning, and humidification; surgical risks; risk of general anesthesia; increased requirements for home care

### COMPLICATIONS OF TRACHEOSTOMY

- *Intraoperative complications:* Hemorrhage, subcutaneous emphysema, pneumomediastinum, pneumothorax
- *Early postoperative complications:* Tracheostomy tube plugging, decannulation, tracheitis
- *Late complications:* Tracheoesophageal fistula, tracheal granulomas, suprastomal collapse. Rarely, tube can erode anterior tracheal wall, which may lead to tracheo-innominate fistula with life-threatening hemorrhage

### TRACHEOSTOMY CARE

- Tracheostomy tube size reflects the inner diameter in millimeters. Outer diameter is variable and depends on manufacturer and/or material
- Cuffless tubes preferred in young children to minimize pressure on tracheal wall. Cuffless tubes also allow inner diameter to be maximized in these small airways, which maximizes ventilation and minimizes risk of occlusion

• Humidified air is supplied to prevent drying of tracheal mucosa
• Trained caregiver, suctioning equipment, and replacement tube should always be available to maintain airway patency

## CHANGING TRACHEOSTOMY TUBES

• Surgeons typically make first change and survey stoma for patency within 1 week of surgery
• Subsequent changes can be made by other caregivers
• All tracheostomy changes best made with neck extended, with good lighting and suction available

## VOCAL CORD PARALYSIS

**Unilateral or bilateral paralysis of the vocal folds**

### EPIDEMIOLOGY

• Accounts for 15–20% of cases of stridor in infants
• Rarely an isolated lesion in children
• Unilateral vocal cord paralysis (VCP) is more common on left

### ETIOLOGY

• Bilateral VCP can be idiopathic, or caused by central nervous system immaturity, various lesions, the Arnold–Chiari malformation, hydrocephalus, or birth trauma
• Unilateral paralysis can be caused by birth trauma, or by previous intervention—Most commonly cardiothoracic surgery (left recurrent laryngeal nerve recurs around aortic arch and ductus arteriosus)

### PATHOPHYSIOLOGY

• Abductors and adductors of vocal cords are controlled by the recurrent laryngeal nerve, a branch of the vagus nerve, which can be damaged anywhere along the path from the brainstem to the larynx
• Unilateral VCP is more commonly due to peripheral nerve injury
• Bilateral VCP is more likely due to CNS cause
• Traumatic or prolonged intubation can directly injure or scar glottic tissues and joints. Vocal cord motion is mechanically restricted, though nerve/muscle function is normal

### CLINICAL MANIFESTATIONS

• *Unilateral VCP*: Weak vocal cord tends to retract away from the midline and glottis fails to close during swallowing and phonation. Result is weak cry, breathy voice, aspiration, and/or feeding difficulties, ineffective cough, recurrent pneumonia, hoarseness
• *Bilateral VCP*: Bilaterally paralyzed vocal cords are often fixed in the midline closed position, causing stridor, and respiratory distress; may have normal cry. Alternatively, weak vocal cords may fall away from the midline and result in aspiration, hoarseness, and/or feeding difficulties, as for unilateral VCP
• *Evaluate severity of respiratory impairment*: Work of breathing, respiratory rate, oxygen saturation
• Search for associated congenital anomalies, surgical history, hydrocephalus, or predisposing trauma

## DIAGNOSTICS

- *Flexible laryngoscopy:* Cornerstone of diagnosis; can usually be done at bedside; sedation is best avoided to allow full assessment of function
- MRI and/or CT in idiopathic cases, to evaluate CNS and course of vagus nerve
- Barium swallow, $+/-$ milk scan, to assess swallowing function and risk of dysphagia or aspiration

## MANAGEMENT

### Three Goals of Management

1. *Safe airway*
   - ✓ *Tracheostomy:* Necessary for 20–50% of bilateral VCP; rarely necessary for unilateral VCP
   - ✓ Spontaneous resolution is common, so period of observation (months in duration) is essential
   - ✓ Surgical management including posterior cricoid graft, lateralization of VC, or cordotomy may be needed for unresolved bilateral VCP
2. *Intelligible speech*
   For unilateral VCP, observation for several months is indicated, to allow for spontaneous nerve regeneration. Also, young children often have gradual voice improvement, due to overcompensation by the opposite VC
   - ✓ Surgical medialization of the paralyzed VC, or nerve reimplantation, may be needed for persistent aspiration or poor vocal quality
3. *Prevention of aspiration*
   - ✓ May require alternate consistency of feedings
   - ✓ May require G-tube temporarily

# Procedures

*Mercedes M. Blackstone, MD*
*Jeannine Del Pizzo, MD*
*Sarah Fesnak, MD*

## BAG VALVE MASK VENTILATION

### INDICATIONS

• Apnea, respiratory depression, hypoxia, cardiac, respiratory or neurologic failure

### EQUIPMENT

• *Appropriate mask size:* An appropriate mask completely covers the patient's nose and mouth without mask edges hanging off the face or covering eyes
• *Bag:* Self-inflating or anesthesia (flow-inflating) bag

### TECHNIQUE

• Position patient's head by either chin lift (stable cervical spine) or jaw thrust (unstable cervical spine) to maximize upper airway diameter
• Place mask over patient's mouth and nose and hold tight against face using C-E hold (see Figure 25-1). The thumb and 2nd finger form a "C" shape over the mask while the 3rd, 4th, and 5th fingers of the same hand form an "E" over the mandible, effectively pulling the patient's jaw up to meet the mask. Be careful not to compress the soft tissues below the mandible
• Squeeze bag to push air into patient's lungs
  ✓ *Self-inflating bag:* Simple to use, pop-off valve limits amount of pressure delivered, no air reaches patient unless bag is squeezed, delivers room air unless attached to an oxygen reservoir
  ✓ *Anesthesia bag:* Requires experienced operator, requires oxygen reservoir, can deliver blow-by oxygen, continuous positive-airway pressure (CPAP), or assisted breaths
• *Goal rate of delivered breaths:* 8–10 breaths per minute
  ✓ *Unsecure airway during one-person CPR:* 2 breaths for every 30 compressions
  ✓ *Unsecure airway during two-person CPR:* 2 breaths for every 15 compressions
  ✓ *Secure airway during CPR:* 8–10 breaths per minute
• Chest wall rise indicates adequate delivery
• Listen for air leak around mask as each breath is delivered. If an air leak is heard, it can be due to hand position, wrong mask size, or fatigue. Try the following—reposition C-E hold, use two hands for C-E hold with a second provider squeezing the bag, or switch providers

## AIRWAY ADJUNCTS: NASOPHARYNGEAL AIRWAY AND ORAL AIRWAY

### NASOPHARYNGEAL (NP) AIRWAY

### INDICATIONS

• Upper airway obstruction in a patient with spontaneous respirations
• Used to stent tongue away from posterior pharynx

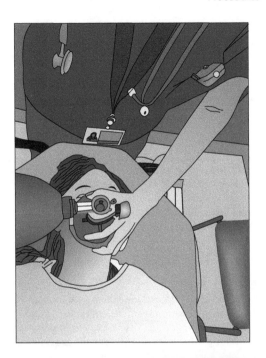

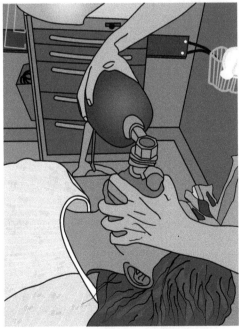

FIGURE 25-1 **A and B: C-E hold for bag valve mask ventilation.**

- Can be used in conscious patients
- *Do not use* in patients with severe head or facial injuries, or concern for basilar skull fracture

## EQUIPMENT

- *Appropriate sized NP airway:* To estimate appropriate NP airway length, measure the distance from nare to tragus
- Lubrication jelly

## TECHNIQUE

- Apply lubrication jelly to insertion end of NP airway
- Insert NP airway into patient's nare with gentle posterior pressure until the flange rests upon the nare edge
- The NP airway should glide in easily. If resistance is encountered, check NP airway size, lubrication, or patency of nasal passage

## ORAL AIRWAY

### INDICATIONS

- Upper airway obstruction in an unconscious patient with spontaneous respirations
- Upper airway obstruction in an unconscious patient receiving bag-assisted ventilations
- Used to stent tongue and pharyngeal soft tissues away from posterior pharynx
- *Do not use* in a conscious patient as it may stimulate the gag reflex, emesis, and aspiration

### EQUIPMENT

- *Appropriate sized oral airway:* To estimate appropriate oral airway length, measure the distance from the corner of the mouth to angle of the mandible
- Wooden tongue depressor

### TECHNIQUE

- Using tongue depressor, push tongue away from palate
- Insert the oral airway along the curve of the tongue so that the innermost edge of the oral airway rests just posterior to the tongue
- The flange of the oral airway should rest on the patient's lips
- Be careful not to push tongue back and cause further upper airway obstruction

## ENDOTRACHEAL INTUBATION

### INDICATIONS

- Airway protection; existing or impending cardiac, respiratory or neurologic failure

### EQUIPMENT

**Mnemonic: "MSOAP"**

- *M-Meds:* Intubation adjuncts, sedatives, paralytics, resuscitation meds, anticonvulsants
  - ✓ See inside back cover for rapid sequence intubation medications
- *M-Monitors:* Cardiorespiratory (CR) monitor, pulse-oximeter, blood pressure (BP), end-tidal $CO_2$ detector
- *S-Suction:* Yankauer (rigid catheter), flexible soft catheter
- *O-Oxygen:* Tank or "wall" supply, delivery tubing

- *A-Airway Equipment:* Endotracheal tubes, stylets, laryngoscope blades, masks, self-inflating bag or anesthesia bag, NP airway, oral airway, laryngeal mask airway, tape, benzoin, syringe for cuff inflation
- *P-Personnel*

## Choosing an Endotracheal Tube

- Beyond the newborn period, cuffed tubes may be safely used
- *Formula for uncuffed ETT diameter:*

$$[Age(years)/4] + 4$$

- *Formula for cuffed ETT diameter:*

  Calculate uncuffed tube size and subtract 0.5

## Choosing a Laryngoscope Blade

- Straight (Miller) and curved (Macintosh) blades are available. Chose blade based on comfort level of laryngoscopist and size of child
- *Some age-related suggestions:*
  - ✓ *Preemie:* Miller 0
  - ✓ *Zero–3 months:* Miller 1
  - ✓ *Three months–3 years:* Miller 1, Miller 2, Wis-Hipple 1.5
  - ✓ *Three–12 years:* Miller 2, Macintosh 2
  - ✓ *Older than 12 years:* Miller 3, Macintosh 3

## TECHNIQUE

- Check all equipment and monitors. Preoxygenate with 100% $O_2$. Administer selected pharmacologic agents (see inside cover)
- Adjust height of bed to accommodate the person performing the intubation
- Position patient's head by either chin lift (stable cervical spine) or jaw thrust (unstable cervical spine) to maximize upper airway diameter. Depending on the age of the child, a towel roll under the head or shoulders may help to achieve the "sniffing" position
- If using stylet, tip should not extend beyond end of ETT
- Consider having an assistant apply gentle cricoid pressure (Sellick maneuver)
- Open mouth using scissor-finger technique with right hand (thumb on mandibular dental ridge, index or middle finger on maxillary dental ridge)
- Holding the laryngoscope in the left hand, insert blade on the right side of the patient's mouth, and sweep tongue toward the midline. Gently but firmly pull up along the axis of the handle of the laryngoscope maintaining a straight wrist. Do not rock back or lever the laryngoscope on the teeth
- Suction and reposition as needed until the glottic opening (characteristic inverted V of vocal cords) is visualized
- While maintaining visualized glottis, introduce ETT with right hand from the right side of mouth and pass tip of tube through the vocal cords
- *Depth of insertion:* Internal diameter of the ETT × 3 (length to corner of mouth), or double lines on tube just past vocal cords
- *Confirmation of proper placement:* Presence of end-tidal $CO_2$, mist in ETT tube, bilateral chest rise, and equal breath sounds
- Temporarily secure ETT to patient with benzoin and tape. Obtain chest x-ray to confirm placement (ideal tip placement is between clavicles and carina). Definitively secure ETT by splitting tape lengthwise; secure one arm to upper lip and wrap second arm around ETT. Repeat with second piece of tape

## LARYNGEAL MASK AIRWAY (LMA)

### INDICATIONS

- Airway protection; cardiac, respiratory, or neurologic failure; difficulty passing endotracheal tube
- Excellent rescue device since fairly easy to use for a variety of providers
- Can serve as a bridge to a more definitive airway

### EQUIPMENT

- *Appropriate sized LMA:* Depends on the patient's weight and the LMA manufacturer. Each LMA will be labeled with a weight range in kilograms that is acceptable for use. Also displayed will be the quantity of air in milliliters that is required to fill the LMA cuff
- Lubrication jelly
- *Equipment as listed in MSOAP pneumonic under "Endotracheal Intubation":* Medications, monitors, suction, oxygen, airway equipment, personnel
- See inside back cover for rapid sequence intubation medications
- If LMA is being placed due to failed intubation, consider calling for additional airway personnel

### TECHNIQUE

- Stand at the head of the bed as if performing intubation
- Check all equipment and monitors. Preoxygenate with 100% $O_2$. Administer selected pharmacologic agents
- Apply lubrication jelly to insertion end of LMA
- Position patient's head by either chin lift (stable cervical spine) or jaw thrust (unstable cervical spine) to maximize upper airway diameter
- With nondominant hand, grasp the patient's mandible and open the mouth
- With the dominant hand, hold the LMA as shown (see **Figure 25-2**) and insert LMA into mouth, skimming along the curve of the tongue into the pharynx until resistance is met

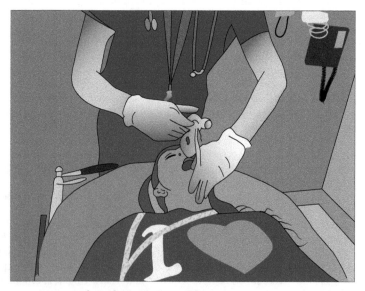

FIGURE 25-2 **Laryngeal mask airway insertion.**

- Once resistance is met, inflate LMA cuff with appropriate amount of air
- In younger patients, consider the rotational approach where the LMA is first inserted with the opening facing the palate and then rotated 180° into position when resistance is felt
- Begin ventilating patient. Ensure appropriate LMA placement by checking for presence of end-tidal $CO_2$, bilateral chest rise, and equal breath sounds

## INTRAOSSEOUS LINE PLACEMENT

### INDICATIONS

- Immediate vascular access for cardiopulmonary arrest or shock; intravenous access difficult or not possible in critically ill patient
- May be used to administer fluids, blood products, medications
- Aspirated blood can be sent for diagnostic studies. Values such as WBC count, potassium, calcium, transaminases, and blood oxygen level are less reliable

### EQUIPMENT

- Gloves, gauze; antiseptic solution (povidone-iodine or chloraprep); 1% lidocaine; syringe; 22- or 25-gauge needles; saline flush in 10-cc syringe; intraosseous (IO) needle
- *If using the battery-powered driver:* Device driver, appropriate IO needle, stabilizer dressing, extension tubing, 2% lidocaine
- If no IO needle is available, a bone marrow aspiration needle with trocar or 20-gauge spinal needle can be used

### PLACEMENT SITES

1. *Proximal tibia:* Tibial plateau (anterior, medial flat surface of tibia), 1–2 cm below the tibial tuberosity. This is the preferred site
2. *Distal femur:* Midline on femoral plateau (lower third of femur), approximately 1–2 cm above the superior border of the patella. Alternative site for infants and young children
3. *Distal tibia:* 1–2 cm above the medial malleolus. Easier to use in children older than 3 years of age
4. *Proximal humerus:* Typically requires battery-powered driver device; greater tubercle of humerus appropriate in the older, skeletally mature child. To access the greater tubercle safely, place patient's arm on their abdomen with elbow flexed. The greater tubercle prominence is about 1 cm above the surgical neck of the humerus or 2 cm below the acromion process

### MANUAL INSERTION TECHNIQUE

- In awake patients, inject 1% lidocaine into skin and periosteum
- Prepare skin with antiseptic solution
- Stabilize extremity with nondominant hand (Keep hand away from opposite side of insertion site to avoid injury!). Identify landmarks for insertion, most commonly at the tibial plateau
- Hold IO needle with hub resting in the palm; stabilize needle with thumb and index finger placed 1–2 cm from the tip
- Insert needle perpendicular to the bony cortex or slightly angled (10–15 degrees) away from the growth plate. Use steady back and forth rotational motion while gradually increasing pressure until a sudden decrease in resistance is felt. Immediately release pressure to prevent piercing opposite end of bone
- Unscrew the needle cap and remove the trocar. If the needle is secure in the bone, it should stand without support

- Confirm intramedullary placement with aspiration of blood or bone marrow and/or easy infusion of fluids without extravasation
  ✓ Flush the needle with 10 mL of normal saline and connect it to conventional IV tubing
- Secure needle with a dressing. Avoid bulky dressings that may make infiltration difficult to detect

### BATTERY-POWERED DRIVER TECHNIQUE

- Battery-powered IO needle and driver sets have become more widely available in prehospital and hospital settings (EZ-IO®, VidaCare Corporation)
- *Needles come in three sizes:*
  ✓ Small (15 mm) = Pink for patients 3–39 kg
  ✓ Medium (25 mm) = Blue for patient ≥40 kg
  ✓ Large (45 mm) = Yellow for patients ≥40 kg with excessive subcutaneous tissues, often needle of choice for humerus site
- Identify appropriate location for insertion and anatomic landmarks. Cleanse insertion site
- Choose the appropriate needle based on the patient's weight and amount of subcutaneous tissue

  *Note:* Weights are rules of thumb; important thing is that one black line is still visible after the needle is through the skin. Due to amount of subcutaneous tissue, pink needle often only helpful in very young patients, blue needle used most widely. If in doubt, go with the longer needle to ensure that the marrow is penetrated!

- Place the needle into the battery-powered driver and remove the safety cap
- Position driver with the needle perpendicular to the bone surface and insert needle until you feel bone. Ensure that at least 5 mm of the needle is visible as indicated by the black line (if not, use a longer needle or alternative site)
- Press trigger to activate the driver applying gentle downward pressure. Release the trigger when you feel a sudden decrease in resistance
- Hold the catheter in place and remove the driver by pulling up. Remove the stylet from the catheter by rotating counterclockwise and safely dispose of the stylet
- Secure the site with the stabilizer dressing
- Connect primed connector and draw labs if necessary
- Flush the catheter quickly with 10 mL of NS (to displace marrow and provide room for infusion)

  *Note:* In an awake or responsive patient, consider infusing 2% lidocaine without epinephrine into IO prior to this step—infusion into the marrow is quite painful

## LACERATION REPAIR

### INDICATION

- Restore integrity and function of injured tissues while minimizing scar formation and infection

### EQUIPMENT

1. *Basics:* Light, mask, sterile gloves, povidone-iodine solution
2. *Irrigation:* 20- to 60-mL syringes, sterile saline, splash guard
3. *Suture tray:* Needle holder, nontraumatic tissue forceps, tissue scissors, hemostats, sterile gauze, sterile drapes
4. *Suture material:*
   ✓ *Nonabsorbable:* Monofilament nylon (Ethilon), polypropylene (Prolene)
   ✓ *Absorbable:* Vicryl, fast-absorbing gut, chromic gut
     - Nonabsorbable sutures have high tensile strength and are typically used on extremities

- Fast absorbing sutures (vicryl rapide, fast-absorbing gut) are frequently used for pediatric facial lacerations
- Chromic gut is useful for intra-oral laceration closure as well as for fingertip/nailbed lacerations

5. *Size:* Face: 6-0 or 5-0; scalp, trunk, extremities: 4-0; sole of foot, over large joints: 4-0 or 3-0

## GENERAL TECHNIQUE

1. *Local Anesthesia:*
   ✓ *"LET" gel:* Contains lidocaine, epinephrine, and tetracaine. Apply for 15–20 minutes up to three times or until skin blanches. Avoid areas where vasoconstriction is contraindicated
   ✓ *1% Lidocaine (10 mg/mL):* Infiltrative anesthetic; maximum dose: 4 mg/kg; onset: 2–5 minutes; duration: 30–120 minutes
   ✓ *1% Lidocaine with epinephrine (1:200,000):* Infiltrative anesthetic, reduces bleeding; maximum dose: 7 mg/kg; onset: 2–5 minutes; duration: 60–180 minutes; contraindicated in digits, penis, pinna, tip of nose
   ✓ *Sodium bicarbonate:* Buffers local anesthetic to improve potency and reduce pain. Mix 1 part $NaHCO_3$ to 9 parts lidocaine or lidocaine with epinephrine

2. *Wound Preparation:*
   ✓ *Exploration:* Provide hemostasis; explore for foreign body
   ✓ *Débridement:* Remove devitalized or heavily contaminated tissue
   ✓ *Hair:* May clip. Alternatively, use petroleum jelly to keep unwanted scalp hair away from wound. Do not shave eyebrows
   ✓ *Irrigation:* Irrigate with normal saline using 20- to 60-mL syringe and splash-guard. Use 100–200 mL for average 2-cm laceration. Clean wound periphery using povidone-iodine solution

3. *Apply Suture Using Needle Holder:*
   ✓ For better control, hold loaded needle holder near the tip. Do NOT keep fingers in rings of the needle holder while sewing
   ✓ Enter skin with needle perpendicular to surface. Retrieve needle after each pass with needle holder or forceps
   ✓ Place just enough sutures so that there are no gaps in the wound

4. *Instrument Tie:* Tighten knot so that skin edges just come together, making sure that wound edges are everted to minimize scar formation (Figure 25-3). Repeat single loop tie, in an over and under manner, for a total of four throws. Cut both ends of suture allowing adequate length (at least 1 cm) to retrieve suture at time of removal

5. *Suture Removal:* Neck: 3–4 days; face: 5 days, scalp: 7–10 days; upper extremities, trunk: 7 days; lower extremities: 8–10 days; joint surface: 10–14 days

## SUTURE TECHNIQUES

1. *Simple Interrupted Sutures:* Most common suture used for uncomplicated wounds. Enter skin with needle directed downward or angled slightly away from wound edge (see Figure 25-3)
2. *Inverted ("Buried") Subcutaneous Sutures:* Used to counteract tension on wound. Insert needle from within wound at fat–dermal junction (Figure 25-4)
3. *Vertical Mattress Sutures:* Combines a deep and superficial stitch into one suture (Figure 25-5). Used in wounds of high tension or where difficult to tie an inverted subcutaneous suture
4. *Horizontal Mattress Sutures:* Reinforces subcutaneous tissue and relieves tension from wound edges. Useful as deep layer in relatively shallow lacerations and in areas with minimal subcutaneous tissue (Figure 25-6)

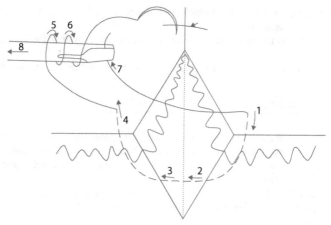

FIGURE 25-3 **Simple interrupted suture.**

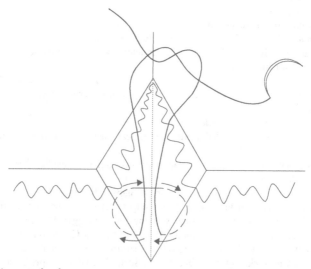

FIGURE 25-4 **Inverted subcutaneous suture.**

5. *Half-buried or Corner Suture:* Useful in flap closure. Enter skin below and just lateral to the point of V-shaped flap (Figure 25-7)
6. *Simple (Continuous) Running Suture:* Limited to linear, clean, low tension wounds. Saves time but breakage unravels entire stitch (Figure 25-8)

## ALTERNATIVES TO SUTURES

### Tape ("Steri-Strips")

• *Indications:* Linear lacerations under minimal tension; useful for reinforcing or refining other repairs; not useful for wounds requiring meticulous approximation or for moist or hairy areas

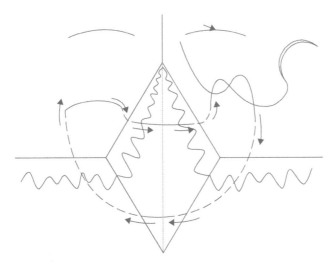

FIGURE 25-5 **Vertical mattress suture.**

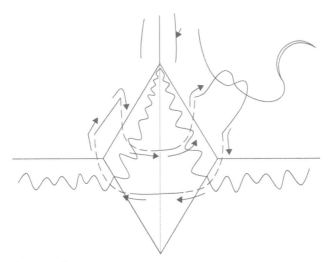

FIGURE 25-6 **Horizontal mattress suture.**

- *Technique:* Clean and dry skin surrounding laceration. Apply adhesive (benzoin) to surrounding skin, and wait 90 seconds for it to become "tacky." Place tape strips perpendicularly across wound leaving some space for oozing. Place extra tape strips across ends of previous strips and parallel to wound

## Staples

- Best for scalp wounds. Requires staple remover
- *Technique:* Prepare wound in same manner as for sutures. Have assistant evert wound edges with tissue forceps or finger pressure. Line up arrow on stapler with center of wound. Place staples by applying steady firm pressure to stapling device. Place staples about 0.5 cm apart

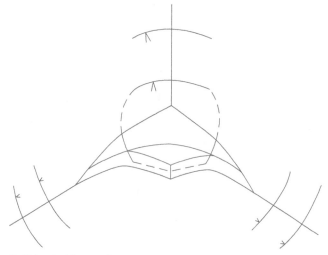

FIGURE 25-7 **Half-buried (corner) suture.**

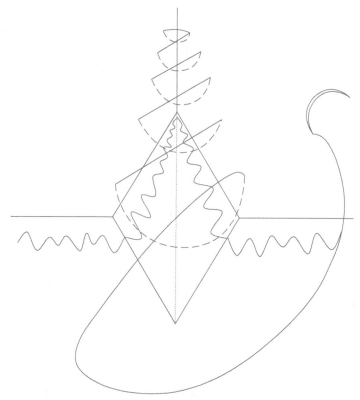

FIGURE 25-8 **Simple (continuous) running suture.**

| TABLE 25-1 Tetanus Prophylaxis | | |
|---|---|---|
| **Prior Tetanus Toxoid Doses** | **Clean, Minor Wound** | **Dirty Wounds** |
| Uncertain or <3 doses | DTaP or Td | DTaP or Td and TIG |
| 3 or more (last >10 years ago) | Td | Td |
| 3 or more (last 5–10 years ago) | None | Td |
| 3 or more (last <5 years ago) | None | None |

DTaP, diphtheria, tetanus, acellular pertussis; Td, tetanus, diphtheria; TIG, human tetanus immune globulin.

## Tissue Adhesives ("Dermabond")

• Best for linear wounds with minimal tension
• Allows rapid, painless closure of wounds. No removal needed
• Do not use in hairy areas, in the mouth, or near the eyes of young children. Do not use on wounds at high risk for infection
• *Technique:* Irrigate wound in same manner as for suture repair. Position patient so that adhesive cannot leak into adjacent structures (particularly important for wounds near the eye). The wound must be completely dry. An assistant should hold the wound edges together with forceps or gloved fingers. Activate tissue adhesive applicator (vials often require crushing to start polymerization process and to soak the foam applicator tip). Apply adhesive along surface of wound creating a thin film. Allow this to dry for a few seconds before applying 2–3 subsequent layers in concentric ovals around the wound (avoid applying adhesive to inside of wound). Hold wound until dry
• In the event that the tissue adhesive needs to be removed, apply petroleum jelly or antibiotic ointment for about 30 minutes
• Wears off in 5–10 days

### POST-LACERATION REPAIR MANAGEMENT

• In general, cover the wound for the first 24 hours and apply topical antibiotic ointment to wounds. In wounds closed with tissue adhesive, however, no cover is necessary and antibiotic ointments should be avoided
• *Antibiotics*—Not indicated for majority of lacerations. Antibiotics may be indicated for "high-risk wounds." Consider first-generation cephalosporin (e.g., cephalexin). Consider erythromycin if penicillin/cephalosporin allergic. Consider amoxicillin/clavulanic acid for mammalian bites
• *High-Risk Wounds:* Highly contaminated wound, wound with foreign body, bite wounds, crush injury, intraoral laceration, wound of hands, feet, or perineum, open fracture, exposed joints and tendons, immunocompromised patient, exposed cartilage, delayed repair, tetanus-prone wounds (Table 25-1)

## LUMBAR PUNCTURE

### INDICATIONS

• Suspicion of CNS infection, suspicion of subarachnoid hemorrhage, measurement of opening pressure, diagnosis and/or treatment of idiopathic intracranial hypertension (pseudotumor cerebri), diagnosis of CNS metastases, suspicion of Guillain–Barré

## CONTRAINDICATIONS

- Increased intracranial pressure (unless likely due to idiopathic intracranial hypertension)
- *Relative contraindications:* Bleeding disorder, cardiopulmonary instability, spinal anomaly

## EQUIPMENT

- Sterile gloves, mask, antiseptic solution (povidone iodine or chlorhexidine), lumbar puncture (LP) tray, CR monitor and pulse-oximeter, topical anesthetic cream (EMLA, LMX4). Resuscitation equipment should also be available
- *Lumbar puncture tray:* Typically includes sterile drapes, sterile gauze, lidocaine 1%, 3-cc syringe for lidocaine injection, gauze, adhesive bandage strip, collecting tubes, manometer; +/− spinal needle
- *Needle size:* Usually 22 gauge; infants: 1.5 inch; 1–12 years: 2.5 inch; >12 years/obese patient: 3.5 inch

## TECHNIQUE

1. *Preparing and positioning the patient:*
   ✓ Apply topical anesthetic cream to puncture site 30+ minutes prior to procedure
   ✓ Begin monitoring, consider sedation in uncooperative older child
   ✓ *Two positions commonly used:*
      - *Lateral recumbent:* Assistant holds infant in fetal position. In an older child, assistant holds patient in knee-chest position. A firm hold is essential to success. In infants, avoid forcefully flexing the neck, which may lead to respiratory compromise
      - *Sitting position:* Patient seated with feet over side of bed with neck/upper body flexed forward over pillow on lap or leaning on bedside tray (does not provide accurate measurement of opening pressure)
   ✓ Locate the puncture site by palpating the superior aspect of the posterior superior iliac crests. A line between the two crests will intersect approximately at top of L4 at midline. The L3–L4 and L4–L5 interspaces are both suitable LP sites
   ✓ Prepare the area with antiseptic solution starting at the intended puncture site and swabbing in enlarging circles. Apply sterile drapes, if possible leaving landmarks visible. Anesthetize the interspace with lidocaine 1%. Studies have shown that local anesthetics decrease pain and increase the success rate of LPs
2. *Inserting the needle:* Ensure the shoulders and hips are perpendicular to the bed. Slowly insert the bevel-up, styletted needle, aiming slightly cephalad, toward the umbilicus. Infants may require a more acute angle of approach. After the needle moves through the epidermal and fat layers, some clinicians remove the stylet before advancing further. Moving beyond the ligamentum flavum/dura into the cerebrospinal fluid (CSF) space, a loss of resistance may be appreciated ("pop"). If the stylet has not been removed, and the "pop" is not appreciated, the physician must remove the stylet every few millimeters to observe for CSF flow
3. *Use of manometer: Obtained in the lateral recumbent position. The manometer should be attached to the needle immediately after CSF flow is seen.* The opening pressure is the highest recorded level the CSF reaches in the column. Normal opening pressure is approximately 5–20 cm $H_2O$. The reading will be falsely high in a struggling patient
4. *Collection and completion:*
   ✓ Collect approximately 1 cc fluid in each tube. Replace stylet and remove needle. Clean site and apply strip bandage or sterile dressing
   ✓ *Send tubes to lab as follows:* Tube 1, Gram stain/culture; tube 2, protein/glucose; tube 3, cell counts; tube 4, any additional studies. If there is concern for subarachnoid hemorrhage, send tube 1 and tube 4 for cell count

## PNEUMOTHORAX: NEEDLE DECOMPRESSION

### INDICATION

- Tension pneumothorax (which may present with deviated trachea, diminished or asymmetric breath sounds, diminished chest wall expansion, or sudden cardiopulmonary decompensation)

### EQUIPMENT

- 16- or 18-gauge angiocatheter; 5- to 10-mL syringe; three-way stopcock; antiseptic solution; lidocaine (1%)

### TECHNIQUE

- Do not delay if tension pneumothorax suspected
- Place patient in supine position and elevate head of bed to 30 degrees
- Swab area with antiseptic solution
- Provide local anesthesia with 1% lidocaine if time permits
- Using a 16- or 18-gauge angiocatheter attached to a syringe, insert needle perpendicular to the midclavicular line on the upper edge of the third rib. Gently pull back on the syringe as the needle is advanced into second intercostal space. A loss of resistance in the syringe indicates evacuation of air
- Advance the catheter over the needle into the pleural space, and remove the needle. Attach a one-way drainage device to the catheter or intermittently draw back on a syringe connected to the catheter with a three-way stopcock
- Obtain immediate chest radiograph, and consider tube thoracostomy

## UMBILICAL VESSEL CATHETERIZATION

### INDICATIONS

- Frequent arterial or venous blood gases, continuous monitoring of arterial or central venous blood pressures, emergency vascular access, prolonged need for administration of fluids and medications, exchange transfusion

### EQUIPMENT

- Umbilical artery catheter (UAC), umbilical vein catheter (UVC), three-way stopcock, radiant warmer, cardiac monitor, pulse oximetry, supplemental oxygen source, antiseptic solution (povidone-iodine), soft restraints, sterile towels, fenestrated drape, sterile gauze, scalpel: no. 11 or 15, forceps: curved, non-toothed (Iris forceps or vessel dilator), forceps: straight, Crile, hemostats: at least four pairs, scissors, suture: 3.0 or 4.0 silk on curved needle, umbilical tape (approximately 15 inches), 3-mL syringes filled with sterile saline (with heparin 0.5–1 U/mL), sterile gown and gloves, mask, hat
- *UAC Sizing:* Generally 3.5F
- *UVC Sizing:* Infants <1 kg: 3.5F; infants >1 kg: 5F

### PREPARATION

- Determine appropriate equation for insertion depth
- Identify appropriate size catheter to be used
- Gently restrain infant in supine, frog-legged position. Keep infant warm with overhead warmers, and place on cardiac monitor/pulse oximetry with supplemental oxygen available
- Perform hand hygiene and don hat, mask, sterile gown, and sterile gloves

- Prepare umbilical lines by connecting a three-way stopcock and 3-mL syringe filled with sterile heparinized saline to each catheter lumen. Flush each lumen with sterile saline and ensure no air bubbles are present. Turn stopcock so that it is "off to baby"

## TECHNIQUE

- Using sterile technique, wash lower 5 cm of umbilical cord and skin surrounding umbilicus with antiseptic solution. Drape with sterile towels
- Loosely tie umbilical tape at base of cord to prevent bleeding. Cut cord with scalpel to length of 1–2 cm above the skin surface. Place fenestrated drape (if available) over cut umbilicus, covering patient completely
- *Stabilize cord with forceps or hemostats:* Grasp one edge of cord with curved hemostat or grasp opposite sides with two hemostats and evert edges
- *Identify the vessels:* One central, cephalad, larger lumen, thin-walled vein; two smaller lumen, thick-walled arteries
- Hold catheter 1 cm from tip with toothless forceps and insert into vessel lumen with gentle pressure. Blood return signifies proper insertion
  - ✓ Catheterization of the umbilical vein does not require dilation. Insert the umbilical venous catheter to predetermined depth, check for blood return and flush the venous line. Turn stopcock handle toward infant to stop flow
  - ✓ Catheterization of the umbilical arteries requires gentle dilation with forceps. Dilate arterial lumen using curved, non-toothed, Iris forceps until the arterial opening is large enough to accommodate the umbilical catheter. It is very easy to cause a false track in the Wharton's jelly if this step is skipped. Insert the umbilical arterial catheter to predetermined depth, check for blood return, and flush the arterial line. Turn stopcock handle toward infant to stop flow
- Secure line placement with 3.0 silk suture through Wharton's jelly of umbilical cord. Wrap suture around the catheter 2–3 times and tie. Repeat wrap and tie a second time. Do not suture line to skin
- Maintaining the sterile field, confirm proper placement with radiograph of chest and abdomen. Once the sterile field is broken, do not advance the catheter. It may be withdrawn
- Secure catheters to skin with tape bridge or tegaderm per unit policy
- *To remove catheter:* Place umbilical tape loosely around stump to control bleeding. Remove catheter gradually over 3–4 minutes, allowing vessels to segmentally constrict and/or clot to form

## POSITIONING AND INSERTION LENGTH

- Guidelines vary by institution

### "High" Umbilical Artery Catheter

- Catheter tip placed just above diaphragm at spinal level T6–T9
- Measure shoulder-to-umbilical length, if less than 13 cm, insert catheter that distance plus 1 cm; if greater than 13 cm, insert catheter that distance plus 2 cm
- Alternatively, UAC length (cm) = [3 × birth weight (kg)] + 9

### "Low" Umbilical Artery Catheter

- Catheter tip positioned below diaphragm, just above aortic bifurcation at spinal level L3–L5
- UAC length (cm) = birth weight (kg) + 7 or alternatively, 2/3 the shoulder-to-umbilicus length (cm) distance + length of remaining umbilical cord

## Umbilical Vein Catheter

- Normally, catheter tip is placed above diaphragm at the junction of the inferior vena cava and right atrium
- In emergent situations, catheter is passed cephalad for 2–3 cm (preterm) or 4–5 cm (term) until blood return obtained (below portal circulation)
- *To estimate normal UVC length:* Length (cm) = 2/3 the shoulder-to-umbilicus length (cm) or alternatively (1.5 × birthweight) + 5.5

**Risks of procedure:**

- Bleeding
- Pericardial effusion/tamponade
- Air embolus
- Vessel perforation
- Arrhythmia
- Thrombosis

# Psychiatry

# 26

*Rahim Rahemtulla, MD*
*Amy Kim, MD*

## AGITATION/AGGRESSION

### ETIOLOGY

*Multiple conditions can cause a patient to act in an agitated or aggressive manner in the inpatient pediatric setting:* alcohol and substance intoxication, primary psychiatric disorders, psychosis, personality disorders, severe conduct disorder, autism, pervasive developmental delay (PDD), mental retardation, delirium, temporal lobe seizure, other "organic" causes (steroid-induced, herpes simplex virus [HSV] encephalitis)

### CLINICAL MANIFESTATIONS

Manifestations depend on the underlying cause:
* *Primary Psychiatric Disorder*
  ✓ Mood/affect lability
  ✓ Irritability
  ✓ Anxiety
  ✓ Impulsivity
  ✓ Psychotic symptoms
  ✓ Suicidal or homicidal ideation
  ✓ Poor insight
  ✓ Impaired judgment
* *Delirium*
  ✓ Altered level of alertness and concentration
  ✓ Hallucinations or delusions
* *Signs of intoxication:*
  ✓ *Alcohol:* Alcohol on breath, dysarthria, incoordination, ataxia
  ✓ *Amphetamines:* Dilated pupils, altered pulse or blood pressure
  ✓ *Cocaine:* Dilated pupils, hypertension, tachycardia
  ✓ *Hallucinogens:* Dilated pupils, tachycardia, sweating, palpitations, tremors, incoordination
  ✓ *Phencyclidine (PCP):* Nystagmus, hypertension, tachycardia, ataxia, dysarthria, muscle rigidity, seizures

### DIAGNOSTICS

* Urine or serum drug screen
* Consider other studies as clinically indicated

### MANAGEMENT

#### Information Gathering

* Interview patient, parents, outpatient psychiatrist/therapist
* Mental status exam and physical exam
* Diagnostic tests if indicated
* Identify and treat the underlying cause of the agitated behavior

### Prevention/De-escalation Strategies

- Provide a safe and nonthreatening environment
- Time-out
- Decrease sensory stimulation (dim lights, speak softly)
- Attempt to redirect patient (talking, offering alternate strategy)
- Consider 1:1 supervision
- Chemical or physical restraints should only be used after less restrictive means have failed and the aggression or behavior is so severe that it places the patient or others in imminent danger

### Chemical Restraints

Refers to the use of medication to achieve behavioral control or sedation. Always attempt to offer oral medications first.

- *Antipsychotic Medications:* Risperidone orally, olanzapine orally, haloperidol orally/IM/IV; may cause side effects (refer to Psychosis: Adverse Effects of Antipsychotics)
- *Benzodiazepines:* Lorazepam orally/IM/IV; in some patients, may cause disinhibition with increased behavioral dyscontrol
- *Antihistamines:* Diphenhydramine orally/IM/IV; may give with antipsychotic as prophylaxis for neuroleptic-induced dystonia. In some patients, may cause disinhibition with increased behavioral dyscontrol

### Physical/Mechanical Restraints

- Should only be used when a patient's behavior becomes so violent or aggressive that it endangers his/her own safety or that of others
- Examples include four-point restraints, papoose board, wrist-to-waist, physical holds by trained staff or security
- While restrained, patient should be continually monitored (checks of vital signs, extremity range of motion, skin integrity, and circulation) and attention given to nutrition, hydration, and elimination needs
- Parents or guardians should be informed as soon as possible
- Restraints should be discontinued as soon as patient's behavior is controlled and is no longer a threat to self or others
- Debrief the patient regarding why restraints were used, future alternative strategies, and provide opportunity for patient to apologize or make amends
- All accredited facilities should have a formal policy regarding the use of restraints that adhere to Joint Commission guidelines. Become familiar with it

## PSYCHOSIS

**Psychotic symptoms include:**

- *Formal thought disorder:* Disorganized or incoherent speech, illogical thought, loose associations
- *Positive symptoms:* Auditory or visual hallucinations, delusions
- *Negative symptoms:* Flattened affect, alogia, avolition

### DIFFERENTIAL DIAGNOSIS

- Mood disorders (depression, bipolar affective disorder)
- Substance-induced
  - ✓ *Intoxicants:* Alcohol, amphetamine, D-lysergic acid diethylamide [LSD], PCP
  - ✓ *Medications:* Stimulants, steroids, anticholinergics

- "Organic" causes
  - ✓ Delirium
  - ✓ Brain tumor
  - ✓ Congenital malformation
  - ✓ Head trauma
  - ✓ Seizure disorder (e.g., temporal lobe epilepsy)
  - ✓ Neurodegenerative disorder
  - ✓ Metabolic disorder
  - ✓ Toxins (heavy metals)
  - ✓ Infections (HSV encephalitis, HIV)
  - ✓ Thyroid disease
  - ✓ Immune mediated (anti-N-methyl-D-aspartate [NMDA] receptor encephalitis, lupus cerebritis, paraneoplastic syndromes)
- Schizophrenia
- Autistic spectrum disorders
- Mental retardation
- Anxiety disorders (posttraumatic stress disorder)

## PATHOPHYSIOLOGY

- Abnormal monoaminergic activity in the central nervous system (CNS)

## CLINICAL MANIFESTATIONS

- Younger children's delusions tend to be less complex, less fixed
- Adolescent's delusions may be paranoid, grandiose, bizarre
- May present agitated or disruptive
- *Mental Status Exam:* Presence of psychotic symptoms, mood and affect (depression, anxiety, irritability, and lability), presence of suicidal or homicidal ideation, impaired judgment
- Signs of intoxication

## DIAGNOSTICS

- Urine or serum drug screen
- Thyroid-stimulating hormone
- Consider EEG, lumbar puncture, head CT or MRI

## MANAGEMENT

### Information Gathering

- See "Agitation/Aggression"

### Evaluate for Safety

- Impaired judgment risks injury of self/others
- Disruptive behavior/agitation risks injury to self/others
- Admit patient if there are safety concerns

### If Patient Requires Admission

- Admit to appropriate level of care until medically stable
- Consider 1:1 supervision of patient for monitoring of safety
- Consult child psychiatrist
- Consider antipsychotic medication
- Evaluate for inpatient psychiatric care

## Antipsychotic Medications

- *Atypical antipsychotic drugs are associated with lower incidence of extrapyramidal symptoms (EPS) and tardive dyskinesia (TD):* Risperidone, olanzapine, quetiapine, aripiprazole
- *Typical antipsychotic drugs:* Haloperidol
- Side effects
  - ✓ *Common side effects:* Sedation, orthostatic hypotension
  - ✓ *Extrapyramidal symptoms:* Acute dystonic reaction (treat with diphenhydramine, benztropine), neuroleptic-induced parkinsonism, akathisia (treat with beta-blocker, benzodiazepine)
  - ✓ *Neuroleptic malignant syndrome:* Life-threatening condition characterized by hyperthermia, muscle rigidity, altered mental status, choreoathetosis, tremors, and autonomic dysfunction (arrhythmias, hypertension, sweating)
  - ✓ Anticholinergic effects (confusion, agitation, constipation, blurred vision, urinary retention)

## SUICIDALITY

**Thoughts, threats, events, or actions characterized by the desire to cause death or harm to oneself. Suicidal ideation (SI) may be ambiguous or strong.**

### EPIDEMIOLOGY

- *In a 2013 nationally representative sample of youth in grades 9–12:*
  - ✓ 17% of students reported that they had seriously considered suicide during the 12 months preceding the survey
  - ✓ 13% of students reported that they had made a plan
  - ✓ 8% reported that they had attempted suicide one or more times
- Second leading cause of death among persons 15–24 years of age, and the third leading cause of death among children and adolescents 10–14 years of age
- While females attempt suicide more often than males, suicide rates among males are four times higher (due to more lethal methods)
- Firearms are the most commonly used method among males (56%)
- Poisoning is the most common method of suicide for females (37%)

### ETIOLOGY/RISK FACTORS

- History of previous suicidal behaviors
- Primary psychiatric disorders; most commonly depression, bipolar affective disorder, conduct disorder
- Developmental and preclinical personality disorders associated with impulsivity or aggression
- Alcohol and substance abuse and/or intoxication
- *Biologic factors:* Often there is a family history of psychiatric illness, suicidal behavior, substance abuse
- *Stressful life events:* Particularly exposure to violence or bullying, physical and sexual abuse, family conflict
- *Sexual orientation:* Lesbian, gay, bisexual, transgender, and questioning (LGBTQ) youth may be more likely to become suicidal because they are at risk for multiple risk factors: depression, substance abuse, sexual victimization, rejection by family, and bullying by peers.
- Access to lethal methods

- Incarceration
- *Suicide contagion effect:* knowing or hearing about someone who recently completed suicide, including news media coverage of an adolescent who completed suicide

## DIFFERENTIAL DIAGNOSIS

- Accidental versus intentional injury
- High versus low risk of injury or lethality

## PATHOPHYSIOLOGY

- *Associated findings include:* Altered serotonergic function, lower cerebrospinal fluid serotonin levels, alterations in hypothalamic-pituitary function, disturbed sleep

## CLINICAL MANIFESTATIONS

- Methods may include drug ingestions, shooting, hanging, suffocation, stabbing, drowning, burning, running into traffic, intentional motor vehicle accidents
- *Mental Status Exam:* Current suicidal ideation/intent/plan, psychotic symptoms, mood and affect (depression, anxiety, irritability, and lability), level of insight, and judgment
- Signs of intoxication

## MANAGEMENT

### Information Gathering

- Interview patient, parents, outpatient psychiatrist/therapist
- Prior history of suicide attempts or self-injurious behaviors
- Accessibility of methods (access to firearms, drugs, alcohol, and medications at home)
- Precipitants/Stressors that preceded the attempt
- *Risk factors:* Substance abuse, new or acute stressors at home or school, family conflict, LGBTQ youth

### Evaluate Suicide Threat/Attempt

- Suicidal intent
- Amount of planning
- Method used
- Potential for lethality
- Desire for death as an outcome
- Awareness of death as a likely outcome
- Likelihood of discovery
- Motivation for the attempt

### If Patient Requires Admission

- Admit to appropriate level of care until medically stable
- Consider 1:1 supervision of patient for monitoring of safety
- Repeated interview and assessment until SI is diminished
- Consult child psychiatrist
- Consider psychiatric medication
- Evaluate for inpatient psychiatric care

### If Stable for Discharge

- Have patient contract for safety
- Parents/caregivers must agree to make guns, firearms, medications, alcohol, and drugs unavailable to patient

- Parents/caregivers must be able to provide appropriate supervision of patient until stable
- Contact outpatient psychiatrist, therapist, and/or pediatrician to coordinate a discharge plan
- Provide references for appropriate outpatient psychiatric resources and/or crisis services
- Instruct family to contact physician/psychiatrist, or return to emergency department if concerned that patient may be at risk for harming self after discharge

# Pulmonology

*Kelly Adams, DO*
*Stamatia Alexiou, MD*
*Howard B. Panitch, MD*

## PULMONARY DISEASES AND SYNDROMES

### ACUTE RESPIRATORY DISTRESS SYNDROME

**An acute, diffuse, inflammatory lung injury that leads to increased pulmonary vascular permeability, increased lung weight, diffuse alveolar damage, and hypoxemia.**
Berlin definition of acute respiratory distress syndrome (ARDS)

#### EPIDEMIOLOGY

• Accounts for approximately 5% of hospitalized and mechanically ventilated pediatric patients
• Incidence in children varies greatly, but in the United States ranges between 2.9 and 9.5 cases/100,000 children per year
• *Mortality depends on age, etiology, pre-morbid conditions, and severity of oxygenation deficit:*
 ✓ Mortality rate in children ranges between 22 and 35%

#### ETIOLOGY

• *Most common etiology:* Sepsis
• Others include systemic inflammatory response syndrome (SIRS), pneumonia, aspiration, smoke inhalation, trauma, drowning, pancreatitis, and massive blood transfusions
• Risk of developing ARDS is higher in adults with a history of alcoholism and obesity

#### PATHOPHYSIOLOGY

• *ARDS follows a predictable progression of histologic and clinical stages:*
 ✓ *Exudative stage:* Release of proinflammatory cytokines and influx of neutrophils lead to epithelial and endothelial injury, noncardiogenic pulmonary edema, impaired gas exchange, surfactant deficiency/deactivation, and diffuse alveolar damage
 ✓ *Proliferative stage:* Proliferation of type II alveolar cells, squamous metaplasia, interstitial infiltration by myofibroblasts, and early deposition of collagen
 ✓ *Fibrotic stage:* Obliteration of normal lung architecture, diffuse fibrosis, collagen deposition

#### CLINICAL MANIFESTATIONS

• The initial presentation can include cyanosis, dyspnea, tachypnea, and diffuse crackles

#### DIAGNOSTICS

• *Arterial blood gas:* Profound hypoxemia, usually refractory to supplemental oxygen administration; elevated alveolar-arterial oxygen gradient. Calculate $PaO_2/FiO_2$ to determine severity of ARDS. Initially the $PCO_2$ is low because of hyperventilation, but later on there is $CO_2$ retention
• *Indicators of end-organ damage and multiorgan failure:* Follow liver enzyme levels, coagulation studies, cardiac enzymes
• *Chest radiograph:* Diffuse bilateral alveolar infiltrates

- *Chest CT scan:* Bilateral patchy airspace opacities in dependent areas of lung
- *Expected changes in lung function and mechanics:* Decreased total lung capacity, decreased functional residual capacity (FRC), large intrapulmonary shunt fraction ($Q_S/Q_T$), decreased pulmonary compliance

## MANAGEMENT

Management involves supportive ventilation and correction of underlying causes while treating comorbidities and limiting complications.

- *Ventilation:* Goal is to achieve adequate (not necessarily normal) alveolar gas exchange while limiting complications by using low tidal volume to avoid alveolar overdistention, low $FiO_2$ to reduce oxidant injury, and high positive end-expiratory pressure (PEEP) to limit barotrauma and maximize lung recruitment:
  - ✓ *Minimize tidal volume:* Goal 4–8 mL/kg
  - ✓ *Permissive hypercapnia:* Smaller tidal volumes result in hypoventilation, therefore an elevation of $PaCO_2$
  - ✓ *PEEP:* 5–15 cm $H_2O$ to prevent or reverse atelectasis
  - ✓ Limit inflating (plateau) pressure (e.g, after an inspiratory hold) to less than 30 cm $H_2O$ if possible
  - ✓ Goal $SpO_2$ 88–95%; attempt to use "nontoxic" $FiO_2$ of less than 60% to keep $PaO_2$ greater than 60 mm Hg
  - ✓ Goal pH 7.25–7.40
- *Adjunctive therapies have not been proven to reduce mortality but include* high-frequency oscillation, inverse inspiratory-to-expiratory ratio ventilation; pressure-regulated volume control (PRVC) ventilation; airway pressure release ventilation (APRV); prone positioning; nitric oxide; exogenous surfactant administration; extracorporeal membrane oxygenation
- *Supportive treatment:*
  - ✓ Limited fluid resuscitation ensures adequate tissue perfusion while limiting alveolar edema. Measures to decrease oxygen demand are helpful
  - ✓ Inotropic support; blood transfusion if necessary; diuretics; sedation; paralysis if necessary; antipyretics
- *Experimental therapies:* Liquid ventilation, dietary antioxidant therapy, granulocyte–monocyte colony stimulating factor, statins, macrolide antibiotics, beta-agonists, steroids
- *Manage comorbidities:* Renal failure, cardiac failure, hepatic failure, CNS failure, disordered coagulation
- *Manage complications:* Ventilator-associated pneumonia, barotrauma, bacterial tracheitis, sepsis, SIRS, chronic respiratory failure, generalized deconditioning, critical illness neuropathy, central line infections, central line thrombosis, decubitus ulcer formation

## CYSTIC FIBROSIS

An autosomal recessive defect in the cystic fibrosis transmembrane conductance regulator (CFTR) gene, located on the long arm of chromosome 7. Abnormal transport of chloride and sodium across an epithelium results in viscid mucus secretions and elevated sweat chloride levels. Progressive chronic pulmonary disease and exocrine pancreatic insufficiency are the primary clinical manifestations.

## EPIDEMIOLOGY

- Carrier frequency in certain white populations as high as 1 in 25
- More than 1900 mutations of the CFTR gene have been identified to date

- F508del-CFTR is the most common mutation in the Northern European-white population and accounts for approximately 70% of CFTR mutations in the United States

## PATHOPHYSIOLOGY

- Failure of epithelial cells to conduct chloride and the associated water transport abnormalities result in tenacious secretions in the respiratory tract, pancreas, gastrointestinal tract, liver/gallbladder, and genitourinary tracts
- Decreased clearance of viscid secretions causes obstruction of progressively larger airways starting with bronchioles
- Chronic airway inflammation and bacterial colonization damage airways. This progresses to bronchiectasis, bronchiectatic cysts, and emphysematous bullae. Loss of normal airway architecture causes secondary obstructive changes with air trapping and hyperinflation
- Long-term treatment goals aim to minimize lung damage and to maintain normal lung function as long as possible, and treatment of acute pulmonary exacerbations are directed at restoring lung function to pre-illness baseline

## CLINICAL MANIFESTATIONS

### Respiratory Tract

- Cough is the most consistent symptom
- *Infants and young children:* Tachypnea, chronic or recurrent episodes of wheezing, respiratory distress with crackles and wheeze, and/or nonproductive cough; recurrent lower respiratory tract infections; respiratory cultures grow *E. coli, Klebsiella pneumoniae, Staphylococcus aureus,* or *Haemophilus influenzae*
- *Older children and adolescents:* Progressive respiratory symptoms including mucopurulent cough worse in morning and with activity, exercise intolerance, recurrent wheezing, and hemoptysis (occasionally massive). Physical exam findings include increased anteroposterior chest diameter, thoracic hyperresonance, persistent crackles, wheezing, and digital clubbing. Respiratory cultures usually grow *Pseudomonas aeruginosa*
- Progressive lung pathology includes bronchiectasis, atelectasis, fibrosis, and occasionally pneumothorax. Right heart failure is usually a late consequence of chronic hypoxemia but can present secondary to acute respiratory failure
- Pansinusitis is common and chronic; acute sinusitis is less common
- Nasal polyps can be a presenting finding
- *Allergic bronchopulmonary aspergillosis (ABPA) can occur:*
  ✓ *Obstructive symptoms and fall in lung function tests that do not respond to aggressive antibiotic and airway clearance therapies. Major diagnostic features include:*
    ▪ Immediate skin test reactivity to Aspergillus antigens
    ▪ Precipitating serum antibodies to *Aspergillus fumigatus*
    ▪ Elevated serum total IgE concentration (>1000 ng/mL)
    ▪ Peripheral blood eosinophilia >500/mm$^3$
    ▪ Elevated specific serum IgE and IgG to *Aspergillus fumigatus*
    ▪ Chest radiograph demonstrates fleeting pulmonary infiltrates while chest CT imaging usually demonstrates central bronchiectasis
  ✓ Treatment for ABPA consists of a prolonged course of systemic corticosteroids and an antifungal agent
- Colonization with select genomovars of *Burkholderia cepacia* correlates with more rapid disease progression

## Gastrointestinal Tract

- *Obstructive symptoms due to paucity of intestinal water and large malabsorptive stools:* 15% of CF newborns present with no passage of stool in the first 24–48 hours of life, abdominal distention, bilious emesis, and meconium ileus. Infants can present with rectal prolapse in association with straining. Children and adolescents can present with constipation, emesis, abdominal distention, and abdominal pain; the constellation of symptoms is referred to as distal intestinal obstruction syndrome (DIOS)
- *Pancreatic insufficiency:* Most (90%) patients with CF have pancreatic insufficiency and suffer from intestinal malabsorption with associated fat-soluble vitamin (A, D, E, K) deficiencies. Recurrent pancreatitis can occur
- About 20% of adolescents and 40–50% of adults patients develop CF-related diabetes which shares features of both Type I and II diabetes
- *Biliary tract:* Persistent neonatal direct hyperbilirubinemia, obstructive biliary cirrhosis
- Failure to thrive
- *Physical exam:* Rectal prolapse, protuberant abdomen, decreased muscle mass, delayed Tanner staging, right lower quadrant stool mass, hepatosplenomegaly

## Genitourinary

- Average delay in sexual maturity of 2 years
- *Males:* Atretic epididymis, vas deferens and seminal vesicles secondary to failure of Wolffian development and inspissation of secretions; obstructive azoospermia and infertility; normal sexual function; higher incidence of anatomic defects including hernia and undescended testes
- *Females:* Increased rate of secondary amenorrhea with pulmonary exacerbations; tenacious cervical mucus leads to increased risk of cervicitis, but does not reduce fertility; pregnancy tolerance is correlated with lung function

## Metabolic Abnormalities

- Higher risk for acute salt and volume depletion with gastroenteritis or dehydration (hyponatremic dehydration) and chronic hypochloremic metabolic alkalosis due to increased losses of sodium and chloride in sweat
- History of "tasting salty" or salt crystallization on forehead

## DIAGNOSTICS

*Both history/physical findings AND laboratory confirmation are required to make the diagnosis of CF* (Table 27-1)

- Tests for abnormal CFTR are used to confirm a diagnosis in a patient with one or more clinical features consistent with the CF phenotype, a history of CF in a sibling, and/or a positive newborn screen
  - ✓ *Sweat test (by pilocarpine iontophoresis):* Sweat chloride concentration of >60 mmol/L on two separate occasions with adequate amounts (>100 mg) of sweat collected; values of 40–60 mmol/L are considered borderline and the test must be repeated
  - ✓ *Identification of two CF mutations:* Finding two CFTR mutations in association with clinical symptoms is diagnostic, but negative results on genotype analyses do not exclude the diagnosis
  - ✓ Nasal potential difference measurements
- Tests suggesting CF (these supporting findings need confirmation with a diagnostic test)
  - ✓ *Positive newborn screen:* Blood test for immunoreactive trypsinogen
  - ✓ Elevated fat content in 72-hour stool collection

| TABLE 27-1 | Diagnostic Criteria for Cystic Fibrosis (Patient must have at least one finding from each column) |
|---|---|
| **Patient History** | **Evidence of CTFR Gene Dysfunction** |
| 1. One or more characteristic phenotypic features. | 1. Elevated sweat chloride. |
| 2. Sibling with cystic fibrosis | 2. Identification of mutation in each CFTR gene known to cause cystic fibrosis. |
| 3. Positive newborn screen | 3. Characteristic abnormalities in ion transport across nasal epithelium. |

✓ Low Vitamin D, A, and E levels

✓ Prolonged prothrombin time and elevated Proteins Induced by Vitamin K Absence (PIVKA)

✓ *Semen analysis:* Obstructive azoospermia

✓ Ultrasound finding of congenital bilateral absence of the vasa deferentia

✓ Bronchoalveolar lavage fluid positive for *Pseudomonas aeruginosa*

✓ Sputum microbiology positive for *S. aureus* or *P. aeruginosa*, especially the mucoid form

• Data used to follow clinical course

  ✓ *Chest radiograph:* Hyperinflation, atelectasis, and peribronchial thickening are initial findings. Advanced findings include bowed sternum, cyst or nodule formation, extensive bronchiectasis, dilated pulmonary artery, pneumothorax, and scarring

  ✓ *Chest CT:* Not recommended for routine monitoring of disease status and progression, but can be considered if patient is not responding to appropriate therapy

  ✓ *Sinus CT:* Pan-opacification + failure of frontal sinus development

  ✓ *Pulmonary function testing:* Initially can be normal. Early changes indicate an obstructive pattern whereas advanced disease displays a combined obstructive and restrictive pattern due to fibrosis or marked air trapping. A decrease of 10% or more from baseline FEV1 may prompt hospital admission

• *Laboratory evaluation during an acute exacerbation:*

  ✓ Fluid balance, renal function, liver enzymes, glucose, magnesium (especially in patients with a history of frequent IV aminoglycoside use)

  ✓ Complete blood cell count with differential

  ✓ PT/international normalized ratio, PIVKA to rule out coagulation disorder secondary to vitamin K deficiency

  ✓ Aminoglycoside levels (after institution of therapy)

  ✓ Serum total IgE level if history of or concern for ABPA

  ✓ Consider vitamin and mineral levels (A, E, zinc, D-25OH)

  ✓ HgbA1c if signs or history of diabetes mellitus

  ✓ Obtain sputum culture, cough swab, or deep throat culture before starting antibiotics. Repeat sputum cultures on day 7 of admission

  ✓ Urinalysis to look for glucosuria, hematuria, proteinuria, and hypercalciuria

## Miscellaneous Diagnostics

• DEXA (bone density scan)

All patients over 18 years of age should have a DEXA scan and it should be repeated every 1–5 years depending on results

  ✓ *Obtain a DEXA if patient is >8 years of age and has any of the following:*

    ▪ Ideal body weight <90%

    ▪ Body Mass Index <50%

    ▪ FEV1 <50% predicted

- Glucocorticoid use of ≥5 mg/day for ≥90 days/year
- Delayed puberty
- Audiology exam (especially in those exposed frequently to aminoglycosides)

## MANAGEMENT

### Respiratory Management of Pulmonary Exacerbation

- *Antibiotics:* Empiric parenteral administration of two antipseudomonal antibiotics for 14–21 days (e.g., aminoglycoside and beta-lactam antibiotic such as tobramycin + imipenem, ticarcillin-clavulanate, or piperacillin-tazobactam). Specific therapy should be based on the identification and susceptibility testing of bacteria isolated from sputum
  - ✓ Administration of chronic aerosolized antibiotics (e.g., tobramycin, aztreonam, colistin) deliver high concentrations of medication directly to the site of infection and can reduce exacerbations, improve lung function and quality of life
  - ✓ Sputum culture should be obtained ideally at every visit, but at least quarterly, along with pulmonary function tests when the patient is able to perform them
- *Non-pharmacologic secretion clearance alternatives:*
  - ✓ Chest physiotherapy with postural drainage
  - ✓ High-frequency chest wall oscillation with an inflatable vest or airway oscillator
  - ✓ Intrapulmonary percussive ventilation
  - ✓ Positive expiratory pressure (PEP) device
  - ✓ Autogenic drainage, directed breathing techniques
- *Pharmacologic secretion clearance:*
  - ✓ Inhaled hypertonic saline can reduce the viscoelasticity of sputum
  - ✓ Inhaled human recombinant DNase can reduce the viscoelasticity of infected sputum
  - ✓ Bronchodilator therapy (beta-2-agonist) can increase ciliary beat frequency, and is also used if there is a history of airway hyperreactivity
- *Anti-inflammatory therapy:*
  - ✓ Azithromycin is used chronically for its anti-inflammatory effects to improve lung function and reduce number of exacerbations
  - ✓ Inhaled corticosteroids are only added when there is a concomitant history of asthma
  - ✓ Ibuprofen can be used as a chronic anti-inflammatory agent in children 6–17 years of age with FEV1 ≥60% predicted, and serum levels should be maintained 50–100 mg/mL
- *CFTR targeted therapy:*
  - ✓ Ivacaftor is a potentiator that activates defective CFTR at the cell surface. It is recommended for individuals with at least one G551D CFTR mutation to improve lung function and quality of life and reduce exacerbations. It also reduces sweat chloride concentrations to near normal levels
  - ✓ Combination therapy with ivacaftor/lumacaftor is approved for all patients who are homozygous for the F508del mutation, which constitutes nearly half of the CF population in the US. Lumacaftor is thought to improve CFTR protein folding and improve trafficking to the cell surface membrane. The combination therapy has been shown to improve FEV1 by up to 4% and more impressively, to reduce the rate of pulmonary exacerbations by nearly 40%

### Nutritional Management

- *Diet:* Most patients have increased caloric needs. Children and adolescents require a high calorie, high protein, and extra salt diet
  - ✓ Oral glucose tolerance test should be done annually after 8 years of age to screen for Cystic Fibrosis-related diabetes (CF-RD)
- Pancreatic exocrine enzyme replacement

✓ Doses should not exceed 2500 lipase units/kg/meal or 10,000 lipase units/kg/day to avoid fibrosing colonopathy and colonic strictures
- Vitamins A, D, E, and K in doses used for malabsorption

## HEMOPTYSIS

**The expectoration of blood or blood-tinged sputum from the lower respiratory tract. The immediate danger is from suffocation, not from exsanguination.**

- *Massive* or *Major:* >200 cc in 24 hours or >100 cc per day for several days
- *Minor:* Smaller volumes
- *Life threatening:* >8 cc/kg/24 hour

### PATHOGENESIS

**The lung contains two separate blood supplies**

- *The pulmonary arterial circulation:* High volume, low-pressure system. Its branches accompany the bronchi down to the level of the terminal bronchioles. Pulmonary vessels branch to supply the capillary bed in the walls of the alveoli and then return to the left atrium via the pulmonary veins
- *The bronchial circulation:* Small volume, systemic pressures. Typically there are three bronchial arteries, two that supply the left lung and one that supplies the right. These arteries usually originate from the aorta or the intercostal arteries and perfuse conducting airways approximately to the level of the terminal bronchioles

### ETIOLOGY

- *Minor hemoptysis:* Direct mucosal injury (e.g., shearing forces dislodging mucus from airway wall, direct trauma from suction catheters)
- *Massive hemoptysis:* Usually from bronchial artery (high-pressure system) to pulmonary artery anastomosis
- Infection is the most common etiology of hemoptysis in children
- Bleeding from tracheostomy
- Foreign body aspiration, especially long standing
- Congenital heart disease with pulmonary vascular obstruction or enlarged collateral bronchial circulation
- Cystic fibrosis (areas of bronchiectasis and inflammation)
- Bronchiectasis
- Tuberculosis
- Nasopharyngeal bleeding (non-pulmonary source of bleeding—not true hemoptysis)
- *Immune-mediated:* Henoch–Schönlein purpura, granulomatosis with polyangiitis, polyarteritis nodosa, Goodpasture syndrome, systemic lupus erythematosus
- *Less frequent:* An infected pulmonary sequestration, pulmonary embolism, tumor, neoplasm, pulmonary arteriovenous malformation, idiopathic pulmonary hemosiderosis

### DIAGNOSTICS

- Assess adequacy of ventilation
- Orthostatic pulse and blood pressure to estimate blood loss
- Chest radiograph
- CBC, PT, PTT
- *If indicated:* serum chemistries, BUN, creatinine, tuberculin skin test (purified protein derivative, PPD), rheumatologic markers including antinuclear antibody, double-stranded DNA,

ESR, CRP, complement levels, anti-neutrophil cytoplasmic antibodies, anti-basement membrane antibodies, IgG levels
- Urinalysis
- Sputum Gram stain and culture
- *Chest CT:* Can help define structural abnormalities including arteriovenous malformations or masses. Spiral CT may be useful if pulmonary embolus is suspected
- Angiography in cases of severe refractory hemoptysis
- *Fiberoptic bronchoscopy:* Performed when bleeding is not acute to identify a source of bleeding and obtain a lavage.
  - ✓ The presence of hemosiderin-laden macrophages from bronchoalveolar lavage confirms pulmonary bleeding; they typically appear 72 hours after the event and last for several weeks
- Rigid bronchoscopy is best for acute bleeding to suction large volumes and control the airway if necessary. Allows better visualization of the airway and removal of a foreign body
- Cardiac evaluation including echocardiogram with visualization of pulmonary veins

## MANAGEMENT

- Management is typically supportive except in the case of massive hemoptysis, and is otherwise directed at treating the underlying cause of bleeding
- Secure the airway and assure adequacy of ventilation; deliver increased PEEP
- Support circulating volume with crystalloid until red cell transfusion is possible
- In the case of massive hemoptysis, emergency bronchoscopy may be required. Sites of bleeding can be slowed by either balloon catheter tamponade or with the use of topical oxymetazoline, epinephrine, or cold saline
- If bleeding cannot be controlled, emergency arteriography may help to localize the area of bleeding and can allow selective embolization

## OBSTRUCTIVE APNEA

**Disorder of breathing during sleep characterized by prolonged partial upper airway obstruction and/or intermittent complete obstruction (obstructive apnea) that disrupts normal ventilation during sleep and normal sleep patterns.**

## EPIDEMIOLOGY

- Occurs at all ages, although may be more common in preschoolers
- Prevalence in school age children from 2% to 12%

## ETIOLOGY

- *Risk factors:* Adenotonsillar hypertrophy, obesity, craniofacial anomalies, neuromuscular disorders, trisomy 21, chronic lung disease, sickle cell disease

## CLINICAL MANIFESTATIONS

- Most common symptom of clinically significant OSA is snoring
- *Other common manifestations:* Labored breathing, restless sleep, apnea while asleep, enuresis, morning headaches, daytime sleepiness, sleeping with neck hyperextended, learning problems, attention-deficit/hyperactivity disorder
- *Severe presentations:* Cor pulmonale, failure to thrive, cognitive impairment
- *Possible exam findings:* Adenotonsillar hypertrophy, adenoidal facies, micrognathia/retrognathia, hypertension, loud pulmonary component of S2, underweight or overweight

## DIAGNOSTICS

- *Full polysomnography* requires overnight admission to a sleep laboratory. It is the only method that quantifies ventilatory and sleep abnormalities, therefore, it is the gold standard
  - ✓ Apnea hypopnea index (AHI) <1.5 events/h is normal, >10 events/h is severe. Severe OSA is not an acute emergency

## DEFINITIONS (BASED ON POLYSOMNOGRAPHIC FINDINGS)

### Obstructive Apnea

- Drop in the peak signal excursion by ≥90% of the pre-event baseline using an oronasal thermal sensor
  - ✓ Lasts at least two breaths during baseline breathing
  - ✓ Respiratory effort present throughout the entire period of absent airflow

### Hypopnea

- Peak signal excursions drop by ≥30% of pre-events baseline using nasal pressure
- Duration of the ≥30% drop lasts for at least two breaths
- Associated with ≥3% desaturation from pre-event baseline or the event is associated with an arousal

### Central Apnea

- *Drop in the peak signal excursion by ≥90% of the pre-event baseline using an oronasal thermal sensor and one of the following conditions:*
  - ✓ The event lasts 20 seconds or longer
  - ✓ The event lasts at least the duration of two breaths during baseline breathing and is associated with an arousal or ≥3% oxygen desaturation
  - ✓ For infants younger than 1 year of age, the event lasts at least the duration of two breaths during baseline breathing and is associated with a decrease in heart rate to less than 50 beats per minute for at least 5 seconds or less than 60 beats per minute for 15 seconds
  - ✓ *If full polysomnography is not available:* Nocturnal pulse oximetry, audio or videotaping, and abbreviated polysomnography or nap sleep study can be done. These all have weaker positive and negative predictive values than full nocturnal polysomnography so a normal study does not rule out sleep disordered breathing
- *Adjunctive tests:* ECG to evaluate for right ventricular hypertrophy; elevated serum bicarbonate reflects chronic hypoventilation

## MANAGEMENT

### Acute

- *Positioning:* Upright, sniffing position. In the case of hypotonia or tracheomalacia, prone positioning may relieve obstruction
- *Nasal airway:* Use preformed nasal trumpet or trimmed down endotracheal tube (ETT). Positive pressure can be delivered through a nasopharyngeal ETT
- *Antibiotics:* If acute infection
- *Anti-inflammatories:* May acutely help reduce swelling, consider dexamethasone.
  - ✓ Intranasal corticosteroids can be used as treatment for mild OSA
- Oxymetazoline nasal spray or nebulized racemic epinephrine can diminish intranasal or extrathoracic airway obstruction
- *Tracheal intubation/tracheostomy placement:* Reserved for refractory cases

## Chronic

- *Adenotonsillectomy:* First line of treatment for pediatric OSA
  - ✓ Reassess OSA signs and symptoms 6–8 weeks after surgery to determine if repeat polysomnogram indicated
- *Continuous positive airway pressure:* Used in patients with specific contraindications to adenotonsillectomy, minimal adenotonsillar tissue, persistent OSA after adenotonsillectomy or for those who prefer nonsurgical alternatives
- *Weight loss:* Improves OSA if patient is obese

## MECHANICAL VENTILATION AND PULMONARY ASSESSMENT

### BLOOD GAS INTERPRETATION

**Step 1: Acidemia or Alkalemia?**
- *Alkalemia:* pH greater than 7.40
- *Acidemia:* pH less than 7.40

**Step 2: Metabolic or Respiratory?**
- *Primary respiratory alkalosis:* pH greater than 7.40 and $PaCO_2$ less than 40
- *Primary metabolic alkalosis:* pH greater than 7.40 and $PaCO_2$ greater than 40
- *Primary respiratory acidosis:* pH less than 7.40 and $PaCO_2$ greater than 40
- *Primary metabolic acidosis:* pH less than 7.40 and $PaCO_2$ less than 40

**Step 3: Is the problem acute or chronic**
- For respiratory acidosis/alkalosis, a 10-mm Hg change in $PaCO_2$ causes a 0.08 change in pH in the acute setting or a 0.03 change in the chronic setting
- For metabolic acidosis/alkalosis, a 10-mEq/L change in $HCO_3^-$ causes a 0.15 change in pH
- For **acute** respiratory acidosis, expect an increase in $HCO_3^-$ of 1 mEq/L for every increase in $PaCO_2$ of 10 mm Hg
- For **acute** respiratory alkalosis, expect a decrease in $HCO_3^-$ of 1–3 mEq/L for every decrease in $PaCO_2$ of 10 mm Hg
- For **chronic** respiratory acidosis, expect an increase in $HCO_3^-$ of 4 mEq/L for every increase in $PaCO_2$ of 10 mm Hg
- For **chronic** respiratory alkalosis, expect a decrease in $HCO_3^-$ of 2–5 mEq/L for every decrease in $PaCO_2$ of 10 mm Hg

**Step 4: Is there a second primary problem?**

In other words, are changes in pH greater than expected from the primary disorder alone? Example: An infant with bronchopulmonary dysplasia is receiving diuretics and is hypochloremic with a pH of 7.42, $PCO_2$ 75, and $HCO_3^-$ 34. The blood gas values reflect not only the patient's chronic respiratory acidosis but also a **second primary** problem (i.e., hypochloremic metabolic alkalosis).

- A compensatory process alone *never* restores pH completely back to normal
- For metabolic acidosis, expect a decrease in $PaCO_2$ of 1–1.5 mm Hg for every decrease in $HCO_3^-$ of 1 mEq/L
- For metabolic alkalosis, expect an increase in $PaCO_2$ of 0.5–1 mm Hg for every increase in $HCO_3^-$ of 1 mEq/L

**Step 5: In metabolic acidosis, calculate the anion gap.**

$$\text{Anion Gap} = Na - (Cl + HCO_3^-)$$

- Normal anion gap is less than 12 mEq/L
- In normal gap metabolic acidosis, hyperchloremic acidosis results from the loss of $HCO_3$ in the gut or kidneys
- Anion-gap acidosis results from addition of nontitratable acid to the system. Etiologies include "MUDPILES": <u>M</u>ethanol, <u>U</u>remia, <u>D</u>iabetic ketoacidosis, <u>P</u>araldehyde/<u>P</u>ropylene glycol, <u>I</u>soniazid/<u>I</u>ron/<u>I</u>nfections, <u>L</u>actic acid<u>o</u>sis, <u>E</u>thanol, <u>S</u>alicylates

**Step 6: If there is an anion-gap metabolic acidosis you should consider the possibility of a second metabolic abnormality.**

- *This is done by calculating the delta–delta gap:*

$$\Delta - \Delta \ Gap = (Measured \ AG - Normal \ AG)/(Normal \ [HCO_3^-] - Measured \ [HCO_3^-])$$

- If $\Delta$-$\Delta$ Gap
  ✓ <1, there is a concurrent non-anion gap acidosis
  ✓ =1, there is a pure anion-gap acidosis
  ✓ >1, there is a concurrent metabolic alkalosis
  ✓ *Example:* A 12-year-old with diabetic ketoacidosis has an anion gap of 22, pH of 7.2, and an $HCO_3^-$ of 17
  ✓ *You calculate the $\Delta$–$\Delta$ gap:* $(22-12)/(24-17) = 1.4$. This tells you that there is a metabolic acidosis with a concurrent metabolic alkalosis (e.g., from vomiting) present

## HYPOXEMIA

### PULMONARY CAUSES OF HYPOXEMIA

- V/Q mismatch
- Hypoventilation
- Shunt
- Diffusion Block
- Low $FiO_2$

### ALVEOLAR-ARTERIAL GRADIENT (A-a GRADIENT)

- A measure of the difference between the alveolar and arterial concentration of oxygen. It is useful in determining the cause of hypoxemia (Table 27-2)

$$A\text{-a Gradient} = PAO_2 - PaO_2$$
$$PAO_2 = FiO_2(P_{atm} - P_{H_2O}) - (PaCO_2/R)$$

| TABLE 27-2 | Determining the Cause of Hypoxemia | | |
|---|---|---|---|
| | $PCO_2$ | Corrected with 100% $O_2$? | A-a Gradient |
| Hypoventilation | ↑ | Y | N |
| V/Q mismatch | ↑, N, or ↓ | Y | ↑ |
| Shunt | N or ↓ | N | ↑ |
| Diffusion block | N or ↓ | Y | ↑ |
| Low $PO_2$ | N or ↓ | Y | N |

where

$PAO_2$ = *partial pressure of oxygen in alveoli.*

$PaO_2$ = *partial pressure of* $O_2$ *measured in arterial blood. Normally 80–100 mm Hg.*

$PCO_2$ = *partial pressure of* $CO_2$ *measured in arterial blood. Normally 35–45 mm Hg.*

$P_{atm}$ *(atmospheric pressure: at sea level) approximately equal to 760 mm Hg, but will vary with altitude*

$P_{H_2O}$ *(water vapor pressure at 37°C)* = *47 mm Hg*

*R (respiratory quotient)* = *0.8 under normal circumstances*

*Normal A-a Gradient: <10 mm Hg*

## MECHANICAL VENTILATION

**A method to mechanically support/assist or replace spontaneous breathing.**

- Common indications for initiating mechanical ventilation are to improve alveolar ventilation, improve arterial oxygenation, prevent or reverse atelectasis, reverse hypoxemic or hypercarbic respiratory failure, and to prevent or reverse respiratory muscle fatigue
- Most ventilators use positive pressure to augment the work of the respiratory muscles, although negative pressure devices are still occasionally used
- A ventilator can use either *pressure control* (PC) or *volume control* (VC) to assist breathing
- *Pressure control:* The clinician sets the desired pressure to be delivered by the ventilator. The tidal volume varies from breath to breath depending on respiratory system compliance and resistance. The inspiratory flow depends on the pressure being delivered and how quickly the peak pressure is set to be achieved. The resulting flow pattern is one of decelerating flow. Because you are able to deliver a uniform pressure over a set inspiratory time, this mode is useful in children with a large leak around a tracheostomy tube or noninvasive interface
- *Volume control:* The clinician sets the volume of the breath to be delivered. Inspiratory flow rate can also be set by the operator; the flow is delivered with a square wave pattern (e.g., flow is constant) to a set tidal volume ($V_T$), allowing the pressure to vary as the compliance and resistance of the system changes
- Breaths are classified according to what triggers (starts) or cycles (stops) inspiration. These events can be either patient or ventilator initiated. Trigger variables include time, pressure, and flow. A few ventilators can also use abdominal movement or diaphragm EMG as trigger variables, but this is less common. Cycle variables can include pressure, volume, flow, or time
- If a positive pressure breath is triggered by the patient and cycled by the patient (or by the inherent mechanical characteristics of the patient's respiratory system as with Pressure Support) the breath is considered to be spontaneous
- If the ventilator triggers OR cycles a breath independent of the patient's effort or mechanics, the breath is considered to be mandatory

## THREE BASIC BREATH SEQUENCES OF A VENTILATOR

- *Intermittent mandatory ventilation (IMV):* Mandatory breaths are interspersed with breaths that are spontaneous. (This would include modes that are commonly referred to as intermittent mandatory ventilation [IMV], synchronized IMV [SIMV], SIMV with pressure support, or APRV)
- *Continuous spontaneous ventilation (CSV):* All breaths are spontaneous. (This would include modes like CPAP or CPAP with Pressure Support). *Pressure Support* (PS) is considered to be a pressure limited, flow or pressure triggered, and flow cycled spontaneous

breath. The breath is supported to a preset pressure by the ventilator and terminated based on characteristics of the patient's respiratory system. This mode enhances the patient's native respiratory drive, reducing respiratory work while allowing the patient to determine respiratory rate as well as the length and depth of breaths. Pressure support is often used in conjunction with mandatory ventilation as a tool for weaning
- *Continuous mandatory ventilation:* No breaths are spontaneous. (This would include modes that are commonly referred to as Control ventilation, Assist/Control ventilation)

## TYPES OF SUPPORTED VENTILATION (ALL BREATHS ARE SPONTANEOUS)

- *Continuous positive airway pressure (CPAP):* Supplies a constant airway pressure above atmospheric pressure during both inspiratory and expiratory phases of spontaneous ventilation. It is often used to overcome upper airway obstruction or to maintain FRC
- *Bi-level positive airway pressure (BLPAP):* Supplies both an inspiratory positive airway pressure (IPAP) and an expiratory positive airway pressure (EPAP). The patient triggers inspiration and cycle variables are set to end inspiration and allow exhalation. BLPAP can also be a form of assisted ventilation if a respiratory rate is set. It is often used to improve ventilation

## TYPES OF MANDATORY VENTILATION (*NO SPONTANEOUS BREATHS*)

- *High-frequency ventilation (high-frequency oscillatory ventilation [HFOV]):* Delivers low tidal volume breaths (1–3 mL/kg) at very high rates (3–15 Hz = 180–900 breaths per minute). HFOV settings are mean airway pressure, frequency (Hz), and amplitude or power. Indications include severe neonatal respiratory distress syndrome (RDS), ARDS, and severe air leak syndromes

## TYPES OF ASSISTED VENTILATION (MIXTURE OF MANDATORY AND SPONTANEOUS BREATHS)

- *Synchronized intermittent mandatory ventilation (SIMV):* The most frequently used mode of ventilation in most pediatric institutions. SIMV allows spontaneous breathing between ventilator breaths that are delivered in either PC or VC mode. Mechanical breaths can be programmed to trigger with patient-initiated breaths or independent of the patient's respiratory effort and are synchronized so as not to occur while the patient is exhaling
- *Pressure-regulated volume control (PRVC):* The delivered tidal volume is set by the practitioner, but the ventilator monitors both the volume delivered and the pressure used to deliver the breath. The pressure is adjusted from breath to breath to meet the targeted tidal volume. Flow is delivered with a decelerating wave form. This allows the ventilator to respond to changes in compliance and resistance in the system, thereby limiting volutrauma and barotrauma
- *Airway pressure release ventilation (APRV):* Allows spontaneous ventilation while maintaining mean airway pressure (MAP) with a high level of CPAP for a preset time (T high) and a "release" that intermittently drops the MAP to a lower CPAP level for a shorter period of time (T low). This is designed to open and maintain collapsed alveoli and enhance ventilation of lungs with poor compliance without excessive PIP

## INITIAL VENTILATOR SETTINGS

*The following should be used as a general guide:* Evaluation of the patient's response and care by physicians experienced with managing the mechanically ventilated child are critical to ensure the settings provide an appropriate level of support.

Initial settings depend on the age and indication.

- In patients with decreased lung or chest wall compliance, a short inspiratory time and higher pressure would be recommended to deliver a set $V_T$. Examples would include premature infants with RDS, or a child with severe interstitial lung disease
- In obstructive lung patterns where the time constant of the lung (the product of resistance and compliance) is long, a slow mandatory rate with a relatively short inspiratory time and longer expiratory time are recommended to allow adequate time for the lungs to empty before inspiration is initiated. Examples would include a child with asthma or patient with CF

## Conventional Ventilation

- *Mode:* In order to pick one of five main modes listed below (VC-continuous mandatory ventilation, VC-IMV, PC-continuous mandatory ventilation, PCIMV, and PC-CSV), you will need to decide if breaths will be mandated, spontaneous, or a combination of the two
- Continuous mandatory ventilation in pressure control (PC-continuous mandatory ventilation) or volume control (VC-continuous mandatory ventilation)
- Intermittent mandatory ventilation in pressure control (PC-IMV) or volume control (VC-IMV)
- Continuous spontaneous ventilation in pressure control (PC-CSV)
- *Mandated respiratory rate (per minute):* Typical starting ventilator rates assuming minimal spontaneous respiration: 30–40 neonates, 20–30 infants, 15–20 children. If allowing for the patient to take some spontaneous breaths, begin supporting at one-half to two-thirds of the normal respiratory rate for age
- *$FiO_2$:* Set at 1.0 (or last known effective $FiO_2$) and wean to desired $SpO_2$
- *Positive end-expiratory pressure (PEEP):* 3–5 cm $H_2O$ is considered "physiologic" and helps to maintain FRC. Neonates with severe lung disease may require much higher levels of PEEP to treat parenchymal disease or to support collapsible airways. Older children with ARDS may require PEEP of 12–15 cm $H_2O$ to recruit surfactant-deficient lung units and prevent injury from recruitment–derecruitment cycling
- *$V_T$:* Set to 8–12 mL/kg; if low tidal volume strategy is desired begin with 4–6 mL/kg as tolerated
- *$T_i$ (inspiratory time):* Neonates 0.3–0.4 seconds; infants 0.4–0.7 seconds; children 0.5–1.0 seconds. Shorter inspiratory times are favored in heterogeneous disease (e.g., ARDS, asthma)
- *I/E ratio:* 1:2, with longer E times in obstructive disease to prevent breath stacking and the development of dynamic hyperinflation
- *Positive inspiratory pressure:* In PC mode, set PC to achieve adequate chest wall movement and desired tidal volume

## High-Frequency Ventilation

- *Frequency:* Set at 10–15 Hz in neonates; may need 5–7 in severe ARDS
- *Mean airway pressure (MAP):* Set 1–4 cm $H_2O$ higher than that needed on conventional ventilation. Wean slowly once recruitment established
- *Amplitude:* Set to level with best chest wall movement

## ADJUSTING VENTILATOR SETTINGS

Ventilator settings are manipulated in order to minimize iatrogenic injury while providing adequate ventilation and oxygenation to support cellular function (Table 27-3).
- *Conventional ventilation:* To increase $CO_2$ exchange, increase either RR or $V_T$. To increase oxygenation, increase MAP or $FiO_2$. MAP increase can be achieved by increasing PEEP, PIP, or inspiratory time
- *High-frequency ventilation:* To increase $CO_2$ exchange, increase amplitude or decrease frequency. Increase oxygenation by increasing $FiO_2$ or MAP

| TABLE 27-3 Some Possible Effects of Ventilator Changes | | |
|---|---|---|
| **Change** | **PaCO$_2$** | **PaO$_2$** |
| ↑ RR | ↓ | No change or ↑ |
| ↑ PIP | ↓ | ↑ |
| ↑ PEEP | ↑, No change, or ↓ | ↑, No change, or ↓ |
| ↑ I time | ↓ | ↑, No change, or ↓ |
| ↑ FiO$_2$ | No change | ↑ |
| ↑ Amp | ↓ | No change |
| ↑ Hz | ↑ | No change |
| ↑ MAP | ↓ | ↑ |

## WEANING VENTILATION

The most common weaning modes are SIMV, PSV, and T-piece trials.

- *Weaning with SIMV:* Gradually wean rate of ventilator as the rate of spontaneous breaths increases. Once all breaths are spontaneous, consider supporting each breath to allow adequate oxygenation and ventilation. This method may increase the metabolic cost of breathing for the patient during the weaning process
- *Weaning with PSV (two options):*
  - ✓ Using SIMV mode with PSV, initiate short trials of only PSV, gradually lengthening the time off SIMV until the patient is maintained only on minimal PSV
  - ✓ Place patient on full PSV mode to produce a fully supported tidal volume. Gradually wean down the PSV until the patient is minimally supported. If tolerated, wean off support

## INDICATORS OF READINESS TO WEAN

*Negative inspiratory force (NIF):* Measures maximum negative deflection during inspiration after occlusion of airway. Used to assess adequacy of spontaneous breaths. A NIF less than $-15$ cm H$_2$O in an adult has 97% sensitivity for weaning failure. There is, however, poor positive predictive value for this test in children.

- *Measured vital capacity:* Adequate vital capacity is 10–15 mL/kg
- *Spontaneous tidal volume:* At least 4 mL/kg
- Able to maintain PaO$_2$ greater than 60 mm Hg in FiO$_2$ less than 0.35
- *Respiratory rate:* Physiologic (lack of rapid shallow breathing); in adults, a respiratory frequency/tidal volume (in liters) ratio <105 during a spontaneous breathing (T-piece) trial is associated with weaning success (rapid shallow breathing index)
- *Rapid shallow breathing index (RSBI):* RSBI adapted for children (*see formula listed below*) of 8 or less has both a sensitivity and specificity of 74% in predicting successful extubation in some studies. In children, RSBI occasionally used in clinical practice

$$\text{RSBI} = \text{RR(breaths}/min)/V_{_T}\,(\text{mL/kg})$$

## PULMONARY FUNCTION TESTS

**Pulmonary function tests (PFTs) are used to diagnose, assess severity, and assess response to therapy in pulmonary disease. To assess reversible airway obstruction or**

bronchodilator responsiveness, the patient is given an inhaled bronchodilator and the test is repeated. Histamine, methacholine, exercise, isocapneic cold dry air, and hypertonic or hypotonic aerosol challenges may also help assess airway reactivity.

## SPIROMETRY

- *Forced vital capacity (FVC):* Volume that can be maximally forcefully exhaled after a complete inspiration
- *FEV1:* Volume of air that is forcefully exhaled in the first second following a complete inspiration
- *FEV1/FVC:* Ratio of FEV1 to FVC, expressed as a percentage
- *FEV 25–75:* Average forced expiratory flow over the mid portion of the FVC
- *Peak expiratory flow (PEF):* Peak expiratory flow rate during forced exhalation

## LUNG VOLUMES (FIGURE 27-1)

A *volume* is the amount that describes a compartment of the lung; when two or more volumes are added together, the new amount is called a *capacity*. All volumes except the residual volume (RV) can be measured by spirometry; any capacity that includes the RV requires specialized equipment for its measurement.

- *Expiratory Reserve Volume (ERV):* Volume that can still be exhaled following normal exhalation
- *Functional residual capacity (FRC):* Volume remaining in the lungs at the end of normal exhalation (RV + ERV)
- *Inspiratory capacity (IC):* Volume in the lungs at full inspiration (IRV + $V_T$)
- *Inspiratory reserve volume (IRV):* Volume that can still be inhaled after normal inspiration
- *Residual volume (RV):* Volume remaining in the lungs after maximal expiration (FRC-ERV, or TLC-VC)
- *Tidal volume ($V_T$):* Volume inhaled and exhaled during normal breathing

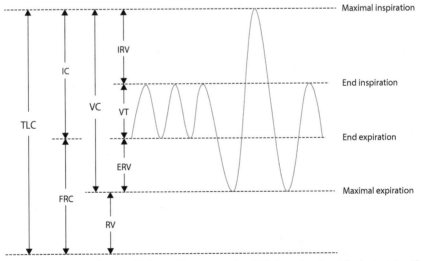

**FIGURE 27-1 Lung volumes.** TLC, total lung capacity; FRC, functional residual capacity; IC, inspiratory capacity; VC, vital capacity; RV, residual volume; IRV, inspiratory residual volume; VT, tidal volume; ERV, expiratory reserve volume.

- *Total lung capacity (TLC):* Total volume of gas in the lungs at full inspiration (VC + RV, or IC + FRC, or IRV + $V_T$ + ERV + RV)
- *Vital capacity (VC):* Maximal volume that can be expired from a full inspiration (IRV + TV + ERV; TLC-RV)

## EQUIPMENT COMMONLY USED TO MEASURE LUNG FUNCTION

- *Body plethysmograph:* Apparatus for measurement of FRC, RV, TLC, and airway resistance. Fractional lung volumes can also be measured with dilution techniques using helium or nitrogen
- *Spirometer:* Apparatus for measuring lung volumes (except RV) and flow rates. Spirometry is used to plot a volume–time curve and a flow–volume loop

## ANTHROPOMETRIC MEASUREMENTS AFFECTING LUNG FUNCTION

- *Height:* Taller individuals have larger lung volumes and airways
- *Age:* Lung volumes change with increasing age in the pediatric population; RV and FRC increase, ERV decreases
- *Sex:* Males have larger lung volumes than females
- *Ethnicity:* TLC is generally lower in African Americans when compared to Caucasians because African Americans have smaller upper-to-lower body segment ratios

## OBSTRUCTIVE LUNG DISEASE

Obstruction to airflow during expiration leads to gas trapping, increased RV, decreased, increased, or normal VC, and increased to normal TLC (Figure 27-1). Common causes include asthma, bronchiolitis, chronic bronchitis, CF, and bronchiectasis. Spirometry demonstrates a low FEV1 (<80% predicted), low FVC (<80% predicted), low FEV1/FVC (<75% predicted), decreased FEF 25–75, and an expiratory flow–volume curve that is concave to the volume axis (Figure 27-2B).

- Small airway obstruction is represented by low FEV 25–75
- Significant response to bronchodilators defined as >12% increase in the FEV1 and/or FVC
- Methacholine challenge that results in a decrease in FEV1 20% or greater from baseline at a dose less than 16 mg/dL, or exercise or cold dry air challenge that results in 15% or greater decrease in FEV1 from baseline are used to diagnose airway hyperreactivity

## RESTRICTIVE LUNG DISEASE

Restrictive lung diseases cause reductions in lung volumes due to decreased lung compliance, decreased chest wall compliance, or muscle weakness. Etiologies include interstitial lung disease, neuromuscular diseases, and chest wall or spine abnormalities. TLC is decreased whereas flow rates are proportionally normal or slightly increased. Spirometry reveals a low FEV1 (<80% predicted), low FVC (<80% predicted), normal FEV1/FVC ratio, and "miniaturized" appearance to flow–volume curve (Figure 27-2C).

## VARIABLE EXTRATHORACIC OBSTRUCTION

During inhalation, narrowing of the extrathoracic airway accentuates any obstruction, and airflow through the narrowed portion of the extrathoracic airway decreases. This results in flattening of the inspiratory flow–volume loop (Figure 27-2D). If the narrowing is not present during exhalation, the expiratory flow–volume curve is normal. Spirometry reveals a normal FVC and FEV1, but the ratio of forced expiratory to inspiratory flow at 50% of vital capacity (FEF50/FIF50) is usually greater than 1. Etiologies include vocal cord dysfunction or vocal cord paralysis.

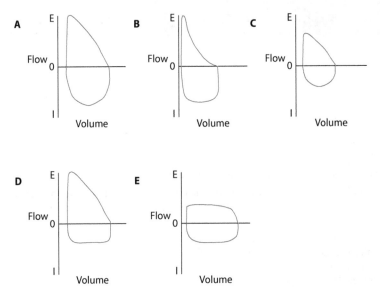

**FIGURE 27-2 Flow–volume loops.** A. Normal flow–volume loop. During expiration (E), the normal loop can be straight or slightly convex to the volume (x-) axis. B. Obstructive flow–volume curve. During expiration, the expiratory loop is concave toward the volume axis. A normal peak flow (as in this case) does not preclude an obstructive process. C. Restrictive flow–volume curve. The flows are normal when corrected for low lung volumes. D. Variable extrathoracic obstruction. The expiratory loop remains normal, but there is flattening of the inspiratory loop. E. Fixed obstruction. Both the expiratory and inspiratory loops reach a plateau at low flows.

## FIXED AIRWAY OBSTRUCTION

There is no change in the caliber of the airway with a fixed intrathoracic or extrathoracic obstruction during the entire respiratory cycle. As a result, airflow limitation through the obstruction is independent of the phase of respiration and results in flattening of both inspiratory and expiratory flow–volume loops (**Figure 27-2E**). Etiologies include tumors, tracheal or subglottic stenosis, and foreign bodies in the airway.

# Rheumatology 28

Elaine Ramsay, MD
Alysha Taxter, MD
Jon Burnham, MD, MSCE

## DERMATOMYOSITIS/JUVENILE DERMATOMYOSITIS (JDM)

### DEFINITION

**Most common pediatric inflammatory myopathy.**

**Bohan and Peter diagnostic criteria** (definite JDM: heliotrope rash or Gottron's papules plus at least three criteria; probable JDM: heliotrope rash or Gottron's papules plus two criteria)

- Heliotrope rash (eyelids) or Gottron's papules (extensor surfaces)
- Progressive symmetric proximal muscle weakness
- Elevated skeletal muscle enzymes (CK, AST, aldolase, LDH)
- EMG consistent with myopathy
- Biopsy evidence of myositis
- Updated criteria will likely include muscle abnormalities on MRI STIR or T2 sequence

### EPIDEMIOLOGY

- *Incidence:* About 2–3 cases/million children
- Peaks at 6 years and 11–12 years of age; female:male is 2:1
- Comparable for blacks and whites, lower in Hispanics
- Unlike in adults, JDM has no definite associations with malignancy

### ETIOLOGY

- *Potential infectious triggers:* Group A beta-hemolytic *Streptococcus*, coxsackie virus B, parvovirus, others
- HLA and TNF-$\alpha$ alleles may predispose a child to JDM
- Molecular mimicry is suspected
- Sun exposure may trigger onset of rash

### DIFFERENTIAL DIAGNOSIS

- *Rheumatologic:*
  - ✓ Juvenile polymyositis is rare in children (2–8% of inflammatory myopathies), has similar age and sex distribution as JDM but includes proximal and distal weakness, muscle atrophy, lacks skin abnormalities, and calcinosis is rare
  - ✓ Systemic lupus erythematosus (SLE) and related conditions (e.g., mixed connective tissue disease, Sjögren syndrome)
  - ✓ Scleroderma
  - ✓ Juvenile idiopathic arthritis (JIA); polyarticular or systemic
  - ✓ Polyarteritis nodosa
  - ✓ Eosinophilic fasciitis
- *Infectious:*
  - ✓ *Viral myopathies:* Influenza A and B, coxsackie, Epstein–Barr virus, herpes, parainfluenza, adenovirus, enterovirus
  - ✓ *Bacterial and parasitic myopathies:* Staph, strep, toxoplasma

- *Metabolic/Genetic:*
  - ✓ Muscular dystrophies
  - ✓ Congenital myopathies
  - ✓ Myotonic disorders
  - ✓ Glycogen storage diseases
  - ✓ Periodic paralysis
  - ✓ Endocrinopathies
- *Other:*
  - ✓ Trauma
  - ✓ Toxins
  - ✓ Drug-induced myopathies
  - ✓ Disorders of neuromuscular transmission

## PATHOPHYSIOLOGY

- Perivascular inflammation, mostly mononuclear cells
- Swelling and blockage of capillaries, tissue infarction, perifasicular atrophy
- Chronic inflammation ensues with fibrosis and microscopic calcification

## CLINICAL MANIFESTATIONS

- *Proximal muscle weakness (neck flexors, shoulders, abdomen, thighs):* Gower sign, difficulty climbing stairs or combing hair
- *Skin:* Heliotrope rash (violaceous rash of eyelids); facial erythema, possibly in malar distribution; papulosquamous eruption on extensor surfaces (Gottron's rash), particularly over interphalangeal joints (Gottron's papules); shawl sign (erythematous rash in a shawl distribution); cutaneous calcinosis and ulceration
- *Nailfolds:* Capillary drop-out, capillary dilation, cuticular hypertrophy
- *Arthritis:* Effusions, limited range of motion, pain, deformity
- *Mucocutaneous:* Oral ulcers, gingival inflammation
- *Pulmonary:* Shortness of breath, cough, crackles can be consistent with interstitial lung disease or aspiration pneumonia
- *Gastrointestinal:* Dysphagia, ulceration, perforation, bleeding, constipation, diarrhea, abdominal pain
- *Other manifestations:* Lipodystrophy, polyneuropathies, retinal exudates, and cotton wool patches
- *Other complications:* Calcinotic lesions may spontaneously drain causing local inflammatory response and superinfection; can form exoskeleton; vasculitic ulcers; rare arrhythmias and cardiomyopathy; complications of chronic corticosteroid exposure (growth failure, hypertension, vertebral compression fractures, striae, avascular necrosis, cataracts, glaucoma)

## DIAGNOSTICS

- *CBC:* Lymphopenia, anemia of chronic inflammation; iron deficiency anemia should raise concern for gastrointestinal blood loss
- *ESR and CRP:* Normal or high
- *Elevated muscle enzymes:* Creatine kinase, aldolase, AST, LDH
- *ANA:* Positive in 10–85% of cases; rheumatoid factor: negative
- *Neopterin and vWF antigen:* Elevations correlate with disease activity
- Anti-RNP (may indicate SLE overlap), anti-PM-SCL (associated with SLE or scleroderma), anti-Jo1 (associated with interstitial lung disease), anti-Mi2 (associated with lung disease)

- Urinalysis to rule out renal involvement (may indicate SLE overlap)
- MRI with T2 or STIR weighted images of muscles: Localizes active disease sites
- *Chest x-ray:* Evaluate for infiltrates
- *High resolution chest CT:* Evaluate for interstitial lung disease
- *Modified barium swallow:* Detect palato-esophageal dysfunction
- *Plain films:* Detect calcinosis, soft tissue, and muscle edema
- *ECG:* May see arrhythmias
- *ECHO:* may detect cardiomyopathy
- *Muscle biopsy:* Myositis, perifascicular necrosis with degenerating and regenerating fibers
- *EMG:* Fibrillations, insertional irritability
- *Pulmonary function tests:* Respiratory muscle weakness or interstitial lung disease cause a restrictive pattern

## MANAGEMENT

- *Mild disease:* Corticosteroids (2 mg/kg/day then taper), methotrexate, +/− hydroxychloroquine if a significant rash is present
- *Moderate–severe disease:* Add pulse corticosteroids (methylprednisolone 30 mg/kg/day, up to 1000 mg) × 3 then oral (2 mg/kg/day then taper), IVIG (2 g/kg IV every 3–4 weeks)
- *Refractory disease:* If active disease persists on a maximal regimen including methotrexate, IVIG, and hydroxychloroquine, other agents such as cyclophosphamide, rituximab, calcineurin inhibitors (cyclosporine A, tacrolimus), intermittent pulse methylprednisolone, and abatacept can be considered
- *Interstitial lung disease:* Cyclophosphamide, pulse corticosteroids
- *Sunscreen:* Minimum SPF 30 with UVA and UVB protection
- *Nutritional supplements:* Vitamin D and calcium
- *Calcinosis:* Decreased with early aggressive therapy, case reports of successful therapy with a variety of agents including bisphosphonates
- Physical and occupational therapy
- *Immunizations:*
  ✓ No live vaccines for individuals on high-dose systemic corticosteroids or other immunosuppressive agents
  ✓ Administer inactivated influenza (annually) and pneumococcal vaccines
  ✓ Delay MMR until 11 months after last IVIG treatment if not otherwise contraindicated (e.g., on other immunosuppressants)

## HENOCH–SCHÖNLEIN PURPURA (HSP)

### DEFINITION

**Small vessel vasculitis affecting the skin, joints, GI tract, and kidneys. EULAR/PRINTO/ PRES 2010 criteria: Purpura or petechiae (mandatory) with lower limb predominance and at least one of the four following criteria: abdominal pain, histopathology, arthritis or arthralgia, or renal involvement.**

### EPIDEMIOLOGY

- Most common childhood vasculitis in the United States
- *Age range:* 3–15 years; peak: 7 years
- *Incidence:* 3–17/100,000
- Typically occurs during winter preceded by upper respiratory tract infection

## DIFFERENTIAL DIAGNOSIS

- *Rheumatologic:*
  ✓ SLE and related conditions
  ✓ ANCA-associated vasculitis
  ✓ Hypersensitivity vasculitis
  ✓ Cryoglobulinemia
  ✓ Urticarial vasculitis
  ✓ Polyarteritis nodosa
  ✓ Sarcoidosis
- *Hematologic/Oncologic:*
  ✓ Immune thrombocytopenic purpura
  ✓ Leukemia
  ✓ Hemophagocytic lymphohistiocytosis
  ✓ Lymphoma
- *Infectious/Post-infectious:*
  ✓ Sepsis
  ✓ Viral and bacterial enterocolitis
  ✓ Post-streptococcal glomerulonephritis
  ✓ Hemolytic-uremic syndrome
- *Gastrointestinal:*
  ✓ Crohn's disease
  ✓ Ulcerative colitis
  ✓ Meckel diverticulum, polyps, lymphoid hyperplasia can cause intussusception

## PATHOPHYSIOLOGY

- Small vessel vasculitis affecting capillaries and pre- and post-capillary vessels
- Mediated by immune complexes (typically IgA, can see IgG and activated complement C3) which are deposited in end-organs causing inflammation
- May be associated with antecedent respiratory infection (group A beta-hemolytic streptococcus, mycoplasma, parvovirus, other viral pathogens)

## CLINICAL MANIFESTATIONS

- Classic presentation includes non-thrombocytopenic purpuric rash, musculoskeletal pain, and colicky abdominal pain
- *Rash:* Most common presenting symptom
  ✓ Non-blanching, purpuric lesions developing in gravity- or pressure-dependent areas, usually distal to the elbows and below the waist
  ✓ Early lesions may appear erythematous, petechial, or urticarial, evolving into hemorrhagic or ecchymotic lesions
  ✓ Lesions may ulcerate
  ✓ Koebner phenomenon may occur (lesions appear at sites of skin injury)
- *Musculoskeletal pain:* Second most common manifestation; symptoms may be persistent or intermittent
  ✓ Periarticular or articular pain with impaired mobility and minimal joint warmth and effusion, typically affecting the ankles, knees, elbows, wrists, digits
- *Gastrointestinal pain:* Occurs in 2/3 of children within a week of rash onset; abdominal pain, hemorrhage, intussusception, bowel perforation possible; presents with colicky pain, vomiting, loose stool, melena, hematemesis; hepatosplenomegaly may be present

- *Renal involvement:* Occurs in 1/3 of patients and usually develops within the first 4–6 weeks; may lead to end-stage renal disease
  - ✓ Manifestations include microscopic or macroscopic hematuria with or without proteinuria, hypertension, glomerulonephritis, ureteritis, urethritis, and cystitis
- *Rare manifestations:*
  - ✓ *GU:* Scrotal swelling/hemorrhage mimicking testicular torsion, testicular torsion (rare)
  - ✓ *CNS:* Headache, seizures, hemorrhage, cerebrovascular thrombosis, focal deficits, and peripheral neuropathies
  - ✓ *Pulmonary:* Interstitial disease, alveolar hemorrhage, and respiratory failure
  - ✓ *CV:* Carditis, myocardial infarction
- *Vital signs:* Low-grade fevers; hypertension due to renal disease; tachycardia due to anemia or pain
- *Duration of symptoms:* Average 4 weeks if untreated, chronic HSP is unusual
- *Recurrence:* Up to 33%, usually within the first year after diagnosis

## DIAGNOSTICS

- WBC (normal to slightly elevated); Hgb (normal to slightly low); platelet count (normal to elevated); PT/PTT (normal)
- *ESR and CRP:* Normal to elevated
- *BUN and creatinine:* Normal or possibly elevated with renal disease or volume depletion
- *Albumin:* Decreased with proteinuria and gastrointestinal losses, malnutrition, and inflammation
- *Urinalysis:* Proteinuria and/or hematuria; RBC casts
- *Stool:* May be hemoccult positive
- *Immunological:*
  - ✓ ANCA should be negative in HSP. If ANCA is positive, consider granulomatosis with polyangiitis (c-ANCA, positive anti-proteinase 3), and microscopic polyangiitis or rarely, Churg–Strauss (p-ANCA, anti-myeloperoxidase)
  - ✓ Elevated IgA levels in 50% (not routinely sent)
  - ✓ Cryoglobulins should be negative (not routinely sent)
- Abdominal x-ray barium studies, ultrasound, and CT may be useful for assessment of abdominal obstruction and intussusception
- *Skin biopsy:* May aid diagnosis in non-classic presentations; light microscopy demonstrates leukocytoclastic vasculitis and IgA deposition on immunofluorescence
- *Renal biopsy:* Useful if proteinuria/hematuria is significant or does not resolve; crescentic glomerulonephritis with IgA deposition may be seen
- *Arthrocentesis:* Perform, if necessary, to exclude infectious arthritis

## MANAGEMENT

- Tylenol for analgesia; avoid NSAIDs if GI or renal involvement
- Monitor for hypertension; hematuria and proteinuria should present within 6 months
- *Corticosteroids:* Indicated for renal involvement, abdominal and musculoskeletal pain
  - ✓ For mild or moderate disease consider prednisone or methylprednisolone 2 mg/kg/day up to 60 mg/day for 1 week with 2-week taper
  - ✓ For severe disease, consider pulse methylprednisolone up to 30 mg/kg/day (maximum 1000 mg/day) up to 3 days then prednisone 2 mg/kg/day up to 60 mg/day for 1 week with a 2-week taper
- Immunosuppressive therapy (cyclophosphamide, azathioprine, methotrexate) should be considered in patients with complicated nephritis, pulmonary, cutaneous, and/or CNS manifestations

- *Supportive care:* Severe pain may require narcotics. Severe GI involvement may require NPO status, NG suction, and TPN, though response to corticosteroids is often dramatic with prompt initiation of therapy

## JUVENILE IDIOPATHIC ARTHRITIS (JIA)

### DEFINITION

**Chronic synovial inflammation of unknown etiology with onset prior to 16 years of age and leading to arthritis in one or more joints for at least 6 weeks. The 2001 International League Against Rheumatism (ILAR) criteria for JIA include seven specific subtypes.**

- *Oligoarthritis:* Arthritis involving one to four joints during the first 6 months of disease. Persistent oligoarthritis affects no more than four joints throughout the course of disease. Extended oligoarthritis affects more than four joints after the first 6 months of disease
- *Polyarthritis (rheumatoid factor negative):* Involvement of five or more joints during the first 6 months of disease; rheumatoid factor test is negative
- *Polyarthritis (rheumatoid factor positive):* Involvement of five or more joints during the first 6 months of disease; two rheumatoid factor tests are positive at least 3 months apart during the first 6 months of disease
- *Enthesitis-related arthritis:* Arthritis and enthesitis (tenderness where a tendon inserts into a bone); or arthritis or enthesitis with at least two of the following: sacroiliac tenderness or inflammatory lumbosacral pain, HLA-B27 positive, onset of arthritis in a male greater than 6 years old, acute (symptomatic) anterior uveitis, history of ankylosing spondylitis, enthesitis-related arthritis, sacroiliitis with inflammatory bowel disease, reactive arthritis, or acute anterior uveitis in a first-degree relative
- *Psoriatic arthritis:* Arthritis and psoriasis, or arthritis with two of the following: dactylitis, nail pitting or onycholysis, or psoriasis in a first-degree relative
- *Systemic arthritis:* Arthritis in one or more joints with or preceded by a fever of 2 weeks' duration with a quotidian fever for at least 3 days plus at least one of the following: evanescent (non-fixed) erythematous rash, generalized lymphadenopathy, hepatomegaly, and/or splenomegaly, or serositis
- *Undifferentiated arthritis:* Arthritis that does not fulfill the above criteria based on subtype-specific exclusion criteria or fulfills criteria in two or more of the above categories

### EPIDEMIOLOGY

- Most common chronic childhood rheumatologic disease
- Sex distribution is subtype-specific
- *Incidence:* 1–20/100,000 in children less than 16 years old
- *Proportion of arthritis subtypes:* Oligoarthritis (50–80%), polyarthritis (20%, of which 85% are rheumatoid factor negative), enthesitis-related arthritis (1–7%), psoriatric arthritis (1–11%), systemic arthritis (5–15%)

### ETIOLOGY

- Genetic and environmental factors suspected
- HLA associations exist
- Associated with immunodeficiencies: IgA deficiency, 22q11 deletion
- Link between infectious triggers and arthritis is not fully established

### DIFFERENTIAL DIAGNOSIS OF CHRONIC ARTHRITIS

- Critical to distinguish acute from chronic arthritis as a first step

- Other rheumatic and inflammatory diseases such as inflammatory bowel disease, sarcoidosis, SLE, and vasculitis can present with an acute or chronic oligo- or polyarthritis with or without fever
- *Oligoarthritis:* Trauma, reactive arthritis, septic arthritis, Lyme disease, foreign body, leukemia, bone or synovial tumor, Legg–Calve–Perthes disease, slipped capital femoral epiphysis, pigmented villonodular synovitis, cystic fibrosis arthropathy, congenital arthropathies, metabolic disorders such as gout
- *Polyarthritis:* Serum sickness, reactive arthritis, septic arthritis (*Neisseria* spp.), parvovirus B19 infection
- *Systemic arthritis:* Kawasaki disease, leukemia, lymphoma, primary hemophagocytic lymphohistiocytosis or secondary to infection or malignancy (e.g., lymphoma), septic arthritis, Lyme disease, Epstein–Barr virus, parvovirus B19, *Bartonella henselae*, mycoplasma, acute rheumatic fever, periodic fever syndromes such as neonatal-onset multisystem inflammatory disease, Langerhans cell histiocytosis, chronic recurrent multifocal osteomyelitis, Kikuchi disease, Castleman disease

## PATHOPHYSIOLOGY

- Synovitis with villous hypertrophy and hyperplasia
- T-cell activation and recruitment into joint synovium leads to release of pro-inflammatory cytokines by multiple cell types
- Pannus formation in late disease, causing progressive erosion of cartilage and bone
- Systemic arthritis is currently considered to be an autoinflammatory condition with interleukin 1 being a key mediator

## CLINICAL MANIFESTATIONS

- *General:* Fatigue, low- or high- grade fevers, anorexia, weight loss, failure to thrive, limp, joint swelling (may be asymptomatic) with morning stiffness, hepatosplenomegaly, pain with inactivity, evanescent urticarial rash, lymphadenopathy
- *Oligoarthritis:* Usually involves knees, ankles, fingers, wrists, elbows; systemic symptoms unusual
- *Polyarthritis:* May involve large and small joints, spares distal interphalangeal joints
- *Systemic arthritis:* High fevers 1–2 times/day for at least 2 weeks, temperature often returns to normal or subnormal accompanied by erythematous macular rash on trunk and proximal limbs; serositis (pericarditis and/or pleuritis); pericardial tamponade may ensue
- *Musculoskeletal:* Swelling/effusion; limited range of motion (including decreased cervical-spine motion); warmth; contracture/deformity; +/− limb length discrepancies and wasting of surrounding muscles (gastrocnemius or quadriceps)
- Arthritis of temporomandibular joint may cause failure to thrive secondary to pain. Micrognathia or jaw deviation may ensue
- *Ophthalmologic:* Pupil irregularities, synechiae, band keratopathy due to anterior uveitis; may lead to visual loss, cataract, glaucoma; uveitis is most common in ANA positive young females
- Macrophage activation syndrome (MAS)/secondary hemophagocytic lymphohistiocytosis is a potentially life-threatening complication seen with systemic arthritis
  - ✓ Symptoms may include unremitting fever, hepatosplenomegaly, lymphadenopathy, bruising, mucosal bleeding, respiratory distress, encephalopathy, and renal involvement progressing to multi-system organ failure
- *Other complications:* Fractures, pseudoporphyria with NSAID use, if untreated can have contractures and limb-length discrepancy

## DIAGNOSTICS

- No laboratory test can confirm the diagnosis of chronic arthritis
- *ESR and CRP:* Normal or high in oligoarthritis or polyarthritis; high with systemic arthritis
- *CBC:* Leukocyte count normal or high; platelets may be elevated
- *ANA:* Highest in younger girls, rarely positive in systemic arthritis; positive ANA associated with increased risk for developing uveitis in subtypes other than systemic arthritis
- *Rheumatoid factor:* Positive in minority of patients with polyarthritis, useful for prognostic purposes only
- *Urinalysis:* Abnormal results may suggest alternative diagnosis
- *Joint fluid aspirate:* Usually 2000–50,000 WBC/mm$^3$ (but may be higher); neutrophils may predominate; glucose normal to slightly low; elevated protein
- Radiologic studies are helpful to rule out other disease processes such as tumors and to establish baseline for evaluation of joint erosions
- If cervical-spine range of motion limited, order cervical lateral flexion and extension spinal films to assess for atlantoaxial instability and subaxial ankylosis prior to surgery, intubation, sports participation
- *Macrophage activation syndrome/secondary hemophagocytic lymphohistiocytosis:* Fall in WBC and platelets, anemia, elevated liver enzymes, hypofibrinogemia, elevated D-dimer, prolonged PT and PTT, hypertriglyceridemia, hyperferritinemia, low ESR, evidence of macrophage hemophagocytosis on bone marrow biopsy

## MANAGEMENT

- *Oligoarthritis:* Treatment of choice is intra-articular corticosteroid injections; NSAIDs (e.g., naproxen 20 mg/kg/day, divided twice per day) for symptomatic relief; if no response to intra-articular corticosteroid injections or manifestations are severe, then use methotrexate and/or biologic therapy
- *Polyarthritis:* Intra-articular corticosteroids, methotrexate, TNF-α inhibitors (e.g., etanercept, adalimumab, infliximab), CTLA-4 Ig (abatacept), IL-6 inhibitor (tocilizumab). Rheumatoid factor positive has poor prognosis and necessitates aggressive therapy
- *Systemic arthritis:* Corticosteroids, IL-1 inhibitors (anakinra or canakinumab), IL-6 inhibitor, cyclosporine (particularly with refractory MAS), intra-articular corticosteroids; cyclophosphamide for refractory disease
- *Regular ophthalmology exams:* Slit-lamp exam to diagnose asymptomatic uveitis
  - ✓ Frequency is every 3–6 months initially, depending on age at onset and ANA status, except in systemic arthritis, in which every 12-month screening is adequate
- *Dietary evaluation:* Ensure adequate calcium, vitamin D
- *Physical and occupational therapy:* To maintain and improve joint function and motion
- *Immunizations:*
  - ✓ Avoid live vaccines (varicella, MMR, intra-nasal influenza) for individuals on high-dose systemic corticosteroids or immunosuppressants
  - ✓ Administer inactivated influenza (annually) and pneumococcal vaccines

## KAWASAKI DISEASE

### DEFINITION

**An acute, febrile vasculitis of childhood defined by at least 5 days of fever and greater than or equal to four of the following: Conjunctivitis, mucous membrane changes,**

**peripheral extremity changes, polymorphous rash, or cervical adenopathy. Incomplete Kawasaki disease may present with fewer than four criteria and coronary artery disease. It is more common in infants less than 6 months old.**

## EPIDEMIOLOGY

- *Incidence:* United States: about 12 per 100,000; Japan: about 112 per 100,000
- Median age = 2 years; 80% of cases occur before 5 years of age and 95% before 10 years
- Recurrence <1% in the United States but 3% in Japan
- Children <1 year have increased likelihood of developing coronary artery aneurysms

## DIFFERENTIAL DIAGNOSIS

- *Viral:*
  ✓ Measles
  ✓ Epstein–Barr virus
  ✓ Adenovirus
  ✓ Enterovirus
  ✓ Parvovirus B19
- *Bacterial:*
  ✓ Scarlet fever
  ✓ Staphylococcal scalded skin syndrome
  ✓ Toxic shock syndrome
  ✓ *Yersinia pseudotuberculosis*
  ✓ Typhoid fever
  ✓ Leptospirosis
  ✓ Rocky Mountain spotted fever
- *Allergic:*
  ✓ Drug reaction
  ✓ Serum sickness
  ✓ Stevens–Johnson syndrome
- *Rheumatologic:*
  ✓ Systemic arthritis
  ✓ Polyarteritis nodosa
  ✓ Reactive arthritis
- *Toxic:*
  ✓ Mercury poisoning

## PATHOPHYSIOLOGY

- Vasculitis of medium-sized arteries
- Edema of endothelial and smooth muscle cells; inflammatory infiltration of vascular wall
- The etiology is unknown, but it may be due to a superantigen stimulation of immune system in genetically susceptible hosts
- Up to 1/3 have an identified infection

## CLINICAL MANIFESTATIONS

- *Three phases:* Acute febrile phase (7–14 days), subacute phase (14–24 days), and convalescent phase (>24 days)
- *Fever:* High (can be >40°C) and spiking
- *Conjunctival injection:* Bilateral, bulbar (Limbic-sparing), generally non-purulent and painless

- *Peripheral extremity changes:* Edema ("sausage-like" digits), erythema; desquamation 2–3 weeks after fever onset
- *Mucous membrane changes:* Injected oropharynx, dry fissured, peeling, cracking lips, strawberry tongue
- *Polymorphous rash:* May be maculopapular, urticarial, scarlatiniform, erythema multiforme, prominence in groin area and groin desquamation may occur by end of first week
- *Cervical adenopathy:* ≥1.5 cm, generally unilateral and may be tender
- *Coronary artery aneurysms:* Develop in 15–25% of patients not treated within 10 days of onset, but in fewer than 5% of treated patients
- *Other manifestations:* Extreme irritability, aseptic meningitis, cranial nerve palsy, transient sensorineural hearing loss, myocarditis, valvular disease, pleural effusions, gallbladder hydrops, hepatitis, jaundice, hepatosplenomegaly, abdominal pain, vomiting, diarrhea, arthralgias, arthritis of small and large joints, urethritis, uveitis, testicular swelling

## DIAGNOSTICS

- Elevated ESR and CRP
- *CBC:* WBC normal or leukocytosis (WBC >15,000/mm³ in 50%); normocytic anemia; thrombocytosis (platelet count up to 1,000,000/mm³) after first week
- Mildly elevated ALT, AST, GGT, bilirubin, alkaline phosphatase but low albumin (<3 g/dL)
- *Urinalysis:* Sterile pyuria in 70% (>10 leukocytes/hpf), catheter sample may miss urethritis
- *CSF:* Pleocytosis with lymphocyte predominance in 25–50% of patients who undergo LP
- *Chest x-ray:* May show pneumonitis, pleural effusion, cardiomegaly
- *ECG:* May show arrhythmia, ischemia, low voltages or ST-segment or T-wave changes
- *Echocardiogram:* Perform at time of diagnosis; may reveal coronary artery ectasia or aneurysms, pericardial effusion, valvular abnormalities, or diminished ventricular function
- *Slit-lamp exam:* Anterior uveitis is common (>85% of patients)
- *Arthrocentesis:* Synovial fluid WBC 50–300,000/mm³, normal glucose, negative Gram stain and culture

## MANAGEMENT

- *Intravenous immunoglobulin (IVIG):* 2 g per kg over 10–12 hours; if still febrile after approximately 36 hours, may consider a repeat dose of 2 g per kg particularly if there is concern for persistent active disease
- *Aspirin:* 80–100 mg/kg/day divided into four oral doses; when afebrile for 48 hours, decrease dose to 3–5 mg/kg daily as a single oral dose for 6–8 weeks. Discontinue aspirin if follow-up echocardiogram and ESR are normal
- *Corticosteroids:* Conflicting clinical trial data on routine addition of corticosteroids to IVIG. Generally not recommended except in refractory cases (i.e., prednisone or methylprednisolone for persistent symptoms after two doses of IVIG)
- Refractory cases with persistent fevers
  ✓ Systemic corticosteroids
  ✓ Anti-TNF drugs such as infliximab
- *Anticoagulants:* Dipyridamole, clopidrogel, warfarin, or low molecular weight heparin, and abciximab can be used for the treatment of coronary aneurysms
- *Other:* Therapeutic apheresis and cyclophosphamide have been examined but data are lacking regarding their role in treatment
- *Disposition:* Close follow-up with pediatric cardiologist. Repeat echocardiogram is routinely performed 6–8 weeks after treatment and depending on the presence of coronary aneurysms

• *Immunizations:* Defer measles and varicella vaccinations for 11 months following high-dose IVIG. Those on long-term salicylate therapy should have an annual influenza vaccination

## RHEUMATIC FEVER

### DEFINITION

**Post-infectious manifestation of group A streptococcal (GABHS) pharyngitis. The diagnosis is based on the Jones criteria** (Table 28-1)

• Should be distinguished from post-streptococcal reactive arthritis, a GABHS-associated reactive arthritis that does not fulfill Jones criteria, and is less likely to cause cardiac disease

### EPIDEMIOLOGY

• Most common in 5–15 year olds
• Annual incidence was less than 1/100,000 until the mid to late 1980s when new outbreaks occurred. Outbreaks are common in overcrowded areas of people with low socioeconomic status
• Carditis more common in young children
• Arthritis more common in adults

### ETIOLOGY

• Usually develops 2–3 weeks following an *untreated* GABHS pharyngitis

### DIFFERENTIAL DIAGNOSIS

• *Bacterial:*
  ✓ Septic arthritis
  ✓ Lyme arthritis
  ✓ Reactive arthritis (including post-streptococcal)
  ✓ Osteomyelitis
  ✓ Endocarditis
  ✓ Mycoplasma pneumonia
• *Viral:*
  ✓ Parvovirus
  ✓ EBV

| TABLE 28-1 | Jones Criteria of Rheumatic Fever | |
|---|---|---|
| **2 Major or 1 Major and 2 Minor PLUS Evidence of Prior GABHS Infection** | | |
| **Major** | **Minor** | **Evidence of Prior GABHS Infection** |
| Carditis | Arthralgias | Throat culture |
| Erythema marginatum | Elevated acute phase reactants (ESR and CRP) | Anti-streptolysin O (ASO)[†] |
| Polyarthritis* | Fever | Anti-deoxyribonuclease B (DNase B) |
| Subcutaneous nodules | Prolonged PR interval | |
| Sydenham chorea | | |

*Can by migratory.
†Peaks at 2–3 weeks.
*Exceptions: Chorea as sole manifestation, indolent carditis; if recurrent need one major or greater than one minor criteria.*

- *Rheumatologic:*
  - ✓ Systemic arthritis
  - ✓ Kawasaki disease
  - ✓ Systemic lupus erythematosus
  - ✓ Antiphospholipid syndrome (primary or secondary)
  - ✓ Behçet disease
- *Immunologic:*
  - ✓ Serum sickness
- *Neurologic:*
  - ✓ Hereditary disorders such as juvenile Huntington disease
  - ✓ Wilson disease
  - ✓ Benign hereditary chorea
  - ✓ Inborn errors or metabolism
  - ✓ Nutritional or electrolyte disturbance
  - ✓ Arteriovenous malformation
- *Oncologic:*
  - ✓ Leukemia
  - ✓ Lymphoma
- *Hematologic:*
  - ✓ Sickle cell arthropathy

## PATHOPHYSIOLOGY

- Immune complexes may cause nondestructive synovitis and reversible reactions in basal ganglia that cause chorea
- Extracellular GAS toxin may target organs such as the heart and brain
- Autoimmunity and cell-mediated cytotoxicity may cause valvular inflammation

## CLINICAL MANIFESTATIONS

- *Arthritis:* Migratory and/or additive, typically affects knees, ankles, elbows; joints may be swollen, warm, tender, limited range of motion; joint involvement more severe and common in teenagers
- *Subcutaneous nodules:* Firm and painless; over extensor surfaces of joints, occipital region, thoracic or lumbar spinous processes
- *Erythema marginatum:* Pink/red blanching rash with raised borders, central clearing, not pruritic or indurated; may worsen with fever
- *Carditis:* Affects mitral valve and aortic valve most commonly. It is a pancarditis that involves the endocardium, myocardium, and pericardium but congestive heart failure, if present, is most commonly due to valvular dysfunction
- *Chorea:* Involuntary, purposeless movements; associated with muscle weakness and emotional lability usually disappears over weeks to months; rarely recurs. "Milkmaid sign": patient's grip strengthens and weakens

## DIAGNOSTICS

- *Evidence of prior infection:* Increased antistreptolysin O, anti-DNase B, positive throat culture, recent history of scarlet fever
- *ESR and CRP:* Usually elevated acutely
- *CBC:* Normocyctic, normochromic anemia
- *Blood culture:* Should be negative
- *Joint fluid:* Sterile, WBC count may be in septic range

- *X-rays of affected joints:* Normal or effusion present
- *Chest x-ray:* May see cardiomegaly
- *ECG:* May see heart block (usually 1st degree)
- *Echocardiogram:* May see mitral and/or aortic valve thickening and regurgitation. Stenotic lesions are associated with chronic valve disease in rheumatic fever

## MANAGEMENT

- GABHS infection treatment (10 days duration)
  - ✓ Penicillin
  - ✓ Erythromycin or other macrolide antibiotic
  - ✓ Clindamycin
  - ✓ Cephalexin
- GABHS prophylaxis
  - ✓ Penicillin G benzathine every 4 weeks
    - Less than 27.3 kg: 600,000 units
    - Greater than or equal to 27.3 kg: 1.2 million units
  - ✓ Penicillin V 250 mg twice per day
  - ✓ Sulfadiazine or sulfisoxazole
    - Less than or equal to 27 kg: 0.5 g daily
    - Greater than 27 kg: 1 g daily
  - ✓ Macrolide if allergic to penicillin and sulfonamide
  - ✓ Duration
    - *Without carditis:* Treat for 5 years after last episode or until age 21, whichever is longer
    - *With carditis:* Treat for 10 years after last episode or until age 21, whichever is longer
    - *With carditis and valvular disease:* Treat for 10 years after last episode or until age 40, whichever is longer. Lifelong prophylaxis may be needed if risk of exposure is high
- *Aspirin:* 90–100 mg/kg/day divided 4 times per day for arthritis and carditis. Naproxen may be used for isolated joint disease
- Corticosteroid therapy may be used in cases of acute carditis and congestive heart failure (prednisone 2 mg/kg/day divided twice per day with slow taper or pulse dosing with methylprednisolone 30 mg/kg/day up to 1000 mg daily for 3 days) if critically ill
- *Chorea:* Diazepam, haloperidol, valproic acid, corticosteroids

## SYSTEMIC LUPUS ERYTHEMATOSUS (SLE)

### DEFINITION

**A multisystem autoimmune disease caused by pathologic production of autoantibodies and tissue deposition of immune complexes, and characterized by global immune dysregulation.**

### EPIDEMIOLOGY

- 15–25% present in first two decades of life, often after puberty
- Female:male = 9:1 after puberty and before menopause, otherwise 3:1
- African American:Caucasian = 3:1
- *Incidence:* 2–8 per 100,000; prevalence: 15–50 per 100,000

### ETIOLOGY

- Genetic predisposition (HLA haplotype associations)
- Immune system dysregulation

- Environmental stimuli (UV light, drugs, herpes virus infections, diet)
- Hormonal factors
- Apoptosis abnormalities

## DIFFERENTIAL DIAGNOSIS

- *Rheumatologic:*
  - ✓ Drug-induced lupus
  - ✓ Cutaneous lupus
  - ✓ Mixed connective tissue disease
  - ✓ Sjögren syndrome
  - ✓ Juvenile dermatomyositis
  - ✓ Scleroderma
  - ✓ JIA (systemic arthritis, polyarthritis)
  - ✓ Henoch–Schönlein purpura
  - ✓ Granulomatosis with polyangiitis
  - ✓ Microscopic polyangiitis
  - ✓ Churg–Strauss syndrome
  - ✓ Hypersensitivity vasculitis
  - ✓ Cryoglobulinemia
  - ✓ Polyarteritis nodosa
  - ✓ Kawasaki disease
  - ✓ Takayasu arteritis
  - ✓ Sarcoidosis
  - ✓ Primary antiphospholipid syndrome
  - ✓ IgG4-related disease
- *Hematologic:*
  - ✓ Thrombotic thrombocytopenic purpura
  - ✓ Immune thrombocytopenic purpura
  - ✓ Autoimmune hemolytic anemia
  - ✓ Evan syndrome
  - ✓ Aplastic anemia
- *Immunologic:*
  - ✓ Common variable immunodeficiency
- *Oncologic:*
  - ✓ Leukemia
  - ✓ Lymphoma
  - ✓ Malignancies metastatic to marrow or causing pleural or pericardial effusions
- *Lymphoproliferative:*
  - ✓ Autoimmune lymphoproliferative syndrome
  - ✓ Castleman disease
- *Cardiac:*
  - ✓ Viral or bacterial pericarditis
  - ✓ Autoinflammatory disease such as Familial Mediterranean Fever
- *Renal:*
  - ✓ Membranoproliferative glomerulonephritis
  - ✓ Minimal change disease
  - ✓ Focal segmental glomerulosclerosis
  - ✓ Tubulointerstitial nephritis

- *Gastroenterologic:*
  - ✓ Autoimmune hepatitis
  - ✓ Inflammatory bowel disease
  - ✓ Celiac disease
  - ✓ Protein-losing enteropathy
- *Endocrine:*
  - ✓ Hypothyroidism
- *Viral:*
  - ✓ Epstein–Barr virus
  - ✓ Cytomegalovirus
  - ✓ Enterovirus
  - ✓ Parvovirus B19
  - ✓ Viral hepatitis
  - ✓ Viral encephalitis
- *Bacterial:*
  - ✓ Lyme disease
  - ✓ Ehrlichiosis
  - ✓ Rocky Mountain Spotted Fever
  - ✓ *Bartonella henselae*
  - ✓ Acute rheumatic fever

## PATHOPHYSIOLOGY

- Autoantibodies are directed against nuclear and cytoplasmic antigens. Organ-specific antibodies to cell surface antigens are also present
- Disease can be secondary to pathogenic autoantibodies (renal disease, thrombocytopenia, antiphospholipid antibody syndrome, neonatal lupus and fetal loss, CNS disease), pathogenic immune complexes (secondary to quantity and size, and tissue tropism), and T lymphocyte dysregulation (skin disease)

## CLINICAL MANIFESTATIONS

Many children have nonspecific symptoms for months before diagnosis, often presenting with fatigue, malaise, easy bruising, arthritis, rash, Raynaud phenomenon, lymphadenopathy, and weight loss before other characteristic findings.

- *Mucocutaneous:* Malar rash, discoid rash, alopecia, photosensitivity, palatal ulceration (usually painless), Raynaud phenomenon, digital ulceration, or vasculitic rash
- *Musculoskeletal:* Arthralgia and arthritis are frequent at presentation. Arthritis is often polyarticular and non-erosive. Myositis may be seen, particularly in cases of mixed connective tissue disease
- *Pleuropulmonary:* Pleural effusion, pneumonitis, interstitial lung disease, shrinking lung syndrome, pulmonary hemorrhage, pulmonary embolus. Consider infection as a cause of pulmonary infiltrates in patients with SLE, particularly when immunocompromised
- *Cardiovascular:* Pericardial effusion, Libman–Sacks endocarditis, myocarditis, myocardial infarction
- *Gastrointestinal:* Hepatosplenomegaly, hepatitis, mesenteric vasculitis, pancreatitis, colitis. Esophageal dysmotility and reflux may be seen as part of mixed connective tissue disease
- *Renal:* Presentation of nephritis is variable and may cause hypertension and edema. It may be associated with interstitial nephritis and renal vein thrombosis

- *Neurologic:* Cognitive dysfunction, seizures, and psychosis are common. Also seen are severe headache, catatonia, chorea, ataxia, stroke (thrombotic or hemorrhagic), cranial nerve palsy, peripheral neuropathy, transverse myelitis. Neuropsychiatric testing may confirm cognitive impairment
- *Hematologic:* Anemia of chronic inflammation, autoimmune hemolytic anemia, microangiopathic hemolytic anemia, thrombocytopenia, and leukopenia (usually lymphopenia), secondary hemophagocytic lymphohistiocytosis, thrombosis (due to secondary antiphospholipid syndrome)
- *Ocular:* Retinal vasculitis, episcleritis, uveitis, optic neuritis, and sicca syndrome secondary to secondary Sjögren syndrome
- *Endocrine:* Autoimmune thyroid disease, short stature, delayed puberty, bone fragility
- *Neonatal lupus:* Congenital heart block, hepatitis, alloimmune cytopenias, erythema annulare

## DIAGNOSTICS (TABLE 28-2)

### Initial Evaluation

- *CBC:* Thrombocytopenia, anemia, leuko/lymphopenia. The following must be used to evaluate for the presence of autoimmune hemolytic anemia:
  - ✓ Peripheral smear: Schistocytes would suggest thrombotic microangiopathy rather than autoimmune hemolytic anemia
  - ✓ Reticulocyte count
  - ✓ Direct antiglobulin test (Coomb's test)
  - ✓ LDH
  - ✓ Bilirubin
- *Metabolic panel:* Elevated creatinine, hypoalbuminemia suggests renal disease with proteinuria; may see hepatitis
- *Urinalysis:* Proteinuria, cellular casts suggests nephritis, gross hematuria suggests renal vein thrombosis
- Amylase/lipase if significant abdominal pain present

**TABLE 28-2** American College of Rheumatology Criteria for the Diagnosis of Systemic Lupus Erythematosus

### Need 4 of 11 Criteria for the Diagnosis (at once or sequentially)

Malar rash

Discoid rash

Oral or nasopharyngeal ulceration (usually painless)

Photosensitivity

Non-erosive arthritis

Serositis (pleuritis or pericarditis)

Renal disorder (persistent proteinuria >0.5 g/day or cellular casts)

Neurologic disorder (seizures or psychosis)

Hematologic disorder (hemolytic anemia with reticulocytosis, leukopenia less than 4000/mm³, lymphopenia less than 1500/mm³, thrombocytopenia less than 100,000/m³)

Immunologic disorder (presence of anti-double stranded DNA, anti-Smith, anti-cardiolipin antibody [IgM or IgG], lupus anticoagulant, false positive RPR)

Antinuclear antibody

- *Complement:* Low CH50, C3, C4
- *ANA profile:* ANA rarely negative in an SLE patient
  - ✓ Anti-double stranded DNA is specific for SLE and suggests renal disease
  - ✓ Anti-Smith is SLE-specific
  - ✓ Anti-ribonuclear protein (RNP) is seen in SLE and in mixed connective tissue disease (high titer)
  - ✓ Anti-SCL 70 is seen in scleroderma and overlap syndromes
  - ✓ Anti-SSA and SSB are seen in Sjögren syndrome
  - ✓ Anti-Jo1 raises suspicion for interstitial lung disease in a variety of autoimmune disorders
- Antiphospholipid syndrome laboratory evaluation
  - ✓ Need an elevated functional lupus anticoagulant (PTT or dilute Russell viper venom time), anticardiolipin antibody or anti-β2-glycoprotein-1 antibody of IgG and/or IgM isotype on one or more occasions at least 12 weeks apart
  - ✓ Thrombosis (clinical or biopsy evidence) or recurrent fetal loss are required to fulfill criteria for antiphospholipid syndrome
- Renal biopsy if significant proteinuria (greater than 1 g/24 hours or a urine protein/creatinine of greater than or equal to 1.0), hematuria, cellular casts, hypertension, or renal function impairment
  - ✓ Allows for characterization of nephritis and choice of therapy based on WHO classification
- Biopsy of skin rash if diagnostic precision required
- Arthrocentesis and culture if concerned about septic arthritis
- Blood culture if febrile. Patient may be functionally immunosuppressed secondary to hypocomplementemia and/or immunosuppressive medications
- Chest x-ray and PFTs if clinical concerns
- ECG and echocardiogram for baseline evaluation or if indicated clinically
- Brain imaging, EEG, and/or lumbar puncture may be required if focal CNS exam, severe headaches, psychiatric symptoms
  - ✓ In addition to routine CSF studies, CSF anti-neuronal antibodies, oligoclonal bands, and IgG synthesis rate are useful. Anti-neuronal antibodies have fair sensitivity and specificity for neuropsychiatric disease. In neuropsychiatric disease: oligoclonal bands may be positive (not specific) and IgG synthesis rate may be increased (evaluated using the IgG index: (CSF IgG/serum IgG)/(CSF albumin/serum albumin))
  - ✓ Serum anti-ribosomal P may be associated with psychosis

## MANAGEMENT

### Pharmacological Management

- Tailor to symptoms and balance benefits of therapy with adverse effects
- *Corticosteroids:* For ongoing disease activity
  - ✓ Initial dose is up to 2 mg/kg/day or 60–80 mg/day with a taper over 3–6 months, usually to maintenance dose or off as tolerated
  - ✓ Life- or organ-threatening disease: High dose (pulse) corticosteroids (30 mg/kg/day up to 1000 mg IV daily for 3 days)
- *Cyclophosphamide:* For severe organ-specific complications such as neuropsychiatric disease and proliferative glomerulonephritis
- *Azathioprine or mycophenolate mofetil:* For maintenance of renal remission or steroid sparing
- *Rituximab (chimeric monoclonal antibody to CD20 on B cells):* For severe, refractory disease or immune cytopenias

- *Belimumab (human antibody targeting B cell activating factor):* Recently approved for treatment, may be helpful in SLE patients in combination with standard therapy
- *Methotrexate:* For arthritis, refractory cutaneous disease, or immune thrombocytopenia
- *IVIG:* For immune thrombocytopenia or autoimmune hemolytic anemia
- *Therapeutic apheresis:* For severe, life-threatening disease such as thrombotic thrombocytopenic purpura or pulmonary hemorrhage
- *NSAIDs:* For arthralgia, arthritis, myalgia, serositis, headache. Use with care in individuals with renal disease
- *Hydroxychloroquine (antimalarial):* For dermatitis, constitutional symptoms, arthralgia, arthritis; regular ophthalmologic exams needed
- *Topical or intralesional steroids:* For skin lesions
- *Angiotensin-converting enzyme inhibitor or angiotensin receptor blocker:* For hypertension and/or proteinuria
- *Low-dose aspirin:* For lupus anticoagulant or presence of antiphospholipid antibodies
- *Anticoagulation:* For thrombotic event (DVT, pulmonary embolus, arterial thrombus, recurrent fetal loss)

## Health Maintenance

- Monitor serum cholesterol, LDL, HDL, and triglycerides
- Encourage regular exercise, weight loss, smoking cessation, and low-fat diet
- Calcium and vitamin D are recommended for patients on chronic corticosteroids. Regular DEXA scans to monitor bone density
- *Obstetric/Gynecologic:* Avoid estrogen-containing oral contraceptives particularly if antiphospholipid antibodies or lupus anticoagulant are present; awareness of neonatal lupus risk, particularly in patients positive for anti-Ro/SSA and anti-La/SSB
- Sun avoidance and protection (minimum SPF 30 with UVA/B protection)—this can flare the disease
- Avoid live vaccines if taking immunosuppressive medications
- Influenza and pneumococcal vaccination are recommended
- Specialized nursing, social work, physical and occupational therapy, psychology, and nutritional counseling

# Surgery

*Jesse D. Vrecenak, MD*
*Michael L. Nance, MD*

## NEONATAL SURGERY

### CONGENITAL DIAPHRAGMATIC HERNIA

**Disorder characterized by pulmonary hypoplasia due to intrauterine compression of the developing lungs by herniated viscera.**

#### EPIDEMIOLOGY

- Incidence is 1000 per year (1:2000–1:5000 live births); female:male 2:1
- 7–10% gestations end in fetal demise
- Defects more common on left side (about 80%)
- Associated with anomalies (10–35%) including: Central nervous system (CNS) lesions, tracheobronchial abnormalities, omphalocele, cardiovascular (CV) lesions, skeletal and syndromes (trisomy 13, 18, 21, Beckwith–Weidemann, Brachmann–de Lange, and Pallister–Killian, among others)

#### ETIOLOGY

- Unknown currently, though several pharmacologic and environmental factors have been implicated, including a possible role for vitamin A deficiency and/or retinoid regulated gene defects
- *Embryologic theory:* Lack of closure of the posterolateral pleuroperitoneal canals in the 8th week of gestation fails to separate the thoracic and abdominal cavities
- Portions of the diaphragm and pulmonary parenchyma arise from thoracic mesenchyme and if disrupted may lead to absence of part of hemidiaphragm and pulmonary hypoplasia
- Most cases are sporadic; familial cases occur (2%)

#### DIFFERENTIAL DIAGNOSIS

- Cystic adenomatoid malformation, cystic teratoma, pulmonary sequestration, bronchogenic cyst, neurogenic tumors, primary lung sarcoma, diaphragmatic eventration

#### PATHOPHYSIOLOGY

- Herniation of abdominal contents into thoracic cavity through posterolateral foramen of Bochdalek
- Diaphragmatic defect may be small or may include entire hemidiaphragm
- Pulmonary vasculature has increased muscularization of pulmonary arterioles and decreased branching of vessels resulting in pulmonary hypertension
- Lungs are hypoplastic due to chronic compression, with decreased numbers of bronchial branches on both ipsilateral and contralateral sides

#### CLINICAL MANIFESTATIONS

- Most patients present with respiratory distress within the first hours of life secondary to severe pulmonary hypoplasia and associated pulmonary hypertension
- 10–20% may have delayed presentation characterized by less severe pulmonary hypoplasia and pulmonary hypertension, as well as gastrointestinal (GI) symptoms (e.g., vomiting, abdominal pain, constipation)

- Pneumothorax
- *On exam:* Absence of breath sounds; bowel sounds in chest; scaphoid abdomen; increased anterior-posterior diameter of chest; shifted heart sounds

## DIAGNOSTICS

- Prenatal ultrasound able to detect defect as early as 11th week, mean gestational age (GA) at diagnosis is 24 weeks; accuracy has been reported to be between 40 and 90%
- Antenatal diagnosis is associated with more severe defects and a worse prognosis; if diagnosed by ultrasound, fetal MRI should be performed
- During fetal period, a lung-head ratio (LHR, area of contralateral lung to fetal head circumference by ultrasound) of <1 indicates severe disease
- Observed-to-expected LHR (O/E LHR) accounts for changes in LHR with GA, and O/E LHR <25% suggests severe CDH
- Echocardiography and amniocentesis to detect other anomalies
- Chest x-ray

## MANAGEMENT

### Initial Medical Management

- Initial resuscitation includes correction of hypoxia, hypercarbia, acidosis, and hypothermia as they increase pulmonary vascular resistance and worsen pulmonary hypertension
- Intubate early to avoid inflation of the stomach with bag-mask ventilation
- Nasogastric decompression to decrease bowel distension
- Umbilical arterial and venous lines should be placed in severe cases
- Peripheral oxygen saturations and/or blood gases should be obtained to determine adequacy of gas exchange
- Echocardiography to determine cardiac anomalies and determine severity of pulmonary hypertension and shunting
- Permissive hypercapnia and gentle ventilation may improve survival and decrease need for extracorporeal membrane oxygenation (ECMO); avoid paralysis
- Surfactant has not been clearly shown to improve outcomes
- Response to nitric oxide is inconsistent
- Persistent right-to-left shunting may require ECMO

### Surgical Management

- Repair typically performed "electively" (age 3–15 days) when/if clinically stable
- Abdominal surgical approach most common. Large defects may require the use of a synthetic patch or muscle flap. Minimally invasive approaches (both laparoscopic and thoracoscopic) have been utilized successfully in selected candidates
- In-utero reduction and repair have been successfully performed but have not consistently shown to benefit survival. Trials of fetoscopic tracheal occlusion are underway

### Prognosis

- Poor prognosis seen with "liver up" CDH, associated major anomaly, symptoms prior to 24 hours, distress requiring ECMO, delivery in nontertiary center and bilateral defects
- Survival 60–97% with initial stabilization, then surgical repair
- Long-term sequelae may include neurodevelopmental problems, gastroesophageal reflux, nutritional deficiencies, skeletal anomalies, and bronchopulmonary dysplasia
- CDH lungs never reach normal alveolar number or structure, leading to persistent risk of emphysema, pneumonia, bronchiolitis, and pulmonary hypertension

## ESOPHAGEAL ATRESIA AND TRACHEOESOPHAGEAL FISTULA

**Anatomic lesions, which may be congenital or acquired and involve a blind pouch of the esophagus, are often associated with a fistula to the trachea.**

### EPIDEMIOLOGY

- Esophageal atresia seen in 1:2500–4500 live births
- 90% of infants with esophageal atresia have an associated tracheoesophageal fistula (TEF)
- Associated with trisomy 18 or 21, DiGeorge, Feingold, Pierre Robin and Potter syndromes, among others
- 30% of affected infants are born prematurely
- *Associated anomalies in greater than 50%:* Musculoskeletal (rib and vertebral anomalies), cardiovascular, GI (duodenal atresia, intestinal malrotation), GU (choanal atresia): *VATER* association (Vertebral and Vascular, Anal, Tracheal, Esophageal, Radial, Renal) or *VACTERL* association (Vertebral, Anal, Cardiac, Tracheal, Esophageal, Renal, Limb), CHARGE association (Coloboma, Heart disease, choanal Atresia, Retarded growth and development, Genital hypoplasia, and Ear anomalies)

### PATHOPHYSIOLOGY (FIGURE 29-1)

- *Esophageal atresia with distal TEF:* Most common type (>85% cases). Proximal esophagus is dilated and thickened, and ends around level of third thoracic vertebra. Fistula at distal esophageal segment enters back wall of lower trachea (Figure 29-1)
- *Pure esophageal atresia (without TEF):* 3–5% of cases. Proximal esophageal pouch ends around third thoracic vertebrae and distal pouch is usually short
- *Isolated TEF without atresia:* 3–6% of cases. "H"-type fistula; level of thoracic inlet. Majority of fistulas are single
- *Esophageal atresia with proximal fistula:* 2% of cases; narrow and short fistula
- *Esophageal atresia with fistulas to upper and lower tracheal segment:* 3–5% of cases. Similar to most common type with additional short, narrow fistula from proximal pouch to trachea

### CLINICAL MANIFESTATIONS

- Association with polyhydramnios, though uncommonly diagnosed prenatally
- May present shortly after birth with excessive secretions and need for frequent suctioning because infant is unable to swallow secretions
- May have aspiration events
- Feeding leads to immediate regurgitation with choking, coughing, and sometimes cyanosis Detection of H-type fistula may be delayed

### DIAGNOSTICS

- Typically noted by the inability to pass a naso/orogastric tube to the level of the stomach
- x-ray will show coiled catheter in upper esophageal pouch
- Air in abdomen on x-ray confirms a distal TEF; gasless abdomen is evidence of esophageal atresia without distal fistula
- Contrast studies of upper esophagus are not routinely necessary, except to diagnose "H"-type
- Echocardiogram and renal ultrasound to evaluate for associated abnormalities
- "H"-type is more difficult to diagnose and often presents (beyond the newborn period) with history of recurrent pneumonia
- Rigid bronchoscopy provides definitive diagnosis

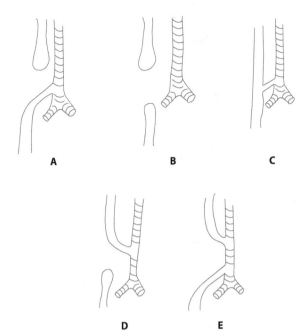

FIGURE 29-1 **Types of trachoesophageal fistulas (TEF).** A. Esophageal atresia with distal TEF (>85%). B. Pure esophageal atresia (without TEF) (3–5%). C. Isolated TEF without atresia (3–6%). D. Esophageal atresia with proximal fistula (2%). E. Esophageal atresia with fistulas to upper and lower tracheal segment (3–5%). (Adapted with permission from Lalwani AK (Ed). *Current Diagnosis & Treatment in Otolaryngology-Head & Neck Surgery*, 3rd ed. New York, NY: McGraw-Hill; 2012.)

## MANAGEMENT

- Avoid pneumonia from aspiration of upper pouch secretions—Use double lumen repogle tube and position patient to maximize drainage
- Surgical repair is either primary or staged
- *Staged repair:* Usually reserved for critically ill or very low birthweight neonates and involves initial ligation of fistula and placement of gastrostomy tube for feeding followed by future esophageal anastomosis
- Contrast swallow should be done 4–7 days after anastomosis to evaluate for anastomotic leak. Oral feedings are then initiated
- *Complications:* Dysphagia, anastomotic stricture, tracheomalacia, airway obstruction, vascular compression, reflex apnea
- Morbidity and mortality in neonates are related to cardiopulmonary comorbidity

## GASTROSCHISIS

Derived from Greek word meaning "belly cleft," a defect in the abdominal wall lateral to the intact umbilical cord

## EPIDEMIOLOGY

- Incidence 2–5:10,000; male>female
- Associated with young maternal age, low socioeconomic status, maternal smoking, alcohol use, medications (aspirin, ibuprofen, acetaminophen, pseudoephedrine)
- Occasionally associated with intestinal atresia, volvulus, and/or perforation; "complicated gastroschisis" carries a worse prognosis

## ETIOLOGY

- Postulated to be result of vascular accident during embryogenesis
- Recent studies suggest a possible inherited tendency

## PATHOPHYSIOLOGY

- In utero, abdominal viscera herniate through abdominal defect lateral to the umbilicus (usually to the right) and float in the amnion
- Contains midgut and may contain stomach and/or gonad
- Normal bowel rotation and fixation do not occur

## CLINICAL MANIFESTATIONS

- Herniation of viscera through lateral abdominal wall, with or without a skin bridge between the cord and the defect
- Intact umbilical cord
- Absence of peritoneal sac covering bowel

## MANAGEMENT

- Delivery may be vaginal or cesarean section
- Protect exposed viscera with saline-moistened sterile wraps or plastic bag immediately
- May need fluids 2.5–3.0 times above maintenance rate because of increased losses
- Up to 75% may be candidates for primary surgical closure performed when clinically stable
- Remaining 25% have prosthetic, extra-abdominal compartment or "silo," which allows for gradual manual reduction
- Postoperative complications include prolonged ileus, parenteral nutrition-related cholestatic liver disease, sepsis, and necrotizing enterocolitis

## PROGNOSIS

- Survival ≥90%

## INTESTINAL ATRESIAS

**Most common cause for neonatal intestinal obstruction, including complete discontinuity of the small bowel, severe stenoses, and webs.**

## EPIDEMIOLOGY

- Duodenal atresia incidence 1:6000–10,000 births
- Jejunoileal atresia incidence 1–2:10,000 births
- Up to 50% of affected infants with duodenal atresias may have another congenital anomaly, compared with 25–35% of those with jejunoileal atresias
- Often associated with trisomy 21, annular pancreas, malrotation, congenital heart disease, esophageal atresia, and anorectal malformations

| TABLE 29-1 | Types of Duodenal and Jejunoileal Atresias | |
|------------|------------------------|-------------|
| **Type** | **Relative Prevalence (%)** | **Description** |
| **Duodenal atresia** | | |
| Type I | 92 | Obstructing septum/web without muscular defect with intact mesentery |
| Type II | 1 | Two blind ends of duodenum connected by a fibrous cord without mesenteric defect |
| Type III | 7 | No connection between two blind ends with v-shaped mesenteric defect. |
| **Jejunoileal atresia** | | |
| Type I | 23 | Obstructing septum without mesenteric defect |
| Type II | 27 | Two blind ends connected by a fibrous cord without mesenteric defect |
| Type IIIa | 18 | No connection between two blind ends with v-shaped mesenteric defect |
| Type IIIb | 7 | "Apple peel" or "Christmas tree"—distal small bowel spirals around vascular supply with large mesenteric defect and significant bowel shortening |
| Type IV | 24 | Multiple atresias |

## ETIOLOGY

- Duodenal atresia thought to result from failure of recanalization following obliteration of the intestinal lumen after the 6th week of gestation—85% occur in second part of duodenum (Table 29-1)
- Jejunoileal atresias likely reflect mesenteric vascular compromise in later gestation (Table 29-1)

## CLINICAL MANIFESTATIONS

- Presentation may be variable depending on level of obstruction; polyhydramnios/emesis more common with proximal obstruction, abdominal distention more common with distal obstruction
- Most prenatally diagnosed atresias are duodenal

## DIAGNOSTICS

- Plain x-ray findings for duodenal atresia include "double bubble" appearance
- Jejunoileal atresias often show dilated proximal loops of bowel with air/fluid levels
- In duodenal atresia, echocardiography and renal ultrasonography should be performed to evaluate for other midline defects

## MANAGEMENT

- Gastric decompression to minimize bowel distention is imperative; note presence of bile in aspirate
- Intravenous fluid resuscitation should be provided and basic laboratory tests obtained

- Operative repair should be undertaken as soon as can safely be performed; duodenoduo-denostomy is routinely performed for duodenal atresia, and treatment of jejunoileal atresia may vary depending on the nature of the bowel defect
- All patients should be evaluated for malrotation and volvulus, and Ladd's procedure should be performed if present. If malrotation cannot be excluded, laparotomy should be pursued
- Tapering enteroplasty may be necessary in the setting of significant size mismatch between proximal and distal limbs
- Evaluate for multiple atresias

## OMPHALOCELE

**A central defect of the umbilical ring through which bowel and abdominal viscera herni-ate. The abdominal contents are covered with a membrane composed of the inner layer of peritoneum fused to outer layer of amnion.**

### EPIDEMIOLOGY

- Occurs in 1:2500–5000 live births
- Up to 30–50% of affected infants have associated karyotypic anomaly (e.g., trisomy 13 or 18)
- Can be associated with Beckwith–Wiedemann and pentalogy of Cantrell (combination of severe defects of the sternum, heart, diaphragm, and abdominal wall)
- *Greater than 50% have other malformations:* cardiovascular anomalies most common; also renal, skeletal, neural tube, sternum, diaphragm, and bladder
- 10% have "giant" omphalocele where liver and intestine herniate through an 8- to 10-cm defect

### PATHOPHYSIOLOGY

- Failure of migration and fusion of embryonic folds
- Most are lateral fold defects, and all involve the umbilicus
- Failure of the gut to migrate from the yolk sac to the abdomen
- Extruded abdominal contents (may contain midgut, liver, spleen, and/or gonad) are covered by a two-layered membrane; umbilical cord inserts into membrane
- Size >4 cm and contents distinguish omphalocele from umbilical cord hernia

### DIAGNOSTICS

- Detected in second trimester ultrasound
- Associated with increased $\alpha$-fetoprotein (AFP) and acetylcholinsesterase in maternal serum and amniotic fluid
- *Amniocentesis:* To evaluate for associated chromosomal abnormalities

### MANAGEMENT

- May be delivered vaginally or via cesarean section
- Cover exposed membranous sac with sterile saline-soaked dressings to prevent heat and fluid losses
- Correct fluid and electrolytes preoperatively
- Extra-uterine echocardiogram before surgical repair to evaluate for cardiac defect
- Surgical primary repair when possible. Staged closure for large defects
- Nonoperative techniques include placement of a "silo" for sequential reduction or use of eschar-producing agents ("paint and wait") when primary repair is not possible due to loss of abdominal domain

## PROGNOSIS

• Survival 70–95%
• Mortality is generally related to comorbidities

## GENERAL SURGERY

## APPENDICITIS

**Inflammation of the appendix caused by obstruction of the appendiceal lumen. Classically difficult to diagnose in children, because typical signs and symptoms may be absent in more than half of the patients presenting to the emergency department.**

### EPIDEMIOLOGY

• Approximately 1 in 12 people will have appendicitis in their lifetime, occurs in 1/1000 children per year
• Peak incidence in adolescence, uncommon in children younger than 5 years of age
• Slight male predominance

### DIFFERENTIAL DIAGNOSIS

• Mesenteric adenitis, bacterial enterocolitis (especially with *Yersinia enterocolitica* and *Campylobacter jejuni*), intussusception, Meckel's diverticulitis, urinary tract infection, right lower lobe pneumonia, testicular torsion, and gynecologic etiologies such as ectopic pregnancy, ovarian torsion, and pelvic inflammatory disease

### PATHOPHYSIOLOGY

• The appendix is a blind pouch that can be obstructed by fecaliths, hypertrophied lymphoid follicles, parasites, or foreign bodies
• Can also have bacterial invasion without previous obstruction
• This closed-loop obstruction causes edema, inflammation, and vasocongestion, which lead to necrosis and perforation
• Once this process starts, children are more prone to earlier perforation and development of peritonitis than adults

### CLINICAL MANIFESTATIONS

• Classically, pain begins in periumbilical region and moves to right lower quadrant (RLQ), nausea, vomiting, anorexia, and fever; presentation can be variable, especially in younger children
• Can have dysuria
• In children, particularly younger than 2 years, clinical signs can be more vague and misleading and can include irritability, upper respiratory infection symptoms, lethargy, abdominal rigidity, or refusal to walk
• Perforation usually occurs 36–48 hours after symptom onset and should be considered in context of patient with persistent symptoms, high fevers, and peritoneal signs
• *Abdominal tenderness:* Typically in the RLQ; can also be diffuse
• Bowel sounds usually normal or hyperactive, occasionally hypoactive but are unreliable
• Coughing, driving over a bump, or standing on the toes and dropping the heels may worsen the pain (indicative of peritonitis)
• Presence of one or more of the following may suggest appendicitis (few pediatric studies):
  ✓ *Rovsing's sign:* Palpation of left lower quadrant (LLQ) causes pain in RLQ
  ✓ *Psoas sign:* Patient flexes right hip against resistance. Increased abdominal pain indicates positive sign

✓ *Obturator sign:* Raise patient's right leg with the knee flexed. Rotate the leg internally at the hip. Increased abdominal pain indicates a positive sign
- Rectal exam can show rectal masses, abdominal abscesses, or right-sided rectal tenderness, but is often nonspecific and not necessary in most cases
- Guarding and rebound more likely with perforation

## DIAGNOSTICS

- Difficult to diagnose, particularly in young children
- 3–6% overall negative appendectomy rate, though rates are considerably higher in children under 5 (15–25%) and somewhat higher in females (5–10%) versus males (1–5%)
- Can be diagnosed on basis of history and physical exam alone, but adjunctive radiologic studies often helpful
  ✓ Abdominal flat plate films have limited utility. Findings include fecalith, localized ileus, soft tissue mass, splinting, loss of peritoneal fat stripe, or free air
  ✓ Ultrasound can be diagnostic; sensitivity and specificity vary among studies. Findings include increased appendiceal diameter or thickened wall, target sign, echogenicity surrounding the appendix, appendicolith, pericecal or perivesical free fluid
  ✓ CT has sensitivity of 87–100% (increased with oral and rectal contrast) and specificity of 83–97%. Findings include fat streaking, increased appendiceal diameter, cecal apical thickening
- Concerns about risk of malignancy following exposure to ionizing radiation during early childhood have led to efforts to reduce the use of CT in diagnosing appendicitis. Recent studies suggest that children evaluated at non-pediatric specialty centers are more likely to undergo CT scans during workup
- No laboratory study sensitive and specific for appendicitis
- Should obtain urine pregnancy test in females of reproductive age
- CBC, urinalysis, CRP frequently ordered
- Often see leukocytosis and high percentage of neutrophils on CBC with differential; one of these is elevated in 90–96% of cases, but specificity of these studies is unclear

## MANAGEMENT

- Patient should have nothing by mouth
- Fluid resuscitation as needed for dehydration or sepsis
- Standard of care is urgent appendectomy in uncomplicated appendicitis; cases with known perforation may require prolonged period of antibiotics
- Patients with uncomplicated cases of acute appendicitis should receive a single dose of preoperative broad-spectrum antibiotic
- Broad-spectrum IV antibiotics that cover enteric aerobes and anaerobes in cases of perforation or sepsis (e.g., ampicillin-sulbactam ± aminoglycoside, ticarcillin-clavulanate, ampicillin + gentamycin + metronidazole, or ciprofloxacin + metronidazole); length of administration should be determined by clinical criteria (fever, pain, bowel function, WBC count) in nonoperative management of perforation
- Following appendectomy, children with evidence of perforation should receive either 5 days of IV antibiotics or 7 days of oral therapy

## EXTRACORPOREAL MEMBRANE OXYGENATION (ECMO)

**Extracorporeal life support may include venoarterial cardiorespiratory support or venovenous access for respiratory support with or without less severe secondary cardiac failure.**

## EPIDEMIOLOGY

- As of 2013, the Extracorporeal Life Support Organization registry lists over 45,000 pediatric patients managed with ECMO, including over 32,000 neonates
- Survival is approximately 85% in neonates with respiratory indications and 55–65% for all other indications and age groups

## MECHANICS

- Circuit comprised of a pump, a membrane oxygenator, and a heat exchanger, along with invasive monitoring devices
- Venoarterial cannulation generally achieved via jugular vein and carotid arteries and/or femoral vein and artery, though when ECMO is employed in patients unable to wean from cardiorespiratory bypass intraoperatively, cannulation may be performed in the chest
- Venovenous access may be achieved via cannulation of two different veins or using a double-lumen venous cannula
- Venovenous configuration preferable (less morbidity) in the absence of cardiac disease
- In children, cannula size to achieve adequate flow may compromise entire vessel lumen, leading to distal ischemia

## INDICATIONS

- Oxygenation Index (OI) = [(Mean airway P × $FiO_2$)/Post ductal $PaO_2$] × 100
- ECMO may be considered for OI >20, and is routinely indicated for OI >40
- Clinical signs of decreased perfusion, including end-organ damage, shock, and cardiac arrest
- Primary diagnoses may include CDH, meconium aspiration syndrome, ARDS, sepsis, congenital cardiac defect, cardiomyopathy, trauma, or cardiac arrest, among others

## CONTRAINDICATIONS

- Prematurity—ECMO should not be used in newborns younger than 30 weeks' gestation or weighing less than 1.5 kg due to a high risk of intracranial bleeding
- Existing intracranial hemorrhage >grade 2
- Profound neurologic impairment, multiple congenital anomalies, or other condition with poor prognosis
- Relative contraindications include prolonged mechanical ventilation (due to high incidence of bronchopulmonary dysplasia and irreversible fibroproliferative pulmonary disease), CDH with severe pulmonary hypoplasia, multiorgan system failure, severe burns, immunodeficiency, or active bleeding

## MANAGEMENT

- Heparin should be titrated to maintain therapeutic anticoagulation during extracorporeal life support
- Generally, activated clotting time should be maintained at 50–60% above normal levels
- Management of the ECMO patient requires a coordinated care team, including surgical/neonatal intensivists, ICU nurses, and ECMO perfusionists
- During ECMO perfusion, ventilator settings should be maintained at low levels to provide lung rest; recruitment maneuvers will generally be required to transition off extracorporeal support
- Blood volume should be titrated to a right atrial pressure of 5–10 mm Hg; fluid management should be aimed at achieving and maintaining dry weight
- Cannula sites should be meticulously cleaned and maintained in accordance with institutional protocols

## COMPLICATIONS

- Bleeding associated with heparinization
- Technical failure (15%); includes circuit thrombus (26%), cannula issues (10%), oxygenator failure (10%), pump malfunction (2%), and air embolus (4%)
- Neurologic sequelae (seizures (10–13%))
- Pneumothorax (5–15%)
- Hemolytic anemia (6–12%)
- Chronic pulmonary disease (60%)
- Growth delay (40%)
- Neurologic abnormalities in up to 50% with detailed testing
- Infection

## HIRSCHSPRUNG DISEASE

**Congenital aganglionic megacolon; abnormal innervation of the bowel beginning in the internal anal sphincter and extending proximally**

### EPIDEMIOLOGY

- Incidence 1:5000 live births; males:females 4:1
- Most common cause of lower intestinal obstruction in neonates
- Associated with Down syndrome, Laurence–Moon–Bardet–Biedl syndrome, Waardenburg syndrome, and cardiovascular abnormalities (especially defects in cardiac septation or Tetralogy of Fallot)

### ETIOLOGY

- Multifactorial genesis and complex pattern of inheritance (up to 25% familial)

### PATHOPHYSIOLOGY

- Absence of ganglion cells in the bowel wall, which extends proximally from the anus for variable distance
- Arrest of neuroblast migration from proximal to distal bowel
- Limited to the rectosigmoid colon in 75% of patients and involves the entire colon in 10% of patients
- Histologically, absence of Meissner and Auerbach plexus and hypertrophied nerve bundles—Increased nerve endings in aganglionic bowel results in increased acetylcholinesterase

### CLINICAL MANIFESTATIONS

- Often presents with delayed passage of meconium; 99% of normal full-term infants pass meconium within 48 hours of birth
- Constipation is presenting symptom later in life
- Bowel dilatation proximal to transition zone leading to increased intraluminal pressure, resultant decreased blood flow and deterioration of the mucosal barrier may lead to stasis and proliferation of bacteria with subsequent enterocolitis
- Patients with enterocolitis (about 10%) may present with fever, abdominal distention and diarrhea, confusing the diagnosis
- Failure to pass stool leads to dilatation of proximal bowel and abdominal distention
- *On exam:* Palpable fecal mass in left lower abdomen but absence of stool in rectum
- Rectal exam reveals normal anal tone but is often followed by massive release of gas and feces

## DIAGNOSTICS

### Roentgenographic (Barium Contrast Enema)

- First-line study for suspected Hirschsprung disease at many centers
- Use water-soluble contrast for neonates
- Transitional zone seen after 1–2 weeks of age as a funnel-shaped area of intestine by barium contrast enema

### Rectal Biopsy

- Obtained no closer than 2 cm to dentate line because there is a normal area of hypoganglionosis at anal verge
- Early rectal biopsy should be avoided in premature infants due to physiologic immaturity of normal ganglion cells
- Need submucosa to accurately evaluate
- Specimen is stained for acetylcholinesterase, which should reveal a characteristic pattern of expression throughout the mucosa and submucosa
- H&E staining shows aganglionosis and hypertrophied nerve bundles
- Positive specimens rarely, if ever, stain for calcitonin

## MANAGEMENT

- Initially, decompression with nasogastric tube; repeated emptying of rectum using rectal tubes and irrigations
- Resuscitation should include IV fluids and broad spectrum antibiotics to cover multiple enteric pathogens
- Associated anomalies should be addressed prior to operative repair
- *Definitive treatment is surgical resection:* Swenson's technique, Duhamel–Grob technique, Soave-endorectal pull-through
- *Postoperative complications:* Recurrent enterocolitis (about 25%), constipation (about 20%), stricture(about 6%), prolapse(2%), fecal soiling (about 5%)

## INGUINAL HERNIA

**A protrusion into the groin of contents of the abdominal cavity, most commonly small bowel, into a persistently patent processus vaginalis. There are three types: indirect, direct, and femoral. Indirect hernias enter the inguinal canal through the internal inguinal ring and are by far the most common in children (>95%). Femoral hernias are rare in children.**

## EPIDEMIOLOGY

- Incidence of approximately 1–5% in children; male:female 3:1–10:1
- More common in premature infants (16–25% incidence); typically present in infancy
- Approximately 10% of inguinal hernias are complicated by incarceration
- Likelihood of incarceration decreases sharply with time; the risk is greatest during the first 6 months of life
- More often right-sided (60%) but bilateral in approximately 10%
- Patients with abdominal wall defects, connective tissue disorders, chronic respiratory disease, or undescended testes are at higher risk. Processes causing increased intra-abdominal pressure such as ascites, ventriculo-peritoneal shunting, or peritoneal dialysis can lead to high incidence of previously unrecognized inguinal hernias

## DIFFERENTIAL DIAGNOSIS

- Lymphadenopathy, lymphoma, undescended or retractile testes, hydrocele, testicular torsion
- May be difficult to differentiate hydrocele from inguinal hernia. Hydroceles typically transillu-minate, but hernias may as well. Unlike hydroceles, neck of hernia can often be felt at the inguinal ring. Also, hydroceles may get larger over the course of the day, but cannot be fully reduced and do not fluctuate in size

## PATHOPHYSIOLOGY

- Embryologically, the processus vaginalis is a diverticular portion of the peritoneum, which herniates through the abdominal wall and into the inguinal canal. The testes descend into the scrotum by the 29th week of gestation external to the processus vaginalis. The processus vaginalis usually fuses and is obliterated by the time a pregnancy reaches term or shortly thereafter. Partial or complete failure to obliterate results in a range of inguinal anomalies from hydroceles to hernias
- With increased intra-abdominal pressure, bowel (or ovary in females) can slip into this communication with risk for possible incarceration (being unable to reduce the hernia), strangulation (compromised blood supply), and subsequent necrosis

## CLINICAL MANIFESTATIONS

- Most children are asymptomatic unless incarceration and/or strangulation occurs
- Characterized by intermittent groin, scrotal, or labial swelling that spontaneously reduces; more prominent with Valsalva
- Examine testes first because retractile testes can be mistaken for hernias
- Classically, an inguinal bulge is noted at the inguinal ring or a scrotal/labial swelling that is reducible or changes in size
- Causing infant to cry or having older child stand can increase intra-abdominal pressure to make diagnosis easier
- Recent evidence indicates that digital photos taken by family members may be useful to document the diagnosis of equivocal cases
- Incarcerated hernia may present with signs of obstruction (emesis, poor feeds, abdominal distention, lack of bowel movements)
- With time, area surrounding an incarcerated hernia will become indurated, tender, and erythematous

## MANAGEMENT

- Once an asymptomatic inguinal hernia is diagnosed, the patient should be scheduled for an elective operative repair; recent data suggests that repair within 2 weeks may decrease the rate of incarceration
- An incarcerated hernia must be immediately reduced to avoid strangulation, necrosis, and perforation. Manual reduction is done by placing a calm child in Trendelenburg position and applying gentle upward pressure while trying to milk herniated tissues back into peritoneal cavity
- Consider analgesia and sedation for difficult or painful reductions. Unsuccessful reductions require immediate surgical repair
- In cases of successful manual reduction, prompt surgical repair can be electively scheduled as outpatient with strict instructions to return to emergency department in case of reincarceration

- In cases where intestinal obstruction is present, patient needs nasogastric tube, laboratory studies, fluid resuscitation, and immediate surgical consultation
- Current data supports the use of trans-inguinal laparoscopic evaluation of the contralateral side in patients with a preoperative diagnosis of unilateral inguinal hernia in younger patients

## INTUSSUSCEPTION

**An invagination of a proximal portion of the bowel and its mesentery (the intussusceptum) into an adjacent distal bowel segment (the intussuscipiens)**

### EPIDEMIOLOGY

- Incidence 1–4:2000
- 2:1 male to female ratio
- Majority of cases occur between 3 months and 2 years with peak incidence between 3 and 9 months of age
- Occasionally associated with cystic fibrosis (CF) and Henoch–Schönlein purpura (HSP)
- Seasonal incidence with peaks in winter and summer
- More common in underweight children
- Occurs in neonates, older children, and adults but usually secondary to a pathologic lead point

### ETIOLOGY

- Cause is unknown in approximately 90% of cases
- Incidence follows peak seasons of viral gastroenteritis. Postulated theory is that Peyer's patches become inflamed secondary to viral infection and serve as a lead point
- Pathologic lead points occur in 1.5–12% of cases; causes include Meckel's diverticulum, intestinal polyps, B cell lymphoma, submucosal hemangioma, carcinoid tumor, and *Ascaris lumbricoides* infestation
- Certain conditions such as CF, HSP, Peutz–Jeghers syndrome, and hemolytic-uremic syndrome predispose to lead points
- Can also occur as a postoperative complication following a laparotomy

### DIFFERENTIAL DIAGNOSIS

- Gastroenteritis, incarcerated hernia, Meckel's diverticulum, malrotation with midgut volvulus
- For patients who present with lethargy, consider vast differential for change in mental status

### PATHOPHYSIOLOGY

- Proximal portion of bowel and its mesentery telescopes into distal portion—Usually ileocolic, but can be ileoileal or colocolic as well
- Constriction of the mesentery causes engorgement of the intussusceptum and venous congestion with eventual bowel necrosis

### CLINICAL MANIFESTATIONS

- Classic triad is intermittent colicky abdominal pain, vomiting, and "currant jelly" stools (due to mucosal sloughing)
- However, this triad is present in less than half of cases and grossly bloody stool is often a late finding
- Pain typically occurs in screaming spells every 20–30 minutes during which the child draws up his/her legs. Children often look healthy and even playful between these episodes

- Emesis becomes bilious as obstruction progresses
- Up to 10% of patients present with only lethargy or hypotonia
- Can be febrile and have other abnormal vital signs
- Even in infants without grossly bloody stools, stools will be guaiac-positive in approximately 75% of cases
- Sausage-shaped mass in the right upper quadrant
- Abdomen often distended; bowel sounds high-pitched or normal
- Up to 20% may reduce spontaneously

## DIAGNOSTICS

- *Plain abdominal x-ray:* Can see paucity of intestinal gas, minimal stool in the colon, small bowel obstruction, and right upper quadrant soft tissue mass; however, plain films may be normal
- *Upright or decubitus film:* Rule out intraperitoneal air
- Ultrasound has recently been shown to be an effective and cost-efficient first test aimed at decreasing the number of negative studies involving radiation; may see pseudokidney sign, target sign, or complex hyperechoic mass
- *Barium or water-soluble contrast enemas:* Gold standard study for diagnosis and treatment of intussusception, which classically has a "coiled spring" appearance. Air contrast enemas have been shown to be as effective as barium enemas in diagnosis and treatment and can decrease the risks associated with a potential perforation
  - ✓ Obtain surgical consultation before attempted reduction because (1) risk of intestinal perforation during reduction and (2) failed reduction attempt requires surgical correction
  - ✓ Barium contraindicated if clinical peritonitis or free air on abdominal x-ray
- May see nonspecific lymphocytosis and electrolyte abnormalities consistent with dehydration

## MANAGEMENT

- Patient should not eat (NPO). Begin antibiotics (e.g., ampicillin-sulbactam, cefazolin) and fluid resuscitation in preparation for barium or air enema
- Surgery and anesthesiology staff should be standing by in case radiologic reduction is unsuccessful. In this event, laparotomy is performed with manual reduction and appendectomy
- Enemas are successful in 60–90% of patients, but are less successful in patients younger than 1 year, those who have had symptoms for more than 48 hours, when bowel obstruction is obvious on plain films or multiple ultrasound findings are present
- Recurrence of intussusception after barium or air reduction can occur in up to 10% of cases, and usually within the first 24 hours
- If the intussusception recurs, repeated radiologic reduction may be attempted once before surgical reduction. Recurrence is rare following surgical resection (about 2%)

## MALROTATION AND MIDGUT VOLVULUS

**Malrotation, an abnormal midgut development, results in anomalous positioning of the small intestine, cecum, and ascending colon. Abnormal bands of tissue are present (Ladd bands) from attempts at colonic fixation. A midgut volvulus occurs when the malrotated intestine twists on the axis of the superior mesenteric artery (SMA) compromising intestinal blood flow.**

## EPIDEMIOLOGY

- Detected in 0.2% of live births, but in 1–2% of autopsy studies
- Approximately 30% of cases detected by 1 week of age, 60% by 1 month, and 90% by 1 year. Remaining 10% may present at any age
- Up to 70% of patients have associated anomalies that include abdominal heterotaxia, omphalocele, gastroschisis, congenital diaphragmatic hernia, intestinal atresia, mesenteric cysts, Hirschsprung disease, anorectal anomalies, situs inversus, atrial septal detect, ventricular septal detect, transposition of the great vessels, dextrocardia, anomalous systemic or pulmonary venous return, asplenia, and polysplenia

## DIFFERENTIAL DIAGNOSIS

*Bilious (green or yellow) emesis in a neonate is a midgut volvulus until proven otherwise!*

- Malrotation is in the differential diagnosis for failure to thrive, cyclic vomiting, chronic abdominal pain, intermittent apnea, testicular torsion, and incarcerated hernia

## PATHOPHYSIOLOGY

- Normally, in the 5th–6th week of development, intestinal size exceeds the space of the abdominal cavity causing them to protrude into the umbilical cord. As the embryo grows, the midgut structures (duodenum, jejunum, ileum, ascending colon, and half of the transverse colon) reposition in the abdominal cavity, rotating 270 degrees around the SMA in a counterclockwise direction
- Malrotation occurs when the normal counterclockwise rotation of the midgut is incomplete; great variation in degree of abnormality in rotation

## CLINICAL MANIFESTATIONS

- Varies from acute intestinal obstruction to chronic, intermittent abdominal pain
- Delayed presentation of a midgut volvulus and significant intestinal necrosis includes shock (septic or hypovolemic) with hematochezia or melena and abdominal distention
- With a midgut intestinal obstruction, the abdomen should be flat or scaphoid. Abdominal distention suggests a more distal small bowel or colonic obstruction
- Abdominal wall distention, edema, erythema, and crepitus suggest gangrenous or necrotic bowel. *Bowel viability is time-dependent*

## DIAGNOSTICS

- *Abdominal radiograph:* Gastric and duodenal dilation with a paucity of distal gas suggests a midgut obstruction. However, a normal film does not exclude the possibility of malrotation with or without volvulus
- *An upper GI series is the best test to diagnose intestinal malrotation:*
  - ✓ To exclude malrotation, the duodenum should be in the retroperitoneal position on lateral projections, the ligament of Treitz should cross the midline to the left of the spine and rise to a level of the pylorus
- Ultrasound and CT scan may be used. A midgut volvulus on ultrasound has a "barber pole" or "whirlwind" appearance of the small intestine wrapping clockwise around the axis of the SMA

## MANAGEMENT

- Given the potential for volvulus and obstruction, with rare exception, a patient with a diagnosis of malrotation requires operative intervention

- *Ladd procedure:* Counterclockwise volvulus reduction, lysis of adhesive bands, conservative (necrotic) bowel resection, *appendix removal,* and repositioning of small intestine to RLQ and cecum to LLQ
- May need repeat operations to assess bowel viability (24–48 hours) if ischemia present at initial operation
- Postoperative course may be complicated by wound infection, shock, sepsis, intra-abdominal abscess, small bowel obstruction, recurrent volvulus, bowel necrosis, intussusception, short gut syndrome, strictures, and dysmotility

## PERIRECTAL ABSCESS

**Infection of the perirectal area via spread from the anal crypts to the anal ducts and glands**

### EPIDEMIOLOGY

- 68–90% of affected children are male
- May be related to androgen levels in infants <12 months of age; in later childhood/adolescence often occur in the setting of inflammatory bowel disease

### ETIOLOGY

- Small tears in the anal mucosa may lead to infection, or infection may arise from the anal glands and extend into the anal crypts
- When cultured, abscesses usually are polymicrobial. Most frequent organisms isolated are *Escherichia coli, Klebsiella pneumoniae, Staphylococcus aureus,* and anaerobes (e.g., *Bacteroides* species)

### CLINICAL MANIFESTATIONS

- 42% of children younger than 2 years of age have history of diarrhea
- Fever (81%), rectal pain (69%), rectal mass (40%), pain on sitting (27%), pain with defecation (21%), abnormal gait (19%)
- On exam, there is erythematous, painful swelling in the perirectal area with or without fluctuance or drainage

### MANAGEMENT

- Most patients require surgical drainage or needle aspiration followed by antibiotic therapy (e.g., cephalexin, amoxicillin-clavulanate, clindamycin) and sitz baths
- 10–20% may progress to fistula-in-ano, for which first-line treatment involves identification and either excision or incisional drainage of the fistulous tract
- MRI may be of use in the setting of Crohn's disease to delineate complex fistulae
- IV antibiotic therapy (e.g., cefazolin, ampicillin-sulbactam) may be required for non-immunosuppressed patients with extensive abscesses or evidence of systemic disease

## PNEUMOTHORAX

**Collection of extrapulmonary air within the chest**

### EPIDEMIOLOGY/ETIOLOGY

- Often due to penetrating or blunt thoracic trauma
- Can result from disruption of pulmonary parenchyma, injury to tracheobronchial tree, bleb or esophageal rupture

- Occurs in 5% of children hospitalized for asthma
- Occurs in 10–25% of patients older than 10 years old with CF
- Spontaneous pneumothorax far more common among males (18–28:100,000/year versus 1.2–6:100,000 females)
- *Iatrogenic:* Tracheotomy, subclavian line placement, thoracentesis, and transbronchial biopsy
- Bilateral pneumothoraces are rare beyond neonatal period
- Tension pneumothorax will develop in up to 20% of patients with simple pneumothorax
- *Other:* Lymphoma or other malignancies, staphylococcal pneumonia

## DIFFERENTIAL DIAGNOSIS

- Localized/generalized emphysema, extensive emphysematous bleb, congenital cystic adenomatoid malformation, diaphragmatic hernia, gaseous distention of stomach

## PATHOPHYSIOLOGY

- *Tension pneumothorax:* A one-way entry of air into the pleural space. This collection of air causes collapse of the ipsilateral lung and compression of the contralateral lung. Mediastinal structures may shift, and there may be a decrease in venous return to the heart and cardiovascular compromise
- *Primary spontaneous pneumothorax:* Occurs in patients without trauma or underlying lung disease (e.g., Ehlers–Danlos disease, Marfan syndrome)
- *Secondary spontaneous pneumothorax:* Arises secondary to underlying lung disorder but without trauma. Examples include pneumonia with empyema, pulmonary abscess, gangrene, infarct, rupture of cyst, rupture of emphysematous bleb, foreign body

## CLINICAL MANIFESTATIONS

- Onset may be abrupt; may be asymptomatic; severity of symptoms depends on extent of lung collapse
- Pain, dyspnea with respiratory distress, cyanosis, splinting on involved side, agitation, increased pulse rate
- *Respiratory distress:* Retractions, tachypnea, cyanosis
- Crepitus
- Decreased breath sounds on auscultation of affected lung
- Percussion of area involved is tympanitic
- Larynx, trachea, and/or heart may be shifted to unaffected side

## DIAGNOSTICS

- *Chest x-ray:* Expiratory views emphasize the contrast between lung markings and area of pneumothorax. Tension pneumothorax limits expansion of contralateral lung

  *Chest CT Scan:* May be obtained after re-expansion of the lung to detect predisposing anatomic abnormalities (e.g., bleb)

## MANAGEMENT

### Medical

- Small (less than 15%) or moderate sized pneumothorax in healthy child may spontaneously resolve within 1 week without intervention
- Because a small pneumothorax can quickly progress to a tension pneumothorax, even asymptomatic trauma patients with pneumothorax should be admitted for observation
- Recent data suggests that blunt trauma patients with occult pneumothorax (visible on CT scan but not on plain x-ray) may be safely observed without intervention despite requirement for positive pressure ventilation

- Administration of 100% oxygen may increase nitrogen pressure gradient between pleural air and blood and shorten time to resolution
- *Analgesia:* Consider respiratory depressant effects of codeine, morphine

### Surgical

- *Tube thoracostomy:* Indicated for symptomatic patients and, generally, those receiving positive pressure ventilation. Tube is placed at the midaxillary line at level of the fifth intercostal space (approximately nipple level) over the top of the rib to avoid the intercostal neurovascular bundle
- *Needle decompression for tension pneumothorax:* Needle is placed in midclavicular, second intercostal space of the ipsilateral side; an immediate release of air is noted, and tube thoracostomy must be performed (see Pneumothorax Needle Decompression in Chapter 25)
- *Recurrent pneumothorax:* May use sclerosing agent that induces an adhesion between the lung and chest wall (tetracycline, talc, silver nitrate), or induce mechanical adhesions via laparoscopic or open approaches
- Video-Assisted Thoracoscopic Surgery (VATS) allows for plication of blebs, closure of fistula, stripping of pleura, basilar pleural abrasion and has largely replaced open thoracotomy in the surgical treatment of recurrent pneumothorax

## PYLORIC STENOSIS

**Enlarged pylorus with increased muscular thickness, which generally leads to gastric outlet obstruction and bilious emesis**

### EPIDEMIOLOGY

- Occurs in approximately 3–6 per 1000 infants
- Male:female 4:1; more common in white infants
- 10–20% of infants of mother with history of pyloric stenosis

### ETIOLOGY

- Hereditary and environmental factors thought to be involved
- *Other factors:* Abnormal muscle innervation, erythromycin therapy during first 2 weeks of life, maternal stress in third trimester, and B and O blood groups
- Underlying defect is thickened pyloric musculature leading to a gradual obstruction

### CLINICAL MANIFESTATIONS

- Typically presents between 2 and 8 weeks of age (most common 3–5 weeks)
- Nonbilious vomiting is initial symptom
- Weight loss and dehydration
- Patients are often hungry and eager to feed
- "Olive-shaped" mass may be palpated in the midepigastrium beneath the liver edge
- Gastric peristaltic wave may be visible in a distended stomach
- Jaundice occasionally present

### DIAGNOSTICS

- Clinical diagnosis possible in 60–80% of patients
- *Electrolyte panel:* Hypokalemic, hypochloremic metabolic alkalosis due to loss of gastric HCl (may be acidotic if severe dehydration)
- *Abdominal x-ray:* Dilated stomach bubble

- *Abdominal ultrasound:* Radiologic study of choice (sensitivity around 90%); positive ultrasound characterized muscle thickness ≥4 mm and/or channel length ≥14 mm
- *Upper GI series:* Sensitive and specific, but risk for aspiration. Barium studies may show elongated pyloric channel, bulge of pylorus into antrum, and parallel streaks of barium in the channel

## MANAGEMENT

### Medical

- *Initial IV fluids:* 5% dextrose with normal saline
  ✓ Risk of hyponatremia if hypotonic saline is used
- Potassium chloride can be added to IV fluids when urine output is established
- Correction of alkalosis to bicarbonate less than 30 essential to prevent postoperative apnea

### Surgical

- Delay surgery until adequate rehydration and electrolyte correction established
- Ramstedt pyloromyotomy is procedure of choice. This involves splitting the pyloric muscle without violating the mucosa
- Can be performed laparoscopically or through small incision
- Families should be counseled preoperatively to expect vomiting after the procedure; in most cases, feeds can begin within a few hours of the procedure and patients should continue to be fed despite vomiting to improve oral tolerance

## UROLOGIC SURGERY

## OVARIAN TORSION

**Twisting of the ovary or adnexa resulting in venous and lymphatic congestion and eventual loss of arterial perfusion with resulting ovarian necrosis**

### EPIDEMIOLOGY

- Incidence 4.9:100,000 in girls 1–20 years old
- Rare in children, occurs predominantly in neonates and early adolescence

### ETIOLOGY

- Torsion typically occurs in the setting of enlarged ovaries containing either follicular cysts or tumors; however, normal ovaries can also torse
- Torsion is the most common complication of ovarian tumors in children occurring in 3–16% of patients. Ovarian tumors that undergo torsion are more commonly benign

### DIFFERENTIAL DIAGNOSIS

- Appendicitis, gastroenteritis, ruptured ovarian cyst, ectopic pregnancy, pelvic inflammatory disease, tubo-ovarian abscess, nephrolithiasis

### PATHOPHYSIOLOGY

- Ovarian mass (follicle, cyst, tumor) acts as a "weight" to promote twisting of the ovary on its vascular pedicle
- Right ovarian torsion is more common than left (3:2)
- Initially, venous and lymphatic drainage are compromised, leading to an enlarged ovary. If prolonged (greater than 8 hours), arterial supply is affected and necrosis, gangrene, and peritonitis can result

• Neonatal ovarian torsion typically occurs in ovaries with large (>5 cm) follicular cysts that are believed to develop in response to exposure to maternal hormones. Torsion can occur either in utero or postnatally

## CLINICAL MANIFESTATIONS

• *Presentation is highly variable:* Abdominal pain (90–100%); nausea/vomiting (70–80%); fever (5–20%); leukocytosis (20%); palpable abdominal mass (20%); dysuria (14%)
• Patients note pain on abdominal (RLQ, LLQ) and pelvic exam

## DIAGNOSTICS

• *Pelvic ultrasound with Doppler:* The preferred imaging modality. Can show complex echogenic pelvic mass and absence of blood flow. Normal US and Doppler flow does not exclude ovarian torsion. If clinical suspicion is high, prompt surgical evaluation
• *Pelvic CT scan:* Helpful if ultrasound unavailable and can help to rule out other abdominal processes
• *B-HCG:* Quantitative to rule out ectopic pregnancy and germ cell tumors
• *α-fetoprotein:* Order if tumor diagnosed; abnormal with teratoma or endodermal sinus tumors

## MANAGEMENT

• Prompt laparoscopy (preferably by 8 hours from onset of symptoms) with detorsion or salpingo-oophorectomy (if necessary)
• Management of a normal torsed ovary should be as conservative as possible; detorsion and careful observation is recommended to preserve fertility in the ovary, and recent literature suggests that up to 70% of adnexae can be salvaged following torsion. If viability is in doubt, consider a second look procedure

## TESTICULAR TORSION

**Surgical emergency of males in which testis and spermatic cord twist, leading to acute ischemia of testis**

### EPIDEMIOLOGY

• Incidence 1:4000 males under 25 years old; not common in newborns
• Peaks at 1 year of age and onset of puberty (weight of testes)

### ETIOLOGY

• Most common in individuals with "bell-clapper deformity" in which the tunica vaginalis extends up to the spermatic cord, suspending the testes freely within the tunica cavity
• Deformity is frequently bilateral and can be detected by examining testes for a horizontal lie
• Undescended testes are ten times more likely to torse
• Intravaginal torsion (associated with bell-clapper deformity) is typically seen in adolescents
• Extravaginal torsion (torsion of the cord and coverings) tends to occur in neonates secondary to highly mobile testes
• Can result from contraction of cremasteric muscle after sex, trauma, cold, or exercise; can occur at rest

### DIFFERENTIAL DIAGNOSIS

• Torsion of appendix testis, epididymitis, orchitis, scrotal trauma, incarcerated inguinal hernia, HSP, idiopathic scrotal edema, varicocele

## PATHOPHYSIOLOGY

- Spermatic cord twists within the tunica vaginalis
- *Arterial blood flow interrupted:* Leads to ischemia
- *Prolonged torsion:* Leads to infarction and necrosis
- Recurrent episodes if spontaneously untwists before significant damage done (one-third of patients have had past transient episodes)
- Can result in abnormal spermatogenesis and infertility

## CLINICAL MANIFESTATIONS

- Acute onset testicular pain (89%); vomiting (39%), dysuria or frequency (5%), history of similar pain or swelling (36%)
- Scrotal pain can radiate to the abdomen, thigh, flank
- Usually afebrile, no dysuria or penile discharge
- *On exam:* Swollen and tender testis, scrotal edema and erythema, high-riding testicle (twisted cord) with horizontal lie, thickened tender spermatic cord, absent cremasteric reflex, palpable secondary hydrocele
- Fever and erythema are late signs

## DIAGNOSTICS

- Doppler ultrasonography is study of choice, but very operator-dependent. Blood flow on Doppler does not rule out torsion
- 99m-Technetium radioisotope scan (rarely available)

## MANAGEMENT

- *Surgical emergency:* Obtain immediate consultation
- *Detorsion:* Cord is untwisted and the testis wrapped in warm saline-soaked gauze while reperfusion is assessed. Necrotic testes are removed, orchiopexy (attach testes to tunica vaginalis) viable testicle. Orchidopexy of the contralateral testis
- Testis removed if not viable because of the risk of infertility secondary to the development of anti-sperm antibodies

# Toxicology 30

*Ruth Abaya, MD, MPH*
*Diane Calello, MD*

## DECONTAMINATION AND ENHANCED ELIMINATION

### ACTIVATED CHARCOAL

- Decreases absorption of some drugs in the stomach, however not routinely recommended unless a potentially toxic amount of poison has been ingested
- Should be used soon after ingestion, ideally within the first hour
- *Technique:* Activated charcoal given orally or by nasogastric (NG) tube at dose of 1 g/kg (maximum, 100 g); repeat dose 0.5–1 g/kg every 4–6 hours, if necessary (see multiple-dose activated charcoal subsequently)
  ✓ Ideally should achieve ratio of at least 10 g charcoal per gram of drug ingested
- Does not bind metals (iron, lithium, lead) or common electrolytes, mineral acids/bases, alcohols, cyanide, solvents, and water-insoluble compounds such as hydrocarbon
- Poses aspiration risk, especially among who vomit or receive charcoal via NG tube
- Contraindicated in caustic or hydrocarbon ingestion and in patients without protected airway (altered mental status or unconscious)

### GASTRIC LAVAGE/GASTRIC EMPTYING

- Gastric lavage still performed, but exceedingly difficult in young children due to size of tube required
- Efficacy not proven, but most effective if done within 1 hour of ingestion
- *Technique:* Place patient on left side with head lower than body. Use large bore orogastric tube
  ✓ Aspirate gastric contents prior to lavage
  ✓ Lavage with normal saline until return of fluid is clear. Fifty to 100 cc per cycle should be used, and up to 200 cc in adolescents
- May delay administration of charcoal
- Contraindicated in patients with altered mental status (inability to protect airway), hydrocarbon or caustic ingestion, cardiac arrhythmia, or possibility of foreign body ingestion
- Syrup of ipecac no longer recommended

### EXTRACORPOREAL REMOVAL

**Includes methods such as hemodialysis, plasmapheresis, and exchange transfusion**

- Reserved for life-threatening poisonings or renal failure; consult pediatric nephrologist
- Hemodialysis is most commonly used. Blood is pumped through dialysis machine and toxins diffuse passively from blood into dialysate solution
- Unstable patients may undergo continuous renal replacement therapy (CRRT, such as continuous veno-venous hemofiltration or CVVH) but the efficacy for poisoning is much less
- Plasmapheresis and exchange transfusion are seldom necessary but may be useful in the neonates or infants

## ENHANCED ELIMINATION

- Urinary alkalinization enhances clearance of certain agents such as salicylates, phenobarbital, chlorpropamide via "ion trapping"
  - ✓ Alkaline environment favors generation of ionized drug species which cannot readily cross the renal tubular membrane, thus preventing reabsorption
  - ✓ Performed with sodium bicarbonate at 1–2 mEq per kg over 1–2 hours with careful monitoring for electrolyte abnormalities
- *Whole bowel irrigation (WBI):*
  - ✓ *Uses:* Iron ingestions, massive ingestions, ingestion of sustained-release or enteric-coated preparations, ingestion of packets of illicit drugs, late presentations when gastric emptying and charcoal will be unlikely to be effective, and when charcoal cannot be used, such as in lithium ingestion
  - ✓ *Technique:* Give preparation via NG tube until stool is clear
  - ✓ Use polyethylene glycol solution, such as GoLYTELY at 500 cc/h in children and 2 L/h in adolescents
  - ✓ Contraindicated in patients with ileus or intestinal obstruction, caustic ingestions, as well as in patients who are unable to protect airway (may require intubation)
  - ✓ Charcoal may be less effective when used together with WBI
- *Multi-dose activated charcoal:*
  - ✓ *Multiple-dose activated charcoal (MDAC):* Some recommend repeat doses after large ingestion (listed in management section for specific drugs)
  - ✓ May improve results by decreasing enterohepatic recirculation
  - ✓ Requires effective peristalsis
  - ✓ *Use caution with sorbitol:* May result in electrolyte abnormalities (sorbitol should not be administered more than every third dose)

## SPECIFIC POISONINGS (TABLE 30-1)

### ACETAMINOPHEN

**Over-the-counter (OTC) analgesics (e.g., Tylenol), OTC cold remedies, prescription combination medications (e.g., Percocet)**

#### TOXICOLOGY/PHARMACOLOGY

- Most common pharmaceutical poisoning exposure
- Hepatic metabolism, including cytochrome p450
- Toxicity via metabolite, N-acetyl-p-benzoquinone-imine (NAPQI), which is normally detoxified by glutathione; in overdose, glutathione is depleted and metabolite causes direct hepatic cell injury and death
- Toxic dose is 150 mg/kg in children or 6–7 g in adults
- Fulminant liver failure develops in 3–4% of children with hepatotoxicity

#### CLINICAL MANIFESTATIONS

- *Early (first 24 hours):* Asymptomatic or nausea, vomiting, malaise
- Initial symptoms may resolve 1–4 days after ingestion despite ongoing hepatotoxicity
  - ✓ Symptoms may include right upper quadrant abdominal pain and jaundice
- Three to 5 days after ingestion those with severe toxicity may develop symptoms or signs of fulminant hepatic failure with encephalopathy or coma; coagulopathy; renal failure; death from liver failure possible

| TABLE 30-1 | Toxins and Their Antidotes | |
|---|---|---|
| **Toxin** | **Antidotes** | **Comments** |
| Acetaminophen | N-acetylcysteine | |
| Anticholinergics | Physostigmine | Can lead to seizures, cholinergic crisis |
| Anticholinesterases/carbamates | Atropine | |
| Organophosphate | Pralidoxime | |
| Benzodiazepines | Flumazenil | Seldom used due to seizure risk |
| Beta-blockers | Glucagon | Causes vomiting |
| Calcium channel blockers | Calcium chloride/calcium gluconate | Use caution with peripheral IV |
| Cyanide | Amyl nitrite + thiosulfate or hydroxocobalamin | Caution with nitrites: methemoglobinemia |
| Digitalis | Digibind | |
| Lead | BAL, EDTA, DMSA | |
| Iron | Deferoxamine | |
| Methanol/ethylene glycol | Fomepizole | |
| Opioids | Naloxone | |
| Tricyclics | Sodium bicarbonate | |
| Beta-blockers, calcium channel blockers, local anesthetics, atypical antipsychotics, tricyclics | Intralipids | Experimental use for cardiovascular collapse |

## DIAGNOSTICS

- Draw acetaminophen (APAP) level 4 hours after ingestion (also at 8 and 12 hours if extended release form or if co-ingestion with medications that delay gastric emptying) (Figure 30-1)
- *Labs:* Aspartate aminotransferase (AST), alanine aminotransferase (ALT), glucose, PT, bilirubin, electrolytes, creatinine (elevated creatinine associated with higher mortality), arterial blood gas, urinalysis (proteinuria and hematuria suggest acute tubular necrosis)
- Single doses of less than 200 mg/kg are unlikely to cause serious harm, however accuracy of ingestion amount and timing may be unreliable in intentional overdose

## MANAGEMENT

- Gastric lavage is controversial; give charcoal if within 4 hours
- For acute ingestions, base need for subsequent treatment on nomogram (see Figure 30-1)
- N-acetylcysteine (NAC, Mucomyst, Acetadote) has greatest benefit in preventing liver toxicity if given within 8 hours of ingestion, but is still beneficial even if initiated many hours to days later
  - ✓ If patient presents 6–8 hours following ingestion, administer N-acetylcysteine while obtaining a level
  - ✓ If patient presents 8 or more hours following ingestion, options include N-acetylcysteine administration while obtaining a level or administration if 4-hour level is above line on nomogram

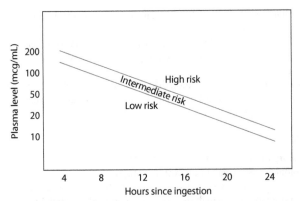

FIGURE 30-1 **Nomogram for estimating severity of acute acetaminophen poisoning.** (Modified with permission from Rumack BH, Matthew H. Acetaminophen poisoning and toxicity, *Pediatrics* 1975 Jun;55(6):871–876.)

- N-acetylcysteine dose
  - ✓ *Oral dose:* Loading dose, 140 mg/kg orally; maintenance dose, 70 mg/kg orally every 4 hours for 17 doses
  - ✓ *IV dose:* Loading dose, 150 mg/kg given over an hour; 2nd dose, 50 mg/kg given over 4 hours; 3rd dose, 100 mg/kg given over 16 hours
  - ✓ Amount of diluent is based on patient age; consider consultation with a pharmacist
  - ✓ Orally N-acetylcysteine can be difficult to tolerate which is avoided by giving the IV form; the greatest risk of IV N-acetylcysteine is anaphylactoid reactions
- Cannot use nomogram to determine need for treatment in chronic ingestions; decision to treat in these cases is based on amount ingested (150–200/kg in 24-hour period) or evidence of hepatotoxicity
- *Criteria for admission:* Admit all patients with 4 hour APAP level above line on nomogram (see Figure 30-1). All intentional ingestions warrant admission

## AMPHETAMINES

**Prescribed for narcolepsy, attention deficit hyperactivity disorder, fatigue, and weight loss; found in OTC diet pills and some nasal decongestants; includes illicit agents such as methamphetamine, which is the most commonly abused amphetamine, and hallucinogenic amphetamine derivatives such as MDMA ("Ecstasy")**

### TOXICOLOGY/PHARMACOLOGY

Increase synaptic concentrations of catecholamines, thereby causing CNS stimulation

- Toxic effects are due to excess sympathetic stimulation as well as dopaminergic effects causing psychosis
- *Toxicity through various routes:* Ingestion, inhalation, or injection
- Tolerance develops with chronic use; low therapeutic index

### CLINICAL MANIFESTATIONS

- *Gastrointestinal:* Nausea, vomiting, anorexia, diarrhea
- *Central nervous system:* Euphoria, agitation, pressured speech, seizures; stroke can occur from either hypertension or vasculitis

- *Cardiac:* Palpitations, chest pain, hypertensive crises, arrhythmias, myocardial infarction, and circulatory collapse
- *Psychiatric:* Psychotic state with hallucinations and paranoia which can be confused with schizophrenia. Hallucinations and altered perception may result with hallucinogenic amphetamine derivatives
- *Other:* Hyperthermia, sweating, tremor, difficulty urinating, dilated pupils, rhabdomyolysis
- *With chronic use may see:* Cardiomyopathy, cerebral vasculitis, weight loss; psychiatric disturbances may be permanent

## DIAGNOSTICS

- Based on history of ingestion and clinical presentation
- Urine toxicologic screen (may not detect all compounds)
- *Laboratory studies:* Electrolytes, glucose, BUN, creatinine, creatine phosphokinase (CPK; to detect rhabdomyolysis), urinalysis (positive "blood" on dipstick in absence of red blood cells suggests rhabdomyolysis)
- ECG, CT of head if concern for cerebrovascular accident

## MANAGEMENT

- *Decontamination:* Activated charcoal; do not induce emesis
- *Symptomatic care:* Hydration; treat seizures or agitation with benzodiazepines; treat hypertension with peripheral vasodilator (nitroprusside, phentolamine); treat hyperthermia
- Treat arrhythmias and rhabdomyolysis if they occur
- *Criteria for hospitalization:* Monitor for at least 6 hours; if symptomatic, admit for observation

## ANTIHISTAMINES

**Over-the-counter and prescription allergy medicines; cold and cough medicines; sleep aids; motion sickness medications**

### TOXICOLOGY/PHARMACOLOGY

- Antihistamines block H1 receptors
- Can cause CNS stimulation or depression
- In overdose can result in anticholinergic symptoms
- Elimination half-lives are variable, ranging from hours to days, depending on the specific drug
- Toxic dose is around three to five times the therapeutic dose

### CLINICAL MANIFESTATIONS

- *Lower doses:* CNS depression-sedative effect
- *Higher doses:* CNS stimulation-agitation, confusion, hallucinations, excitement, tremors
- *Neurologic:* Seizures (diphenhydramine only)
- *Cardiac:* QRS widening with diphenhydramine (Benadryl)
- *Anticholinergic toxidrome:* Delirium, flushed skin, dry mouth, fever, tachycardia, hypertension, dilated pupils

### DIAGNOSTICS

- Diagnosis based on history and presence of anticholinergic syndrome
- Can be detected on comprehensive urine toxicologic screen
- *Laboratory studies:* Electrolytes, glucose, blood gas; ECG

## MANAGEMENT

- Charcoal and/or gastric emptying; WBI may be helpful when antihistamine is in sustained-release form
- Manage hyperthermia with external cooling
- Manage agitation or seizures with benzodiazepines
- If symptoms are severe and life-threatening, can use physostigmine to treat anticholinergic effects—not routinely recommended because of toxicity
  - ✓ *Physostigmine dose:* 0.02 mg/kg given over 1–2 minutes every 5 minutes to a maximum dose of 2 mg; can repeat if needed in 20 minutes
  - ✓ PERFORM ECG before physostigmine to rule out conduction delays
  - ✓ DO NOT use in tricyclic overdose
  - ✓ GIVE SLOWLY—Can precipitate seizures or asystole
  - ✓ Have atropine ready if needed for cholinergic cardiac effects (bradycardia and hypotension)
  - ✓ Atropine dose is half of the amount of physostigmine given

## BETA-BLOCKERS

Most common use is for cardiac disorders, such as hypertension, angina, and arrhythmia; noncardiac uses include migraines, essential tremor, thyrotoxicosis, glaucoma, and anxiety.

### TOXICOLOGY/PHARMACOLOGY

- In treatment doses, drugs are beta-receptor-specific; in overdose, this specificity is lost
- Sustained release preparations exist
- Can be fatal in doses of only two to three times the therapeutic dose

### CLINICAL MANIFESTATIONS

- *Cardiac:* Bradycardia, hypotension, atrioventricular block; asystole can occur but is rare
- *Central nervous system:* Coma
- *Bronchospasm:* Mostly seen in patients who have asthma
- Labs may show hypoglycemia in young children; children require serial glucose checks to assess for fasting hypoglycemia
- ECG may show prolonged PR interval or wide QRS if severe; sotalol ingestion can result in a prolonged QT interval and torsades de pointes

### DIAGNOSTICS

- Diagnosis based on history and vital signs
- *Laboratory studies:* Electrolytes, glucose, BUN, creatinine, blood gas
- ECG

### MANAGEMENT

- *Decontamination:* Gastric lavage if large ingestion or immediate presentation; activated charcoal; can consider WBI for sustained-release preparations
- *Hypotension:* Treat with fluids; vasoactive pressor infusions may be needed
- *Bradycardia:* Atropine; isoproterenol can be used if no response to atropine
- Glucagon can also be used to treat hypotension and bradycardia that do not respond to previous measures
- Magnesium for torsades de pointes
- Bronchodilators for bronchospasm

- Cardiac pacing or extracorporeal membrane oxygenation (ECMO) is reserved for patients not responding to medical management
- *Criteria for hospitalization:* Must perform ECG monitoring for 6 hours after ingestion; all pediatric ingestions and ingestions with sustained-release preparation should be admitted

## CALCIUM CHANNEL BLOCKERS

Medication for treatment of hypertension, atrial fibrillation, angina, migraines

### TOXICOLOGY/PHARMACOLOGY

- Toxicity due to vasodilatory effects on both coronary and peripheral vessels, decreased myocardial contractility, slowing of the conduction system both at sinus node and through AV node
- Toxicity can occur from therapeutic use or in overdose
- Can be fatal in small doses
- Most severe toxicity seen with verapamil or diltiazem
- Sustained release preparations available

### CLINICAL MANIFESTATIONS

- May be asymptomatic for hours after ingestion with sustained-release preparations
- *Cardiac:* Hypotension, bradycardia (verapamil, diltiazem), reflex tachycardia followed by bradycardia as poisoning worsens (amlodipine, nifedipine)
- Neurologic compromise (altered mental status, convulsions, coma) may result from impaired cerebral perfusion, but late in clinical picture. Mental status usually preserved at initial presentation
- *Other symptoms:* Hyperglycemia, metabolic acidosis; serum calcium may be normal

### DIAGNOSTICS

- Based on history and clinical presentation
- *Laboratory studies:* Electrolytes, BUN, creatinine, glucose (risk for hyperglycemia, hypokalemia, metabolic acidosis), blood gas
- ECG shows prolonged PR interval with normal QRS
- Troponin or other cardiac biomarkers may help differentiate drug-induced from ischemic causes of bradycardia
- Urine toxicology screen (to detect co-ingested drugs)

### MANAGEMENT

- *Decontamination:*
  - ✓ *Gastric lavage:* Only if within 1 hour and will not delay charcoal administration
  - ✓ *Activated charcoal:* Consider multiple-dose (MDAC) in large sustained-release ingestions
  - ✓ WBI for sustained-release preparations
- *Treating hypotension:*
  - ✓ IV fluids (normal saline bolus)
  - ✓ Calcium chloride (20 mg/kg IV) or calcium gluconate (50–75 mg/kg IV)
  - ✓ Dopamine, epinephrine, or norepinephrine for refractory hypotension
- High-dose insulin (Up to 1 U/kg/h) and glucose (to maintain euglycemia) infusions
- Atropine for bradycardia
- *Last-resort therapies:* ECMO, cardiac pacing, intra-aortic balloon

- Some evidence exists in support of intravenous lipid emulsion
- *Criteria for hospitalization:* (1) Observe for 24 hours; (2) monitor for at least 24 hours if large ingestion or sustained release

## CARBAMAZEPINE

Medication used for seizures (Tegretol, Carbatrol), neuropathic pain, some psychiatric disorders

### TOXICOLOGY/PHARMACOLOGY

- Blocks sodium channels in the brain, preventing high-frequency firing; at high doses, also blocks cardiac sodium channels
- Mild anticholinergic activity
- Absorption can be erratic due to anticholinergic-induced delayed gastric emptying
- Peak level reached from 4 to 24 hours
- Metabolized via P450 to active compound, so drug level may not reflect magnitude of clinical toxicity

### CLINICAL MANIFESTATIONS

- *Central nervous system:* Ataxia, mydriasis, nystagmus, altered mental status, nausea, vomiting, dystonic posturing, coma, seizures; status epilepticus indicates poor prognosis
- *Cardiac:* Sinus tachycardia, hypotension from myocardial depression, atrioventricular block, bradycardia, QRS or QT prolongation, ventricular dysrhythmias
- *Chronic toxicity:* Syndrome of inappropriate antidiuretic hormone secretion, leukopenia, thrombocytopenia
- Symptom onset may be delayed due to delayed absorption

### DIAGNOSTICS

- Based on history and clinical signs
- Obtain immediate carbamazepine level; repeat levels every 4–6 hours; levels above 40 mg/L associated with severe toxicity in adults; toxic level is even lower in children
- *Laboratory studies:* CBC, electrolytes, glucose, ABG
- ECG

### MANAGEMENT

- Treatment based on clinical status, not drug levels
- Supportive care
- Recognize that carbamazepine can significantly slow GI motility and that neurological status may warrant early airway management
- Activated charcoal
- *Massive ingestion:* Can consider MDAC or WBI
- *Life-threatening toxicity:* Hemodialysis
- Treat seizures with benzodiazepines and phenobarbital, NOT phenytoin (has same intracellular mechanism as carbamazepine)
- *Criteria for hospitalization:* Observe asymptomatic patients for 6 hours; admit symptomatic patients to monitored bed if levels or clinical picture are concerning

## CARBON MONOXIDE

**Fire (indoor charcoal or house fire), automobile exhaust, gasoline engines operating in enclosed spaces (car or generator in garage), faulty furnaces or gas stoves, woodburning stoves, inhaled spray paint; also, the main ingredient in paint remover is metabolized to carbon monoxide**

### TOXICOLOGY/PHARMACOLOGY

- Children are at higher risk from CO because of their higher metabolic and respiratory rates
- Toxicity results from CO binding hemoglobin with higher affinity than oxygen, which results in decreased oxygen saturation tissue delivery
- CO also can bind myoglobin, resulting in cardiac toxicity by decreasing contractility
- Mild symptoms of toxicity can be seen at carboxyhemoglobin levels of 5% and death at levels of 50%

### CLINICAL MANIFESTATIONS

- Most mild exposures present with flu-like symptoms, headache, visual changes, dizziness, nausea, and/or weakness
- More severe exposure can present with syncope, seizures, coma, cardiac ischemia or infarction, dysrhythmias, pulmonary edema, or death
- Physical exam findings can include tachycardia, hypotension or hypertension, tachypnea, and pallor; skin and soft tissue also more susceptible to trauma with pressure points most affected
- Classic description of cherry red skin is actually a late finding
- Delayed neurologic sequelae may develop days to weeks after exposure; symptoms include headache, disorientation, dementia, apraxia, peripheral neuropathy, ataxia, chorea, or Parkinson-like signs
  ✓ 25% of patients with delayed neurologic sequelae may have permanent neurologic findings

### DIAGNOSTICS

- *Carbon monoxide hemoglobin (COHgb) levels:* Remember, pulse-oximetry may be normal
- CBC, BUN, creatinine, cardiac enzymes, glucose, pregnancy test
- Chest x-ray
- ECG to look for ischemia or dysrhythmias
- Obtain history of risk factors for CO poisoning (e.g., fuel-burning space heaters, charcoal grills, portable generators)

### MANAGEMENT

- Give 100% oxygen to reduce half-life of carboxyhemoglobin
- *Consider hyperbaric oxygen in several situations:* COHgb greater than 25%, pregnancy, or significant cardiac or neurologic symptoms
  ✓ Hyperbaric oxygen may decrease the likelihood neurologic sequelae
- Continue therapy until COHgb less than 5–10%
- Monitor for metabolic acidosis, which may require therapy with sodium bicarbonate in extreme cases
- *Criteria for hospitalization:* (1) Adults with COHgb greater than 25%; (2) children with COHgb greater than 15%; (3) metabolic acidosis; (4) ECG changes; (5) neuropsychiatric symptoms; (6) abnormal thermoregulation; (7) PaO$_2$ less than 60 mm Hg

## CAUSTICS

**Acids or alkali; oven or drain cleaner; powdered laundry and dishwasher detergents; hair relaxers; industrial products**

### TOXICOLOGY/PHARMACOLOGY

- Causes burns when inhaled or ingested, but also with skin and eye contact
- Acids result in coagulation necrosis, and alkalis cause liquefaction necrosis
  - ✓ Although liquefaction necrosis is deeper, the clinical course is similar in both acid and alkali ingestions

### CLINICAL MANIFESTATIONS

- Stridor, hoarseness, dyspnea, aphonia, vomiting, or drooling
- May initially be asymptomatic
- Symptoms do not reliably predict presence or absence of esophageal injury
- Usually present with burning of exposed areas
- Airway edema and obstruction can be delayed up to 48 hours in alkali exposures
- Acids and alkali both can cause esophageal injury
  - ✓ Acid ingestions usually also cause damage to stomach with risk for gastric perforation and peritonitis
  - ✓ Alkali ingestions are more likely to damage esophagus with possibility of perforation and resulting mediastinitis
- May present with acute GI bleed or acute gastric perforation
- Third-degree esophageal burns at risk for developing strictures

### DIAGNOSTICS

- Based on history of exposure and symptoms
- Determine if substance was only irritant or if actually a corrosive
  - ✓ Determined by pH, concentration, and viscosity
  - ✓ Contact poison center for information
- *Laboratory studies:* CBC, type and screen, electrolytes, glucose, blood gas
- Chest x-ray and abdominal x-rays to look for free air

### MANAGEMENT

- *Stabilize airway:* May need intubation under direct visualization (fiberoptic)
  - ✓ Blind intubation can worsen damage or cause perforation
- IV access; keep patient NPO, perform a CXR
- No GI decontamination, No ipecac, No lavage. Simple dilution may pose the risk of fluid leakage into surrounding tissues in the event of perforation, may worsen damage depending on the pH of administered fluids, and eliminates NPO status
- Perform endoscopy as soon as possible to determine extent of burn
- Surgery consult in all patients with significant burns
- Careful examination of the eyes with irrigation if indicated
- Corticosteroids may be beneficial in some esophageal burns to prevent strictures (controversial)
- Pain control
- *Antibiotics:* If evidence of perforation or if steroids are used
- Histamine-2 blocker to reduce gastric acid formation
- *Criteria for hospitalization:* All symptomatic patients with caustic ingestions

## CLONIDINE

**Imidazoline class, along with dexmedetomidine (Precedex®), tetrahydrozoline (Visine®), oxymetazoline (Afrin®), guanfacine (Tenex®, Intuniv®)**

**Medication to treat hypertension and attention deficit hyperactivity disorder; has been used to treat withdrawal symptoms from opioids and nicotine**

### TOXICOLOGY/PHARMACOLOGY

- Agonist at central alpha-2 receptors resulting in decreased sympathetic outflow
- Binds to peripheral alpha-1 receptors resulting in vasoconstriction and hypertension early in the course
- Can cause significant toxicity in small doses
- Rapidly absorbed and distributed, so symptoms appear soon after ingestion

### CLINICAL MANIFESTATIONS

- *Neurologic:* Altered mental status with irritability, lethargy, or coma
- Respiratory depression, occasionally necessitating endotracheal intubation, apnea
- *Cardiac:* Most commonly see hypotension and bradycardia, but can also see tachycardia, transient hypertension, or AV nodal blockade
- *Other:* Miosis, pallor, hypothermia
- Clinical effects typically last 8–24 hours

### DIAGNOSTICS

- Based on history and physical finding
- Drug levels not available
- *Laboratory studies:* Electrolytes, glucose, blood gas
- ECG

### MANAGEMENT

- Activated charcoal
- Treatment primarily supportive
- *Hypotension:* Give fluids; if refractory can also use dopamine or epinephrine
- *Bradycardia:* Treat with atropine
- Hypertension, when present, rarely needs treatment
- Naloxone is sometimes effective in reversing respiratory, cardiac, and neurologic effects. Initial dose is usually 1–2 mg though larger amounts may be necessary
- *Criteria for hospitalization:* Observe asymptomatic patients for 6 hours; admit all symptomatic patients

## COCAINE

**Used medically as local anesthetic; popular street drug**

### TOXICOLOGY/PHARMACOLOGY

- Toxic effects are via CNS stimulation and inhibited catecholamine uptake
- Toxicity develops though multiple routes (ingestion, inhalation, or injection)
- Toxic dose is highly variable, however toxicity usually decreased with ingestion given time for absorption

- "Body packers" swallow many tightly wrapped packets or condoms of cocaine in attempt to hide or smuggle drugs
  - ✓ Toxicity results when packets break open, releasing drugs into GI tract with potentially fatal effect
- "Body stuffers" hastily ingest smaller packets sold on the street to avoid detection by law enforcement
  - ✓ Body stuffing associated with a higher risk of rupture because drugs are not securely enclosed
  - ✓ Risk of mortality, however, is lower than with body packing because relatively small quantities are typically ingested

## CLINICAL MANIFESTATIONS

- *Central nervous system:* Euphoria, agitation, psychosis, seizures, stroke
- *Cardiac:* Hypertension, tachycardia, arrhythmias including ventricular fibrillation, myocardial ischemia, and infarction
- *Respiratory:* Bronchospasm, pneumothorax, pneumomediastinum, hemoptysis
- *Other:* Dilated pupils, hyperthermia, rhabdomyolysis, renal failure, nasal septum perforation
- Cocaine adulterants may cause otherwise unexpected toxicity
  - ✓ For example, levamisole, a veterinary antihelminthic, has caused outbreaks of fever and agranulocytosis in cocaine users

## DIAGNOSTICS

- Based on history of use and clinical presentation
- *Urine toxicologic screen:* Metabolites may be found up to 3 days after exposure
- *Laboratory studies:* Electrolytes, glucose, BUN, creatinine, CPK, urinalysis
- ECG
- Chest x-ray if respiratory symptoms present
- Head CT if suspect stroke
- Abdominal x-rays if suspect body packing; body stuffer packets not well visualized on radiographs

## MANAGEMENT

- *Decontamination:* Give activated charcoal if cocaine taken orally; if suspect body packer give MDAC and consider WBI or surgical removal, given high mortality associated with cocaine packet rupture
- *Supportive care:* Benzodiazepines are used to decrease agitation, tachycardia, and hypertension, and treat seizures
- *Severe hypertension:* DO NOT use beta-blocker, which can cause unopposed alpha-adrenergic effect leading to increase in blood pressure and increased coronary vasospasm
- Treat hyperthermia
- Consider co-ingestions
- Treat arrhythmias and rhabdomyolysis
- *Criteria for hospitalization:* Admit patient with ECG changes, seizures, or neurologic deficits; "body packers"

## CYANIDE

**Naturally occurring in some plants but also present in car exhaust and cigarette smoke in small amounts; toxic exposure usually from the burning of cyanide containing natural or synthetic products, and industrial exposure**

## TOXICOLOGY/PHARMACOLOGY

- Cyanide inhibits electron transport in mitochondria, impairing aerobic metabolism and causing metabolic acidosis
- Small amounts are metabolized under normal circumstances, symptoms occur when these systems are overwhelmed

## CLINICAL MANIFESTATIONS

- *Cardiac:* Tachycardia, hypertension, myocardial toxicity, bradycardia, arrythmias, and cardiovascular collapse
- *Respiratory:* Tachypnea, dyspnea, no cyanosis (cherry-red skin is classically described but not reliably seen)
- *Neurologic:* Headaches, lightheadedness, ataxia, posturing, seizures
- Patients may have a "bitter almond" odor

## DIAGNOSTICS

- *Blood gas with lactate:* Often reveals high mixed venous saturation and severe lactic acidosis
- Lactate
- Electrolytes
- CBC
- ECG

## MANAGEMENT

- Decontamination by removal of wet clothes in the appropriate context (environmental exposure)
- *Supportive care:* 100% oxygen, support of circulation with fluids and pressors if needed, correction of acidosis with sodium bicarbonate, and treatment of seizures with benzodiazepines
- *Antidotes:*
  - ✓ *Older therapy:* Nitrites (amyl and sodium nitrite) and sodium thiosulfate. Nitrites can cause hypotension and affect oxygen-carrying capacity by inducing methemoglobinemia
    - In pediatric patients thiosulfate alone may be used; thiosulfate dose is 400 mg/kg for children <25 kg with a maximum of 12.5 g
  - ✓ *Newer therapy:* Involves use of hydroxocobalamin without attendant side effects of nitrites
    - Dose is 70 mg/kg IV given over 15 minutes; dose may need to be repeated
    - Side effects include hypertension and reddish discoloration of skin, mucous membranes, and urine
    - May be given with or without thiosulfate

## DIGOXIN

**Medication used to treat congestive heart failure and supraventricular tachycardias; digitoxin also found in plants (oleander, rhododendron, foxglove)**

## TOXICOLOGY/PHARMACOLOGY

- Inhibits sodium–potassium ATP pump, increases vagal tone, and slows AV conduction
- Toxicity can occur from chronic use or with overdose, symptoms may be more striking in patients with chronic toxicity
- Doses as small as 1 mg can be toxic in children
- Absorption and redistribution occur rapidly; therefore, digoxin levels can decrease rapidly after ingestion
- Elimination half-life is 30–50 hours, renal clearance is the major mode of elimination

## CLINICAL MANIFESTATIONS

- Symptoms include nausea, vomiting, lethargy, visual changes (halos or changes in color vision)
- Higher levels of intoxication can cause lethargy, mental status changes, electrolyte abnormalities (the most prognostic of which is hyperkalemia), bradycardia, ventricular dysrhythmias, and cardiac arrest

## DIAGNOSTICS

- Stat digoxin level; therapeutic level is 0.9–1.2 ng/mL
- Laboratory findings include hyperkalemia or with chronic toxicity may see hypokalemia if concurrent diuretic use
- *Other laboratory studies:* Electrolytes, calcium, magnesium, BUN, creatinine
- ECG changes may vary; most common ECG abnormalities are sinus bradycardia and AV block
  - ✓ Ventricular dysrhythmias may occur precipitously so early treatment advised in the patient with ECG abnormalities and elevated serum digoxin concentration

## MANAGEMENT

- Decontamination; activated charcoal may be of benefit
- Correction of hyperkalemia will not prevent dysrhythmias. Digoxin-specific Fab (Digibind) will correct hyperkalemia and rhythm disturbances: consider in any patient with ECG abnormalities, high serum digoxin concentration, and/or hyperkalemia (>5 mEq/L, depending on source)
- *Calculating Digibind dosing:*
  - ✓ *If amount of digoxin ingested is known:* 38 mg Digibind to bind 0.5 mg digoxin
  - ✓ *If amount unknown:* Number of vials = [(serum digoxin level in ng/mL) × (body weight in kg)]/100
  - ✓ Potential side effects include hypersensitivity reactions, decreased potassium, worsening of heart failure
  - ✓ Recognize that serum digoxin level may increase after administration, but this reflects inactive drug
- Additional treatment of hyperkalemia
  - ✓ Calcium salts are CONTRAINDICATED and may cause cardioplegia ("stone heart")
  - ✓ Adjunctive therapies such as insulin/glucose and sodium bicarbonate may be useful
- *Criteria for hospitalization:* Admit patients with (1) symptoms of digoxin toxicity, (2) ECG abnormalities, (3) hypokalemia, (4) hyperkalemia, (5) elevated serum digoxin concentration, (6) any patient getting Digibind
  - ✓ Patients with normal digoxin levels, no electrolyte abnormalities, and a normal ECG can be discharged after 6 hours of observation

## ETHANOL

**Beer, wine, liquors; used as solvent, topical antiseptic; ingredient in perfume, cologne, mouthwash; used as antidote in treatment of methanol and ethylene glycol overdoses**

### TOXICOLOGY/PHARMACOLOGY

- Acts as a direct CNS depressant by binding to GABA receptors
- Ethanol can also have effects on cardiac muscle, thyroid, and liver
- Ethanol is metabolized by the liver

- Dose-independent fasting hypoglycemia in children results from ethanol-inhibiting gluconeogenesis
- Levels at which symptoms appear are highly variable

## CLINICAL MANIFESTATIONS

- *Mild acute toxicity:* Nausea, vomiting, euphoria, incoordination, ataxia, nystagmus, impaired judgment; hypoglycemia and seizures seen in younger age group
- *More severe acute toxicity:* Coma, respiratory depression, metabolic acidosis; can have death from apnea
- Presentation in infants and children includes hypothermia, hypoglycemia, metabolic acidosis, and coma
  ✓ These occur at levels of 50–100 mg/dL

## DIAGNOSTICS

- Blood glucose STAT
- *Laboratory studies:* Electrolytes, BUN, creatinine, liver enzymes, PT, blood gas
- Ethanol level
- Chest x-ray if suspicious for aspiration

## MANAGEMENT

- *Supportive care:* Assess airway and establish access; treat hypoglycemia, seizures, hypothermia
- *Decontamination:* Gastric lavage if presenting within 2 hours of ingestion; activated charcoal should be given only if concern for co-ingestion
- Hemodialysis effective, but rarely needed (consider in patients with hepatic impairment or very high blood alcohol levels)
- *Criteria for hospitalization:* In acute ingestions, observe until mental status is at baseline
  ✓ Admit those with ethanol level greater than 100 mg/dL (toddlers), or greater than 200 mg/dL (adolescents) and those with hypoglycemia

## ETHYLENE GLYCOL

**Main ingredient in antifreeze; occasionally used by alcoholics in place of ethanol**

### TOXICOLOGY/PHARMACOLOGY

- Metabolized by alcohol dehydrogenase to toxic glycoaldehyde, glycolic, glyoxylic, and oxalic acids, causing metabolic acidosis and acute renal failure
- Oxalic acid chelates serum calcium, causing hypocalcemia and calcium oxalate precipitation in renal tubules

### CLINICAL MANIFESTATIONS

- Initially, patients will have CNS depression and coma from direct intoxicating effect
- As compound is metabolized, anion-gap metabolic acidosis ensues with tachycardia and hyperpnea, elevated WBC count, GI distress, and hypocalcemia
  ✓ Cardiovascular compromise may result from metabolic derangements and dysrhythmias from hypocalcemia
- Acute kidney injury appears as calcium oxalate crystals precipitate in the kidney, causing direct tubular injury beginning approximately 24 hours after exposure

### DIAGNOSTICS

- Anion-gap metabolic acidosis, elevated osmolar gap
- Hypocalcemia

- Ethylene glycol levels are available, but may be low if already converted to toxic metabolite
- *Other laboratory studies:* Electrolytes, glucose, BUN, creatinine, liver enzymes, urinalysis (which may demonstrate oxalate crystals), blood gas
- ECG
- *Urine:* Some antifreeze contains fluorescein, so urine may fluoresce under Wood's lamp; can see calcium oxalate crystals on microscopic urinalysis

## MANAGEMENT

- *Supportive:* Cardiac monitoring; correct hypocalcemia with IV calcium salts; correct acidosis with sodium bicarbonate
- *Decontamination:* NO charcoal (ineffective); consider gastric lavage if presents within 1 hour
- *Antidote:* Fomepizole and ethanol bind ADH with higher affinity than ethylene glycol and thereby prevent formation of toxic metabolites
  ✓ Treat with fomepizole (preferred) for ethylene glycol level greater than 20 mg/dL or patients with presumed ingestion and metabolic acidosis
  ✓ IV ethanol infusion is a second-line option that is effective but difficult to administer
  ✓ Other options include pyridoxine, folate, and thiamine prevent toxic metabolite formation
- Hemodialysis can be used to enhance elimination; indicated in renal failure or in cases of severe metabolic derangement
- *Criteria for hospitalization:* Any known ingestion of ethylene glycol; clinical or laboratory abnormalities suggestive of ethylene glycol toxicity

## HYDROCARBONS

**Solvents, degreasers, fuels, pesticides, gasoline, kerosene, lighter fluid, torch fuels**

### TOXICOLOGY/PHARMACOLOGY

- Three categories of hydrocarbons
  ✓ Aliphatic (petroleum distillates, furniture polish, lamp oils, lighter fluid)
  ✓ Aromatic (benzene, toluene, xylene, camphor found in glues, solvents, and nail polish)
  ✓ Otherwise "toxic" (halogenated, hydrocarbons that serve as a vehicle for other substances)
- Toxicity can be due to inhalation, skin absorption, or ingestion with systemic toxicity (in aromatic, halogenated hydrocarbons or those with toxic additives)
- As little as 1 mL of fluid aspirated can lead to severe pneumonitis

### CLINICAL MANIFESTATIONS

- *Respiratory symptoms are the primary consequence of most aliphatic hydrocarbon ingestions, due to spillage into tracheobronchial tree:* Tachypnea, dyspnea, cyanosis, grunting, cough
  ✓ Severe pneumonitis and acute respiratory distress syndrome may develop
- Lower viscosity associated with higher aspiration risk
- *Neurologic symptoms usually result from systemic toxicity:* Seizures, lethargy, coma (usually with aromatic hydrocarbons)
- *Gastrointestinal symptoms usually result from ingestion:* Nausea, vomiting, liver failure (carbon tetrachloride)
- *Hematologic:* Hemolysis, hemoglobinuria
- *Cardiac:* Dysrhythmias (with halogenated hydrocarbons)
- Fever
- Skin or eye contact can result in burns or corneal injury

## DIAGNOSTICS

- Based on history of exposure
- If respiratory symptoms, check ABG and chest x-ray
  - ✓ Repeat CXR may be needed in 4–6 hours if initially negative
- If concern over significant ingestion, check electrolytes, glucose, BUN, creatinine, liver enzymes, and an ECG

## MANAGEMENT

- In general, No charcoal, No lavage, and No induction of emesis
  - ✓ Aspiration poses the greatest risk and prevention of aspiration is a mainstay of management
  - ✓ *Exceptions to above "No" rules:* (1) Consider charcoal if hydrocarbon contains a toxic substance (e.g., heavy metal, insecticide, camphor); (2) consider lavage (after intubating to protect airway) if massive amount is ingested
- *Supportive respiratory care:* Supplemental oxygen, continuous positive airway pressure, intubation as needed
- ECMO has been used successfully in some patients
- Antibiotics and steroids are not routinely indicated
- Epinephrine is contraindicated (increased risk of ventricular fibrillation)
- *Criteria for hospitalization:* All symptomatic patients and those with abnormal chest x-rays; monitor for at least 6 hours if asymptomatic
  - ✓ Symptoms can begin up to 24 hours after exposure therefore appropriate discharge instructions are needed

## IRON

**Ingredient in both pediatric and adult multivitamins; adult preparations have greater toxicity due to more elemental iron per tablet**

## TOXICOLOGY/PHARMACOLOGY

- In overdose, transferrin becomes saturated and unbound iron causes injury to cells
- Toxicity can be due to direct corrosive injury or to impaired cellular metabolism
- Toxic dose is 20–30 mg/kg of elemental iron

## CLINICAL MANIFESTATIONS

- Four stages
  - ✓ Direct injury to GI mucosa results in vomiting and diarrhea, both of which can be bloody. Massive blood loss resulting in shock and death may result
  - ✓ Gastrointestinal symptoms are seen to resolve over the next 12–24 hours. In mild ingestions, this may indicate recovery. However, may represent a brief quiescence prior to phase III and patients should be monitored closely
  - ✓ Up to 48 hours after ingestion, systemic symptoms may begin with GI bleeding, metabolic acidosis, coagulopathy, liver failure, seizures, shock, and possibly death
  - ✓ Pyloric stenosis may occur from scarring 4–6 weeks after ingestion

## DIAGNOSTICS

- Based on history of exposure and symptoms
- *Laboratory studies:* STAT iron level if possible, should be done 4–6 hours after ingestion and then repeated 8–12 hours after ingestion to evaluate possibility of delayed absorption
  - ✓ Level greater than 350 μg/dL likely to have toxicity
  - ✓ Level greater than 500 μg/dL suggests more severe toxicity

- CBC, electrolytes, glucose, BUN, creatinine, liver function tests, PT/PTT, type and cross-match
  ✓ Elevated WBC (>15,000 mm³) and glucose (>150 mg/dL) are consistent with ingestion
  ✓ Acidosis is most concerning for toxicity
- Abdominal radiograph at presentation and again after WBI, though a negative x-ray does not necessarily preclude a significant ingestion

## MANAGEMENT

- *Decontamination:* If less than 30 minutes since ingestion, consider gastric lavage; WBI if iron tablets seen on abdominal films (DO NOT use phosphate-containing solutions); activated charcoal is NOT EFFECTIVE
- *Supportive care:* Treat hypotension with fluids; may need to give blood products to treat GI blood loss
- Chelation with continuous IV deferoxamine for severe toxicity
  ✓ Dose is 10–15 mg/kg/h with maximum dose of 6 g/day
  ✓ Chelation treatment results in pink/orange appearance of urine (helpful to forewarn patient and family)
  ✓ Discontinue when asymptomatic with normal laboratory studies and normal appearance of urine
  ✓ Hypotension is a well-described side effect
- *Criteria for hospitalization:* Symptomatic patients; patients with iron level greater than 500 or if iron tablets seen on abdominal radiographs; asymptomatic patients should have iron levels repeated at 8–12 hours—if levels normal and still asymptomatic, can be discharged

## ISOPROPYL ALCOHOL

**Solvent, antiseptic, disinfectant; main ingredient in rubbing alcohol; often ingested by alcoholics as a substitute for liquor**

### TOXICOLOGY/PHARMACOLOGY

- Less toxic than other alcohols
- Toxicity can result from ingestion, inhalation, or via absorption through skin
- Causes CNS depression; large doses can also cause direct vasodilation resulting in hypotension
- Metabolized via alcohol dehydrogenase to acetone, which is also a CNS depressant

### CLINICAL MANIFESTATIONS

- *Gastrointestinal:* Abdominal pain, vomiting, hemorrhagic gastritis
- *Central nervous system:* Slurred speech, ataxia, stupor, coma, respiratory arrest
- *Cardiac:* Myocardial depression
- *Respiratory:* Tracheobronchitis

### DIAGNOSTICS

- Based on history of ingestion, presence of osmolar gap without metabolic acidosis (unlike other toxic alcohols)
- Odor of acetone may be detected
- Ketones (acetone) present in blood and urine

### MANAGEMENT

- Supportive care
- Activated charcoal adsorbs alcohols poorly

- For large, recent ingestions, may consider gastric lavage
- Hemodialysis indicated for hemodynamic instability (very rare)
- *Criteria for hospitalization:* Any patient with symptomatic isopropanol ingestion; symptoms do not rely as heavily on toxic metabolites as other alcohols so symptoms emerge soon after ingestion

## LEAD

**Most common source is chipping paint in homes built before the 1970s; also found in pipes, electric cable, munitions, batteries, glaze used for ceramics, imported toys, jewelry, cosmetics, and food**

### TOXICOLOGY/PHARMACOLOGY

- Majority of toxicity results from chronic exposure
- Toxicity from enzyme inhibition, resulting in blocked heme synthesis
- Can also effect neurotransmitter functioning

### CLINICAL MANIFESTATIONS

- Most children are actually asymptomatic
- *Gastrointestinal:* Can be nonspecific; abdominal pain, vomiting, constipation, anorexia
- *Neurologic:* Seen at higher lead levels ($>70\,\mu g/dL$); irritability, lethargy, ataxia, seizures, encephalopathy or death; may have increased intracranial pressure
- *Renal:* Clinical picture similar to Fanconi; aminoaciduria and glycosuria

### DIAGNOSTICS

- Venous whole blood lead level
- CBC will show microcytic anemia with basophilic stippling
- Elevated free erythrocyte protoporphyrin
- *Long bone radiograph:* May see metaphyseal "lead lines"
- *Abdominal radiographs:* May see opacities
- Avoid lumbar puncture if possible due to potential of increased ICP

### MANAGEMENT

**Symptomatic patients and asymptomatic patients with elevated BLL are at increased risk of CNS involvement**

- *Prevention:* Screening should start at 9–12 months of age at well-child visit
- *Decontamination:* For acute ingestion, consider inducing vomiting or doing gastric lavage
  - ✓ Activated charcoal does not bind lead
  - ✓ Perform WBI if there are findings (paint chips) on abdominal radiographs
- Identify and remove the source
- *Need for subsequent treatment based on blood lead levels:* Should be less than $5\,\mu g/dL$
  - ✓ *Level $>20\,\mu g/dL$:* Consider chelation
  - ✓ *Level $>45\,\mu g/dL$:* start oral chelation with succimer or with IV CaEDTA
  - ✓ *Level $>69\,\mu g/dL$ or signs of encephalopathy:* Hospitalize for two-drug chelation therapy with BAL and CaEDTA (give BAL first and then both together 4 hours later) or BAL and succimer
- Chelation dosing
  - ✓ *Succimer (DMSA):* Dose is $1050\,mg/m^2/day$ (or $30\,mg/kg/day$) divided every 8 hours for 5 days, then $700\,mg/m^2/day$ (or $20\,mg/kg/day$) divided every 12 hours for 14 days

✓ *Edetate Calcium Disodium (CaNa$_2$ EDTA):* 1000 mg/m$^2$/day IV divided every 12 hours for 3–5 days; for lead level greater than 69 μg/dL or signs of encephalopathy, use 1500 mg/m$^2$/day as a continuous infusion for first 48 hours; maintain adequate hydration

✓ *Dimercaprol or British anti-Lewisite (BAL):* Used if lead level greater than 69 μg/dL or signs of encephalopathy; dose is 75 mg/m$^2$ per dose IM every 4 hours for 3–5 days; give first dose alone, then give BAL with CaEDTA; at 48 hours get lead level to decide whether to continue chelation

  ▪ DO NOT use BAL in patients with hepatic insufficiency, peanut allergy, or glucose-6-phosphate dehydrogenase deficiency

  ▪ Use cautiously in patients with hypertension or renal insufficiency

• *Criteria for hospitalization:* Lead level greater than 69 μg/dL or signs of encephalopathy; if only option for removing child from source of lead exposure

• *Supportive care (in lead encephalopathy):* Anticonvulsants; manage increased ICP, adequate hydration to maintain urine output

## METHANOL

**Windshield washer fluid; sterno fuel; solvents, paint remover, antifreeze; used by alcoholics as substitute for ethanol**

### TOXICOLOGY/PHARMACOLOGY

• Metabolized by alcohol dehydrogenase to formaldehyde and formic acid, which are responsible for the toxicity

• Metabolism is slow and symptoms may be delayed for hours. though in large ingestions CNS depression and acidosis may manifest more acutely

• In children, small ingestions (5 mL of 100% methanol) can result in death

### CLINICAL MANIFESTATIONS

• *Ophthalmologic:* "Snowfield vision," retinal toxicity, papilledema, ophthalmoplegia, loss of pupillary light reflex, blindness

• *Central nervous system:* Inebriation, CNS depression, seizures, coma, death

• *Cardiovascular:* Hypotension, reflex tachycardia

• These findings may not appear for up to 24–30 hours

### DIAGNOSTICS

• Based on history and symptoms

• Fundus exam may show optic disc hyperemia, venous engorgement, or papilledema

• Anion-gap metabolic acidosis may be preceded by an elevated osmolar gap

• *Other laboratory studies:* Electrolytes, glucose, BUN, creatinine, serum osmolality, blood gas, methanol level, lactate level

### MANAGEMENT

• *Decontamination:* Do not induce emesis; activated charcoal is NOT effective

  ✓ May perform gastric lavage

  ✓ Treat metabolic acidosis with IV sodium bicarbonate

• *Antidote:* Fomepizole and ethanol bind alcohol dehydrogenase with higher affinity than ethylene glycol and thereby prevent formation of toxic metabolites

  ✓ Treat with fomepizole (preferred) for methanol level greater than 25 mg/dL or patients with presumed ingestion and metabolic acidosis

  ✓ If not available, IV ethanol infusion is also effective but difficult to administer

- Folic acid helps conversion of formic acid to carbon dioxide and water
- Hemodialysis is indicated in cases of severe metabolic acidosis or blood methanol concentrations greater than 50 mg/dL
- *Criteria for hospitalization:* Any known methanol ingestion or clinical and lab findings suggestive of methanol ingestion

## OPIOIDS

**Can be natural or synthetic; most commonly used to treat severe pain, can also be used as antitussive; opioid abuse can result from use of prescription medication or illegal street drugs.**

### TOXICOLOGY/PHARMACOLOGY

- Opioid effects result from binding directly to opioid receptors in CNS
- Tolerance develops with chronic use, except for miosis, constipation
- Buprenorphine is an opioid partial agonist with low potential for abuse, which can also block the effect of full opioid agonists at high doses; prescribed for opioid addiction
- Rising common accidental pediatric ingestion with increased toxicity in children

### CLINICAL MANIFESTATIONS

- Classic triad of pinpoint pupils, coma, and respiratory depression
- *Gastrointestinal:* Decreased motility and increased sphincter tone can result in constipation; effects on biliary sphincter may cause RUQ pain that mimics other biliary conditions
- *Cardiac:* Hypotension; propoxyphene may cause arrhythmias
- *Central nervous system:* Lethargy, respiratory depression, coma, seizures (primarily with meperidine)
- *Pulmonary:* Pulmonary edema
- Diphenoxylate results in delayed onset of symptoms secondary to formulation that includes atropine

### DIAGNOSTICS

- Can be based on clinical findings
- Can perform urine or blood toxicologic screen, though methadone, fentanyl, and oxycodone may not be detected on routine drug screens
- *Laboratory studies:* Electrolytes, glucose, BUN, creatinine, blood gas
- Chest x-ray

### MANAGEMENT

- *Decontamination:* Activated charcoal for oral ingestion; consider MDAC or WBI for "body stuffers"
- *Supportive care:* May need to intubate to maintain airway; treat hypotension, seizures, pulmonary edema if they occur
- Naloxone is an opioid antagonist; dose is 0.4–2 mg IV; may repeat if no response after 2–3 minutes
  ✓ May need to use repeat doses or an infusion to maintain response
  ✓ May precipitate withdrawal in addicted patients; therefore, detoxification of an addicted patient is usually done with methadone
- *Criteria for hospitalization:* In general, patients should be admitted for observation; length of observation is based on half-life of specific drug

## ORGANOPHOSPHATES

**Insecticides; ingredient in chemical warfare agents**

### TOXICOLOGY/PHARMACOLOGY

- Toxicity is a result of inhibition of acetylcholinesterase; clinical findings are result of accumulation of acetylcholine at muscarinic, nicotinic, and CNS receptors
  - ✓ Enzyme inhibition can become irreversible with increasing time of exposure, a process known as "aging"
- Can be from inhalation, ingestion, or absorption from skin
- Rapid onset of symptoms after exposure
- Children and pregnant women are at increased risk of toxicity due to lower baseline cholinesterase levels
- Note that carbamate insecticides act similarly on acetylcholinesterase but do not cause irreversible inhibition ("aging")

### CLINICAL MANIFESTATIONS

- *Central nervous system:* Headache, agitation, seizures, coma
- *Nicotinic:* Weakness, fasciculations, increased heart rate and blood pressure; can result in death from respiratory muscle paralysis
- *Muscarinic:* Abdominal pain, vomiting, diarrhea, urinary and fecal incontinence, bronchospasm, decreased heart rate and blood pressure (opposite from nicotinic effects), salivation, diaphoresis, miosis
- Can occasionally see a delayed, permanent, peripheral neuropathy

### DIAGNOSTICS

- Diagnosis based on history of exposure and classic clinical presentation
- Not detected on urine toxicologic screens
- Can measure plasma pseudocholinesterase levels or red blood cell cholinesterase activity, but this is not very helpful unless baseline levels have been obtained
- *Laboratory studies:* Electrolytes, glucose, BUN, creatinine, liver function tests, blood gas
- ECG

### MANAGEMENT

- Avoid contact with contaminated clothing, skin, or gastric aspirates
- *Decontamination:* Contaminated clothing must be removed and discarded as toxic waste, skin should be cleaned with soap and water
  - ✓ No ipecac, gastric lavage for recent ingestions, activated charcoal
- *Antidote:* Atropine in doses of 0.05–0.1 mg/kg should be repeated until asymptomatic; administer either IV or IM
  - ✓ Pralidoxime (used in conjunction with atropine) is used specifically to treat muscle weakness and prevent "aging"—dose is 20–40 mg/kg either IV or IM; doses can be repeated every hour as needed until muscle weakness and other cholinergic signs and symptoms resolve
- Avoid any concurrent therapy with drugs that affect acetylcholine uptake (i.e., phenothiazines)
- *Criteria for hospitalization:* Any patient requiring treatment

## PHENOTHIAZINES (ANTIPSYCHOTICS)

**Used for depression, psychosis, aggression, emotional instability, sleep disturbance, and acute management of agitation and delirium**

## TOXICOLOGY/PHARMACOLOGY

- *Typical antipsychotics:* Phenothiazines/butyrophenones—chlorpromazine, thioridazine, haloperidol, droperidol
  - ✓ Toxicity is due to effects on CNS, anticholinergic effects, alpha-adrenergic blocking effects
  - ✓ Have variable antagonism at the D2 dopamine receptor but cause nonspecific blockade throughout the brain leading to side effects
  - ✓ Toxicity can be seen with therapeutic doses
- Atypical antipsychotics (risperidone, clozapine, olanzapine, quetiapine)
  - ✓ Serotonin receptor antagonists or partial agonists in addition to dopamine receptor blockade
  - ✓ Lower risk of extrapyramidal side effects
  - ✓ Can bind with high affinity leading to long lasting adverse effects

## CLINICAL MANIFESTATIONS

*Typical antipsychotics:*

- Toxicity
  - ✓ *Mild toxicity:* CNS: sedation, ataxia, slurred speech; anticholinergic symptoms include constipation, urinary retention, dry mouth (except clozapine causes hypersalivation); orthostatic hypotension, tachycardia
  - ✓ *Severe toxicity:* CNS: hypothermia or hyperthermia, coma, seizures, respiratory arrest; cardiac: QRS or QT prolongation, dysrhythmias, hypotension; extrapyramidal effects: torticollis, rigidity, tremor, cogwheel rigidity
- *Dystonic reactions:* Can be seen regardless of amount ingested
- *Neuroleptic malignant syndrome:* Rigidity, hyperthermia, rhabdomyolysis, lactic acidosis

*Atypical antipsychotics:*

- *Mild toxicity:* Sialorrhea (clozapine), orthostasis, sedation, metabolic and endocrinologic abnormalities, nausea and vomiting, urinary retention, sleep abnormalities, blurred vision
- *Severe toxicity:* Coma, respiratory depression, seizures, movement disorders, hypotension, myocardial depression, QT prolongation, hepatic toxicity, severe allergic reactions, delirium, agranulocytosis, neuroleptic malignant syndrome

## DIAGNOSTICS

- Based on history of ingestion and symptoms
- *Drug levels not generally available:* Some cause a false positive tricyclic screen
- *Laboratory studies:* Electrolytes, BUN, creatinine, glucose, CPK, blood gas, liver function tests
- *Abdominal x-ray:* Pills can be radio-opaque
- ECG to look for conduction delays

## MANAGEMENT

- *Decontamination:* Activated charcoal, WBI for some sustained-release formulations. In specific cases a lipid emulsion may be helpful in consultation with local poison control
- *Supportive care:* Treat dystonic reactions with either diphenhydramine (0.5–1.0 mg/kg IV or IM) or benztropine (0.02 mg/kg IV or IM for children over 3 years)
  - ✓ Be alert for other sequelae such as arrhythmias (requires cardiac monitoring), seizures, and hypotension

- Neuroleptic malignant syndrome
  - ✓ Cooling blankets for hyperthermia
  - ✓ Benzodiazepines for muscular rigidity
  - ✓ Intubation and paralysis if needed
  - ✓ Dantrolene or bromocriptine for severe cases
- *Criteria for hospitalization:* Admit patients with signs of toxicity; observe asymptomatic ingestions for 6 hours

## PHENYTOIN (ANTICONVULSANT)

### TOXICOLOGY/PHARMACOLOGY

- Phenytoin increases brain concentrations of GABA, reduces high-frequency neuronal firing, and affects cardiac conduction through Class Ib antidysryhthmic effect (sodium channel blockade)
- Toxicity can be seen at doses of 20 mg/kg
- Erratic oral absorption
- Drug is highly protein bound and toxicity can develop from decreased protein binding or displacement of drug by other drugs
- With IV preparations, toxicity may be due to diluent, propylene glycol

### CLINICAL MANIFESTATIONS

- *Cardiac:* Can see tachycardia or bradycardia; hypotension (ventricular fibrillation and asystole can be seen with IV overdose)
- *Neurologic:* Ataxia, encephalopathy, tremor, agitation, nystagmus, confusion, hallucinations; seizures are rare (must rule out co-ingestion)
- *Gastrointestinal:* Nausea, vomiting, hepatitis
- Can also see hypersensitivity reactions
- Rapid intravenous administration can result in hypotension (due to propylene glycol) and arrhythmias

### DIAGNOSTICS

- Diagnosis based on history of ingestion
- STAT phenytoin concentration (10–20 mg/L considered therapeutic); need to recheck due to possibility of delayed absorption
- *Laboratory studies:* Electrolytes, BUN, creatinine, glucose, albumin
- ECG if drug was given IV

### MANAGEMENT

- *Decontamination:* Activated charcoal, may consider MDAC
- *Supportive care:* Treat hypotension, manage dysrhythmias (ACLS/PALS guidelines)
- *Criteria for hospitalization:* Cardiac or neurologic symptoms; unable to tolerate fluids due to severity of nausea and vomiting, fall risk due to ataxia

## SALICYLATES (ASPIRIN)

**Over-the-counter analgesics and cold medications; Pepto-Bismol (bismuth subsalicylate); liniments, oil of wintergreen (methyl salicylate)**

## TOXICOLOGY/PHARMACOLOGY

- Direct CNS stimulation of respiration resulting in respiratory alkalosis
- Uncouples oxidative phosphorylation and inhibits Krebs cycle, causing elevated anion-gap metabolic acidosis
- *A unique mixed acid–base disorder ensues:* Concomitant respiratory alkalosis and metabolic acidosis
  - ✓ Young children are more likely to present with acidosis
- 60% of cases of salicylism are from acute ingestion
- Start to see toxicity at doses of 150 mg/kg
- Elimination half-life can be as high as 36 hours in cases of overdose because of loss of first-order kinetics as drug concentrations increase

## CLINICAL MANIFESTATIONS

- Acute toxicity
  - ✓ Mild symptoms include vomiting, tinnitus, lethargy, tachypnea
  - ✓ Moderate symptoms include agitation, diaphoresis, fever
  - ✓ Severe symptoms include seizures, coma, pulmonary edema, death results from CNS toxicity and inhibition of cardiorespiratory centers in the brain
- *Chronic toxicity:* Symptoms can appear at much lower serum concentrations
- Can be nonspecific with only confusion or dehydration
- Can see metabolic acidosis and pulmonary and cerebral edema

## DIAGNOSTICS

- *Salicylate level:* Therapeutic level is 15–30 mg/dL
  - ✓ Mild toxicity (tinnitus) at levels of 30–40 mg/dL
  - ✓ CNS depression at levels greater than 80 mg/dL
  - ✓ Severe toxicity at levels greater than 100 mg/dL
- Chronic toxicity may manifest at lower levels
- Obtain serial salicylate levels (every 2–4 hours) and blood gases until level falling into nontoxic range
- Other
  - ✓ Electrolytes (repeat every 2 hours during alkalinization and then every 12 hours until acid–base disturbances resolve; early hyperglycemia followed by hypoglycemia and hypokalemia)
  - ✓ Arterial blood gas (combined respiratory alkalosis and anion gap metabolic acidosis)
  - ✓ Liver function tests
  - ✓ CBC, PT, and PTT (coagulopathy may occur)
  - ✓ Urinalysis (every 2 hours; for pH and specific gravity; maintain urine pH of 7.5–8)
  - ✓ ECG

## MANAGEMENT

- Activated charcoal where appropriate
- Treat fluid deficits (often profound) and electrolyte abnormalities
- *Alkalinize to enhance salicylate excretion and maintain serum pH greater than 7.4:* Give 100–150 mEq sodium bicarbonate/L of D5W at two times maintenance; goal urine pH is 7.5–8.0
- Maintain normal serum potassium (>4.0 mEq/L)
- If intubation needed, attempt to mimic the patient's own respiratory rate as depression of their spontaneous rate may worsen neurological outcomes

- Hemodialysis should be considered for metabolic acidosis not easily reversed with alkalinization, CNS dysfunction impairing patient's ability to maintain hyperpnea, salicylate levels >100 mg/dL, renal failure, pulmonary edema, or deterioration despite therapy
- *Criteria for hospitalization:* Admit all symptomatic patients; observe asymptomatic patients for at least 6 hours

## SELECTIVE SEROTONIN UPTAKE INHIBITORS/SELECTIVE SEROTONIN-NOREPINEPHRINE UPTAKE INHIBITORS

**Used to treat depression and obsessive compulsive disorder and other behavioral disorders; examples include fluoxetine, paroxetine, and sertraline (SSRIs) and venlafaxine, duloxetine (SNRIs)**

### TOXICOLOGY/PHARMACOLOGY

- Caused by CNS depression
- Safer than tricyclic or monoamine oxidase inhibitor (MAOI) antidepressants; death from overdose is uncommon
- Trazodone is an SARI (serotonin antagonist/reuptake inhibitor) and can cause SIADH and priapism

### CLINICAL MANIFESTATIONS

- *Neurologic:* Confusion, sedation, coma
- Respiratory depression can occur, more likely after co-ingestion with other sedatives
- *Cardiac:* Usually mild, can get tachycardia and hypotension or hypertension, arrhythmias due to QT prolongation
- *GI:* Nausea, vomiting, and anorexia
- *Serotonin syndrome:* Can be seen after starting drug, switching drugs, increasing dose, or overdose; presents with rigidity, hyperreflexia, autonomic instability, alteration in mental status, restlessness, hyperthermia; may resemble neuroleptic malignant syndrome

### DIAGNOSTICS

- Drug levels are not useful
- *Laboratory studies:* Electrolytes, glucose, CPK, UA, blood gas; ECG

### MANAGEMENT

- Decontamination
- *Supportive care:* Hydration; alkalinize urine if signs of rhabdomyolysis; manage seizures with benzodiazepine, manage hyperthermia with external cooling, neuromuscular paralysis, and intubation
- In some reports, serotonin syndrome has been successfully treated with cyproheptadine, a serotonin receptor antagonist

## TRICYCLIC ANTIDEPRESSANTS

**Used to treat depression, enuresis, neuropathic pain**

### TOXICOLOGY/PHARMACOLOGY

- Due to anticholinergic effects, peripheral alpha blocking effects, sodium channel blockade causing ventricular conduction delay and myocardial depression, and inhibition of norepinephrine and serotonin reuptake
- Large volumes of distribution

## CLINICAL MANIFESTATIONS

- *Anticholinergic syndrome:* Urinary retention, delayed gastric emptying, flushed and dry skin, delirium, dilated pupils, hyperthermia
- Extreme hyperthermia can result in rhabdomyolysis
- *Cardiac:* Hypotension from peripheral vasodilation; sinus tachycardia; conduction abnormalities (prolongation of PR, QRS, or QT intervals); QRS interval greater than 0.1 seconds is predictive of significant morbidity; various arrhythmias including PVCs, ventricular tachycardia, ventricular fibrillation
- *Neurologic:* Can range from lethargy to seizures to coma

## DIAGNOSTICS

- Drug levels are usually not helpful
- Most can be detected on urine screening
- *Laboratory studies:* Electrolytes, BUN, creatinine, glucose, blood gas, CPK, urinalysis
- *ECG:* Width of QRS interval >100 milliseconds is predictive of ventricular dysrhythmias and seizures

## MANAGEMENT

- *Decontamination:* Consider lavage, activated charcoal
- Sodium bicarbonate reverses cardiac sodium channel blockade and narrows QRS complex, by alkalinizing the blood (thereby trapping the drug in the circulation and not the myocardium) and overcoming channel blockade with sodium loading. 1 mEq/kg bolus dosing to narrow QRS, repeat PRN for wide complex. Consider infusion if repeated doses needed
- *Supportive care:* Treat seizures with benzodiazepines. Norepinephrine can be used for persistent hypotension. Lidocaine can be used for persistent arrhythmias. Prevent hyperthermia
- Physostigmine SHOULD NOT be given and will worsen cardiac toxicity
- *Criteria for hospitalization:* Observe all ingestions at least 6 hours. If any signs of toxicity, admit for 24 hours of observation

## DESIGNER DRUGS

**Can refer to any synthetic form of a controlled substance**

### TOXICOLOGY/PHARMACOLOGY

**Synthetic cannabinoids**

- Similar to THC in function by binding to cannabinoid receptors
- *Common names:* "Spice," "yucatan fire," "aroma," "incense," "potpourri," "K2"
- Attractive to users because they are not typically detected by drug screens and are advertised as "safe and legal"
- Limited data on human toxicity and high variability in preparations contribute to danger
- Common effects include nausea, vomiting, tachycardia, and hypertension; chest pain and ischemia occur in more severe cases, psychiatric effects include anxiety, depression, and psychosis; seizures reported

**Synthetic stimulants**

- Can be marketed as "bath salts" or "plant food"
- Derivatives of a stimulant called cathinone, a controlled substance
- Can be taken orally, intranasally, or intravenously

- Inhibit dopamine and norepinephrine reuptake
- Common effects include tachycardia and hypertension, agitation, diaphoresis, psychosis, and hallucinations. Dysphoric reactions causing panic and anxiety have also been described

## DIAGNOSTICS

- Chemistry (synthetic cannabinoids have been reported to cause hypokalemia), ECG
- Drug screens may identify co-ingestions and high performance liquid chromatography/tandem mass spectroscopy might identify more rare drugs but is rarely useful in the immediate setting

## MANAGEMENT

- Recognize that even designer drugs of the same name can have unreliable chemical compositions and can cause variable reactions
- Management consists largely of supportive care and close cardiorespiratory monitoring. Patients may benefit from benzodiazepines for psychiatric symptoms

### FOREIGN BODY INGESTIONS

**Includes button batteries, detergent pods, magnet toys, and expanding toys**

## TOXICOLOGY/PHARMACOLOGY

- *Button batteries:*
  - ✓ Increased number of objects powered by button batteries (toys, remote controls, children's books with musical push buttons) with a resultant increase in ingestions
  - ✓ Injury occurs primarily from direct electrical current and caustic alkaline injury with liquefactive necrosis, heavy metal leaching, and direct pressure can also be a factor
  - ✓ Increasing number of fatal cases in recent years, most of which are associated with 20 mm 3V lithium disc battery
- *Detergent pods:*
  - ✓ Agents thought to contribute to symptomatology include propylene glycol, ethoxylated alcohols, and highly concentrated detergents
- *Magnet toys:*
  - ✓ Increasing incidence as magnets are more common in toys and household objects
- *Expanding toys:*
  - ✓ Commonly balls made of superabsorbent polymers that expand when exposed to water
  - ✓ Generally attractive to toddlers because of their size and color, easy to swallow
  - ✓ Superabsorbent polymer technology more common now in household products and gardening supplies in addition to toys

## CLINICAL MANIFESTATIONS

- Button battery ingestions may be asymptomatic or might cause respiratory symptoms, pain, drooling, or dysphagia
- *Detergent pods:*
  - ✓ Detergent pods may cause drooling, coughing or gagging, respiratory distress, vomiting, and mental status changes which may be profound
- *Magnet toys:*
  - ✓ Number of magnets is important as more than one may attract and cause intestinal obstruction, necrosis, and perforation
  - ✓ Magnet ingestions are often asymptomatic but may cause abdominal obstruction or fistulas

- *Expanding toys:*
  - ✓ Ingestion of expanding toys may also be initially asymptomatic but can rapidly cause symptoms of GI obstruction including nausea/vomiting, abdominal distension, and pain

## DIAGNOSTICS

- Plain film of the chest and abdomen (does not rule out foreign body as many are radiolucent)
- For detergent pods, a blood gas, metabolic panel, glucose, ECG, and CBC might be helpful in the differential diagnosis of the mental status changes

## MANAGEMENT

- Supportive care including close airway monitoring, in patients with worsening respiratory distress or mental status changes securing the airway early might be indicated
- For proximal foreign bodies (esophageal and pre-pyloric) involve GI/ENT to discuss removal (always indicated for button batteries and multiple magnets, highly recommended for expanding toys)
- *Admission criteria:* Any symptomatic patient should be admitted for serial exams and monitoring, patients requiring intervention, unknown type, or quantity of ingested object

| TABLE 1A | Range of Normal Values for Respiratory Rate and Heart Rate in Childhood | |
| --- | --- | --- |
| **Age** | **Respiratory Rate (Per Minute)** | **Heart Rate (Per Minute)** |
| Neonate | 35–66 | 93–154 |
| 1 month | 34–64 | 121–182 |
| 3 months | 32–61 | 106–186 |
| 6 months | 30–56 | 109–169 |
| 12 months | 27–49 | 89–151 |
| 5 years | 16–31 | 65–133 |
| 10–18 years | 12–20 | 60–120 |

| TABLE 1B | Range of Blood Pressure Values for Children of Average Height* | | |
| --- | --- | --- | --- |
| **Age** | | **BP Percentile** | **Value or Range**** |
| Neonate (term) | Systolic | 5th | 63 |
| | | 50th | 78 |
| | | 95th | 92 |
| | Diastolic | 5th | 30 |
| | | 50th | 45 |
| | | 95th | 60 |
| 1–5 years | Systolic | 50th | 85–95 |
| | | 95th | 103–112 |
| | Diastolic | 50th | 37–53 |
| | | 95th | 56–72 |
| 6–10 years | Systolic | 50th | 96–102 |
| | | 95th | 114–119 |
| | Diastolic | 50th | 55–61 |
| | | 95th | 74–80 |
| 11–18 years | Systolic | 50th | 104–118 |
| | | 95th | 121–136 |
| | Diastolic | 50th | 61–67 |
| | | 95th | 80–87 |

Abbreviations: BP, blood pressure.

*Please consult alternate sources for more precise classification of normal blood pressure since the values vary slightly by gender, age, and height. Data derived in part from (1) American Academy of Pediatrics. The fourth report on the diagnosis, evaluation, and treatment of high blood pressure in children and adolescents. *Pediatrics.* 2004;114:555–576; (2) Zubrow AB, et al. Determinants of blood pressure in infants admitted to neonatal intensive care units: a prospective, multicenter study. *J Perinatol.* 1995;15:470–479; and (3) Rusconi F, et al. Reference values for respiratory rate in the first 3 years of life. *Pediatrics.* 1994;94:350–355.

**By convention, the inflatable bladder width of an appropriate size cuff covers at least 40% of the arm circumference at a point midway between the olecranon and the acromion (for more information consult the American Heart Association or search their website at www.americanheart.org).

### Pediatric Septic Shock Algorithm

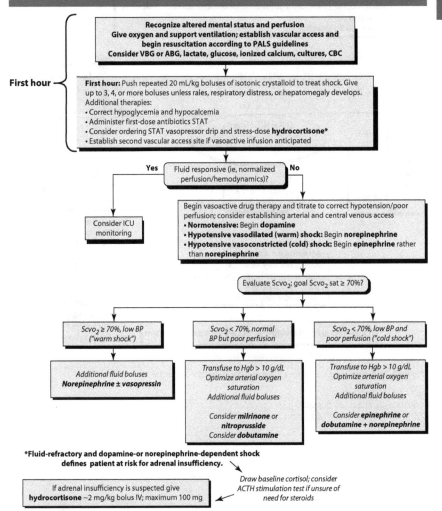

**First hour**

**Recognize altered mental status and perfusion**
**Give oxygen and support ventilation; establish vascular access and begin resuscitation according to PALS guidelines**
**Consider VBG or ABG, lactate, glucose, ionized calcium, cultures, CBC**

**First hour:** Push repeated 20 mL/kg boluses of isotonic crystalloid to treat shock. Give up to 3, 4, or more boluses unless rales, respiratory distress, or hepatomegaly develops.
Additional therapies:
- Correct hypoglycemia and hypocalcemia
- Administer first-dose antibiotics STAT
- Consider ordering STAT vasopressor drip and stress-dose **hydrocortisone***
- Establish second vascular access site if vasoactive infusion anticipated

**Yes** — Fluid responsive (ie, normalized perfusion/hemodynamics)? — **No**

Consider ICU monitoring

Begin vasoactive drug therapy and titrate to correct hypotension/poor perfusion; consider establishing arterial and central venous access
- **Normotensive: Begin dopamine**
- **Hypotensive vasodilated (warm) shock: Begin norepinephrine**
- **Hypotensive vasoconstricted (cold) shock: Begin epinephrine** rather than **norepinephrine**

Evaluate $Scvo_2$; goal $Scvo_2$ sat ≥ 70%?

| $Scvo_2$ ≥ 70%, low BP ("warm shock") | $Scvo_2$ < 70%, normal BP but poor perfusion | $Scvo_2$ < 70%, low BP and poor perfusion ("cold shock") |

Additional fluid boluses
**Norepinephrine ± vasopressin**

Transfuse to Hgb > 10 g/dL
Optimize arterial oxygen saturation
Additional fluid boluses

Consider **milrinone** or **nitroprusside**
Consider **dobutamine**

Transfuse to Hgb > 10 g/dL
Optimize arterial oxygen saturation
Additional fluid boluses

Consider **epinephrine** or **dobutamine + norepinephrine**

**\*Fluid-refractory and dopamine-or norepinephrine-dependent shock defines patient at risk for adrenal insufficiency.**

*Draw baseline cortisol; consider ACTH stimulation test if unsure of need for steroids*

If adrenal insufficiency is suspected give **hydrocortisone** ~2 mg/kg bolus IV; maximum 100 mg

**Figure 1.** Pediatric Septic Shock Algorithm. Modified from Brierley J, Carcillo JA, Choong K, Cornell T, Decaen A, Deymann A, Doctor A, Davis A, Duff J, Dugas MA, Duncan A, Evans B, Feldman J, Felmet K, Fisher G, Frankel L, Jeffries H, Greenwald B, Gutierrez J, Hall M, Han YY, Hanson J, Hazelzet J, Hernan L, Kiff J, Kissoon N, Kon A, Irazuzta J, Lin J, Lorts A, Mariscalco M, Mehta R, Nadel S, Nguyen T, Nicholson C, Peters M, Okhuysen-Cawley R, Poulton T, Relves M, Rodriguez A, Rozenfeld R, Schnitzler E, Shanley T, Kache S, Skippen P, Torres A, von Dessauer B, Weingarten J, Yeh T, Zaritsky A, Stojadinovic B, Zimmerman J, Zuckerberg A. Clinical practice parameters for hemodynamic support of pediatric and neonatal septic shock: 2007 update from the American College of Critical Care Medicine. *Crit Care Med.* 2009;37(2): 666-688.

## Pediatric Bradycardia With a Pulse and Poor Perfusion Algorithm

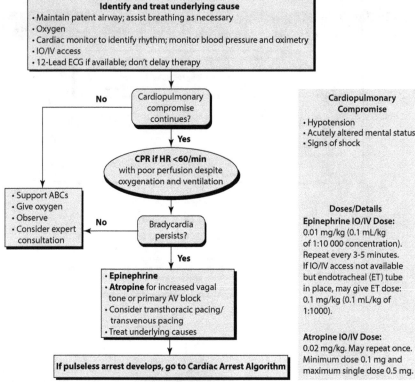

**Identify and treat underlying cause**
- Maintain patent airway; assist breathing as necessary
- Oxygen
- Cardiac monitor to identify rhythm; monitor blood pressure and oximetry
- IO/IV access
- 12-Lead ECG if available; don't delay therapy

Cardiopulmonary compromise continues?

**No**

**Cardiopulmonary Compromise**
- Hypotension
- Acutely altered mental status
- Signs of shock

**Yes**

**CPR if HR <60/min** with poor perfusion despite oxygenation and ventilation

- Support ABCs
- Give oxygen
- Observe
- Consider expert consultation

**No**

Bradycardia persists?

**Yes**

- **Epinephrine**
- **Atropine** for increased vagal tone or primary AV block
- Consider transthoracic pacing/ transvenous pacing
- Treat underlying causes

**Doses/Details**
**Epinephrine IO/IV Dose:**
0.01 mg/kg (0.1 mL/kg of 1:10 000 concentration). Repeat every 3-5 minutes. If IO/IV access not available but endotracheal (ET) tube in place, may give ET dose: 0.1 mg/kg (0.1 mL/kg of 1:1000).

**Atropine IO/IV Dose:**
0.02 mg/kg. May repeat once. Minimum dose 0.1 mg and maximum single dose 0.5 mg.

**If pulseless arrest develops, go to Cardiac Arrest Algorithm**

© 2010 American Heart Association

**Figure 2.** Pediatric Bradycardia With a Pulse and Poor Perfusion Algorithm.

Reprinted with permission
Pediatric Advanced Life Support
©2011, American Heart Association, Inc.

## Pediatric Tachycardia With a Pulse and Adequate Perfusion Algorithm

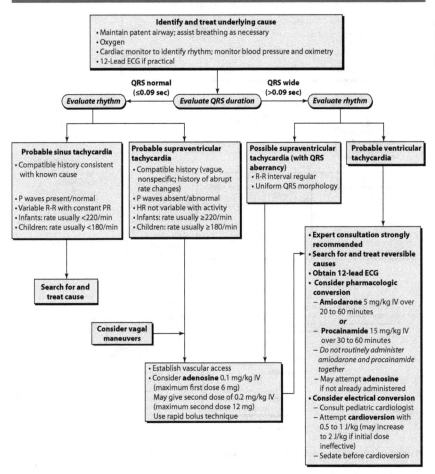

**Figure 3.** Pediatric Tachycardia With a Pulse and Adequate Perfusion Algorithm.

## Pediatric Tachycardia With a Pulse and Poor Perfusion Algorithm

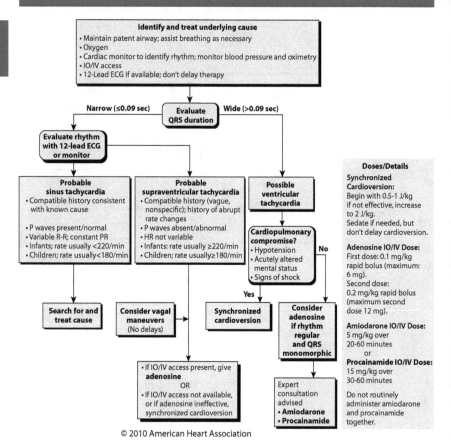

© 2010 American Heart Association

**Figure 4.** Pediatric Tachycardia With a Pulse and Poor Perfusion Algorithm.

Reprinted with permission
Pediatric Advanced Life Support
©2011, American Heart Association, Inc.

# Pediatric Cardiac Arrest

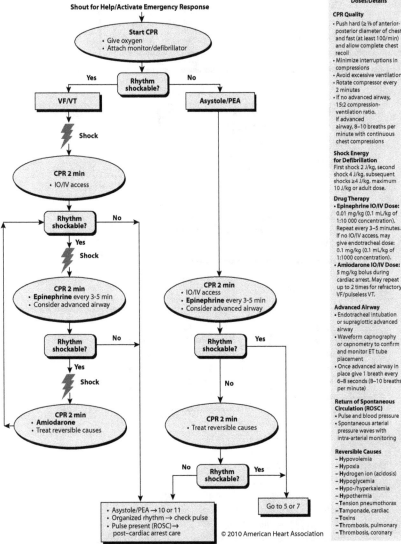

Shout for Help/Activate Emergency Response

**Start CPR**
• Give oxygen
• Attach monitor/defibrillator

**Rhythm shockable?** — Yes → **VF/VT** / No → **Asystole/PEA**

**VF/VT**

⚡ Shock

**CPR 2 min**
• IO/IV access

**Rhythm shockable?** No →

Yes
⚡ Shock

**CPR 2 min**
• **Epinephrine** every 3-5 min
• Consider advanced airway

**Rhythm shockable?** No →

Yes
⚡ Shock

**CPR 2 min**
• Amiodarone
• Treat reversible causes

**Asystole/PEA**

**CPR 2 min**
• IO/IV access
• **Epinephrine** every 3-5 min
• Consider advanced airway

**Rhythm shockable?** Yes →

No

**CPR 2 min**
• Treat reversible causes

**Rhythm shockable?** No / Yes →

• Asystole/PEA → 10 or 11
• Organized rhythm → check pulse
• Pulse present (ROSC) → post–cardiac arrest care

**Go to 5 or 7**

© 2010 American Heart Association

## Doses/Details

**CPR Quality**
• Push hard (≥ ⅓ of anterior-posterior diameter of chest) and fast (at least 100/min) and allow complete chest recoil
• Minimize interruptions in compressions
• Avoid excessive ventilation
• Rotate compressor every 2 minutes
• If no advanced airway, 15:2 compression-ventilation ratio. If advanced airway, 8–10 breaths per minute with continuous chest compressions

**Shock Energy for Defibrillation**
First shock 2 J/kg, second shock 4 J/kg, subsequent shocks ≥4 J/kg, maximum 10 J/kg or adult dose.

**Drug Therapy**
• **Epinephrine IO/IV Dose:** 0.01 mg/kg (0.1 mL/kg of 1:10 000 concentration). Repeat every 3–5 minutes. If no IO/IV access, may give endotracheal dose: 0.1 mg/kg (0.1 mL/kg of 1:1000 concentration).
• **Amiodarone IO/IV Dose:** 5 mg/kg bolus during cardiac arrest. May repeat up to 2 times for refractory VF/pulseless VT.

**Advanced Airway**
• Endotracheal intubation or supraglottic advanced airway
• Waveform capnography or capnometry to confirm and monitor ET tube placement
• Once advanced airway in place give 1 breath every 6–8 seconds (8–10 breaths per minute)

**Return of Spontaneous Circulation (ROSC)**
• Pulse and blood pressure
• Spontaneous arterial pressure waves with intra-arterial monitoring

**Reversible Causes**
– Hypovolemia
– Hypoxia
– Hydrogen ion (acidosis)
– Hypoglycemia
– Hypo-/hyperkalemia
– Hypothermia
– Tension pneumothorax
– Tamponade, cardiac
– Toxins
– Thrombosis, pulmonary
– Thrombosis, coronary

**Figure 5.** Pediatric Cardiac Arrest Algorithm.

Reprinted with permission
Pediatric Advanced Life Support
©2011, American Heart Association, Inc.

## Management of Shock After Return of Spontaneous Circulation (ROSC)

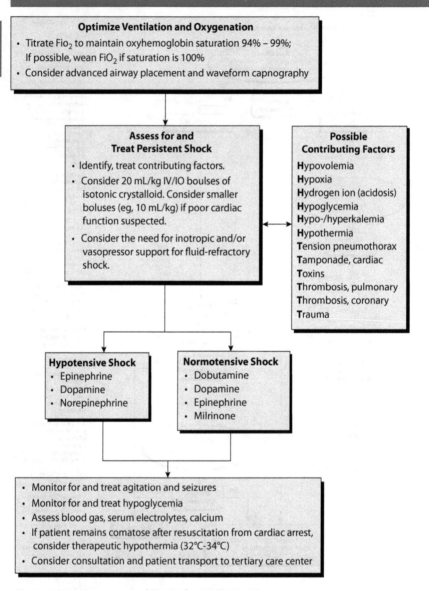

**Optimize Ventilation and Oxygenation**
- Titrate $Fio_2$ to maintain oxyhemoglobin saturation 94% – 99%; If possible, wean $FiO_2$ if saturation is 100%
- Consider advanced airway placement and waveform capnography

**Assess for and Treat Persistent Shock**
- Identify, treat contributing factors.
- Consider 20 mL/kg IV/IO boluses of isotonic crystalloid. Consider smaller boluses (eg, 10 mL/kg) if poor cardiac function suspected.
- Consider the need for inotropic and/or vasopressor support for fluid-refractory shock.

**Possible Contributing Factors**
**H**ypovolemia
**H**ypoxia
**H**ydrogen ion (acidosis)
**H**ypoglycemia
**H**ypo-/hyperkalemia
**H**ypothermia
**T**ension pneumothorax
**T**amponade, cardiac
**T**oxins
**T**hrombosis, pulmonary
**T**hrombosis, coronary
**T**rauma

**Hypotensive Shock**
- Epinephrine
- Dopamine
- Norepinephrine

**Normotensive Shock**
- Dobutamine
- Dopamine
- Epinephrine
- Milrinone

- Monitor for and treat agitation and seizures
- Monitor for and treat hypoglycemia
- Assess blood gas, serum electrolytes, calcium
- If patient remains comatose after resuscitation from cardiac arrest, consider therapeutic hypothermia (32°C-34°C)
- Consider consultation and patient transport to tertiary care center

**Figure 6.** PALS Management of Shock After ROSC Algorithm.

# Index

*Note: Page numbers with an f and/or t indicate a figure or table on the designated page.*

A-a gradient, 34, 500–501
Abdominal masses, 417
Abnormal red reflex, 436–437
Abnormal uterine bleeding, 4–6
ABO blood group incompatibility, 337–338
Abscess, 244
  intra-abdominal, 253t
  perirectal, 542
  peritonsillar, 273–275
  retropharyngeal, 273–275
Absolute neutrophil count (ANC), 34
Acalculous cholecystitis, 140
ACE inhibitors, 54
Acetaminophen, 27, 575t
Acetaminophen poisoning, 549–551
Acidemias, 317–319
Acquired heart disease, 54–60
Acquired hypothyroidism, 111–112
Acquired immune deficiency syndrome
    (AIDS), 189
Acquired neurologic disease, 366–382
Activated charcoal, 548
Activated partial thromboplastin time (aPTT),
    176, 182t
Acute angioedema, 13
Acute bacterial sinusitis, 278–279
Acute cerebellar ataxia, as differential dx for
    Guillain-Barré syndrome, 371
Acute chest syndrome, 174
Acute cholecystitis, 140
Acute cutaneous lupus erythematosus, as
    differential dx for DRESS, 79
Acute disseminated encephalomyelitis,
    366, 368, 368t
  as differential diagnosis for ataxia, 362
Acute generalized exanthematous pustulosis, as
    differential dx for DRESS, 79
Acute kidney injury (AKI), 348–349
Acute leukemia, 411–414
Acute lymphoblastic leukemia (ALL), 412–414
Acute mastoiditis, 263–265
Acute myeloid leukemia (AML), 414
Acute myopathy, 368–369
Acute obstructive apnea, 498
Acute otitis media (AOM), 270–272
  as differential dx for hearing loss, 462
Acute pancreatitis, 152–153

Acute paroxysmal vertigo, as differential
    diagnosis for ataxia, 362
Acute recurrent pancreatitis, 152
Acute respiratory distress syndrome (ARDS),
    490–491
Acute rheumative fever, as differential dx for
    fever of unknown origin, 253t
Acute symptomatic hypocalcemia, 117
Acute tubular necrosis (ATN), as differential dx
    for hematuria, 344
Acute urticaria, 13
Acute urticarial hypersensitivity, 80–82, 81t
  compared to erythema multiforme, 81t
Acute weakness, 359–361, 360t
Adenotonsillar hypertrophy, 454–456, 455f
Adenovirus, 255t, 260
Adolescent medicine, 1–10
Adrenal disorders, as differential dx for
    abnormal uterine bleeding, 4
Adrenal insufficiency, 106–108
Afterload reducing agents, 54–55
Aggression, 484–485
Agitation, 484–485
Airway adjuncts, 468–474
Airway pressure release ventilation (APRV), 502
Airway stabilization, 90
Akinetic mutism, as differential dx for coma, 364
Alagille syndrome, 162
Albuterol, for asthma, 22
Allergic transfusion reaction, 188
Allergy, 11–20
Allogeneic transplantation, 403–404
Alpha-1 antitrypsin deficiency, 135–136
Alpha-thalassemia, 175
Altered mental status, 361–362
Alveolar-arterial gradient (A-a gradient), 34,
    500–501
Amino acid metabolism defects, 312–315
Amniotic band syndrome, 157
Amphetamine poisoning, 551
Analgesia, 25–29
  non-pharmacologic methods of, 28
  patient-controlled, 28–29
Analgesics
  narcotic, 26–27
  non-narcotic, 27–28
  for sedation, 31

Anaphylaxis, 11–13
Anaplasmosis, 295
Anemia, 169–170, 170t
  as differential dx for apparent life-threatening
    event, 329
  iron-deficiency, 169, 172–173
  macrocytic, 170
  microcytic, 169
  normocytic, 169
Anesthesia
  allergic reaction to, 18
  local, 25–26
Angioedema, 13–15
  hereditary forms, 15–16
Anion gap (serum), 35
Anorexia nervosa, 1–4, 3t
Anovulatory cycles, as differential dx for
    abnormal uterine bleeding, 4
Antibacterial agents, antimicrobial spectra of,
    243f
Antibiotics
  for acute otitis media, 271
  for bite wounds, 239t
  drug allergies caused by, 17
  for sepsis, 98t
  for suspected sepsis, 98t
Anticholinergics, 575t
Anticholinesterases, 575t
Anticholinesterase test, 376
Anticoagulation, medications for, 181–183
Anticonvulsants, poisoning, 570–571
Antidepressant poisoning, 573
Antidiuretic hormone (ADH), syndrome of
    inappropriate, 114–115
Antihistamine poisoning, 552
Antiphospholipid antibody syndrome, as
    differential dx for multiple sclerosis, 374
Antipsychotic poisoning, 569–570
Antiretroviral medications, 189t
Antiviral medications, 189t
Anxiolysis, 29
Anxiolytics, 31
Aortic stenosis, 41–42
Aortic valve stenosis, 41, 42
Apgar scores, 327, 327t
Aplastic anemia, as differential dx for severe
    congenital neutropenia, 234
Aplastic crisis, 174
Apnea of infancy, as differential dx for apparent
    life-threatening event, 329
Apparent life-threatening event (ALTE),
    328–330

Appendicitis, 533–534
Arginase deficiency (argininemia), 310
Argininosuccinic acid lyase deficiency, 311
Argininosuccinic acid synthetase deficiency
    (citrullinemia), 311
Arrhythmias, 64–72
  atrial fibrillation, 64–65
  atrial flutter, 65
  atrial ventricular block, 65–66
  long QT syndrome, 66–67
  premature atrial contraction, 67
  premature ventricular contraction,
    67–68
  supraventricular tachycardia, 68–69
  syncope, 69–70
  ventricular fibrillation, 70
  ventricular tachycardia, 71
  Wolff-Parkinson-White syndrome (WPW),
    71–72
Arterial ischemic stroke, 380–381
Arterial oxygen content (CaO₂), 35
Arterial switch operation (ASO), 50
Arterial switch operation (of JATENE), 53
  for congenital heart disease, 53
Arterial thrombosis, 184
Arthritis
  juvenile idiopathic, 513–515
  septic, 276–278, 453
Asparaginase, 404t
  allergic reaction to, 18
Aspergillosis, 201t, 211t
Aspirin, 28
  allergic reaction to, 18
  poisoning, 571–572
Asthma, 20–24, 22t, 23f
Astrocytoma, 427t
Astrovirus, 255t
Ataxia, 362–363
Ataxia-telangiectasia, 230–231
  as differential diagnosis for ataxia, 362
Atopic dermatitis, 87–89
Atrial fibrillation, 64–65
Atrial flutter, 65
Atrial septal defect, 42–43
Atrial switch operation, 50
Atrioventricular block (AV block),
    65–66
Atrioventricular nodal reentry tachycardia, 68
Atrioventricular reentry tachycardia, 68
Autoimmune hepatitis (AIH), 136–137
Autoimmune pancreatitis, 153
Autoimmune urticaria, 14

*Bacillus cereus*, 255t
Bacteria
  gram negative, 299f
  gram positive, 299f
Bacterial meningitis, 265–267, 266t
Bacterial pericarditis, 58
Bag valve mask ventilation, 468, 469f
Balloon atrial septostomy (Rashkind procedure), 50
Barbiturates, 31
Barium contrast enema, 537
Barth syndrome, 320
*Bartonella*, 199t, 207t
Basilar migraine, as differential diagnosis for ataxia, 362
B cell disorders, 219t, 220t
Beckwith-Wiedemann syndrome (BWS), 164–165
Benzodiazepines, 31, 575t
Beta-blocker poisoning, 552–553
Beta-blockers, 575t
Beta-ketothiolase deficiency, 305t
Beta-thalassemia, 174–175
Bicarbonate, for diabetic ketoacidosis, 104
Bidirectional Glenn shunt, 53
Bilateral stroke, as differential dx for Guillain-Barré syndrome, 371
Bi-level positive airway pressure (BLPAP), 502
Biliary atresia, 138–139
Bilirubin nomogram, 336f
Biostatistics, 35–36
Birth defects, 155–158
Bite wound infections, 237–238, 239t
β-ketothiolase deficiency, 308
Blalock-Taussig shunt, 53
Blalock-Taussig shunt, modified, 53
Bleeding
  abnormal uterine, 4–6
  gastrointestinal, 146–148
Bleeding disorders, 176–179
  coagulation studies, 176
  hemophilia, 177–178
  vitamin K deficiency, 178
  von Willebrand disease, 178–179
Bleeding time, 176
Blistering disorders, 73–78
  necrotizing fasciitis, 73–74
  staphylococcal scalded skin syndrome, 74–76
  Stevens-Johnson syndrome (SJS), 76–78
  toxic epidermal necrolysis, 76–78
Blood gas interpretation, 499–500
Body composition, 121

Body mass index (BMI), 36, 390
Body surface area (BSA), 36
  percent by age, 93t
Bone marrow transplantation, 403–404
Bone tumors, 421
*Bordetella pertussis*, 294
*Borrelia burgdorferi*, 288–289
Botulism, 369–371
Brain death, 363–364
Brainstem glioma, 427t
Branchial cleft anomalies, 456–457
Bronchiolitis, 238–241
Brucellosis, as differential dx for fever of unknown origin, 253t
Burn debridement, sedation for, 33
Burns, 92–93

Calcium channel blocker poisoning, 553–554
Calcium channel blockers, 575t
Calcium deficiency, in rickets, 117t, 119
Calcium homeostasis, 116–120
  hypercalcemia, 118
  hypocalcemia, 116–117
  rickets, 117t, 118–120
Calculations, 34–40
  for absolute neutrophil count, 34
  for alveolar-arterial oxygen gradient (A-a gradient), 34
  for anion gap (serum), 35
  for arterial oxygen content ($CaO_2$), 35
  for biostatistics, 35–36, 35t
  for blood volume to exchange, 340
  for body mass index, 36
  for body surface area, 36
  for cerebral perfusion pressure, 37
  for change in serum sodium, 37
  for conversion of units, 37–38
  for corrected QT interval, 38
  for corrected serum sodium, 38
  for correct serum calcium, 38
  for creatinine clearance (from timed urine specimen), 38
  for creatinine clearance (Schwartz method), 39
  for fractional excretion of sodium, 39
  for free water deficit, 39
  for glucose infusion rate, 39, 396
  of maintenance electrolyte, 1222–1223
  for mean arterial pressure, 40
  for osmolality (serum), 40
  for P/F ratio, 40
  for Winter's formula, 40

Calories, guidelines for daily, 391t
*Campylobacter jejuni*, 255t
Cancer, 401–433
    acute leukemia, 411–414
    fever and neutropenia in, 405–406
    in immunocompromised host, 405
    lymphadenopathy and lymphoma, 415–417
    oncologic emergencies, 405–411
    pancytopenia, 411–412
    principles of treating, 401–404
    solid tumors, 417–428
    supportive care, 429–433
*Candida* infections, 202t
*Candida* mucocutaneous infections, 211t–212t
Carbamates, 575t
Carbamazepine poisoning, 554–555
Carbamoyl phosphate synthetase deficiency, 311
Carbohydrate metabolism defects, 315–319
Carbon monoxide poisoning, 93, 555–556
Carboplatin, 404t
Carcinoma, 428t
Cardiac arrest, 93–94
Cardiac catheterization
    for aortic stenosis, 41
    for atrial septal defect, 43
    for coarctation of the aorta, 44
    for endocardial cushion defect, 45
    for hypoplastic left heart syndrome, 46
    for tetralogy of Fallot, 47
    for total anomalous pulmonary venous
        return, 49
    for transposition of the great arteries, 49
    for ventricular septal defect, 52
Cardiac syncope, 69, 70
Cardiology, 41–72
Cardiomyopathies, 55–56, 159–161
Carnitine/acylcartinine translocase deficiency,
    305t, 306
Carnitine palmitoyltransferase I deficiency,
    305t, 306
Carnitine palmitoyltransferase II deficiency,
    305t, 306
Carnitine transporter defect, 305t, 306
Cartilage hair hypoplasia, as differential dx for
    IgA deficiency, 226
Cataracts, as differential dx for leukocoria, 437
Catatonia, as differential dx for coma, 364
Catch-up growth, 392–393
Cat-scratch disease, 283–284
    as differential dx for fever of unknown
        origin, 253t
Caustics poisoning, 556–557

Celiac disease, 143–144
    as differential dx for eosinophilic
        esophagitis, 20
Cellulitis, 244
    orbital, 272–273
    periorbital, 272–273
    preseptal, 272–273
Central α2 adrenergic agonists, 32
Central apnea, 498
Central fever, as differential dx for fever of
    unknown origin, 253t
Central-line associated bloodstream infection,
    241–242
Central nervous system tumors, 424–426,
    427t–428t
Central venous line, sedation for, 33
Cerebellar hemorrhage, as differential diagnosis
    for ataxia, 362
Cerebellitis, as differential diagnosis for
    ataxia, 362
Cerebral edema, in diabetic ketoacidosis, 104
Cerebral perfusion pressure, 37
Cerebral salt wasting (CSW), 113–114, 113t
Cerebral sinovenous thrombosis, 184
Cerebrospinal fluid profiles, meningitis, 267t
Cervical spine stabilization, 90
Cervicitis, as differential dx for abnormal uterine
    bleeding, 4
Change in serum sodium, 37
CHARGE syndrome, 162–163
    as differential dx for 22q11.2 deletion
        syndrome, 228
Chediak-Higashi syndrome, as differential dx for
    severe congenital neutropenia, 234
Chemotherapy, 401, 402t, 431t
    allergic reaction to, 17
    emetogenic potential of, 431t
Chest x-ray, for aortic stenosis, 41
*Chlamydia trachomatis*, 7t
Chloral hydrate, 31
Cholecystitis, 139
Choledocholithiasis, 139, 140
Cholelithiasis, 139, 140
Cholesteatoma, as differential dx for hearing
    loss, 462
Cholesterol, in anorexia nervosa, 3t
Cholesterol gallstones, 139
Chromosomal abnormalities, incidence at live
    birth, 156t
Chromosome 10p deletions, as differential dx for
    22q11.2 deletion syndrome, 228
Chronic cholecystitis, 140

Chronic granulomatous disease (CGD), 231–232
Chronic hyponatremia, 115
Chronic mastioditis, 263–265
Chronic meningococcemia, as differential dx for fever of unknown origin, 253t
Chronic obstructive apnea, 498
Chronic pancreatitis, 152, 153
Chronic progressive external ophthalmoplegia (CPEO), 320
Chronic renal failure, in rickets, 117t, 119
Chronic rhabdomyolysis, 358
Chronic sinusitis, 278–279
Chronic suppurative otitis media (CSOM), 270–272
Chronic urticaria/angioedema, 13
Circulation, 90
Cisplatin, 404t
Citrullinemia, 311
Clavicle fractures, 445–446
Cleft lip/palate, 457–458
Clonidine poisoning, 557–558
*Clostridium botulinum*, 369
*Clostridium difficile*, 256t
*Clostridium difficile* infection, 284–285
CNS infection
    as differential dx for fever of unknown origin, 253t
    as differential dx for multiple sclerosis, 374
Coagulation studies, 176
Coarctation of the aorta, 43–44
Coats disease, as differential dx for leukocoria, 437
Cocaine poisoning, 558–559
Coccidioidomycosis, 203t, 212t
Codeine, 26
Colitis
    food protein-induced, 18
    intermittent, 149
    ulcerative, 148–149
Collagen vascular diseases, as differential dx for fever of unknown origin, 253t
Collagen vascular pericarditis, 58
Coloboma, as differential dx for leukocoria, 437
Coma, 364–365
Common variable immunodeficiency (CVID), 222–223
Community-acquired MRSA, 291–292
Community-acquired pneumonia, 245–246, 247t
Compartment syndrome, 451
Complement disorders, 221t
Complete blood count, in anorexia nervosa, 3t

Complicated hemangiomas, 83–87, 84t–85t
Complications, sedation-related, 32
Computed tomography (CT) scan, sedation for, 32
Concussion
    management, 96
    signs of, 96
Congenital adrenal hyperplasia (CAH), 108–109
Congenital diaphragmatic hernia, 526–527
Congenital disorders of glycosylation, 325–326
Congenital heart disease, 41–53, 161–163
    aortic stenosis, 41–42
    atrial septal defect, 42–43
    coarctation of the aorta, 43–44
    endocardial cushion defect, 44–45
    hypoplastic left heart syndrome, 45–46
    surgeries for, 53
    tetralogy of Fallot, 46–48
    total anomalous pulmonary venous return, 48–49
    transposition of the great arteries, 49–50
    tricuspid atresia, 50
    truncus arteriosus, 51
    ventricular septal defect, 51–52
Congenital hyperthyroidism, 110–111
Congenital hypothyroidism, 110
Conjugated hyperbilirubinemia, 334–337
Conjunctivitis, neonatal, 267–268
Constipation, 144–146
Constrictive pericarditis, 58
Contact dermatitis, as differential diagnosis for atopic dermatitis, 88
Continuous feeds, 393
Continuous mandatory ventilation (CMV), 502
Continuous positive airway pressure (CPAP), 502
Continuous spontaneous ventilation (CSV), 501
Contraception, emergency, 6–8, 7t
Conversions of units, 37–38
Convulsive status epilepticus, 387
Corneal clouding, 435–436
Corner sutures, 478, 478f
Corrected QT interval ($QT_c$), 38
Corrected serum calcium (for hypoalbuminemia), 38
Corrected serum sodium (for hyperglycemia), 38
Corticosteroids, for asthma, 24
Cortisol, in Cushing syndrome, 109
Costello syndrome, 160, 162

Coumadin, for anticoagulation, 182–183
Counter-regulatory hormone deficiency, 104
Cranial nerves, 366
Craniopharyngioma, 428t
Creatinine clearance
    Schwartz method, 39
    from timed urine specimen, 38
Critical aortic stenosis, 41
Crohn's disease, 148, 149
    as differential dx for eosinophilic
        esophagitis, 20
Croup, 246, 248
Cryoprecipitate transfusion, 185
Cryptococcosis, 203t–204t, 213t
Cryptosporidiosis, 205t, 215t, 259t
Cushing syndrome, 109–110
Cutaneous drug hypersensitivity, evaluation and
    management of, 84t–85t
Cyanide, 575t
Cyanide poisoning, 93, 559–560
Cyclic neutropenia
    as differential dx for leukocyte adhesion
        deficiency, 233
    as differential dx for severe congenital
        neutropenia, 234
Cyclophosphamide, 404t
Cyclosporiasis, 259t
Cystic fibrosis, 491–495, 494t
Cystic masses, 457f
Cystitis, as differential dx for hematuria, 344
Cytomegalovirus (CMV), 200t–201t, 209t–210t,
    260, 343
    as differential dx for HSV, 293
Cytotoxic edema, 372

Daily recommended intake for protein, 391t
Daunorubicin, 404t
Decontamination, 548–549
Deep sedation, 29
Deep tendon reflexes, scale strength for, 359t
Deep vein thrombosis (DVT), low-molecular-
    weight, 184
Dehydration, 124
    hypernatremic, 126–127
    hyponatremic, 126
Dermabond, 479
Dermatitis
    atopic, 87–89
    exfoliative, 79
    seborrheic, 88
Dermatology, 73–89
Dermatomes, 366, 367f

Dermatomyositis, 508–510
    as differential dx for fever of unknown origin,
        253t
Designer drugs, 574
Diabetes insipidus (DI), 115–116
Diabetes mellitus (DM), 100–103, 102t
Diabetic embryopathy, 158
Diabetic ketoacidosis (DKA), 103–104
Diabetic mother, infant of a, 330–333
Diarrhea-associated hemolytic uremic
    syndrome, 353–354
Diastolic blood pressure (DBP), 345
Diazepam, 28
Dietary reference intake (DRI), 390
Digitalis, 575t
Digoxin
    for heart failure, 54
    poisoning, 560–561
Dilated cardiomyopathy, 55, 160
Diphtheria, as differential dx for Guillain-Barré
    syndrome, 371
Diuretics, for heart failure, 54
Diverticulum, Meckel's, 151–152
Down syndrome, 161–162, 166–167
Doxorubicin, 404t
DRESS. See Drug reaction with eosinophilia and
    systemic symptoms (DRESS)
Drowning, 94–95
Drug allergy, 16–18
Drug fever, as differential dx for fever of
    unknown origin, 253t
Drug-induced hypersensitivity syndrome
    (DIHS), 78–80
Drug reaction with eosinophilia and systemic
    symptoms (DRESS), 78–80, 85t
DSM-V criteria, for anorexia nervosa, 1
Duodenal atresias, 530–532, 531t
Dysautonomia, as differential dx for fever of
    unknown origin, 253t
Dyskeratosis, as differential dx for severe
    congenital neutropenia, 234

Echocardiography
    for aortic stenosis, 41
    for atrial septal defect, 43
    for coarctation of the aorta, 44
    for endocardial cushion defect, 45
    for heart failure, 54
    for hypoplastic left heart syndrome, 46
    for myocarditis, 57
    for pericarditis, 58
    for tetralogy of fallot, 47

for total anomalous pulmonary venous
return, 48
for transposition of the great arteries, 49
for tricuspid atresia, 50
for truncus arteriosus, 51
for ventricular septal defect, 52
Ectopic pregnancy, as differential dx for
abnormal uterine bleeding, 4
Eczema herpeticum, 88
Edwards syndrome, 162
Ehrlichiosis, 295
Elbow fractures, 446–447, 447f
Electrocardiography, 61–64
for aortic stenosis, 41
axis, 61, 62f
for coarctation of the aorta, 44
for endocardial cushion defect, 45
for heart failure, 54
for hypoplastic left heart syndrome, 46
left ventricular hypertrophy, ECG signs, 64
for myocarditis, 57
for pericarditis, 58
precordial lead placement, 61
PR interval, 61
P-wave, 61
QRS complex, 61, 63t
QT interval, 63
R and S voltage norms, 64t
rate, 61
rhythm, 61
right ventricular hypertrophy, ECG signs, 64
segment and intervals, 62f
ST segment, 63
for tetralogy of Fallot, 47
for total anomalous pulmonary venous
return, 48
for transposition of the great arteries, 49
for tricuspid atresia, 50
for truncus arteriosus, 51
T-wave, 64
for ventricular septal defect, 52
Electrolytes
abnormalities, 127–131
basic requirements, 122t
for diabetic ketoacidosis, 103
maintenance calculation, 122–123
Emergency contraception, 6–8, 7t
Emergency medicine, 90–99
airway and cervical spine stabilization, 90
breathing/ventilation, 90
burns, 92–93
cardiac arrest, 93–94

circulation, 90
disability (rapid neurologic evaluation) and
dextrose, 90
drowning, 94–95
evaluation and interventions, 91f
exposure/decontamination, 90
head injury, 95–96
hypoglycemia, 96–97
hypothermia, 97
initial approach to sick child, 90
obtain brief history, 90
sepsis, 97–99
trauma, 99
Emetogencity, 430, 431t
EMLA. See Eutectic mixture of local anesthetics
(EMLA)
Encephalitis, 248–251, 250t–251t
Endemic fungi, as differential dx for fever of
unknown origin, 253t
Endemic typhus, 295
Endocardial cushion defect, 44–45
Endocarditis, 59–60
as differential dx for fever of unknown
origin, 253t
Endocrinology, 100–120
acquired hypothyroidism, 111–112
adrenal insufficiency, 106–108
calcium homeostasis, 116–120
cerebral salt wasting, 113–114
congenital adrenal hyperplasia, 108–109
congenital hyperthyroidism, 110–111
congenital hypothyroidism, 110
Cushing syndrome, 109–110
diabetes insipidus, 115–116
diabetes mellitus, 100–103
diabetic ketoacidosis, 103–104
glucose homeostasis, 100–106
Graves disease, 112–113
hypoglycemia, 104–106
hypothalamic-pituitary-adrenal axis,
106–110
salt and water homeostasis, 113–116
syndrome of inappropriate antidiuretic
hormone, 114–115
thyroid disease, 110–113
Endometriosis, as differential dx for abnormal
uterine bleeding, 5
Endomyocardial biopsy, for myocarditis, 57
Endotracheal intubation, 470–471
Enhanced elimination, 548–549, 549
Entamoeba histolytica, 259t
Enteral nutrition, 393–395, 394t, 396t, 397t–398t

Enteritis, as differential dx for fever of unknown origin, 253t
Enteroaggregative *E. coli* (EAEC), 256t
Enterocolitis, food protein-induced. *See* Food protein-induced enterocolitis (FPIES)
Enteroinvasive *E. coli* (EIEC), 256t
Enteropathogenic *E. coli* (EPEC), 256t
Enterotoxigenic *E. coli* (ETEC), 256t
Enthesitis-related arthritis (ERA), 513
Eosinophilic esophagitis, 19–20
  as differential dx for dermatomyositis, 508–509
Eosinophilic gastroenteritis, as differential dx for eosinophilic esophagitis, 20
Ependymoma, 427t
Epidermolysis bullosa
  as differential dx for HSV, 293
  as differential dx for staphylococcal scalded skin syndrome, 75
Epilepsy, 382–383, 386–387
Epinephrine, for asthma, 24
Epistaxis, 458–459
Epstein-Barr virus (EBV), 260
Erythema multiforme, 82–83, 84t
  compared to acute urticarial hypersensitivity, 81t
  as differential diagnosis for acute urticarial hypersensitivity, 81
  as differential dx for staphylococcal scalded skin syndrome, 75
Erythema toxicum, as differential dx for HSV, 293
*Escherichia coli*, 256t
Esophageal atresia, 528–529
Esophagitis, eosinophilic, 19–20
Esophagus, 132–135
Ethanol poisoning, 561
Ethylene glycol, 575t
Ethylene glycol poisoning, 561–562
Etomidate, 32
Etoposide, 404t
Eutectic mixture of local anesthetics (EMLA), 25
Ewing sarcoma, 422–423
Exanthems, 78–83
  acute urticarial hypersensitivity, 80–82, 81t
  drug-induced hypersensitivity syndrome (DIHS), 78–80
  drug reaction with eosinophilia and systemic symptoms (DRESS), 78–80
  erythema multiforme, 82–83
Exfoliative dermatitis, as differential dx for DRESS, 79

Extracorporeal membrane oxygenation (ECMO), 534–536
Extracorporeal removal, 548

Faces scale, 25
Factitious fever, as differential dx for fever of unknown origin, 253t
Failure to thrive (FTT), 19
Familial hypophosphatemic rickets, 119
Fanconi pancytopenia, as differential dx for severe congenital neutropenia, 234
Fatty acid oxidation disorders, 303–307, 305t
Febrile nonhemolytic transfusion reaction, 188
Febrile seizures, 383–384
Femur fractures, 449
Fentanyl, 26, 29, 31
Fetal movement, decreased, 157
Fever
  in cancer, 405–406
  in neonates and young infants, 251–252
  of unknown origin, 253–254, 253t
Fibrillation, ventricular, 70
First-degree AV block, 65
First-degree burns, 92
Fixed airway obstruction, 507
Flow-volume loops, 507f
Fluid administration rate, 121
Fluids and electrolytes, 121–131
Fluid therapy, 121–127
  maintenance, 121–122
  replacement, 123–127
Flumazenil, 32
Fontan procedure (2-4 years), 53
Food allergy, non-IgE-mediated, 18–20
Food protein-induced colitis, 18
Food protein-induced enterocolitis (FPIES), 19
Foot fractures, 450
Forearm fractures, 447–448
Foreign body aspiration, 460–461
Foreign body ingestions, 460–461, 574–576
  as differential dx for apparent life-threatening event, 329
Fourth-degree burns, 92
FPIES. *See* Food protein-induced enterocolitis (FPIES)
Fractional excretion of sodium ($FE_{NA}$), 39
Fracture reduction, sedation for, 33
Fractures, 444–450
  clavicle, 445–446
  elbow, 446–447
  femur, 449
  foot, 450

forearm, 447–448
hand, 448–449
lower extremity, 449–450
orbital, 439–441
of the physis, 444–445
proximal humerus, 446
tibia, 449–450
upper extremity, 445–449
Free water deficit (FWD), 39
Fresh-frozen plasma transfusion, 185
Friedreich ataxia, 362
Full-thickness burns, 92
Functional constipation, 145
Fundoplication, 133–134

Galactosemia, 315–316
Gallbladder disease, 139–140
Gallstones, 139
Gastric emptying, 548
Gastric lavage, 548
Gastroenteritis, 254, 255t–259t, 260
Gastroenterology, 132–154
    celiac disease, 143–144
    constipation, 144–146
    esophagus and stomach, 132–135
    gastroesophageal reflux disease, 132–134
    gastrointestinal bleeding, 146–148
    hepatobiliary system, 135–136
    inflammatory bowel disease, 148–151
    Meckel's diverticulum, 151–152
    pancreatitis, 152–154
    peptic ulcer disease, 134–135
    small and large intestines, 143–152
Gastroesophageal reflux (GER), 132
Gastroesophageal reflux disease (GERD), 19,
    132–134
Gastrointestinal bleeding, 146–148
Gastroschisis, 529–530
Gel-Coombs Classification of Hypersensitivity
    Reactions, 16t
General anesthesia, 29
General surgery, 533–545
Genetic approach to evaluation
    of cardiomyopathy, 159–161
    of growth disturbances, 158–159
    of hypotonia, 163–164
    of infant with dysmorphic features of multiple
        anomalies, 155–158
    of structural congenital heart disease, 161–163
Genetics, 155–168
Germinoma, 428t
Giardia lamblia, 259t

Glasgow coma scale, 90, 365t
Glaucoma, 435–436
Glioblastoma, 427t
Glomerular diseases
    glomerulonephritis, 349
    IgA nephropathy, 351
    nephrotic syndrome, 351–353
    postinfectious glomerulonephritis, 349–350
Glomerulonephritis, 349
    as differential dx for hematuria, 344
    postinfectious, 349–350
Glucocorticoids, for adrenal insufficiency,
    107–108
Gluconeogenesis, disorders of, 104
Glucose-6-phosphate dehydrogenase deficiency,
    170–171
Glucose correction, rule of 50s for, 97t
Glucose homeostasis, 100–106
    diabetes mellitus, 100–103
    diabetic ketoacidosis, 103–104
    hypoglycemia, 104–106
Glucose infusion rate (GIR), 39, 396
Glutaric aciduria type II, 307
Glycogen storage disease (GSD), 104, 105,
    141–142, 141t
Glycosylation, congenital disorders of, 325–326
Goldenhar syndrome, 158
Graft-versus-host disease, 227
    as differential dx for eosinophilic
        esophagitis, 20
Gram negative bacteria, 299f
Gram positive bacteria, 299f
Graves disease, 112–113
Griscelli syndrome type 2, as differential dx for
    severe congenital neutropenia, 234
Group B Streptococcus, as differential dx for
    HSV, 293
Growth disturbances, 158–159
Growth velocity, 390t
Grunting baby syndrome, 145
Guillain-Barré syndrome, 371–372
    as differential diagnosis for ataxia, 362

Half-buried (corner) sutures, 478, 478f
Hand fractures, 448–449
Head injury, 95–96
Head trauma, as differential diagnosis for
    ataxia, 362
Hearing loss, 461–462
Heart disease
    acquired, 54–60
    congenital, 41–53, 161–163

Heart failure, 54–55, 57
Heart transplantation, for hypoplastic left heart
 syndrome, 46
*Helicobacter pylori*, in peptic ulcer disease, 134
Hemangiomas
 complicated, 83–87, 84t–85t
 complications related to, 81t
Hematocrit (HCT), 169
 normal, by age, 170t
Hematology, 169–188
 anemia, 169–170
 bleeding disorders, 176–179
 glucose-6-phosphate dehydrogenase
  deficiency, 170–171
 hereditary spherocytosis, 171–172
 iron-deficiency anemia, 172–173
 sickle cell disease, 173–174
 thalaseemias, 174–176
 thrombocytopenia, 180–181
 thrombotic disorders, 181–185
 transfusion medicine, 185–188
Hematuria, 344–345
Hemifacial microsomia, 158
Hemi-Fontan (4-6 months), 53
Hemoglobin, normal, by age, 170t
Hemolytic disease
 ABO incompatibility, 337–338
 Rh incompatibility, 338–339
Hemolytic transfusion reaction, 187
Hemophilia, 177–178
Hemoptysis, 496–497
Hemorrhagic stroke, 380–381
Henoch-Schönlein purpura (HSP), 510–513
Heparin
 for anticoagulation, 181–182, 182t
 low-molecular-weight, 182
Heparin-induced thrombocytopenia (HIT), 182
Hepatic glycogen storage disease, 142
Hepatitis
 autoimmune, 136–137
 as differential dx for fever of unknown
  origin, 253t
Hepatitis A virus (HAV), 285–286
Hepatitis B virus (HBV), 286–287, 287t
Hepatitis C virus (HCV), 288
Hepatobiliary system, 135–143
 alpha-1 antitrypsin deficiency, 135–136
 autoimmune hepatitis, 136–137
 biliary atresia, 138–139
 gallbladder disease, 139–140
 glycogen storage disease, 141–142
 Wilson disease, 142–143

Hereditary fructose intolerance, 316–317
Hereditary pancreatitis, 153
Hereditary spherocytosis, 171–172
Hereditary tyrosinemia type 1, 312–313
Hermansky-Pudlak type 2, as differential dx for
 severe congenital neutropenia, 234
Herpes zoster, 300–302
High-frequency ventilation, 502
Highly active antiretroviral treatments
 (HAART), 189, 189t, 193
Hirschsprung's disease, 536–537
Histoplasmosis, 204t, 213t–214t
Hodgkin lymphoma (HL), 415–416
Holliday-Segar method, 121–122
Horizontal mattress sutures, 475, 477f
Hospital-acquired MRSA, 291–292
Human immunodeficiency virus (HIV)
 infection, 189–218, 192f, 195t–196t, 197t
 as differential dx for 22q11.2 deletion
  syndrome, 228
 as differential dx for fever of unknown
  origin, 253t
 as differential dx for IgA deficiency, 226
 as differential dx for multiple sclerosis, 374
 as differential dx Wiskott-Aldrich
  syndrome, 229
 infectious mononucleosis and, 260
 inflammatory syndromes, management
  of, 198
 medication side effects, 197t
 opportunistic infections, management of, 198,
  199t–216t
 opportunistic infections, primary prophylaxis
  of, 197–198
 pediatric classification system,
  195t–196t
 post-exposure prophylaxis, 217, 217t, 218f
 testing algorithm, 192f
Hydrocarbon poisoning, 562–563
Hydrocephalus, as differential diagnosis for
 ataxia, 362
Hydromorphone, 26, 29
Hydrostatic edema, 373
Hyperbilirubinemia, neonatal,
 334–337
Hypercalcemia, 118, 130
Hypercalciuria, as differential dx for
 hematuria, 344
Hypereosinophilic syndrome, as differential dx
 for eosinophilic esophagitis, 20
Hyperglycemia, corrected serum sodium
 for, 38

Hyper IdE syndrome
  as differential dx for chronic granulomatous
    disease, 231
  as differential dx for leukocyte adhesion
    deficiency, 233
Hyper-IgE syndrome (STAT3 deficiency),
    235–236
Hyperinsulinemia, 104
Hyperinsulinism, 105, 106
Hyperkalemia, 129–130
Hyperleukocytosis, 407
Hypernatremia, 128
Hypernatremic dehydration, 126–127
Hyperoxia test, for transposition of the great
    arteries, 49
Hyperprolactinemia, as differential dx for
    abnormal uterine bleeding, 4
Hypersensitivity reactions, classification
    of, 16t
Hypertension, 345–347
Hypertensive emergency, 346, 347
Hypertensive urgency, 346, 347
Hyperthyroidism, 112
  congenital, 110–111
  as differential dx for fever of unknown
    origin, 253t
Hypertrophic cardiomyopathy, 55, 159–160
  in infant of a diabetic mother, 331
Hyphema, 438–439
Hypnotics, 31–32
Hypoalbuminemia, correct serum calcium
    for, 38
Hypocalcemia, 116–117, 130
  as differential dx for apparent life-threatening
    event, 329
  in infant of a diabetic mother, 331
Hypoglycemia, 96–97, 104–106
  as differential dx for apparent life-threatening
    event, 329
  in infant of a diabetic mother, 331, 332
Hypoglycemic reactions, 103
Hypokalemia, 129
Hyponatremia, 127–128
  iatrogenic, in hospitalized children, 128
Hyponatremic dehydration, 126
Hypoparathyroidism, 117
Hypophosphatasia, 119, 120
Hypoplastic left heart syndrome, 45–46
Hypopnea, 498
Hypothalamic-pituitary-adrenal (HPA) axis,
    106–110
  adrenal insufficiency, 106–108

congenital adrenal hyperplasia, 108–109
  Cushing syndrome, 109–110
Hypothalamic tumors, 115
Hypothermia, 97
Hypothyroidism
  acquired, 111–112
  congenital, 110
Hypotonia, 163–164
Hypoxemia, 500–501, 500t

Iatrogenic hyponatremia, in hospitalized
    children, 128
Idarubicin, 404t
IgA deficiency, 225–226
IgA neprhopathy, 351
Imatinib, 404t
Immune reconstitution inflammatory
    syndrome (IRIS), as differential dx in HIV
    infection, 198
Immune thrombocytopenia (ITP), 180–181
  as differential dx Wiskott-Aldrich
    syndrome, 229
Immunodeficiency
  22q11.2 deletion syndrome, 227–229
  ataxia-telangiectasia, 230–231
  chronic granulomatous disease, 231–232
  common variable, 222–223
  as differential diagnosis for atopic
    dermatitis, 88
  hyper-IgE syndrome, 235–236
  IgA deficiency, 225–226
  leukocyte adhesion deficiency, 232–233
  primary, 219, 219t, 220t–221t
  severe combined, 226–227
  severe congenital neutropenia, 233–235
  transient hypogammaglobulinemia of infancy,
    224–225
  Wiskott-Aldrich syndrome (WAS),
    229–230
  x-linked agammaglobulinemia, 221–222
Immunology, 219–236
Inborn errors of metabolism, 104–105, 160
  as differential dx for apparent life-threatening
    event, 329
  hereditary fructose intolerance, 316–317
  phenylketonuria, 314–315
Incision and drainage, sedation for, 33
Increased intracranial pressure, 372–374
Infantile spasms, 384–385
Infant of diabetic mother (IDM), 330–333
Infants, fever in, 251–252
Infected preauricular cyst/sinus, 463

Infectious diseases, 237–302
abscess, 244
bite wound infections, 237–238
bronchiolitis, 238–241
cat-scratch disease, 283–284
cellulitis, 244
central-line associated bloodstream infection, 241–242
*Clostridium difficile* infection, 284–285
community-acquired pneumonia, 245–246, 247t
croup, 246, 248
encephalitis, 248–251, 250t–251t
fever in neonates and young infants, 251–252
fever of unknown origin, 253–254, 253t
gastroenteritis, 254, 255t–259t, 260
hepatitis A, 285–286
hepatitis B, 286–287, 287t
hepatitis C, 288
infectious mononucleosis, 260–262
Lyme disease, 288–290
lymphadenitis, 262–263
lymphadenopathy, 262–263
malaria, 290–291
mastoiditis, 263–265
meningitis, 265–267, 266t
methicillin-resistant *Staphylococcus aureus*, 291–292
neonatal conjunctivitis, 267–268
neonatal herpes simplex, 292–293
osteomyelitis, 268–270
otitis media, 270–272
periorbital/preseptal and orbital cellulitis, 272–273
peritonsillar abscess, 273–275
pertussis, 294–295
retropharyngeal abscess, 273–275
rickettsial diseases, 295–296
sepsis, 275–276
septic arthritis, 276–278
sinusitis, 278–279
toxic shock syndrome, 280–281
tuberculosis, 296–300, 299f
urinary tract infection, 281–283
varicella zoster, 300–302
Infectious mononucleosis, 260–262
as differential dx for fever of unknown origin, 253t
Infectious prophylaxis, 429
Inflammatory bowel disease, 148–151
as differential dx for eosinophilic esophagitis, 20

as differential dx for fever of unknown origin, 253t
Inflammatory syndromes, 198
Inguinal hernia, 537–539
Injectable local anesthetic, 26
Injuries
head, 95–96
trauma, 99
Insulin
for diabetic ketoacidosis, 104
subcutaneous insulin pharmacodynamics, 102t
Interferon gamma release assay (IGRA), 298
Intermediate-acting insulin, 102t
Intermittent (bolus) feeds, 393, 394t
Intermittent colitis, 149
Intermittent mandatory ventilation (IMV), 501
Interstitial edema, 373
Interstitial nephritis, as differential dx for hematuria, 344
Intestinal atresias, 530–532, 531t
Intra-abdominal abscess, as differential dx for fever of unknown origin, 253t
Intracranial hemorrhage, as differential dx for apparent life-threatening event, 329
Intraosseous line placement, 473–474
Intrauterine device (IUD), 7t
Intravenous afterload reducing agents, 55
Intravenous inotropic agents, 55
Intussusception, 539–540
Inverted subcutaneous suture, 475, 476f
Ipratropium bromide, for asthma, 22
Iron, 575t
Iron-deficiency anemia, 169, 172–173
Iron poisoning, 563–564
Isonatremic dehydration, 125–126
Isopropyl alcohol poisoning, 564–565

Jackson Canyon (JC) virus, 201t, 211t
Jaundice, 334
Jejunoileal atresias, 530–532, 531t
Jones criteria, for rheumatic fever, 518t
Juvenile dermatomyositis (JDM), 508–510
Juvenile idiopathic arthritis (JIA), 513–515
as differential dx for dermatomyositis, 508
Juvenile rheumatoid arthritis, as differential dx for fever of unknown origin, 253t

Kaposiform hemangioendothelioma, as differential dx for hemangiomas, 86
Kasai procedure, 138–139

Kawasaki disease (KD), 515–518
  as differential dx for DRESS, 79
  as differential dx for fever of unknown
    origin, 253t
  as differential dx for staphylococcal scalded
    skin syndrome, 75
Kearns-Sayre syndrome, 320
Kernicterus, 334
Ketamine, 28, 31
Ketone metabolism, disorders of, 305t
Ketone utilization defects, 307–308
Ketosis without acidosis, 102
Ketotic hypoglycemia, 104, 105
Koebner phenomenon, 83
Kussmaul's sign, 58

Labyrinthitis, as differential diagnosis for
    ataxia, 362
Laceration repair, 474–475, 476f, 477f, 478,
    478f, 479f
  alternatives to sutures, 478–480
Lactic acidosis, primary, 320–323
Langerhans cell histiocytosis, as differential dx
    for HSV, 293
Large for gestational age (LGA), in infant of a
    diabetic mother, 331
Large intestines, 143–152
Laryngeal mask airway (LMA), 472–473, 472f
Laryngomalacia, 463–465
Late-dumping syndrome, 106
Latent tuberculosis infection (LTBI), 296
Latex allergy, 18
Lead, 575t
Lead poisoning, 565–566
Left ventricular hypertrophy, ECG signs, 64
Leptospirosis, as differential dx for fever of
    unknown origin, 253t
Leukemia, acute, 411–414
Leukocoria, 436–437
Leukocyte adhesion deficiency (LAD), 232–233
  as differential dx for chronic granulomatous
    disease, 231
Lidocaine, 31
  viscous, 26
Lidocaine, epinephrine, tetracaine (LET), 25
Lidocaine jelly, 26
Liver function tests, in anorexia nervosa, 3t
Liver transplantation, 139
Local anesthesia, 25–26
Locked-in state, as differential dx for coma, 364
Long-acting insulin, 102t
Long-chain fatty acid oxidation disorders, 306–307

Long QT syndrome, 66–67
Loop diuretics, for heart failure, 54
Lower extremeties, fractures of, 449–450
Low-molecular-weight heparin, 182
Lumbar puncture, 480–481
  sedation for, 33
Lung disease
  obstructive, 506
  restrictive, 506
Lung function
  anthropometric measurements affecting, 506
  equipment used to measure, 506
Lung volumes, 505–506, 505f
Lyme disease, 288–290
  as differential dx for fever of unknown origin,
    253t
  as differential dx for multiple sclerosis, 374
Lymphadenitis, 262–263
Lymphadenopathy, 262–263, 415–417
Lymphoma, 415–417

Macrocytic anemia, 170
Macrosomia, in infant of a diabetic mother, 331
Magnesium sulfate, for asthma, 24
Magnetic resonance imaging (MRI)
  for coarctation of the aorta, 44
  for myocarditis, 57
  sedation for, 32–33
  for total anomalous pulmonary venous
    return, 49
Maintenance fluid therapy, 121–122
Major anomalies, genetic approach to evaluation
    of, 155–158
Malaria, 290–291
  as differential dx for fever of unknown
    origin, 253t
Malignancy, as differential dx for fever of
    unknown origin, 253t
Mallampati classification of pharyngeal
    structures, 30f
Malnutrition, 390
Malrotation, 540–542
Maple syrup urine disease (MSUD),
    313–314
Mastoiditis, 263–265
Maternal to child transmission (MTCT), of HIV,
    189, 191
Maturity onset diabetes of the young
    (MODY), 100
Mean airway pressure (MAP), 502
Mean arterial pressure (MAP), 40
Mean corpuscular hemoglobin (MCH), 169

Mean corpuscular hemoglobin concentration (MCHC), 169
Mean corpuscular volume (MCV), 169
 normal, by age, 170t
Mechanical ventilation, 501–504
Meckel's diverticulum, 151–152
Meconium aspiration syndrome, 333–334
Medium-chain acyl CoA dehydrogenase (MCAD) deficiency, 304, 305t
Medulloblastoma, 427t
Meningitis, 265–267, 266t, 267t
 as differential diagnosis for ataxia, 362
Mental status, altered, 361–362
Meperidine, 27
6-Mercaptopurine, 404t
Metabolism, 303–326
 carbohydrate metabolism defects, 315–319
 congenital disorders of glycosylation, 325–326
 defects of amino acid metabolism, 312–315
 fatty acid oxidation disorders, 303–307
 ketone utilization defects, 307–308
 peroxisomal disorders, 323–325
 primact lactic acidosis, 320–323
 urea cycle defects, 308–312
Methadone, 27
Methanol, 575t
Methanol poisoning, 566–567
Methicillin-resistant Staphylococcus aureus (MRSA), 291–292
Methotrexate, 404t
Methylacetoacetyl-CoA thiolase deficiency, 308
MHC class I or II deficiency, as differential dx for IgA deficiency, 226
Microcytic anemia, 169
Microsporidiosis, 205t, 215t
Middle ear effusion (OME), as differential dx for hearing loss, 462
Midgut volvulus, 540–542
Miliaria, as differential dx for HSV, 293
Miliary tuberculosis, 297
Mineralocorticoid replacement, for adrenal insufficiency, 108
Minimal sedation, 29
Mitochondrial depletion syndromes, 321–322
Mitochondrial trifunctional protein deficiency and long-chain-3-hydroxyacyl CoA dehydrogenase deficiency, 305t, 306–307
Mitochondrial encephalomyelopathy with lactic acidosis and stroke (MELAS), 320
Mitoxantrone, 404t
Moderate sedation, 29

Modular supplements, 397t–398t
Moebius syndrome, 158
Monitoring, of enteral nutrition, 393–394
Mononucleosis, infectious, 260–262
Monosomy X, 162
Morbilliform eruptions, 84t
Morning cortisol level, in anorexia nervosa, 3t
Morphine, 27, 28, 31
Mosteller method, 36
MSOAP mnemonic, 470–471
Mucositis, 83, 429
Multi-dose activated charcoal (MDAC), 549
Multiple acyl CoA dehydrogenation deficiency, 305t, 307
Multiple sclerosis, 374–375
Munchausen syndrome by proxy, as differential dx for fever of unknown origin, 253t
Murphy's sign, 140
Muscle glycogen storage disease, 142
Muscle relaxants, allergic reaction to, 18
Mustard and Senning procedure, 50, 53
Myasthenia gravia, 376–377
Mycobacterium avium complex (MAC), in HIV, 197
Mycobacterium avium intracellulare (MAI), 200t
Mycobacterium avium intracellulare (MAI), 208t–209t
Mycobacterium tuberculosis, 199t, 208t
Myocarditis, 56–57
Myoclonic epilepsy with ragged red fibers (MERRF), 320
Myoneurogastrointestinal disorder and encephalomyopathy (MNGIE), 320
Myopathy, as differential dx for Guillain-Barré syndrome, 371
Myositis, as differential dx for Guillain-Barré syndrome, 371

Nalbuphine, 27
Naloxone, 32
Narcotic analgesics, 26–27
Nasopharyngeal (NP) airway, 468, 470
Natural rubber latex, allergic reaction to, 18
Nausea and vomiting, in cancer patients, 430
Necrotizing fasciitis, 73–74
Negative inspiratory force (NIF), 504
Neisseria gonorrhoeae, 7t
Neonatal conjunctivitis, 267–268
Neonatal diabetes, 100
Neonatal herpes simplex virus infection, 292–293
Neonatal hyperbilirubinemia, 334–337
Neonatal lupus, as differential dx for HSV, 293

Neonatal resuscitation, 327–328
Neonatal seizures, 385–386
Neonatal surgery, 526–533
Neonates, fever in, 251–252
Neonatology, 327–343
Nephritic syndrome, 349
Nephrology, 344–358
Nephrotic syndrome, 351–353
Neuroblastoma, 419–420
    as differential diagnosis for ataxia, 362
Neurocardiogenic syncope, 69, 70
Neurology, 359–388
Neuropathic pain, 432
Neuropathy, ataxia, and retinitis pigmentosa
    (NARP), 320
Neuropsychiatric syncope, 69
Neurosarcoidosis, as differential dx for multiple
    sclerosis, 374
Neutropenia, 405–406
Nitrogen scavenging agents, 311t
Nitrous oxide, 31
Nonconvulsive status epilepticus, 387
Non-germunomatous germ cell tumors, 428t
Non-Hodgkin lymphoma (NHL), 416–417
Non-IgE-mediated food allergy, 18–20
Non-involuting congenital hemangioma
    (NICH), 86
Non-narcotic analgesics, 27–28
Nonoccupational post-exposure prophylaxis, for
    HIV, 217, 218f
Non-pharmacologic methods of analgesia, 28
Nonsteroidal anti-inflammatory drugs
    (NSAIDs), 28
    allergic reaction to, 18
Non-typhoidal *Salmonella*, 257t
Noonan syndrome, 162, 165–166
Normocytic anemia, 169
Norovirus, 255t
Norwood procedure, 53
    for hypoplastic left heart syndrome, 46
Nummular dermatitis, as differential diagnosis
    for atopic dermatitis, 88
Nutrition, 389–400
    enteral, 393–395
    estimating needs, 390–391, 392t
Nutritional status, assessment o, 389–393
Nutritional support, in cancer patients, 430–431

Obese population, 392
Obstructive apnea, 497–498
Obstructive lung disease, 506
Ocular exposure, 434

Oligoarthritis, 513, 514
Oligodendroglioma, 427t
Omenn syndrome, as differential dx for
    hyper-IgE syndrome, 235
Omphalocele, 532–533
Oncologic emergencies, 405–411
Oncology, 401–433
    *See also* Cancer
    bone marrow transplantation, 403–404
    chemotherapy, 401, 402t
    radiation therapy, 401, 403
    supportive care, 429–433
    surgery, 403
Ophthalmology, 434–443
Ophthalmology consultation, when to consider,
    442–443
Opioid agonists, 31
Opioid poisoning, 567–568
Opioids, 575t
Opportunistic infections, 199t–216t
    management of, 198
    primary prophylaxis of, 197–198
Oral airway, 470
Oral rehydration, 124–125
Orbital cellulitis, 272–273
Orbital fracture, 439–442
Organic acidemias, 317–319
Organophosphates, 575t
Organophosphates poisoning, 568–569
Ornithine carbamoyltransferase deficiency,
    311–312
Ornithine transcarbamylase deficiency, 311
Orthopedics, 444–453
Orthotopic heart transplantation, for hypoplastic
    left heart syndrome, 46
Osmolality (serum), 40
Osmotic edema, 373
Osteomyelitis, 268–270
    as differential dx for fever of unknown origin,
    253t
Osteopenia, 4
Osteosarcoma, 421–422
Otitis media, 270–272
Otitis media with effusion (OME), 270–272
Otolaryngology, 454–467
OUCHER scale, 25
Ovarian torsion, 545–546
Overnight dexamethasone suppression test, 109
Oxycodone, 27

Packed red cell transfusions, 432
*P. aeruginosa*, as differential dx for HSV, 293

Pain
  assessment, 25
  in cancer patients, 431–432
  neuropathic, 432
  somatic, 431–432
  visceral, 431–432
Painful procedures, sedation for, 33
Palliative surgery, for tetralogy of Fallot, 48
Pancreatitis, 152–154
Pancytopenia, 411–412
Papilloma, 428t
Parenteral nutrition, 395–400
Parenteral rehydration, 125
Paroxysmal hypercyanotic attacks, 47
Partial exchange transfusion (PET), 340
Patau syndrome, 162
Patient-controlled analgesia, 28–29
Pearson syndrome, 320
Pediatric infection, of HIV, 189
Pelvic inflammatory disease (PID), 8–10
  as differential dx for abnormal uterine
    bleeding, 4
PELVIS/SACRAL syndrome, 86
Penicillin, allergic reaction to, 17
Peptic ulcer disease (PUD), 134–135
Pericardiocentesis, 58
Pericarditis, 57–58
Perinatal asphyxia, in infant of a diabetic
    mother, 331
Periodic fever syndrome, as differential dx for
    fever of unknown origin, 253t
Periodontal abscess, as differential dx for fever of
    unknown origin, 253t
Periorbital cellulitis, 272–273
Perirectal abscess, 542
Peritonsillar abscess, 273–275
Peroxisomal biogenesis disorders, 323–324
Peroxisomal disorders, 323–325
Pertussis, 294–295
P/F ratio, 40
PHACES syndrome, 86
Phagocyte disorders, 219t, 221t
Pharyngeal structures, Mallampati classification
    of, 30f
Phenylketonuria (PKU), 314–315
Phenytoin poisoning, 570–571
Phosphorus, for diabetic ketoacidosis, 104
Phosphorus deficiency, in rickets, 117t, 119
Physis, fractures of the, 444–445, 445t
PID. See Pelvic inflammatory disease (PID)
Pigment gallstones, 139
Pineoblastoma, 427t

Platelet transfusion, 185–186, 432
Pneumocystis pneumonia (PCP), 198,
    204t–205t, 214t, 429
Pneumonia
  community-acquired, 245–246, 247t
  pneumocystis, 204t–205t, 214t, 429
Pneumothorax, 542–544
  needle decompression, 481–482
Poisoning, 549–570
Poliomyelitis, as differential dx for Guillain-
    Barré syndrome, 371
Polyarteritis nodosa, as differential dx for
    dermatomyositis, 508
Polyarthritis, 513, 514
Polycystic ovary syndrome (PCOS), as differential
    dx for abnormal uterine bleeding, 4
Polycythemia, 339–340
Portoenterostomy, 138–139
Positive end-expiratory pressure (PEEP), 503
Positive pressure ventilation, for asthma, 24
Posterior fossa lesion, as differential dx for
    Guillain-Barré syndrome, 371
Post-exposure prophylaxis, for HIV, 217
Postinfectious glomerulonephritis, 349–350
Post-pericardiotomy syndrome, 58
Postprandial hypoglycemia, 106
Post-sedation recovery and discharge, 32
Potassium, for diabetic ketoacidosis, 103–104
Prader-Willi syndrome, 166
  as differential dx for hypotonia, 163
Premature atrial contraction (PAC), 67
Premature ventricular contraction (PVC), 67–68
Premixed insulin, 102t
Prenatal ultrasound, for hypoplastic left heart
    syndrome, 46
Pre-sedation assessment, 29, 30t
Preseptal cellulitis, 272–273
Pressure-regulated volume control (PRVC), 502
Pressure support (PS), 501
Primary adrenal insufficiency, 106–107
Primary glaucoma, 435
Primary immunodeficiency
  approach to, 219, 220t–221t
  classification of, 219t
Primary lactic acidosis, 320–323
Procedures, 468–483
  airway adjuncts, 468–474
  bag valve mask ventilation, 468, 469f
  endotracheal intubation, 470–471
  intraosseous line placement, 473–474
  laceration repair, 474–480
  laryngeal mask airway, 472–473, 472f

lumbar puncture, 480–481
nasopharyngeal airway, 468, 470
oral airway, 470
pneumothorax: needle decompression, 481–482
umbilical vessel catheterization, 482–483
Progressive multifocal leukodystrophy (PML),
201t, 211t
Prolactin, in anorexia nervosa, 3t
Prophylaxis
dental and oral procedures, 60
endocarditis, 60
infectious, 429
of opportunistic infections, 197–198
post-exposure, 217
rabies post-exposure, 238
recommendations, 60
tetanus, 238, 480t
Protein intake, daily recommended, 391t
Prothrombin time (PT), 176
Proton pump inhibitor (PPI)-responsive
esophageal eosinophilia, as differential dx
for eosinophilic esophagitis, 20
Proximal humerus fractures, 446
Pseudotumor cerebri, 377–378
Psittacosis, as differential dx for fever of
unknown origin, 253t
Psoriatic arthritis, 513
Psychiatric support, for cancer patients, 432
Psychiatry, 484–489
Psychosis, 485–487
Psychosocial support, for cancer patients, 432
Puberty, Tanner staging, 120t
Pulmonary artery banding, 53
Pulmonary assessment, 499–500, 504–507
Pulmonary diseases/symptoms, 490–498
Pulmonary embolism, 184
Pulmonary function tests (PFTs), 504–507
Pulmonology, 490–507
Pulsus paradoxus, 58
Pyelonephritis, as differential dx for
hematuria, 344
Pyloric stenosis, 544–545
Pyridoxine dependency, 386
Pyruvate dehydrogenase (PDH) deficiency,
322–323

Q fever, 295
as differential dx for fever of unknown
origin, 253t

Rabies post-exposure prophylaxis, 238
Radiation therapy (RT), 401, 403

Radiocontrast media, allergic reaction to, 18
Rapid-acting insulin, 102t
Rapidly involuting congenital hemangioma
(RICH), 86
Rapid neurologic evaluation, 90
Rapid shallow breathing index (RSBI), 504
Rashkind procedure, 50
RDA guidelines for daily calories, 391t
Recommended daily allowances (RDA),
390–391
Rectal biopsy, 537
Red blood cell (RBC) indices, 169
Red blood cell transfusion, 186–187, 186t
Red cell distribution width (RDW), 169
Red reflex testing, 436–437
Refeeding syndrome, 2
Renal tubular acidosis (RTA), 354–355
Renal vein thrombosis, 184
Replacement fluid therapy, 123–127
dehydration, 124
hypernatremic dehydration, 126–127
hyponatremic dehydration, 126
isonatremic dehydration, 125–126
ongoing losses, 124, 124t
oral rehydration, 124–125
parenteral rehydration, 125
Respiratory chain defects, 320–321
Respiratory distress syndrome (RDS), in infant
of a diabetic mother, 331
Respiratory syncytial virus (RSV), as differential
dx for apparent life-threatening event, 329
Respiratory tract infection, as differential dx for
fever of unknown origin, 253t
Resting energy expenditure (REE), 391, 392t
Restrictive lung disease, 506
Resuscitation, neonatal, 327–328
Retentive encopresis, 145
Reticular dysgenesis, as differential dx for severe
congenital neutropenia, 234
Reticulocyte count, 169
Retinal detachment, as differential dx for
leukocoria, 437
Retinal dysplasia, as differential dx for
leukocoria, 437
Retinoblastoma, as differential dx for
leukocoria, 437
Retinopathy, as differential dx for
leukocoria, 437
Retropharyngeal abscess, 273–275
Rhabdomyolysis, 357–358
Rhabdomyosarcoma, 423–424
Rheumatic fever, 518–520, 518t

Rheumatology, 508–525
Rh incompatibility, 338–339
Rickets, 117t, 118–120
Rickettsial diseases, 295–296
  as differential dx for fever of unknown
    origin, 253t
Rickettsialpox, 295
Right ventricular hypertrophy, ECG signs, 64
Rocky Mountain spotted fever (RMSF), 295
Roentgenographic (barium contrast enema), 537
Ross procedure, 53
Rotavirus, 255t
Rubella, 342–343

Salicylates (aspirin), poisoning, 571–572
Salmonella typhil, 257t
Salt and water homeostasis, 113–116
  cerebral salt wasting, 113–114
  diabetes insipidus, 115–116
  syndrome of inappropriate antidiuretic
    hormone, 114–115
Salt-wasting, 108, 113–114
Sapovirus, 255t
Scabies, as differential diagnosis for atopic
    dermatitis, 88
Schwartz method, 39
Scleroderma
  as differential dx for dermatomyositis, 508
  as differential dx for fever of unknown
    origin, 253t
Seborrheic dermatitis, as differential diagnosis
    for atopic dermatitis, 88
Secondary adrenal insufficiency, 106, 107
Secondary glaucomas, 435
Second-degree AV block, Mobitz type II, 65
Second-degree AV block, Mobitz type I
    (Wenckebach), 65
Second-degree burns, 92
Sedation, 29–33, 30t
Sedation-related complications, 32
Sedative antagonists, 32
Sedative drugs, 31–32
Seizures, 382–388
  as differential diagnosis for ataxia, 362
  febrile, 383–384
  neonatal, 385–386
  unprovoked, first, 387–388
  unprovoked, second, 388
Selective serotonin-norepinephrine uptake
    inhibitors (SNRIs), poisoning, 572–573
Selective serotonin uptake inhibitors (SSRIs),
    poisoning, 572–573

Senning technique, 50
Sepsis, 97–99, 275–276
Septic arthritis, 276–278, 453
Serious bacterial infection (SBI), 251
Serum chemistries, in anorexia nervosa, 3t
Serum sickness, as differential diagnosis for
    acute urticarial hypersensitivity, 81
Serum sodium, change in, 37
Severe combined immunodeficiency (SCID),
    226–227
Severe congenital neutropenia (SCN), 233–235
  as differential dx for chronic granulomatous
    disease, 231
  as differential dx for leukocyte adhesion
    deficiency, 233
Severe cutaneous adverse reactions (SCAR),
    76–78
  severe congenital neutropenia, 76–78
Sexually transmitted infection (STI), as
    differential dx for abnormal uterine
    bleeding, 4
Shiga-toxin producing E. coli (STEC), 256t
Short-acting insulin, 102t
Short-chain acyl CoA dehydrogenase (SCAD)
    deficiency, 305, 305t
Short-chain L-3-hydroxyacyl CoA
    dehydrogenase deficiency, 305t, 306
Short/medium-chain fatty acid oxidation
    disorders, 304–306
Shwachman-Diamond syndrome, as differential
    dx for severe congenital neutropenia, 234
Sickle cell disease, 173–174
  as differential dx for hematuria, 344
Simple (continuous) running sutures, 478, 479f
Simple interrupted suture, 475, 476f
Sinus aspiration, 279
Sinusitis, 278–279
Sjögren syndrome, as differential dx for multiple
    sclerosis, 374
Slipped capital femoral epiphysis (SCFE),
    451–452, 452f
Small intestines, 143–152
Sodium, for diabetic ketoacidosis, 104
Solid neck masses, 457f
Solid tumors, 417–428
Somatic pain, 431–432
Sorafenib, 404t
Spinal cord compression, 407–408
  as differential dx for Guillain-Barré syndrome,
    371
Spinal cord emergency, 378–379
Spirometry, 505

Spironolactone, for heart failure, 54
Splenic sequestration, in sickle cell disease, 173–174
Splints, 448f
Staphylococcal scalded skin syndrome (SSSS), 74–76
*Staphylococcus aureus*
  in atopic dermatitis, 88
  as differential dx for HSV, 293
  methicillin-resistant, 291–292
  in toxic shock syndrome, 280–281
Staples, as alternative to sutures, 478
STAT3 deficiency, 235–236
Status epilepticus, 386–387
Steri-strips, 478
Stevens-Johnson syndrome (SJS), 76–78, 84t
  as differential dx for DRESS, 79
  as differential dx for staphylococcal scalded skin syndrome, 75
Stock intravenous solutions, terminology and conversions for, 123t
Stokes-Adams syndrome, 69
Stomach, 132–135
Strabismus, as differential dx for leukocoria, 437
*Streptococcus mitis*, 429
*Streptococcus pyogenes*, in atopic dermatitis, 88
Stroke, 379–381
  in sickle cell disease, 174
Structural congenital heart disease, 161–163
Stunting, 390
Subacute sinusitis, 278–279
Subaortic stenosis, 42
Subvalvular stenosis, 41
Succinyl-CoA:3-oxoacid CoA transferase (SCOT) deficiency, 308
Suicidality, 487–489
Sulfa antibiotics, allergic reaction to, 17
Superior mediastinal syndrome, 408–409
Superior vena cava syndrome, 184, 408–409
Supravalvular stenosis, 41, 42
Supraventricular tachycardia (SVT), 68–69
Surgery
  for cancer, 403
  for congenital heart disease, 53
  general, 533–545
  neonatal, 526–533
  for tetralogy of Fallot, 48
  for transposition of the great arteries, 50
  urologic, 545–547
Sutures, 474–475, 476f, 477f, 478, 478f, 479f
  alternatives to, 478–480
Symptomatic hyponatremia, 114

Synchronized intermittent mandatory ventilation (SIMV), 502
Syncope, 69–70
Syndrome of inappropriate antidiuretic hormone (SIADH), 113t, 114–115
Synovial fluid findings, 277t
Syphilis, 207t–208t, 342
  as differential dx for fever of unknown origin, 253t
  as differential dx for multiple sclerosis, 374
Systemic arthritis, 513, 514
Systemic lupus erythematosus (SLE), 520–525, 523t
  as differential dx for dermatomyositis, 508
  as differential dx for fever of unknown origin, 253t
  as differential dx for multiple sclerosis, 374
Systemic viral syndrome, as differential dx for fever of unknown origin, 253t
Systolic blood pressure (SBP), 345

T2 deficiency, 308
Tamponade, 58
Tanner staging, 120t
T cell disorders, 219t, 220t
Terbutaline, for asthma, 24
Testicular torsion, 546–547
Tetanus prophylaxis, 238, 480t
Tetralogy of Fallot, 46–48
Tet spells, 47
Thalassemias, 169, 174–176
Thermal burn, as differential dx for staphylococcal scalded skin syndrome, 75
Thiazide diuretics, for heart failure, 54
Thioguanine, 404t
Third-degree AV block, 66
Third-degree burns, 92
Thrombin time, 176
Thrombocytopenia, 180–181
  differential diagnosis, 180
  immune, 180–181
Thrombolytic therapy, for anticoagulation, 183
Thrombosis, 183–185, 184t
Thrombotic disorders, 181–185
Thyroid disease, 110–113
  acquired hypothyroidism, 111–112
  congenital hyperthyroidism, 110–111
  congenital hypothyroidism, 110
  as differential dx for abnormal uterine bleeding, 4
  Graves disease, 112–113
Thyroid function tests, in anorexia nervosa, 3t

Thyroid storm, 112
Tibia fractures, 449–450
Tissue adhesives, 479
Tonsils, adentonsillar hypertrophy, 454–456, 455f
TORCH infections, 340–343
Total anomalous pulmonary venous return, 48–49
Total body water (TBW), 121
Toxic epidermal necrolysis (TEN), 76–78, 85t
  as differential dx for staphylococcal scalded skin syndrome, 75
Toxicology, 548–576
Toxic shock syndrome, 280–281
  as differential dx for DRESS, 79
  as differential dx for staphylococcal scalded skin syndrome, 75
Toxin-mediated perineal erythema, as differential dx for staphylococcal scalded skin syndrome, 75
*Toxoplasma gondii*, 198, 260
Toxoplasmosis, 206t, 215t–216t, 341
Tracheoesophageal fistula (TEF), 528–529, 529f
Tracheostomy, 465–466
Transfusion medicine, 185–188
  for cancer patients, 432–433
  complicated hemangiomas, 187t
  complications, 187–188
  cryoprecipitate transfusion, 185
  fresh-frozen plasma transfusion, 185
  packed red cell transfusions, 432
  platelet transfusion, 185–186, 432–433
  red blood cell transfusion, 186–187, 186t
Transient hypogammaglobulinemia of infancy, 224–225
Transient ischemic attack (TIA), 379–380
Transient synovitis, 453
Transposition of the great arteries, 49–50
Transverse myelitis, 381–382
  as differential dx for Guillain-Barré syndrome, 371
Trauma, 99
Treponema pallidum, as differential dx for HSV, 293
Tricuspid atresia, 50
Tricyclic antidepressants, 575t
  poisoning, 573
Triglyceride, in anorexia nervosa, 3t
Trisomy 13, 162
Trisomy 18, 162
Trisomy 21, 161–162, 166–167
  as differential dx for hypotonia, 163

Truncus arteriosus, 51
Tube feeding, 393
Tuberculosis, 296–300, 299f
  as differential dx for fever of unknown origin, 253t
Tularemia, as differential dx for fever of unknown origin, 253t
Tumor lysis syndrome, 410–411, 410t–411t
Tumors
  abdominal masses, 417
  bone, 421–423
  central nervous system, 424–426, 427t–428t
  hypothalamic, 115
  neuroblastoma, 419–420
  rhabdomyosarcoma, 423–424
  solid, 417–428
  Wilms tumor, 417–419
Turner syndrome, 162
22q11.2 deletion syndrome, 162, 164, 227–229
  as differential dx for IgA deficiency, 226
25-hydroxylase deficiency, in rickets, 117t Type 1 diabetes, 100–103
Type 2 diabetes, 100–103

Ulcerative colitis, 148–149
Ulcers, peptic ulcer disease, 134–135
Umbilical vessel catheterization, 482–483
Unconjugated hyperbilirubinemia, 334–336
Undifferentiated arthritis, 513
Unit conversions, 37–38
Unprovoked seizure, first, 387–388
Unprovoked seizure, second, 388
Upper extremities, fractures of, 445–449
Urea cycle defects, 308–312
Urethritis, as differential dx for hematuria, 344
Urinalysis, in anorexia nervosa, 3t
Urinary alkalinization, 549
Urinary tract infection, 281–283
  as differential dx for fever of unknown origin, 253t
  as differential dx for hematuria, 344
Urine culture results, 282t
Urolithiasis, 355–357
  as differential dx for hematuria, 344
Urologic surgery, 545–547
Urticaria, 13–15, 84t
Uveitis, 437–438

Vaccination
  in cancer patients, 433
  in HIV patients, 198

VACTERL association, 157
Vaginitis, as differential dx for abnormal uterine
 bleeding, 4
Variable extrathoracic obstruction, 506–507
Varicella, 300
 as differential dx for HSV, 293
Varicella zoster infections, 300–302
Vascular access, 433
Vascular malformations, as differential dx for
 hemangiomas, 86
Vascular phenomena, 83–89
 atopic dermatitis, 87–89
 complicated hemangiomas, 83–87, 84t–85t
Vascular tumor mimics, as differential dx for
 hemangiomas, 86
Vasculitis, as differential dx for fever of
 unknown origin, 253t
Vasogenic edema, 372
Venous sinus thrombosis, 380–381
Ventilation
 mechanical, 501–504
 positive pressure, 24
Ventricular fibrillation, 70
Ventricular septal defect, 51–52
Ventricular tachycardia, 71
Verbal numeric pain rating, 25
Vertical mattress sutures, 475, 477f
Very long-chain acyl CoA dehydrogenase
 deficiency, 305t, 307
*Vibrio cholerae*, 258t
Vinblastine, 404t
Vincristine, 404t
Viral exanthems, as differential dx for DRESS, 79
Viral hepatitis, as differential dx for fever of
 unknown origin, 253t
Viral meningitis, 265–267
Viral pericarditis, 58
Visceral pain, 431–432

Viscous lidocaine, 26
Vitamin $B_{12}$ deficiency, as differential dx for
 multiple sclerosis, 374
Vitamin D deficiency, in rickets, 117t, 118, 119
Vitamin K deficiency, 178
Vocal cord paralysis, 466–467
Vomiting, in cancer patients, 430
Von Willebrand disease, 178–179

Warfarin (coumadin), for anticoagulation,
 182–183
Wasting, 390
Waterlow criteria for grading malnutrition, 390
Wheezing, differential diagnosis of, 21
WHIM syndrome, as differential dx for severe
 congenital neutropenia, 234
Whole bowel irrigation (WBI), 549
Williams syndrome, 162, 167–168
Wilms tumor, 417–419
Wilson disease, 142–143
Winter's formula, 40
Wiskott-Aldrich syndrome (WAS), 229–230
 as differential dx for IgA deficiency, 226
Wolff-Parkinson-White syndrome (WPW), 68,
 71–72
Wound care, burns, 93

X-linked adrenoleukodystrophy, 324–325
X-linked agammaglobulinemia (XLA),
 221–222
 as differential dx for severe congenital
 neutropenia, 234
X-linked hyper IgM syndrome, as differential dx
 for severe congenital neutropenia, 234

*Yersinia enterocolitica*, 258t
*Yersinia pseudotuberculosis*, 258t
Yuzpe regimen, 7t

# Notes

# Notes

# Notes

# Notes

# Notes

# Notes

# Notes

# Notes

# Notes

# Notes

# Notes

## TABLE 1 Medications for Rapid Sequence Intubation

| Step | Medication | IV Dose | Max dose | Comments |
|---|---|---|---|---|
| 1. Premedication | Atropine | 0.02 mg/kg | 1 mg | Min dose 0.1 mg. Prevents bradycardia during intubation. |
| 2. Sedatives | Etomidate | 0.2 - 0.3 mg/kg | 20 mg | Decreases ICP. Minimal myocardial depression. May cause myoclonus. |
| | Fentanyl | 1 - 2 mcg/kg | 100 mcg | May cause chest wall rigidity (reversible with naloxone or muscle relaxant). |
| | Ketamine | 1 - 2 mg/kg | 100 mg | Dissociative anesthetic. Consider for status asthmaticus. Sympathetic stimulant. |
| | Midazolam | 0.1 - 0.2 mg/kg | 10 mg | Titrate to effect. May cause hypotension. Reversible with flumazenil. |
| | Propofol | 2.5 - 3.5 mg/kg | — | Reduces airway resistance and bronchospasm. Can cause hypotension. |
| | Thiopental | 3-7 mg/kg | — | Decreases ICP. In hypovolemia, use 1mg/kg. Can cause bronchospasm. |
| 3. If increased ICP | Lidocaine | 1 mg/kg | — | Decreases ICP elevation associated with intubation. |
| 4. Paralytics | Pancuronium | 0.1 mg/kg | — | Avoid in cases of renal failure or tricyclic antidepressant use. |
| | Rocuronium | 0.6 - 1.2 mg/kg | 70 mg | Minimal effect on heart rate or blood pressure. |
| | Succinylcholine | 1 - 2 mg/kg | 150 mg | Avoid in cases of hyperkalemia, severe burn or myopathy with increased CPK. |
| | Vecuronium | 0.1 - 0.2 mg/kg | 10 mg | Minimal effect on heart rate or blood pressure. |

## TABLE 2 Airway Medications

| Route | Medication | Dose | Max Dose | Comments |
|---|---|---|---|---|
| Nebulized | Albuterol* | 0.25 - 1 mL | 1 mL | 0.5% solution (5 mg/ml). May give as continuous neb up to 4 mL/hr. |
| | Ipratropium bromide | 0.025 mg - 0.5 mg | 0.5 mg | May help prevent need for hospitalization if given in the ED. |
| | Racemic epinephrine | 0.25 - 0.5 mL | 0.5 mL | 2.25% solution. |
| Subcutaneous | Epinephrine | 0.01 mL/kg | 0.5 mL | 1:1000 solution. May repeat q15 minutes x 3 doses. |
| | Terbutaline | 0.005 – 0.01 mg/kg | 0.4 mg | Usual adult dose = 0.25 mg. |
| Intravenous | Dexamethasone | 0.6 mg/kg | 8 mg | May be given IV, IM, and/or PO. Often used for airway edema/croup. |
| | Magnesium sulfate | 50 mg/kg | 2 grams | May cause hypotension, apnea, or complete heart block. Infuse over 20 minutes |
| | Methylprednisolone | 2 mg/kg | — | After loading dose, give 1 mg/kg q12 hours. |
| | Terbutaline: Bolus | 2 – 10 mcg/kg | — | Initial bolus usually followed by continuous infusion. |
| | Infusion | 0.08 – 0.4 mcg/kg/min | 3 mcg/kg/min | Titrate to effect in increments of 0.1 mcg/kg/min q30 minutes. |

*Mix with 2.5 mL normal saline or with ipratropium bromide.

**TABLE 1** Emergency Medications

| Medication | | Dose (IV) | Max dose | Comments |
|---|---|---|---|---|
| Adenosine: | 1st dose | 0.1 mg/kg | 6 mg | Rapid IV push followed immediately by 5-10 mL normal saline flush. |
| | 2nd dose | 0.2 mg/kg | 12 mg | May repeat every 2 minutes. |
| Calcium Gluconate | | 30-100 mg/kg | 3.7 g | For hypocalcemia, administer q6 hours. 1g CaGluc = 4.5 mEq elemental Ca. |
| Dobutamine | | 2-15 mcg/kg/min | 40 mcg/kg/min | Titrate to desired effect. |
| Dopamine | | 1-20 mcg/kg/min | 50 mcg/kg/min | 2-5 mcg/kg/min increases renal blood flow with minimal cardiac effect. |
| Epinephrine: | Initial dose | 0.1 mL/Kg, 1:10,000 | 1 mg | May be given IV, IO. May repeat every 3-5 minutes PRN up to max dose. |
| | High dose | 0.1 mL/Kg, 1:1,000 | 5 mL = 5 mg | May be given IV, IO, and ETT. May repeat every 3-5 min PRN. |
| | Infusion | 0.05-1 mcg/kg/min | — | Lower doses may be considered in neonates. |
| Flumazenil | | 0.01 mg/kg | 0.2 mg | May repeat every 1 minute to max cumulative dose of 1 mg. |
| Glucagon | | 0.025-0.1 mg/kg | 1 mg | May repeat in 20 minutes.  May be given IV, IM, SC. |
| Glucose: | Neonate | 2-4 mL/kg of D10W | — | Then start continuous infusion of D10W at 6-8 mg/kg/min and titrate. |
| | Child | 2-4 mL/kg of D25W | — | — |
| Hydrocortisone: | Stress dose | 0.3-0.6 mg/kg | 100 mg | Alternative dose: 25-100 mg/m² IV or 50 mg/m²/dose IM q12 hours. |
| | Acute adrenal insufficiency | 1-2 mg/kg | | May be given IV, IM. |
| Insulin infusion for DKA | | 0.1 unit/kg/hour | — | Only regular insulin should be given IV. Consider 0.1 unit/kg initial bolus. |
| Lidocaine: | Loading dose | 1 mg/kg | — | Antiarrhythmic dose. May be given IV, IO.  ETT dose is 2-2.5 times higher. |
| | Infusion | 20-50 mcg/kg/min | 2-4 mg/min | — |
| Mannitol Increased ICP | | 1.5-2 g/kg | — | Decreases ICP in approximately 15 minutes and lasts 4-6 hours. 20% solution given over at least 30 minutes. |
| Naloxone | | 0.1 mg/kg | 2 mg | May be given IV, IM, ETT, SC. May repeat every 2-3 minutes. |
| Prostaglandin E1 | | 0.01-0.1 mcg/kg/min | 0.1 mcg/kg/min | Start at 0.05 – 0.1 mcg/kg/min and reduce to lowest effective dose. |
| Sodium Bicarbonate | | 1-2 mEq/kg | — | Use ½ strength formulation (0.5 mEq/ml) in neonates. |

**TABLE 2** Defibrillation and Cardioversion

| | Pediatric | Adult |
|---|---|---|
| Defibrillation | 2 J/kg, 4 J/kg, 4 J/kg | 200 J, 200-300 J, 360 J |
| Synchronized Cardioversion | 0.5-1 J/kg, 2 J/kg | 50 - 200 J |

CPSIA information can be obtained
at www.ICGtesting.com
Printed in the USA
FFHW021835300519
52744843-58257FF